# ESSENTIALS OF
# HEALTH CARE
# FINANCE

## EIGHTH EDITION

### WILLIAM O. CLEVERLEY, PhD
Chairman and Founder
Cleverley & Associates
Worthington, Ohio

### JAMES O. CLEVERLEY, MHA
President
Cleverley & Associates
Worthington, Ohio

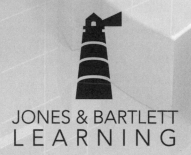

JONES & BARTLETT
LEARNING

*World Headquarters*
Jones & Bartlett Learning
5 Wall Street
Burlington, MA 01803
978-443-5000
info@jblearning.com
www.jblearning.com

Jones & Bartlett Learning books and products are available through most bookstores and online booksellers. To contact Jones & Bartlett Learning directly, call 800-832-0034, fax 978-443-8000, or visit our website, www.jblearning.com.

Substantial discounts on bulk quantities of Jones & Bartlett Learning publications are available to corporations, professional associations, and other qualified organizations. For details and specific discount information, contact the special sales department at Jones & Bartlett Learning via the above contact information or send an email to specialsales@jblearning.com.

10919-1

**Production Credits**

VP, Executive Publisher: David D. Cella
Publisher: Michael Brown
Associate Editor: Lindsey M. Sousa
Associate Editor: Danielle Bessette
Senior Production Editor: Amanda Clerkin
Senior Marketing Manager: Sophie Fleck Teague
Manufacturing and Inventory Control Supervisor: Amy Bacus

Composition: Integra Software Services Pvt. Ltd.
Cover Design: Scott Moden
Rights & Media Specialist: Merideth Tumasz
Media Development Editor: Shannon Sheehan
Cover Image (Title Page, Chapter Opener): © A1Stock/Shutterstock
Printing and Binding: Edwards Brothers Malloy
Cover Printing: Edwards Brothers Malloy

**Library of Congress Cataloging-in-Publication Data**

Names: Cleverley, William O., author. | Cleverley, James O., author.
Title: Essentials of health care finance / William O. Cleverley and James O. Cleverley.
Description: Eighth edition. | Burlington, Massachusetts : Jones & Bartlett Learning, [2018] | Includes bibliographical references and index.
Identifiers: LCCN 2016047263 | ISBN 9781284094633
Subjects: | MESH: Costs and Cost Analysis | Financial Management | Health Services—economics
Classification: LCC RA971.3 | NLM W 74.1 | DDC 362.11068/1—dc23
LC record available at https://lccn.loc.gov/2016047263

6048

Printed in the United States of America
23 22 21 20 19   10 9 8 7 6 5 4 3

# Contents

# Preface

This book represents the eighth edition of a book published originally in 1978, entitled *Essentials of Hospital Finance*. The text has evolved from a book containing seven chapters that dealt largely with understanding and interpreting hospital financial statements into a comprehensive financial text. The *Eighth Edition* has 23 chapters that cover most of the major areas of financial decision making that healthcare executives deal with on a daily basis.

This book has been widely used over the years for many reasons. No other textbook so fully melds the best of current financial theory with the tools needed in day-to-day practice by healthcare managers. The textbook also encompasses virtually the whole spectrum of the healthcare industry, including hospitals, pharmaceutical companies, health maintenance organizations, home health agencies, skilled nursing facilities, surgical centers, physician practices, hospital departments, and integrated healthcare systems.

Building on the strong foundation of the previous editions, the *Eighth Edition* introduces a number of enhancements. We have continued the inclusion of learning objectives at the beginning of each chapter. The learning objectives orient students to the material in the chapter and highlight some particular concepts and skills they should acquire by studying the chapter. Following the learning objectives, each chapter has a real-world scenario, which places the material in the chapter into the context of how the concepts and tools are used in practice. As with previous editions, each chapter concludes with a summary, followed by a large number of problems with related solutions. We believe the application of finance theory to real-world financial problems is the best way to accomplish learning. One of the primary enhancements of the *Eighth Edition* is the addition and updating of supporting data tables that provide tangible benchmarking information for students and practitioners in a larger number of areas. In summary, the chapters are designed to provide a framework for understanding healthcare financial issues as well as resources for implementing appropriate operational strategies.

Before discussing the coverage of this book, it is important to understand the objective, which has not changed in more than 30 years. This text is intended to provide a relevant and readable resource for healthcare management students and executives. This is important to understand because *Essentials of Health Care Finance* is neither a traditional financial textbook nor a traditional management or financial accounting textbook. It attempts to blend the topics of both accounting and finance that have become part of the everyday life of most healthcare executives. This textbook does not provide as much coverage of cost of capital, capital structure, and capital budgeting topics as is present in most financial management textbooks. *Essentials of Health Care Finance* likewise does not provide major coverage of management control and budgeting systems that are present in most cost accounting and management accounting textbooks. Instead, this text tries to cover those types of financial decisions with which healthcare executives are most likely to be involved and provides the necessary materials to help them understand the conceptual basis and mechanics of financial analysis and decision making as they pertain to the healthcare industry sector.

# Content of the Book

The general basis of financial decision making in any business is almost always built on understanding three critical elements. First, most financial decisions are based on the use of accounting information. It is difficult to make intelligent decisions without having at least a basic understanding of accounting information. The user does not need to be a CPA, but it is essential to have a little understanding of what accounting is and is not. Second, all business units operate within an industry. The healthcare industry is a huge, complex industry that in many areas is unlike any other industry. Unless the student has an appreciation for these critical differences, major mistakes can be made. Finally, both accounting and finance are, in many ways, subsets of economics. The principles of economics form the conceptual basis upon which many types of business decisions are made.

Chapter 1 provides an introduction to the role of information in decision making. Chapter 2, "Billing and Coding for Health Services," recognizes the increasing importance that billing and coding play in financial decision making. Chapter 3 provides detailed information about the economic environment of healthcare firms. Specific coverage of payment methods for all types of providers, from hospitals to physicians, is included. Much of Chapter 3 was rewritten for this edition because payment rules are constantly changing. This edition covers current Medicare prospective payment systems for outpatient, home health, and skilled nursing facilities. Chapter 4 provides coverage of the numerous legal and regulatory provisions that affect today's healthcare manager.

Chapter 5, "Measuring Community Benefit," provides expanded coverage of a topic that has gained more attention with the recent passage of healthcare reform. Nonprofit healthcare providers increasingly are being asked to document the community benefits they provide to their communities. Chapter 6, "Revenue Determination," devotes specific attention to pricing and managed-care contract negotiations. Extensive coverage of managed care, its definition, concepts, organizational structures, and its financial implications is included in Chapter 7 and woven throughout the remainder of the text. Managed-care

contracting is covered extensively in this edition along with coverage of "bundled payments."

Chapters 8, 9, and 10 cover financial reporting for healthcare firms. Specific discussions of accounting jargon are included. Perhaps of more importance, the accounting terms are related to healthcare issues, such as self-insurance of professional liability.

Chapters 11, 12, and 13 cover financial analysis and financial planning. Chapter 11 has been thoroughly revised to reflect the best analytical tools and techniques available for financial statement analysis. Chapter 12 provides specific coverage of healthcare firms other than hospitals. Comparative financial and operating benchmark values are included for hospitals, and benchmark values are included for hospitals, health maintenance organizations, nursing homes, and medical groups. These benchmark values are used later to evaluate the financial position of a number of different kinds of healthcare firms.

Chapters 14 through 16 cover cost finding, pricing, break-even analysis, and budgeting, and other managerial-care examples and concepts have been added in this edition. This edition also features more extensive coverage of relative value units. Chapter 17 includes material on the application of variance analysis techniques to both healthcare providers and payers.

Chapters 18 through 21 include coverage of capital budgeting, consolidations, valuation, and capital formation topics as they pertain to healthcare firms. Special attention is given to capital formation in both taxable and voluntary nonprofit situations. Chapter 20 covers the increasingly important topics of consolidations, mergers, and acquisitions. In that chapter we offer detailed coverage of several valuation techniques. Chapter 21 includes extensive coverage of sources of capital used by healthcare providers, especially tax-exempt revenue bonds. Chapters 22 and 23 cover the topics of working capital management and cash budgeting.

Building from the practical educational approach of prior editions, we believe that the enhancements made to the text will provide students and practitioners with a greater understanding of financial application in the complex and changing healthcare industry.

# About the Authors

**William O. Cleverley, PhD,** is the chairman and founder of Cleverley & Associates, which was started in January 2000. Before forming Cleverley & Associates, Dr. Cleverley was the president and founder of CHIPS (Center for Healthcare Industry Performance Studies). United Healthcare acquired the firm in March 1998, and Dr. Cleverley remained on staff as a part-time employee until December 1999. Dr. Cleverley is also professor emeritus at The Ohio State University where he taught courses in healthcare finance starting in 1973.

Dr. Cleverley was the original author of *Essentials of Healthcare Finance* in 1978. In addition, he has authored over 250 articles on healthcare financial issues in a wide variety of both academic and professional journals.

**James O. Cleverley, MHA,** is the president of Cleverley & Associates, where he has worked since September 2003. Mr. Cleverley consults with hospital and healthcare organizations to identify financial and operating opportunities, as well as related strategies for performance improvement. Before joining the firm, he directed a statewide health services program for a medical association.

Mr. Cleverley has authored over 50 books and articles dealing with healthcare financial analysis and application, including the annual Community Value Index* hospital survey, the State of the Hospital Industry, and *Essentials of Health Care Finance*. He is a two-time recipient of the Healthcare Financial Management Association's Yerger/Seawell Best Article award.

Mr. Cleverley received his master of health administration from The Ohio State University in 2004. He received his bachelor of science in business administration from The Ohio State University in 1999.

# Contributor

**Peter A. Pavarini, Esq.**
Squire, Sanders & Dempsey, LLP
Columbus, Ohio

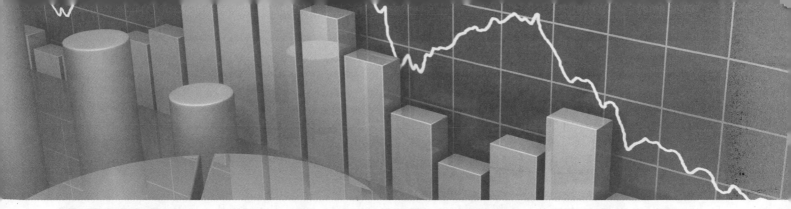

# CHAPTER 1

# Financial Information and the Decision-Making Process

## REAL-WORLD SCENARIO

In 1946, a small band of hospital accountants formed the American Association of Hospital Accountants (AAHA). They were interested in sharing information and experiences in their industry, which was beginning to show signs of growth. First published in 1947, a small educational journal was created in an attempt to disseminate information of interest to their members. Ten years later, in 1956, the AAHA's membership had grown to over 2,600 members. The real growth, however, was still to come with the advent of Medicare financing in 1965.

With the dramatic growth of hospital revenues came an escalation in both the number and functions delegated to the hospital accountant. Hospital finance had become much more than just billing patients and paying invoices. Hospitals were becoming big businesses with complex and varied financial functions. They had to arrange funding of major capital programs, which could no longer be supported through charitable campaigns. Cost accounting and management control were important functions for the continued financial viability of their firms. Hospital accountants soon evolved into hospital financial managers, and so in 1968 the AAHA changed its name to the Hospital Financial Management Association (HFMA).

The hospital industry continued to boom through the late 1960s and 1970s. Third-party insurance became the norm for most of the American population. Patients either received insurance through governmental programs such as Medicare and Medicaid or obtained it as part of the benefit program at their place of employment. Hospitals were clearly no longer quite as charitable as they once were. There was money, and plenty of it, to finance the growth required through increased demand and the new evolving medical technology. By 1980, HFMA was a large association with 19,000 members. Primary offices were located in Chicago, but an important office was opened in Washington, DC, to provide critical input to both the executive and legislative branches of government. On many issues that affected either government payment or capital financing, HFMA became the credible voice that policymakers sought.

The industry adapted and evolved even more in the 1980s as fiscal pressure hit the federal government. Hospital payments were increasing so fast that new systems were sought to curtail the growth rate. Prospective payment systems were introduced in 1983, and alternative payment systems were developed that provided incentives for treating patients in an ambulatory setting. Growth in the hospital industry was still rapid, but other sectors of health care began to experience colossal growth rates, such as ambulatory surgery centers. More and more, health care was being transferred to the outpatient setting. The hospital industry was no longer the only large corporate player in health care. To acknowledge this trend, the HFMA changed its name in 1982 to the Healthcare Financial Management Association to reflect the more diverse elements of the industry and to better meet the needs of members in other sectors.

---

In 2015, HFMA had over 39,000 members in a wide variety of healthcare organizations (HCOs). The daily activities of their members still involve basic accounting issues—patient bills must still be created and collected, payroll still needs to be met—but strategic decision-making is much more critical in today's environment. It would be impossible to imagine any organization planning its future without financial projections and input. Many HCOs may still be charitable from a taxation perspective, but they are too large to depend upon charitable giving to finance their business future. Financial managers of healthcare firms are involved in a wide array of critical and complex decisions that will ultimately determine the destiny of their firms.

This text is intended to improve decision makers' understanding and use of financial information in the healthcare industry. It is not an advanced treatise in accounting or finance but an elementary discussion of how financial information in general and healthcare industry financial information in particular are interpreted and used. It is written for individuals who are not experienced healthcare financial executives. Its aim is to make the language of healthcare finance readable and relevant for general decision makers in the healthcare industry.

Three interdependent factors have created the need for this text:

1. Rapid expansion and evolution of the healthcare industry
2. Healthcare decision makers' general lack of business and financial background
3. Financial and cost criteria's increasing importance in healthcare decisions

The healthcare industry's expansion is a trend visible even to individuals outside the healthcare system. The hospital industry, the major component of the healthcare industry, consumes about 6.3% of the gross domestic product; other types of healthcare systems, although smaller than the hospital industry, are expanding at even faster rates. **TABLE 1-1** lists the types of major healthcare institutions and indexes their relative size.

### Learning Objective 1

Describe the importance of financial information in healthcare organizations.

The rapid growth of healthcare facilities providing direct medical services has substantially increased the numbers of decision makers who need to be familiar with financial information. Effective decision making in their jobs depends on an accurate interpretation of financial information. Many healthcare decision makers involved directly in healthcare delivery—doctors, nurses, dietitians, pharmacists, radiation technologists, physical therapists, inhalation therapists—are medically or scientifically trained but lack education and experience in business and finance. Their specialized education, in most cases, did not include courses such as accounting. However, advancement and promotion within HCOs increasingly entails assumption of administrative duties, requiring almost instant, knowledgeable reading of financial information. Communication with the organization's financial executives is not always helpful. As

| TABLE 1-1 Healthcare Expenditures 2008–2024* | | | | | | |
|---|---|---|---|---|---|---|
| **Type of Expenditure** | **2008** | **2010** | **2012** | **2014** | **2016** | **2024** |
| Hospital care | 728.9 | 814.9 | 898.5 | 978.3 | 1,087.3 | 1,755.1 |
| Physician and clinical services | 486.5 | 519.0 | 565.3 | 615.0 | 666.5 | 1,034.8 |
| Other professional services | 64.0 | 69.8 | 76.8 | 85.5 | 96.0 | 155.4 |
| Dental services | 102.4 | 105.4 | 110.0 | 114.5 | 123.5 | 183.4 |
| Other health, residential, and personal care | 113.5 | 128.5 | 140.1 | 153.0 | 167.1 | 251.1 |
| Home health care | 62.3 | 71.2 | 77.1 | 81.9 | 91.7 | 156.0 |
| Nursing care facilities and continuing care retirement communities | 132.6 | 143.0 | 152.2 | 160.2 | 176.1 | 274.4 |
| Prescription drugs | 242.7 | 256.2 | 264.4 | 305.1 | 343.2 | 564.3 |
| Durable medical equipment | 34.9 | 37.0 | 41.3 | 44.2 | 48.2 | 76.9 |
| Other non-durable medical products | 49.5 | 51.2 | 53.7 | 58.4 | 62.6 | 98.7 |
| **Personal Health Care** | **2,017.3** | **2,196.2** | **2,379.4** | **2,596.1** | **2,862.2** | **4,550.1** |
| Government administration | 29.4 | 30.5 | 34.2 | 39.9 | 45.5 | 82.2 |
| Net cost of private health insurance | 140.7 | 152.3 | 165.3 | 200.4 | 235.4 | 384.3 |
| Government public health activities | 71.5 | 75.5 | 74.8 | 78.7 | 86.2 | 137.7 |
| **Health Consumption Expenditures** | **2,258.9** | **2,454.5** | **2,653.6** | **2,915.3** | **3,229.3** | **5,154.2** |
| Research | 44.0 | 48.7 | 48.0 | 45.9 | 48.7 | 72.0 |
| Structures and equipment | 111.2 | 101.0 | 115.7 | 118.9 | 124.7 | 198.9 |
| **National Health Expenditures** | **2,414.1** | **2,604.1** | **2,817.3** | **3,080.1** | **3,402.6** | **5,425.1** |
| **Gross Domestic Product** | **14,718.6** | **14,964.4** | **16,163.2** | **17,418.9** | **18,821.2** | **27,648.0** |
| **National Health Expenditures to GDP** | **16.4%** | **17.4%** | **17.4%** | **17.7%** | **18.1%** | **19.6%** |
| **Hospital Care to GDP** | **5.0%** | **5.4%** | **5.6%** | **5.6%** | **5.8%** | **6.3%** |

*Values are in US$ in billions.

Centers for Medicare and Medicaid Services, Office of the Actuary a result, nonfinancial executives often end up ignoring financial information.

Governing boards, which are significant users of financial information, are expanding in size in many healthcare facilities, in some cases to accommodate demands for more consumer representation. This trend can be healthy for both the community and the facilities. However, many board members, even those with backgrounds in business, are being overwhelmed by financial reports and statements. There are important distinctions between the financial reports and statements of business organizations, with which some board members are familiar, and those of healthcare facilities. Governing board members must recognize these differences if they are to carry out their governing missions satisfactorily.

The increasing importance of financial and cost criteria in healthcare decision making is the third factor creating a need for more knowledge of financial information. For many years, accountants and others involved with financial matters have been caricatured as individuals with narrow vision, incapable of seeing the forest for the trees. In many respects, this may have been an accurate portrayal. However, few individuals in the healthcare industry today would deny the importance of financial concerns, especially cost. Payment pressures from payers, as described in the beginning-of-chapter scenario, underscore the need for attention to costs. Careful attention to these concerns requires *knowledgeable* consumption of financial information by a variety of decision makers. It is not an overstatement to say that inattention to financial criteria can lead to excessive costs and eventually to insolvency.

The effectiveness of financial management in any business is the product of many factors, such as environmental conditions, personnel capabilities, and information quality. A major portion of the total financial management task is the provision of accurate, timely, and relevant information. Much of this activity is carried out through the accounting process. An adequate understanding of the accounting process and the data generated by it are thus critical to successful decision making.

## ▶ Information and Decision Making

The major function of information in general and financial information in particular is to oil the decision-making process. Decision making is basically the selection of a course of action from a defined list of possible or feasible actions. In many cases, the actual course of action followed may essentially be no action; decision makers may decide to make no change from their present policies. It should be recognized, however, that both action and inaction represent policy decisions.

**FIGURE 1-1** shows how information is related to the decision-making process and gives an example to illustrate the sequence. Generating information is the key to decision making. The quality and effectiveness of decision making depend on accurate, timely, and relevant information. The difference between data and information is more than semantic: data become information only when they are useful and appropriate to the decision. Many financial data never become information because they are not viewed as relevant or are unavailable in an intelligible form.

For the illustrative purposes of the ambulatory surgery center (ASC) example in Figure 1-1, only two possible courses of action are assumed: to build or not to build an ASC. In most situations, there may be a continuum of alternative courses of action. For example, an ASC might vary by size or by facilities included in the unit. In this case, prior decision making seems to have reduced the feasible set of alternatives to a more manageable and limited number of analyses.

Once a course of action has been selected in the decision-making phase, it must be accomplished. Implementing a decision may be extremely complex. In the ASC example, carrying out the decision to build the unit would require enormous management effort to ensure that the projected results are actually obtained. Periodic measurement of results in a feedback loop, as in Figure 1-1, is a method commonly used to make sure that decisions are actually implemented according to plan.

As previously stated, results that are forecast are not always guaranteed. Controllable factors, such as

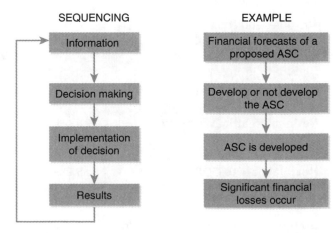

**FIGURE 1-1 Information in the Decision-Making Process**

| **TABLE 1-2** Results Matrix for the ASC | | | |
|---|---|---|---|
| | **Possible Events (Utilization Percentages)** | | |
| **Alternative Actions** | **25% Usage** | **50% Usage** | **75% Usage** |
| Build the ASC | $400,000 loss | $10,000 profit | $200,000 profit |
| Do not build the ASC | 0 profit | 0 profit | 0 profit |

failure to adhere to prescribed plans, and uncontrollable circumstances, such as a change in reimbursement, may obstruct planned results.

Decision making is usually surrounded by uncertainty. No anticipated result of a decision is guaranteed. Events may occur that have been analyzed but not anticipated. A results matrix concisely portrays the possible results of various courses of action, given the occurrence of possible events. **TABLE 1-2** provides a results matrix for the sample ASC; it shows that approximately 50% utilization will enable this unit to operate in the black and not drain resources from other areas. If forecasting shows that utilization below 50% is unlikely, decision makers may very well elect to build.

A good information system should enable decision makers to choose those courses of action that have the highest expectation of favorable results. Based on the results matrix of Table 1-2, a good information system should, specifically, do the following

- List possible courses of action.
- List events that might affect the expected results.
- Indicate the probability that those events will occur.
- Estimate the results accurately, given an action/event combination (e.g., profit in Table 1-2).

One thing an information system does not do is evaluate the desirability of results. Decision makers must evaluate results in terms of their organizations' preferences or their own. For example, construction of an ASC may be expected to lose $400,000 per year, but it could provide a needed community service. Weighing these results and determining criteria is purely a decision maker's responsibility—not an easy task, but one that can be improved with accurate and relevant information.

### Learning Objective 2

Discuss the uses of financial information.

## ▶ Uses and Users of Financial Information

As a subset of information in general, financial information is important in the decision-making process. In some areas of decision making, financial information is especially relevant. For our purposes, we identify five uses of financial information that may be important in decision making:

1. Evaluating the *financial condition* of an entity
2. Evaluating *stewardship* within an entity
3. Assessing the *efficiency* of operations
4. Assessing the *effectiveness* of operations
5. Determining the *compliance* of operation with directives

### Financial Condition

Evaluation of an entity's financial condition is probably the most common use of financial information. Usually, an organization's financial condition is equated with its viability or capacity to continue pursuing its stated goals at a consistent level of activity. Viability is a far more restrictive term than solvency; some HCOs maybe solvent but not viable. For example, a hospital may have its level of funds restricted so that it must reduce its scope of activity but still remain solvent. A reduction in payment rates by a major payer may be the vehicle for this change in viability.

Assessment of the financial condition of business enterprises is essential to our economy's smooth and efficient operation. Most business decisions in our economy are directly or indirectly based on perceptions of financial condition. This includes the largely nonprofit healthcare industry. Although attention is usually directed at organizations as whole units, assessment of the financial condition of organizational divisions is equally important. In the ASC example, information on the future financial condition of the unit is valuable. If continued losses from this operation are projected, impairment of the financial condition of other divisions in the organization could be in the offing.

Assessment of financial condition also includes consideration of short-run versus long-run effects. The relevant time frame may change, depending on the decision under consideration. For example, suppliers typically are interested only in an organization's short-run financial condition because that is the period in which they must expect payment. However, investment bankers, as long-term creditors, are interested in the organization's financial condition over a much longer time period.

## Stewardship

Historically, evaluation of stewardship was the most important use of accounting and financial information systems. These systems were originally designed to prevent the loss of assets or resources through employees' malfeasance. This use is still very important. In fact, the relatively infrequent occurrence of employee fraud and embezzlement may be due in part to the deterrence of well-designed accounting systems.

## Efficiency

Efficiency in healthcare operations is becoming an increasingly important objective for many decision makers. Efficiency is simply the ratio of outputs to inputs, not the quality of outputs (good or not good) but the lowest possible cost of production. Adequate assessment of efficiency implies the availability of standards against which actual costs may be compared. In many HCOs, these standards may be formally introduced into the budgetary process. Thus a given nursing unit may have an efficiency standard of 4.3 nursing hours per patient day of care delivered. This standard may then be used as a benchmark to evaluate the relative efficiency of the unit. If actual employment were 6.0 nursing hours per patient day, management would be likely to reassess staffing patterns.

## Effectiveness

Assessment of the effectiveness of operations is concerned with the attainment of objectives through production of outputs, not the relationship of outputs to cost. Measuring effectiveness is much more difficult than measuring efficiency because most organizations' objectives or goals are typically not stated quantitatively. Because measurement of effectiveness is difficult, there is a tendency to place less emphasis on effectiveness and more on efficiency. This may result in the delivery of unnecessary services at an efficient cost. For example, development of outpatient surgical centers may reduce costs per surgical procedure and thus create an efficient means of delivery. However, the necessity of those surgical procedures may still be questionable.

## Compliance

Finally, financial information may be used to determine whether compliance with directives has taken place. The best example of an organization's internal directives is its budget, an agreement between two management levels regarding use of resources for a defined time period. External parties may also impose directives, many of them financial in nature, for the organization's adherence. For example, rate-setting or regulatory agencies may set limits on rates determined within an organization. Financial reporting by the organization is required to ensure compliance.

| *Learning Objective 3* |
| --- |

List the users of financial information and their uses for it.

**TABLE 1-3** presents a matrix of users and uses of financial information in the healthcare industry. It identifies areas or uses that may interest particular decision-making groups. It does not consider relative importance.

Not every use of financial information is important in every decision. For example, in approving a HCO's rates, a governing board may be interested in only two uses of financial information: (1) evaluation of financial condition and (2) assessment of operational efficiency. Other uses may be irrelevant. The board wants to ensure that services are being provided efficiently and that the rates being established are sufficient to guarantee a stable or improved financial condition. As Table 1-3 illustrates, most healthcare decision-making groups use financial information to assess financial condition and efficiency.

## ▶ Financial Organization

It is important to understand the management structure of businesses in general and HCOs in particular. **FIGURE 1-2** outlines the financial management structure of a typical hospital.

**TABLE 1-3**  Users and Uses of Financial Information

| Users | Uses of Financial Information | | | | |
|---|---|---|---|---|---|
| | **Financial Condition** | **Stewardship** | **Efficiency** | **Effectiveness** | **Compliance** |
| **External** | | | | | |
| Healthcare coalitions | X | | X | X | |
| Unions | X | | X | | |
| Rate-setting organizations | X | | X | X | X |
| Creditors | X | | X | X | |
| Third-party payers | X | | X | X | |
| Suppliers | X | | | X | |
| Public | X | | X | X | |
| **Internal** | | | | | |
| Governing board | X | X | X | X | X |
| Top management | X | X | X | X | X |
| Departmental management | | | X | | |

---

### Learning Objective 4

Describe the financial functions within an organization.

---

Financial Executives International has categorized financial management functions as either controllership or treasurership. Although few HCOs have specifically identified treasurers and controllers at this time, the separation of duties is important to the understanding of financial management. The following describes functions in the two categories designated by Financial Executives International, along

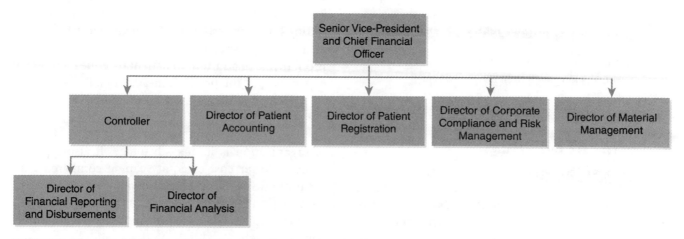

**FIGURE 1-2  Financial Organization Chart of a Typical Hospital**

with an example of the type of activities conducted within each of these functions:

1. Controllership
   (a) Planning for control: Establish budgetary systems (Chapters 13 and 16)
   (b) Reporting and interpreting: Prepare financial statements (Chapter 9)
   (c) Evaluating and consulting: Conduct cost analyses (Chapter 14)
   (d) Administrating taxes: Calculating payroll taxes owed
   (e) Reporting to government: Submit Medicare bills and cost reports (Chapter 2 and 6)
   (f) Protecting assets: Develop internal control procedures
   (g) Appraising economic health: Analyze financial statements (Chapters 11 and 12)

2. Treasurership
   (a) Providing capital: Arrange for bond issuance (Chapter 21)
   (b) Maintaining investor relations: Assist in analysis of appropriate dividend payment policy (for-profit firms) (Chapters 20 and 21)
   (c) Providing short-term financing: Arrange lines of credit (Chapters 22 and 23)
   (d) Providing banking and custody: Manage overnight and short-term funds transfers (Chapters 22 and 23)
   (e) Overseeing credits and collections: Establish billing, credit, and collection policies (Chapters 2 and 22)
   (f) Choosing investments: Analyze capital investment projects (Chapter 19)
   (g) Providing insurance: Managing funds related to self-insurance program

---

### *Learning Objective 5*

Discuss the common ownership forms of healthcare organizations, along with their advantages and disadvantages.

---

# ▶ Forms of Business Organization

More so than in most other industries, firms in the healthcare industry consist of a wide array of ownership and organizational structures. In health care, there are three main types organizations (adapted from the American Institute of Certified Public Accountants' Audit and Accounting Guide *Health Care Organizations*, 2015):

- Not-for-profit, business-oriented organizations
- For-profit healthcare entities
  - Investor-owned
  - Professional corporations/professional associations
  - Sole proprietorships
  - Limited partnerships
  - Limited liability partnerships/limited liability companies
- Governmental healthcare organizations

These three main types of firms differ in terms of ownership structure. Additionally, different HCOs require slightly different sets of financial statements.

## Not-for-Profit, Business-Oriented Organizations

Not-for-profit HCOs are owned by the entire community rather than by investor–owners. Unlike its for-profit counterpart, the primary goal of a not-for-profit (also referred to as a nonprofit) organization is not to maximize profits, but to serve the community in which it operates through the healthcare services it provides. Not-for-profit HCOs must be run as a business, however, in order to ensure their long-term financial viability. With an annual budget of more than $20 billion, Ascension Healthcare is an example of one of the largest not-for-profit HCOs.

Not-for-profit organizations (described in Sec. 501(c)(3) of the Internal Revenue Code) usually are exempt from federal income taxes and property taxes. In return for this favorable tax treatment, not-for-profit organizations are expected to provide **community benefit**, which often comes in the form of providing more uncompensated care (vis-à-vis for-profit firms), setting lower prices, or by offering services that, from a financial perspective, might not be viable for for-profit firms. In addition to patient revenue in excess of expenses, not-for-profits can additionally be funded by tax-exempt debt, grants, donations, and investments by other nonprofit firms.

The primary advantage of the not-for-profit form of organization is its tax advantage. It also typically enjoys a lower cost of equity capital compared with for-profit firms. The main disadvantage of this form of organization is that not-for-profits have more limited access to capital. Nonprofits cannot raise capital in the equity markets.

While for-profit firms are becoming increasingly prevalent in many sectors of health care, not-for-profits still dominate the hospital sector. About 80% of hospitals are not-for-profit. In the future, however, this sector may witness the growth of investor-owned organizations, owing mainly to their easier access to capital that will be necessary for adapting to the rapid changes in the healthcare system.

## For-Profit Healthcare Entities

The main objective of most for-profit firms is to earn profits that are distributed to the investor–owners of the firms or reinvested in the firm for the long-term benefit of these owners.

For-profit hospital management must strike a balance between their fiduciary responsibilities to the owners of the company and their other mission of providing acceptable-quality healthcare services to the community. For-profit firms have a wide variety of organization and ownership structures. For-profit firms that buy and sell shares of their company stocks on the open market are referred to as **publicly traded companies**. A major advantage of being publicly traded is the ability to raise equity capital through the sale of company stocks. Publicly traded firms are subject to reporting requirements and regulation by the Securities and Exchange Commission (SEC). For-profit firms may also be **privately held**, meaning the shares of the company are held by relatively few investors and are not available to the general public. Privately held companies also have far few reporting requirements to the SEC. Large for-profit firms are typically publicly traded. However, there are exceptions. For example, HCA, Inc. is a national for-profit healthcare services company headquartered in Nashville, Tennessee. Prior to 2005, HCA was the largest publicly traded hospital company. In 2005, HCA was purchased by a private equity firm and converted from a publicly traded to privately held company. HCA, Inc. returned to publicly traded status in 2010 and remains the largest for-profit hospital company, with 16 hospitals and 43,275 licensed beds. In its fiscal year ending December 31, 2015, the company had after-tax income of $2.1 billion.

Both publicly traded and privately held for-profit firms are often referred to as "investor-owned" firms. **Investor-owned** firms are owned by risk-based equity investors who expect the managers of the corporation to maximize shareholder wealth. Most large for-profit firms use this legal form. Investor-owned firms have a relative advantage in terms of financing. In addition to debt, for-profit firms can raise funding through risk-based equity capital. They enjoy limited liability, but their earnings are taxed at both the corporate level and the shareholder level (so-called double taxation). The company pays corporate income tax and the shareholder pays both tax on dividends paid by the company and gains made on the sale of the company's stock.

A **professional corporation (PC)**, also called a professional association (PA), is a corporate form for professionals who wanted to have the advantages of incorporation. A PC does not, however, shield its owners from professional liability. PCs and PAs have been widely used by physicians and other healthcare professionals.

**Sole proprietorships** are unincorporated businesses owned by a single individual. They do not necessarily have to be small businesses. Solo practitioner physicians often are sole proprietors. The main advantages are easy and inexpensive to set up, no sharing of profits, total control, few government regulations, no special income taxes, and that they are easy and inexpensive to dissolve. Its two main disadvantages are unlimited liability and limited access to capital.

**Partnerships** are unincorporated businesses with two or more owners. Group practices of physicians sometimes were set up using this form. There are now a wide variety of partnership forms. They are easy to form, are subject to few government regulations, and are not subject to double taxation. On the downside, partnerships have unlimited liability, are difficult to dissolve, and create potential for conflict among the partners.

In a **limited partnership (LP)** there is at least one general partner who has unlimited liability for the LP's debts and obligations. LPs offer limited liability to the limited partners along with tax flow-through treatment. The disadvantage to LPs is that they require a general partner who remains fully liable for the LP's debts and obligations.

A **limited liability company (LLC)**, also called a **limited liability partnership (LLP)**, is a business entity that combines the tax flow through treatment characteristics of a partnership (i.e., no double taxation) with the liability protection of a corporation. In an LLC, the liability of the general partner is limited. LLCs are flexible in the sense that they permit owners to structure allocations of income and losses any way they desire, so long as the partnership tax allocation rules are followed.

## Governmental Healthcare Organizations

Governmental HCOs are public corporations, typically owned by a state or local government. They are operated for the benefit of the communities they serve. A variation on this type of ownership is the **public benefit**

**organization**. Assets (and accumulated earnings) of a nonprofit public benefit corporation belong to the public or to the charitable beneficiaries the trust was organized to serve. In 1999, for example, the Nassau County Medical Center (NCMC), a 1,500-bed healthcare system on Long Island, New York, converted from county ownership to a public benefit corporation. The purpose of the conversion was to give NCMC greater autonomy in its governing board and decision making so that it could compete more effectively with the area's large private hospitals and networks.

In some cases, governmental HCOs may have access to an additional revenue source through taxes—an option not available to other not-for-profit HCOs. Similar to other not-for-profits, government HCOs are not able to raise funds through equity investments and they are exempt from income taxes and property taxes.

Governmental HCOs can face political pressures if their earnings become too great. Rather than reinvesting their surplus in productive assets, the hospital might be pressured to return some of the surplus to the community, to reduce prices, or to initiate programs that are not financially advisable.

## ▶ SUMMARY

The healthcare sector of our economy is growing rapidly in both size and complexity. Understanding the financial and economic implications of decision making has become one of the most critical areas encountered by healthcare decision makers. Successful decision making can lead to a viable operation capable of providing needed healthcare services. Unsuccessful decision making can and often does lead to financial failure. The role of financial information in the decision-making process cannot be overstated. It is incumbent on all healthcare decision makers to become accounting-literate in our financially changing healthcare environment.

## ASSIGNMENTS

1. Only in recent years have hospitals begun to develop meaningful systems of cost accounting. Why did they not begin such development sooner?
2. Your hospital has been approached by a major employer in your market area to negotiate a preferred provider arrangement. The employer is seeking a 25% discount from your current charges. Describe a structure that you might use to summarize the financial implications of this decision. Describe the factors that would be critical in this decision.
3. What type of financial information should be routinely provided to board members?

## SOLUTIONS AND ANSWERS

1. Prior to 1983, most hospitals were paid actual costs for delivering hospital services. With the introduction of Medicare's prospective payment system for inpatient care in 1983 and outpatient care in 2000, hospitals now receive prices based on diagnosis-related groupings and ambulatory patient classifications that are fixed in advance. Cost control and, therefore, cost accounting are critical in a fixed-price environment. The expansion of managed care has further restricted revenue and fostered greater interest in costing.
2. This problem could be set up in a results matrix (see Table 1-2). The two actions to be charted are to accept or to reject the preferred provider arrangement opportunity. Possible events would center on the magnitude of volume changes, for example, to lose 1,000 patient days or to gain 500 patient days. A key concern in estimating the financial impact would be the hospital's incremental revenue and incremental cost positions. In short, how large would the revenue reduction and cost reduction be if significant volume were lost? Actuarial gains or losses of business would be functions of the hospital's market position.
3. Board members do not need to see detailed financial information that relates to their established plans to ensure that the plans are being met. If significant deviations have occurred more details may be necessary to take corrective action or to modify established plans.

## References

Nicholson, S., Pauly, M. V., Burns, L. R., Baumritter, A., & Asch, D. A. (2000). Measuring community benefits provided by for-profit and nonprofit hospitals. *Health Affairs, 19*(6), 168.

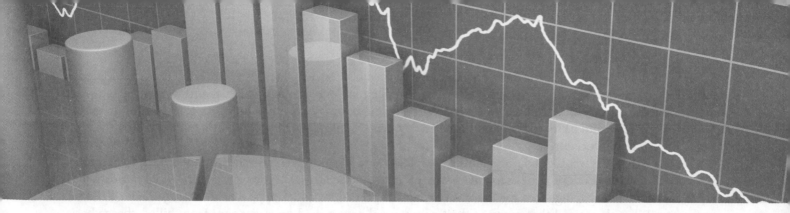

# CHAPTER 2
# Billing and Coding for Health Services

## REAL-WORLD SCENARIO

Riley Ilene, the Chief Financial Officer of Campbell Hospital, was concerned by the reduction in revenue during the last 3 months. The revenue reduction was most pronounced in the outpatient arena and represented a 15% reduction from prior-year levels. Loss of this revenue had eroded Campbell's already thin operating margins, and the hospital was now operating with losses.

Riley's first thought was that volume may be down from prior-year levels. She asked her controller, Michael Dean, to report on comparative volumes for last year and this year. Michael's report showed that total numbers of outpatient visits were actually above last year. Furthermore, the increases in volumes appeared relatively uniform across all product line groupings. Riley then directed Michael to review "revenue and usage" summaries for the current year and last year. A revenue and usage summary would show the quantity of items billed by charge code and payer. The summaries would also break out the volumes by inpatient and outpatient areas.

After reviewing these data Michael reported back to Riley with some startling news. Volumes for several procedures in the hospital's "charge master" were well below prior-year levels. Specifically, the numbers of drug administration codes that are reported when an injectable or infusible drug is administered were well below prior-year levels. This was surprising because the number of injectable and infusible drugs had actually increased.

Riley thought she had discovered the problem and reported back to her CEO, Meredith Lynn. However, Meredith asked Riley whether this could have caused the revenue reduction. Meredith believed that a heavy percentage of the hospital's payment was related to either case payment for inpatients or APC (ambulatory patient classification) groups for outpatients. Meredith believed that these bundled payments would not be impacted by a failure to document the drug administration procedures.

Riley said that this was a good point and she would do some additional research and report back to Meredith. Riley found that Medicare provides separate payment for the drug administration procedure when performed in outpatient visits. The average loss for the undocumented procedure codes appeared to average about $150 per occurrence. Riley also found that many of their commercial payers paid on a discount from billed charge basis. Failure to report these procedures for these payers would result in lost revenue. The only remaining task was to discover why charges for drug administration procedures for outpatient procedures were not being recorded.

---

Healthcare firms are for the most part business-oriented organizations. Their ultimate financial survival depends on a consistent and recurring flow of funds from the services they provide to patients. Without an adequate stream of revenue these firms would be forced to cease operations. In this regard, healthcare firms are similar to most business entities that sell products or services in our economy. **FIGURE 2-1** depicts the stages involved in the revenue cycle for a healthcare firm. The critical stages in the revenue cycle for healthcare firms are the provision and documentation of services to the patient, the generation of charges for those services, the preparation of a bill or **claim**, the submission of the bill or claim to the respective payer, and the collection of payment.

A simple review of the six stages of the revenue cycle in Figure 2-1 hides the significant degree of complexity involved in revenue generation for healthcare providers. No other industry in our nation's economy experiences the same level of billing complexity that most healthcare firms face. Part of this complexity is related to the nature and importance of the services provided. Regulation is also a factor that further complicates documentation and billing for healthcare services. Finally, the existence of different payment methods and rates for multiple payers further complicates the revenue cycle for most healthcare firms. Payment complexity is addressed in Chapter 3.

## ▶ Generating Healthcare Claims

**FIGURE 2-2** provides more detail to the steps and processes involved in the actual generation of a healthcare bill or claim. The process and steps mirror those in Figure 2-1 except additional detail unique to healthcare firms is included. The process often begins with the collection of information about the patient before the delivery of services in the patient registration function. Information about the patient, including address, date of birth, and insurance data, is collected to facilitate bill preparation after services are provided. Once

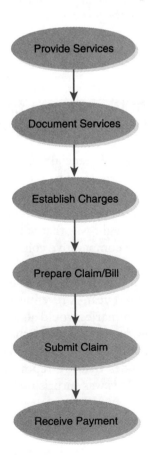

**FIGURE 2-1  Revenue Cycle**

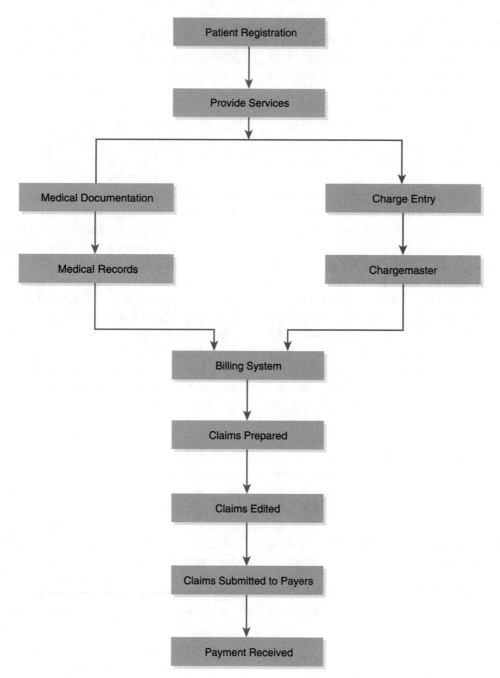

**FIGURE 2-2  Detailed Revenue Cycle**

services have been provided, data from that encounter(s) flow into two areas: medical documentation and charge capture.

Although the primary purpose of the data accumulated in the medical record may be related to clinical decision making, a substantial proportion of the information may also be linked to billing. For example, the assignment of diagnosis and procedure codes within the medical record by physicians plays a key role in diagnosis-related group (DRG) assignment. Many healthcare payers provide payment for inpatient care related to a DRG-constructed assignment. Data

in the medical record are also the primary source for documenting the provision of services. For example, if a patient's bill listed a series of drugs used by the patient but the medical record did not show those drugs as being used, the claim would not be supported. The primary linkage between the claim and the medical record is related to the documentation of specific services provided and their reporting in a series of clinical codes. We explore the categories of coding and their importance to billing shortly.

Data from the provision of services also flow directly to billing through the capture of charges. The posting of charges to a patient's account is usually accomplished through the issuance and collection of "charge slips" in a manual mode or through direct order entry or bar code readers in an automated system. The critical link here is the firm's price list, often referred to as its "charge master" or **charge description master (CDM)**. The CDM is simply a list of all items for which the firm has established specific prices. In a hospital setting it is not unusual to find more than 20,000 items on its charge master.

Information from the medical record and the charge master then flow into the actual claim. For most healthcare firms there are two basic categories of claims: the Uniform Bill 2004 (UB-04) and the Centers for Medicare and Medicaid Services (CMS) 1500. The UB-04 is the claim form used by most hospitals to report claims for both inpatient and outpatient services. The CMS-1500 is used primarily for physician and professional claims. **Appendix 2-A** provides samples of these two claim forms.

The final step before actual claim submission is claims editing. Although all healthcare firms may not perform this step, for many it is critical. During this editing process several key areas are reviewed. First, does the claim have enough information to trigger payment by the patient's payer? For example, perhaps the claim is missing the patient's social security number or healthcare plan identification number. Second, does the claim meet logical standards and is it complete? For example, a claim may have a charge for laboratory panel but no charge for a blood draw to collect the sample. Editing is critical for accurate and timely payment by third-party payers. Now that we have a general overview of how the revenue cycle works to generate a claim to receive payment, we will discuss the various stages (Figure 2-2) in more detail.

## ▶ Scheduling and Registration

In most cases a patient or their representative provides a basic set of information regarding the patient before the actual delivery of services. In a physician's office this may be done just before performance of medical services. For an elective hospital inpatient admission, it may be done a week or more before admission. A number of clinical and financial sets of information are collected at this point. From the financial perspective, three activities are especially important in the billing and collection process.

Perhaps the most important activity is *insurance verification*. If the patient has indicated they have third-party insurance coverage, it is important to have this coverage verified from the payer. The

patient may also have secondary coverage from another health plan. Verification of that coverage is also critical to accurate and timely billing. The critical piece of information to collect from the patient in this regard is their health plan identification number, which may sometimes be their social security number. Queries to the health plan before service can validate the type of coverage provided by the health plan and the eligibility of the patient for the scheduled service. In today's environment insurance verification is often done online. Sometimes prior approval for elective services is required by the health plan before a claim can be submitted. This prior verification is often referred to as **precertification**. Information regarding coverage for large governmental programs such as Medicare and Medicaid is often not needed because the benefit structure is standardized. It is important, however, to verify the existence of current coverage.

The second activity in registration is often related to the computation of **copayment** or **deductible** provisions that may be applicable for the patient. Once insurance coverage has been determined, it is usually possible to calculate the required amount that may still be due from the patient. For example, a Medicare patient without supplemental coverage may report to a hospital for a scheduled computed tomography. It is possible for the registration staff to calculate the amount of copayment due by the patient. The registration staff can then advise the patient regarding the amount of payment due and try to make arrangements for payment at the point of service.

The third activity in this registration process relates to **financial counseling**. Patients who have no coverage may be eligible for some discount through the healthcare firm's charity care policy. Any residual that may still be due can be discussed with the patient, and financing may be arranged before the point of service. It is also possible that an uninsured patient may be eligible for some governmental programs, especially Medicaid. Staff at the healthcare firm can advise the patient regarding eligibility and help them to complete the necessary documents required for coverage. It is important to note that the reasons for delays in payment to the provider are often the result of inaccurate information or inappropriate processes in the scheduling and registration phase.

## ▶ Provide Services

As services are being provided to the patient, information is being recorded. Some of this information will require additional human interaction to generate an appropriate claim. This information will be reviewed and processed through the Medical Documentation and Health Information Management (HIM)/Medical Records phases of the revenue cycle. This information will eventually meet up with data that has been recorded electronically and does not require additional professional review (collected through charge entry and the charge master). Let's first discuss the areas that will require additional professional review.

## ▶ Medical Documentation and HIM/Medical Records

Information regarding the services provided to the patient is recorded in the patient's medical record. Critical pieces of information contained in that record are used in the billing process and are communicated to the payers to trigger payment. The Health Insurance Portability and Accountability Act (HIPAA) of 1996 designated two specific coding systems to be used in reporting to both public and private payers:

1. International Classification of Diseases. As of October 1, 2015, version 10 is the edition used in the United States.
2. Healthcare Common Procedure Coding System (HCPCS)

HIPAA requires that two categories of information be reported to payers: diagnosis codes and procedure codes. The **ICD-10** has sets of codes that provide information for both diagnoses and procedures. For diagnosis codes, ICD-10-CM (Clinical Modification) is utilized and for procedure codes, ICD-10-PCS (Procedure Coding System). ICD-10-CM is the United States' clinical modification of the ICD-10 code set created by the World Health Organization. ICD-10-PCS is maintained and updated by CMS. This coding system is primarily used in the United States. The HCPCS provides information in the procedure area but does not provide information regarding diagnoses. HIPAA therefore requires

that ICD-10 codes be used for diagnosis reporting for all healthcare providers, including hospitals and physicians. ICD-10 procedure codes are required for procedure reporting for hospital inpatients, whereas HCPCS codes are used for procedure reporting by hospitals for outpatient services and also by physicians (**TABLE 2-1**).

ICD-10-CM reflects a significant improvement over ICD-9-CM. ICD-10-CM is an expanded code set to include health-related conditions and offer a higher level of specificity by including separate codes for laterality and additional characters for greater detail. The ICD-10-CM code set can be three to seven characters in length, compared to ICD-9 diagnosis codes, which comprise three digits that may be followed by a decimal point with up to two additional digits. Each code in ICD-10-CM provides greater specificity at the sixth and seventh character level. The hierarchical structure is similar, where the first three characters are the category of the codes and all codes with the same category have similar traits. For example, all ICD-10-CM codes that start with I50 (letter I followed by number 50) represent heart failure. Additional characters further specify the patient's exact condition. For example, I50.31 refers to acute diastolic (congestive) heart failure. **TABLE 2-2** provides a listing of the top 10 inpatient diagnoses reported by participating hospitals in 2015.

ICD-10-PCS codes are used to report hospital inpatient procedures. ICD-10-PCS codes are challenging, yet flexible. ICD-10-PCS codes each have a unique definition and procedures are assigned to only one code, unlike ICD-9 procedure codes. The process of constructing procedure codes in ICD-10-PCS is logical and consistent. The ICD-10-PCS code set has expanded to always include seven characters, whereas the ICD-9 procedure codes could be three to four digits long with a decimal point placed after the second digit. To represent an open right heart catheterization (previously ICD-9 procedure code 37.21), one would consult section 4 (measurement and monitoring), body system A (physiological systems), root operation

| **TABLE 2-1** HIPAA-Designated Coding | | | | |
|---|---|---|---|---|
| | **Inpatient** | | **Outpatient** | |
| **Provider** | **Diagnosis** | **Procedure** | **Diagnosis** | **Procedure** |
| Professional | ICD-10-CM | CPT/HCPCS | ICD-10-CM | CPT/HCPCS |
| Facility | ICD-10-CM | ICD-10-PCS | ICD-10-CM | CPT/HCPCS |

**TABLE 2-2** 2015 Primary Diagnosis Frequency

| Dx1 | Definition | Frequency | Percentage of Total |
|------|------------|-----------|---------------------|
| Z3800 | Single liveborn infant, delivered vaginally | 26,558 | 6.6% |
| A419 | Sepsis, unspecified organism | 15,732 | 3.9% |
| Z3801 | Single liveborn infant, delivered by cesarean | 12,953 | 3.2% |
| J189 | Pneumonia, unspecified organism | 6,456 | 1.6% |
| N179 | Acute kidney failure, unspecified | 5,719 | 1.4% |
| O3421 | Maternal care for scar from previous cesarean delivery | 5,560 | 1.4% |
| I214 | Non-ST elevation (NSTEMI) myocardial infarction | 5,264 | 1.3% |
| J441 | Chronic obstructive pulmonary disease w (acute) exacerbation | 5,262 | 1.3% |
| I5023 | Acute on chronic systolic (congestive) heart failure | 3,889 | 1.0% |
| N390 | Urinary tract infection, site not specified | 3,711 | 0.9% |

Courtesy of Cleverley & Associates

0 (measurement), body part 2 (cardiac), approach 0 (open), function/device N (sampling and pressure), and qualifier 6 (right heart). The final code selection would be 4A020N6. **TABLE 2-3** shows a listing of the top 10 inpatient ICD-10 procedure codes reported by participating hospitals in 2015.

ICD-10 diagnosis and procedure codes are very important in the assignment of a DRG. DRG

**TABLE 2-3** 2015 Primary Procedure Frequency

| Px1 | Definition | Frequency | Percentage of Total |
|------|------------|-----------|---------------------|
| 10E0XZZ | Delivery of Products of Conception, External Approach | 20,305 | 8.0% |
| 10D00Z1 | Extraction of POC, Low Cervical, Open Approach | 13,464 | 5.3% |
| 3E0234Z | Introduction of Serum/Tox/Vaccine into Muscle, Perc Approach | 13,100 | 5.1% |
| 0VTTXZZ | Resection of Prepuce, External Approach | 10,578 | 4.1% |
| 02HV33Z | Insertion of Infusion Dev into Sup Vena Cava, Perc Approach | 4,630 | 1.8% |
| 4A023N7 | Measure of Cardiac Sampl and Pressure, L Heart, Perc Approach | 4,490 | 1.8% |
| 30233N1 | Transfuse Nonaut Red Blood Cells in Periph Vein, Perc | 4,003 | 1.6% |
| 0SRC0J9 | Replace of R Knee Jt with Synth Sub, Cement, Open Approach | 3,799 | 1.5% |
| 0SRD0J9 | Replace of L Knee Jt with Synth Sub, Cement, Open Approach | 3,795 | 1.5% |
| 5A1D60Z | Performance of Urinary Filtration, Multiple | 3,463 | 1.4% |

Courtesy of Cleverley & Associates

payment is widely used by many payers, especially Medicare. Coding therefore has a critical link to provider payment. **TABLE 2-4** provides a list of the top 10 DRGs reported by Medicare in fiscal year (FY) 2015.

Physicians and other clinical professionals use HCPCS codes for reporting both inpatient and outpatient procedures. HCPCS codes are also used by facilities for reporting outpatient procedures; however, they use ICD-10-PCS procedure codes for reporting inpatient procedures. There are two tiers used in HCPCS coding, Level I and Level II. Level I codes are referred to as current procedure terminology (CPT) codes; these codes have been developed and maintained by the American Medical Association. Level I and CPT are used interchangeably to describe these sets of codes. Six main categories of CPT codes are currently used:

- Evaluation and Management (99201 to 99499)
- Anesthesia (01000 to 01999)
- Surgery (10021 to 69979)
- Radiology (70010 to 79999)
- Pathology and Laboratory (80047 to 89398)
- Medicine (90281 to 99607)

The five-digit CPT code may also contain a "modifier" that is a two-digit numeric or alphanumeric code that may provide additional information essential to process a claim. For example, modifier 91 is used to indicate that a laboratory procedure was repeated. **TABLE 2-5** provides a list of the top 10 hospital outpatient CPT codes reported to Medicare in FY 2015.

Level II HCPCS codes were developed by CMS to report services, supplies, or procedures that were not present in the Level I (CPT) codes. There are two groups within the Level II HCPCS codes: permanent and temporary. Permanent codes are five-digit codes that begin with an alpha character. **TABLE 2-6** provides a list of the top 10 Level II permanent HCPCS codes reported to Medicare in FY 2015 for hospital outpatients.

Level II temporary HCPCS codes are used to meet a temporary need for a new code. These codes are also five-digit codes that begin with an alpha character. These codes can exist for a long time, but they may be replaced with a permanent code. **TABLE 2-7** provides a list of the top 10 Level II temporary HCPCS codes reported to Medicare in FY 2015 for hospital outpatients.

HCPCS/CPT codes have a significant effect on provider payment for both facilities and physicians. CPT codes are often linked to fee schedules for many physicians by a large number of payers, which makes coding by medical groups especially critical. CPT

### TABLE 2-4  2015 Public Data: DRG Frequency

| DRG | Definition | Frequency | Percentage of Total |
|-----|------------|-----------|---------------------|
| 871 | Septicemia or severe sepsis w/o MV 96+ hours w MCC | 698,326 | 5.2% |
| 470 | Major joint replacement or reattachment of lower extremity w/o MCC | 648,919 | 4.8% |
| 291 | Heart failure and shock w MCC | 305,874 | 2.3% |
| 292 | Heart failure and shock w CC | 273,563 | 2.0% |
| 392 | Esophagitis, gastroent and misc digest disorders w/o MCC | 265,473 | 2.0% |
| 872 | Septicemia or severe sepsis w/o MV 96+ hours w/o MCC | 212,543 | 1.6% |
| 683 | Renal failure w CC | 210,497 | 1.6% |
| 690 | Kidney and urinary tract infections w/o MCC | 208,193 | 1.5% |
| 194 | Simple pneumonia and pleurisy w CC | 203,574 | 1.5% |
| 190 | Chronic obstructive pulmonary disease w MCC | 199,499 | 1.5% |

Courtesy of Cleverley & Associates

**TABLE 2-5**  2015 Public Data: CPT Frequency

| CPT | Definition | Frequency | Percentage of Total |
|---|---|---|---|
| 36415 | Drawing blood | 33,143,861 | 8.2% |
| 85025 | Automated hemogram | 23,390,665 | 5.8% |
| 80053 | Comprehen metabolic panel | 20,227,551 | 5.0% |
| 85610 | Prothrombin time | 12,772,008 | 3.1% |
| 80048 | Metabolic panel total Ca | 11,100,899 | 2.7% |
| 93005 | Electrocardiogram, tracing | 9,100,359 | 2.2% |
| 80061 | Lipid panel | 8,984,219 | 2.2% |
| 84443 | Assay thyroid stim hormone | 7,585,005 | 1.9% |
| 84484 | Assay of troponin, quant | 6,198,958 | 1.5% |
| 85027 | Automated hemogram | 6,134,892 | 1.5% |

Courtesy of Cleverley & Associates

**TABLE 2-6**  2015 Public Data: Level II (Permanent) Frequency

| Level II (Perm) | Definition | Frequency | Percentage of Total |
|---|---|---|---|
| J0878 | Daptomycin injection | 46,996,523 | 8.2% |
| J1442 | Inj, filgrastim g-csf 1 mcg | 26,933,441 | 4.7% |
| J2704 | Inj, propofol, 10 mg | 23,561,098 | 4.1% |
| J1756 | Iron sucrose injection | 21,799,458 | 3.8% |
| J1453 | Fosaprepitant injection | 18,895,315 | 3.3% |
| J2405 | Ondansetron HCl inj 1 mg | 16,283,351 | 2.8% |
| J0897 | Denosumab injection | 15,014,923 | 2.6% |
| J0881 | Darbepoetin alfa, inj, non-ESRD, 1 mcg | 14,266,565 | 2.5% |
| J0583 | Bivalirudin | 13,296,583 | 2.3% |
| J0131 | Acetaminophen injection | 13,242,289 | 2.3% |

Courtesy of Cleverley & Associates

and Level II HCPCS codes are also used by Medicare to define payment for many hospital outpatient services in the ambulatory patient classification (APC) system.

## Learning Objective 3

Define the basic characteristics of charge masters.

**TABLE 2-7** 2015 Public Data: Level II (Temporary) Frequency

| Level II (Temp) | Definition | Frequency | Percentage of Total |
|---|---|---|---|
| Q9967 | LOCM 300–399 mg/ml iodine, 1 ml | 80,292,567 | 54.1% |
| G0463 | Hospital outpt clinic visit | 25,487,287 | 17.2% |
| Q0138 | Ferumoxytol, non-ESRD | 13,707,635 | 9.2% |
| Q9966 | LOCM 200–299 mg/ml iodine, 1 ml | 4,527,896 | 3.1% |
| Q9963 | HOCM 350–399 mg/ml iodine, 1 ml | 2,318,546 | 1.6% |
| G0378 | Hospital observation per | 2,111,162 | 1.4% |
| G0277 | Hbot, full body chamber, 30 m | 1,737,553 | 1.2% |
| Q9965 | LOCM 100–199 mg/ml iodine, 1 ml | 1,692,373 | 1.1% |
| Q9958 | HOCM <=149 mg/ml iodine, 1ml | 1,433,080 | 1.0% |
| Q0162 | Ondansetron 1 mg, oral | 1,155,710 | 0.8% |

Courtesy of Cleverley & Associates

# ▶ Charge Entry and Charge Master

Performing actual medical services is the lifeblood of a healthcare firm's revenue cycle. Without the provision of services there is no revenue, but it is imperative that charges for those services are captured. A service that is performed but not billed does not produce revenue. The three greatest concerns in billing are the following:

- Capture of charges for services performed
- Incorrect billing
- Billing late charges

**Charge capture** is usually accomplished in one of two ways. Historically, many providers have used actual paper documents or charge slips to identify services performed.

These charge slips were then posted to a patient's account in a batch-processing mode by data processing or the business office. However, with the implementation of the electronic health record (EHR), providers more frequently are applying charges to accounts through an order entry system. This method may involve direct entry of charges to the patient's account through a computer terminal. Scanning of bar codes may also be used.

Sometimes healthcare firms use a "**charge explosion**" system to better organize charge entry for selective services. For example, a specific type of surgery may routinely require a standardized set of supplies. Rather than entering all of these supplies, one code may be used that then explodes into the list of supply codes used for that surgery.

The key link between charge capture and the billing process is the "**charge code**" that is reflected in the order entry system or the charge slips and also represented on the firm's charge master (also known as CDM). There is a unique charge code for each service procedure, supply item, or drug in the CDM. As a result, many thousands of items are present in the typical hospital charge master. Every charge master usually has the following six common elements:

- Charge code
- Item description
- Department number
- Charge/price
- Revenue code
- CPT/HCPCS code

**TABLE 2-8** provides a sample of selected codes in a hospital's charge master. The first column in the charge master is the charge code or item code for the specific service or product to be billed. The second

**TABLE 2-8** Partial Charge Master File

| Item Code | Item Description | Dept Num | Standard Price ($) | Revenue Code | HCPCS |
|-----------|-----------------|----------|--------------------|--------------|-------|
| 3023001 | DAILY CARE FOURTH NORTH | 13030 | 665.50 | 111 | |
| 3120000 | DAILY CARE ICU | 13120 | 1,172.50 | 200 | |
| 4156159 | MINERAL OIL 30 ML | 13190 | 11.50 | 250 | |
| 4400206 | SINGLE TOWEL | 14430 | 2.25 | 270 | |
| 4440302 | HEP C ANTIBODIES-0288 | 14440 | 53.50 | 300 | 86803 |
| 4470220 | HAND XRAY-0183 | 14470 | 102.50 | 320 | 73130 |
| 4472538 | C/T PELVIS W & W/O ENHANCEMENT | 14302 | 1,069.75 | 350 | 72194 |
| 4416000 | LASIK SURGERY—PER EYE | 13190 | 2,105.25 | 360 | 66999 |
| 4416013 | O.R. MINOR CHARGE—0.5 HOUR | 13190 | 556.75 | 360 | |
| 4416014 | O.R. MINOR CHARGE—1 HOUR | 13190 | 770.75 | 360 | |
| 4416015 | O.R. MINOR CHARGE—1.5 HOURS | 13190 | 983.00 | 360 | |
| 4416016 | O.R. MINOR CHARGE—2 HOURS | 13190 | 1,197.25 | 360 | |
| 4416017 | O.R. MINOR CHARGE—2.5 HOURS | 13190 | 1,409.25 | 360 | |
| 4416018 | O.R. MINOR CHARGE—3 HOURS | 13190 | 1,622.25 | 360 | |
| 4520013 | ANESTHESIA MINOR—0.5 HOUR | 14520 | 110.25 | 370 | |
| 4520014 | ANESTHESIA MINOR—1 HOUR | 14520 | 151.25 | 370 | |
| 4520015 | ANESTHESIA MINOR—1.5 HOURS | 14520 | 192.75 | 370 | |
| 4520016 | ANESTHESIA MINOR—2 HOURS | 14520 | 233.00 | 370 | |
| 4520017 | ANESTHESIA MINOR—2.5 HOURS | 14520 | 274.75 | 370 | |
| 4520018 | ANESTHESIA MINOR—3 HOURS | 14520 | 317.00 | 370 | |
| 3167020 | BLOOD TRANSFUSION | 13160 | 303.25 | 391 | 36430 |
| 4532057 | MASSAGE, 8 MINS | 14532 | 21.00 | 420 | 97124 |
| 3050717 | EVALUATION—OT | 13050 | 130.00 | 430 | 97003 |
| 3160001 | EMERG DEPT OBSERVATION 0–3 HRS | 13160 | 241.25 | 450 | 99218 |
| 3160002 | EMERG DEPT OBSERVATION 3–6 HRS | 13160 | 406.00 | 450 | 99218 |
| 3160003 | EMERG DEPT OBSERVATION 6–12 HRS | 13160 | 492.00 | 450 | 99219 |

| 3160004 | EMERG DEPT OBSERV. OVER 12 HRS | 13160 | 592.75 | 450 | 99220 |
|---------|-------------------------------|-------|--------|-----|-------|
| 4465350 | OUTPAT VISIT LEVEL 1 (NEW) | 14465 | 78.50 | 510 | 99201 |
| 4465351 | OUTPAT VISIT LEVEL 2 (NEW) | 14465 | 92.25 | 510 | 99202 |
| 4465352 | OUTPAT VISIT LEVEL 3 (NEW) | 14465 | 112.50 | 510 | 99203 |
| 4465353 | OUTPAT VISIT LEVEL 4 (NEW) | 14465 | 159.75 | 510 | 99204 |
| 4465354 | OUTPAT VISIT LEVEL 5 (NEW) | 14465 | 209.00 | 510 | 99205 |

column provides a short description of the specific item code. For example, item code 3023001 is "Daily Care Fourth North." The third column is the *department number* and may reference a specific department within the firm that might also relate to their accounting system or general ledger. The fourth column is the *current price* or standard price for the service or product. In some cases there may be multiple prices for a given code. For example, a hospital might price a laboratory procedure at one rate for inpatient care and at another for outpatient care. These differences may reflect differences in cost or competitive price pressure. Competition for outpatient laboratory procedures may be intense, and the hospital may believe that it must discount its price if it wants to maintain its market share for outpatient laboratory services.

The fifth column is the revenue code. *Revenue codes* are a required field in any hospital claim that is submitted on a UB-04. The current categories used have been mandated by CMS, and the current list is presented in **TABLE 2-9**. The last column included in many charge masters is the field for the HCPCS code.

| **TABLE 2-9** Revenue Code Categories | |
|---|---|
| | **Accommodation Revenue Codes** |
| 010X | All-Inclusive Rate |
| 011X | R&B—Private (Medical or General) |
| 012X | R&B—Semiprivate (2 Beds) (Medical or General) |
| 013X | Semiprivate (3 and 4 Beds) |
| 014X | Private (Deluxe) |
| 015X | R&B—Ward (Medical or General) |
| 016X | Other R&B |
| 017X | Nursery |
| 018X | LOA |
| 019X | Subacute Care |
| 020X | Intensive Care |
| 021X | Coronary Care |

*(continues)*

**TABLE 2-9** Revenue Code Categories *(continued)*

| | Ancillary Services Revenue Codes |
|---|---|
| 022X | Special Charges |
| 023X | Incremental Nursing Care Rate |
| 024X | All-Inclusive Ancillary |
| 025X | Pharmacy (See also 063X, an extension of 025X) |
| 026X | IV Therapy |
| 027X | Medical/Surgical Supplies and Devices (See also 062X, an extension of 027X) |
| 028X | Oncology |
| 029X | DME (Other than Renal) |
| 030X | Laboratory |
| 031X | Laboratory Pathological |
| 032X | Radiology—Diagnostic |
| 033X | Radiology—Therapeutic and/or Chemotherapy Administration |
| 034X | Nuclear Medicine |
| 035X | Computed Tomographic (CT) Scans |
| 036X | Operating Room Services |
| 037X | Anesthesia |
| 038X | Blood and Blood Products |
| 039X | Blood and Blood Component Administration, Processing and Storage |
| 040X | Other Imaging Services |
| 041X | Respiratory Services |
| 042X | Physical Therapy |
| 043X | Occupational Therapy |
| 044X | Speech-Language Pathology |
| 045X | Emergency Room |
| 046X | Pulmonary Function |
| 047X | Audiology |

| 048X | Cardiology |
|------|-----------|
| 049X | Ambulatory Surgical Care |
| 050X | Outpatient Services |
| 051X | Clinic |
| 052X | Freestanding Clinic |
| 053X | Osteopathic Services |
| 054X | Ambulance |
| 055X | Skilled Nursing |
| 056X | Home Health—Medical Social Services |
|      | **Ancillary Services Revenue Codes** |
| 057X | Home Health—Home Health Aide |
| 058X | Home Health—Other Visits |
| 059X | Home Health—Units of Service |
| 060X | Home Health—Oxygen |
| 061X | Magnetic Resonance Technology (MRT) |
| 062X | Medical/Surgical Supplies (Extension of 027X) |
| 063X | Pharmacy (Extension of 025X) |
| 064X | Home IV Therapy Services |
| 065X | Hospice Service |
| 066X | Respite Care |
| 067X | Outpatient Special Residence Charges |
| 068X | Trauma Response |
| 069X | Pre-hospice/Palliative Care Services |
| 070X | Cast Room |
| 071X | Recovery Room |
| 072X | Labor Room/Delivery |
| 073X | EKG/ECG (Electrocardiogram) |

*(continues)*

**TABLE 2-9** Revenue Code Categories   *(continued)*

|  | Ancillary Services Revenue Codes |
|---|---|
| 074X | EEG (Electroencephalogram) |
| 075X | Gastrointestinal Services |
| 076X | Treatment or Observation Room |
| 077X | Preventive Care Services |
| 078X | Telemedicine |
| 079X | Extra-Corporeal Shock Wave Therapy |
| 080X | Inpatient Renal Dialysis |
| 081X | Acquisition of Body Components |
| 082X | Hemodialysis—Outpatient or Home |
| 083X | Peritoneal Dialysis—Outpatient or Horne |
| 084X | CAPD—Outpatient or Home |
| 085X | CCPD—Outpatient or Home |
| 086X | Magnetoencephalography (MEG) |
| 087X | Reserved for Dialysis |
| 088X | Miscellaneous Dialysis |
| 089X | Reserved |
| 090X | Behavioral Health Treatments/Services (See also 091X, an extension of 090X) |
| 091X | Behavioral Health Treatments/Services (Extension of 090X) |
| 092X | Other Diagnostic Services |
| 093X | Medical Rehabilitation Day Program |
| 094X | Other Therapeutic Services |
| 095X | Other Therapeutic Services—Extension of 094X |
| 096X | Professional Fees (See also 097X and 098X) |
| 097X | Professional Fees (Extension of 096X) |
| 098X | Professional Fees (Extension of 096X and 097X) |
| 099X | Patient Convenience Items |

| 100X | Behavioral Health Accommodations |
|------|----------------------------------|
| 101X–209X | Reserved |
| 210X | Alternative Therapy Services |
| 211X–300X | Reserved |
| 310X | Adult Care |
| 311X–999X | Reserved |

In our sample charge master not all entries have an HCPCS code. For example, the first two entries that relate to room and board charges do not have an HCPCS code. Also notice that surgery and anesthesia do not have HCPCS codes. For a great majority of their surgeries, most hospitals bill on a time/level basis. A trained coding professional from the health information management department assigns a CPT code or an ICD-10 procedure code to the procedure at a later point in time before billing. Where an HCPCS code is present in the charge master, less time is required in coding claims at the back end, but care needs to be taken that appropriate charge codes are used at charge entry. Utilizing the time/level billing approach with HIM assignment of appropriate procedure codes permits additional oversight for accuracy, as well as an efficiency for the maintenance of the charge master. Consider surgery where there are almost unlimited combinations of types of procedures and variable time. To have a unique line for each variation would literally explode the size of the charge master.

Direct coding of HCPCS codes into the charge master is referred to as **static coding** or "hard coding." When codes are left off the charge master and entered later by HIM personnel, the process is referred to as **dynamic coding** or "soft coding." Many ancillary procedures, such as laboratory or radiology procedures, can be coded statically; that is, HCPCS codes can be placed in the charge master. In contrast, many surgery codes are dynamically coded and HIM staff will assign the appropriate HCPCS code after the procedure based on documented and authenticated medical record information.

## Learning Objective 4

Define the two major bill types used in healthcare firms.

## ▶ Billing and Claims Preparation

For most healthcare providers, medical claims fall into one of two types: CMS-1500 and CMS-1450 (UB-04). Noninstitutional providers and suppliers use the CMS-1500 form to submit claims to Medicare and many other payers. Institutional providers use the HCFA-1450 or UB-04 to submit claims to Medicare and most other payers. Sample copies of both a CMS-1500 and a UB-04 are shown in Appendix 2-A.

Most claims in today's environment are submitted in an electronic format. Usually, claims are submitted directly to the payer or indirectly to a "clearinghouse" where the claims are grouped and then sent to the appropriate payer. The HIPAA administrative simplification provisions direct the Secretary of Health and Human Services to adopt standards for administrative transactions, code sets, and identifiers as well as standards for protecting the security and privacy of health data. After October 16, 2003, all providers who were not small providers (institutional organizations with fewer than 25 full-time employees or physicians with fewer than 10 full-time employees) had to send all claims electronically in the HIPAA format.

The electronic format required under HIPAA is 837I for the UB-04 and 837P for the CMS-1500. These formats specify both the nature of data exchange and the required data fields. There have been a few additional data elements included in the 837I and 837P protocols that were not in the current CMS-1500 and UB-04 claim forms.

Two primary payment grouping algorithms are DRGs and APCs, both of which are used by Medicare for hospital payment and also many commercial payers. Both DRGs and APCs are assigned based on data in the UB-04. A DRG is often assigned depending on values found in the UB-04 for ICD-10-PCS procedure codes and ICD-10-CM diagnosis codes. Surgical procedures require an ICD-10-PCS procedure code and may also require an ICD-10-CM diagnosis code. A medical DRG requires one or more ICD-10-CM diagnosis codes. Note that in the UB-04 form in Appendix 2-A there are spaces allowed for up to 25 diagnosis and 25 procedure codes. Many diagnosis and procedure codes may group to more than one DRG. A complete review of the DRG title is necessary to understand the correct DRG assignment. To illustrate this concept, let's examine the following related DRGs:

- DRG 689 Kidney and Urinary Tract Infections with Major Complications or Comorbidities (MCC)
- DRG 690 Kidney and Urinary Tract Infections without Major Complications or Comorbidities (MCC)

Both of the above DRGs have a common set of diagnosis codes, one of which must be present to assign a patient to one of these DRGs. ICD-10-CM N39.0 (Urinary tract infection, site not specified) is one of a list of diagnosis codes that would qualify. If the patient did not present with any complications or comorbidities, he or she would be grouped to MS-DRG 690, which carries a lower weight and payment. Examples of common complications or comorbidities would be specific types of congestive heart failure, certain diabetes conditions, and specific anemia cases. If the patient did present with a complication or comorbidity approved by Medicare, then the patient would receive the higher weighted MS-DRG assignment (MS-DRG 689), which would provide greater reimbursement for the hospital. A list of MS-DRG weights can be found in Appendix 3-A.

In 2000, Medicare payment for hospital outpatient services shifted to APC payment. Each APC is related to one or more HCPCS/CPT codes. The assignment of HCPCS/CPT codes is presented in the UB-04 claim form in field locator (FL) #44 HCPCS/Rates. For many inpatient claims there may be no HCPCS/CPT codes presented. The sample claim in Appendix 2-A is for an inpatient claim, and no HCPCS codes are presented. Items are aggregated at the revenue code level. For example, all laboratory procedures are grouped under Revenue Code 300. Outpatient claims, however, show detailed procedures, and HCPCS/CPT codes will be present. For example, APC 5493 (Level 3 Intraocular Procedures) may be assigned if one of the following CPT codes is present: 65770 (Revise cornea with implant) or 67027 (Implant eye drug system). The key point to remember is that for an APC to be assigned, an HCPCS code must be present. Multiple HCPCS codes may map to one APC code, but any given HCPCS code maps to one and only one APC.

Appreciate the role of claims editing in the bill submission process.

## ▶ Claims Editing

Both providers and payers use claims editing software to detect possible errors in claim submission. From the provider's perspective they are interested in two major objectives. First, they want to ensure they receive the maximum payment for the medical services delivered to their patients. Second, providers want to shorten the amount of time from claim submission to actual payment. Payers have a similar set of incentives except they are reversed. Payers do not want to make payment in an amount that is greater than the amount of their obligation. Payers also would like to delay payment for as long as possible without violating state payment laws or contract discount terms.

Most large providers use some type of automated software for editing claims that are to be submitted to payers. These software packages check for a large number of possible errors. First, the software determines whether the requisite information for submitting a "clean claim" is present in the claim, such as the correct spelling of the patient's name and the presence of the social security or healthcare plan identification, diagnosis and procedure codes, and the date of service as well as many other possible conditions. The second set of conditions that are often tested deal with the internal validity of the claim. Is the procedure consistent with the gender of the patient? Was there an injection procedure included in the claim but no injectable drug listed? Many of these edit checks may be internally developed, but a large number of them may also be related to uniform claim edits developed by Medicare.

CMS developed the National Correct Coding Initiative (NCCI) to promote national correct coding methodologies and to control improper coding that leads to inappropriate payment of Part B health insurance claims. The coding policies developed are based on coding conventions defined in the American Medical Association's CPT codes, national and local policies and edits, coding guidelines developed by national societies, analysis of standard medical and surgical practice, and review of correct coding practice. CMS has designated a series of specific edit checks that are used in determining hospital outpatient claim status. These edit checks are referred to as outpatient code edits (OCE) and at the time of this writing include 98 specific edit checks.

The OCE uses claim-level and line item–level information in the editing process. The claim-level information includes such data elements as "from" and "through" dates, ICD-10-CM diagnosis codes, type of bill, age, gender, and so on. The line-level information includes such data elements as HCPCS code with up to two modifiers, revenue code, and service units.

Each OCE results in one of six different dispositions. The dispositions help to ensure that all FI/MACs (Fiscal Intermediary/Medicare Administrative Contractor) are following similar procedures. There are four claim-level dispositions:

- Rejection: Claim must be corrected and resubmitted.
- Denial: Claim cannot be resubmitted but can be appealed.
- Return to provider: Problems must be corrected and claim resubmitted.
- Suspension: Claim requires further information before it can be processed.

There are two line item–level dispositions:

- Rejection: Claim is processed but line item is rejected and can be resubmitted later.
- Denial: Claim is processed but line item is rejected and cannot be resubmitted.

The NCCI edits, a subset of the OCE, identify pairs of services that normally should not be billed by the same physician for the same patient on the same day. The NCCI includes two types of edits:

- Comprehensive/component edits identify code pairs that should not be billed together because one service inherently includes the other.
- Mutually exclusive edits identify code pairs that, for clinical reasons, are unlikely to be performed on the same patient on the same day. For example, a mutually exclusive edit might identify two different types of testing that yield equivalent results.

This area of coding edits is very complex but extremely important to the provider's ultimate payment. Sometimes the code edits appear to be inconsistent. For example, OCE edit #43 specifies that when a blood transfusion procedure code is present in the claim but there was no related blood product present, the claim is returned to the provider. There is no related OCE to detect the reverse situation, however. A blood product may be present but no transfusion procedure included. In this situation Medicare pays for the blood product, but the provider loses payment for the transfusion procedure. This is an example of an edit that is most likely added to many hospital claims editing programs.

## ▶ Claim Payment

Everything we have described so far provides context for the complexities that healthcare providers face in documenting and charging for patient services. However, just because the patient claim has exited the facility does not necessarily mean the provider will be paid, paid in full, or paid quickly. In order to receive payment, providers must submit claims in a timely manner (Medicare requires claims be submitted no later than 12 months from the date of service) and address any challenges and questions that payers may pose. In these situations, claims are often sent back to HIM and other administrative staff to address concerns, and potentially resubmit claims, prior to payments being made. While obtaining payment for services can be protracted and challenging, providers that manage the coding and billing process well are better positioned to receive timely payments.

## ▶ SUMMARY

Accurate billing and coding are essential to a healthcare firm's financial survival. This is a very complex area that requires the input of billing and coding professionals. In many healthcare firms, the billing and coding functions may report to the chief financial officer because of their integral relation to revenue generation. Failure to capture all charges associated with a patient encounter can result in significant lost revenue. Some estimates of lost charges run as high as 5% of total charges. Given the relatively low margins for most healthcare firms, this could be a catastrophic loss.

Most claims are submitted electronically to payers and must now be consistent with HIPAA provisions that govern electronic data interchange submissions. Healthcare claims are unique in many respects, but coding is an area of special importance. In most other business settings, a bill simply lists the items purchased or services rendered. In healthcare firms the charge codes describing the services or products must be related to standard procedure codes and supplemented with diagnosis codes to document the legitimacy of the services. These codes can and do have a major role in not only the amount of payment received, but also the timeliness of that payment. Claims editing software is widely used by healthcare providers to ensure the accuracy of their claims before submission.

## ASSIGNMENTS

1. A hospital submitting an outpatient claim would use a UB-04 claim form. What source of coding information is used to report diagnosis codes? What source of coding information is used to report procedures?
2. Elective procedures often require prior approval from the patient's insurance company. What is this approval process often called?
3. From what types of coding information must the following codes be derived:
   - H00.11, Chalazion right upper eyelid
   - 0D160ZA, Open gastric bypass surgery to jejunum
   - 69090 Ear Piercing
   - G0283 Electrical Stimulation
4. Including an HCPCS/CPT code directly in the charge master is called what?
5. Many DRGs are in "families" that differ by severity. There are three levels of severity: (1) MCC—Major Complication/Comorbidity, which reflects the highest level of severity; (2) CC—Complication/Comorbidity, which is the next level of severity; and (3) Non-CC—Non-Complication/Comorbidity, which do not significantly affect severity of illness and resource use. The DRG that has the MCC is usually paid at a higher rate. What can cause a DRG without MCC to be changed to a DRG with MCC?
6. A payer may delay or deny payment because of inaccurate or missing information in a submitted claim. Many contracts require payment within a specified period of time (e.g., 30 days) from submission of a "clean claim." How can providers of healthcare services avoid submitting claims that may be rejected?
7. The Medicare intermediary has returned a claim to a hospital because of OCE violation #1: invalid diagnosis code. This would imply that the procedure performed is not supported by the diagnosis code. What action can the provider take to get this claim paid?

## SOLUTIONS AND ANSWERS

1. ICD-10 diagnosis codes are used to report diagnosis information on a UB-04 for both hospital inpatient and outpatient claims. HCPCS codes are used to report procedure codes for hospital outpatient claims.
2. Precertification.
3. H00.11 (ICD-10-CM Diagnosis Code), 0D160ZA (ICD-10-PCS Procedure Code), 69090 (Level I HCPCS/CPT Code), G0238 (Level II HCPCS Code).
4. Static coding.
5. Although a number of factors may lead to the designation of "with MCC," the presence of additional diagnosis codes that reflect the severity of the patient's health status (such as UTI, kidney failure, or sepsis) can often change the coding to a "with MCC" designation. This illustrates the importance of good physician documentation in the medical record and accurate transcription from the medical record to the claim form.
6. Insurance of clean claim submission often starts at registration. Accurate collection of patient and related insurance information is critical in the claims submission process. Claims editing software can also check for issues that may result in claims denial before submission.
7. Because this is an OCE violation where the claim is returned to the provider, the provider can correct the diagnosis code and resubmit for payment. Ideally, a good claims editing system would have caught this problem before submission.

# Appendix 2-A

## Sample UB-04 Form and Sample CMS-1500 Form

### SAMPLE UB-04 FORM

| | | |
|---|---|---|
| **1** ABC Medical Center<br>PO Box 1713<br>Columbus, OH 43210<br>614-722-9614 | **2** | **3a PAT. CNTL #** 13504295    **4 TYPE OF BILL** 111<br>**b. MED. REC. #** 404390000003<br>**5 FED. TAX NO.** 311054871   **6 STATEMENT COVERS PERIOD FROM** 080010 **THROUGH** 081410 **7** |

| 8 PATIENT NAME | a | Brutus Buckeye | 9 PATIENT ADDRESS | a | 00 Buckeye Lane, Columbus, OH 43210 |
|---|---|---|---|---|---|
| b | | | b | c d e | |

| 10 BIRTHDATE | 11 SEX | 12 DATE | 13 HR | 14 TYPE | 15 SRC | 16 DHR | 17 STAT | 18 | 19 | 20 | 21 | 22 | 23 | 24 | 25 | 26 | 27 | 28 | 29 ACDT STATE | 30 |
|---|---|---|---|---|---|---|---|---|---|---|---|---|---|---|---|---|---|---|---|---|
| 01301960 | M | 080906 | 06 | 8 | 1 | 14 | 01 | | | | | | | | | | | | | |

| 31 OCCURRENCE CODE DATE | 32 OCCURRENCE CODE DATE | 33 OCCURRENCE CODE DATE | 34 OCCURRENCE CODE DATE | 35 OCCURRENCE SPAN CODE FROM THROUGH | 36 OCCURRENCE SPAN CODE FROM THROUGH | 37 |
|---|---|---|---|---|---|---|
| | | | | | | |

| 38 Brutus Buckeye<br>00 Buckeye Lane<br>Columbus, OH 43210 | | 39 CODE VALUE CODES AMOUNT | 40 CODE VALUE CODES AMOUNT | 41 CODE VALUE CODES AMOUNT |
|---|---|---|---|---|
| | a | 01   444 00 | | |
| | b | | | |
| | c | | | |
| | d | | | |

| 42 REV. CD. | 43 DESCRIPTION | 44 HCPCS / RATE / HIPPS CODE | 45 SERV. DATE | 46 SERV. UNITS | 47 TOTAL CHARGES | 48 NON-COVERED CHARGES | 49 |
|---|---|---|---|---|---|---|---|
| 1 | 110 | Room board, pvt | 447 00 | | 5 | 2,235.00 | 15.00 | 1 |
| 2 | 250 | Pharmacy | | | 61 | 674.87 | | 2 |
| 3 | 253 | Drugs, take home | | | 65 | 88.75 | 88.75 | 3 |
| 4 | 259 | Other Pharmacy | | | 27 | 151.38 | | 4 |
| 5 | 270 | Medsur supplies | | | 40 | 1,603.82 | | 5 |
| 6 | 278 | Supply Implants | | | 5 | 2,969.55 | | 6 |
| 7 | 300 | Laboratory | | | 3 | 228.50 | | 7 |
| 8 | 310 | Path Lab | | | 6 | 589.00 | | 8 |
| 9 | 360 | OR services | | | 29 | 7,662.00 | | 9 |
| 10 | 370 | Anesthesia | | | 3 | 1,108.05 | | 10 |
| 11 | 410 | Respiratory Services | | | 1 | 8.65 | | 11 |
| 12 | 710 | Recovery Room | | | 2 | 391.00 | | 12 |
| 13 | 999 | Pt convenience | | | 1 | 7.20 | 7.20 | 13 |
| 23 | 001 | **PAGE 1 OF 1**   **CREATION DATE** 081910   **TOTALS →** | | | | 17,697.77 | 110.96 | 23 |

| 50 PAYER NAME | 51 HEALTH PLAN ID | 52 REL. INFO | 53 ASG. BEN. | 54 PRIOR PAYMENTS | 55 EST. AMOUNT DUE | 56 NPI | |
|---|---|---|---|---|---|---|---|
| A Central Benefits | 230147 | Y | Y | | | 57 OTHER PRV ID | A |
| B | | | | | | | B |
| C | | | | | | | C |

| 58 INSURED'S NAME | 59 P.REL | 60 INSURED'S UNIQUE ID | 61 GROUP NAME | 62 INSURANCE GROUP NO. | |
|---|---|---|---|---|---|
| A Brutus Buckeye | 08 | 000 00 0000 | | | A |

| 63 TREATMENT AUTHORIZATION CODES | 64 DOCUMENT CONTROL NUMBER | 65 EMPLOYER NAME | |
|---|---|---|---|
| A | | | A |
| B | | | B |
| C | | | C |

| 66 DX | 52469 | 5180 | 52461 | 72210 | | | | | 68 |
|---|---|---|---|---|---|---|---|---|---|
| 69 ADMIT DX | 52469 | 70 PATIENT REASON DX | a | b | c | 71 PPS CODE | 72 ECI | a b c | 73 |

| 74 PRINCIPAL PROCEDURE CODE DATE | OTHER PROCEDURE CODE DATE | OTHER PROCEDURE CODE DATE | 75 | 76 ATTENDING NPI TZ AC 198x |
|---|---|---|---|---|
| 765 081410 | 247 081410 | | | QUAL   LAST   FIRST |
| OTHER PROCEDURE CODE DATE | OTHER PROCEDURE CODE DATE | OTHER PROCEDURE CODE DATE | | 77 OPERATING NPI QUAL LAST FIRST |
| 80 REMARKS | 81CC a b c d | | | 78 OTHER NPI QUAL LAST FIRST<br>79 OTHER NPI QUAL LAST FIRST |

UB-04 CMS-1450   © 2005 NUBC    OMB APPROVAL PENDING    **NUBC** National Uniform Billing Committee LIC9213257    THE CERTIFICATIONS ON THE REVERSE APPLY TO THIS BILL AND ARE MADE A PART HEREOF.

F245-367-000

Reproduced from Centers for Medicare and Medicaid Services

**SAMPLE CMS-1500 FORM**

## HEALTH INSURANCE CLAIM FORM

| 1. MEDICARE | MEDICAID | CHAMPUS | CHAMPVA | GROUP HLTH PLAN | FECA BLK LUNG | OTHER | 1a. INSURED'S I.D. NUMBER (FOR PROGRAM IN ITEM 1) |
|---|---|---|---|---|---|---|---|
| ☐ (Medicare #) | ☐ (Medicaid #) | ☐ (Sponsor SSN) | ☐ (VA File #) | ☐ (SSN or ID) | ☐ (SSN) | ☐ (ID) | |

**2. PATIENT'S NAME (Last, First, MI)**

**3. PATIENT'S DATE OF BIRTH**
MM DD YY   SEX
M ☐  F ☐

**4. INSURED'S NAME (Last, First, MI)**

**5. PATIENT'S ADDRESS (No., Street)**

**6. PATIENT RELATIONSHIP TO INSURED**
Self ☐   Spouse ☐   Child ☐   Other ☐

**7. INSURED'S ADDRESS (No., Street)**

CITY                      STATE

**8. PATIENT STATUS**
Single ☐   Married ☐   Other ☐

CITY                      STATE

ZIP CODE   TELEPHONE (Incl Area Code)

Employed ☐   Full-Time ☐   Part-Time ☐
Student        Student

ZIP CODE   TELEPHONE (Incl. Area Code)

**9. OTHER INSURED'S NAME (Last, First, MI)**

**10. IS PATIENT'S CONDITION RELATED TO:**

**11. INSURED'S POLICY GROUP OR FECA NUMBER**

**a. OTHER INSURED'S POLICY OR GROUP NUMBER**

**a. EMPLOYMENT?** (Current or Previous)
YES ☐   NO ☐

**a. INSURED'S DATE OF BIRTH**
MM DD YY   SEX
M ☐  F ☐

**b. OTHER INSURED'S DATE OF BIRTH**
MM DD YY   SEX
M ☐  F ☐

**b. AUTO ACCIDENT?**        PLACE (State)
YES ☐   NO ☐

**b. EMPLOYER'S NAME OR SCHOOL NAME**

**c. EMPLOYER'S NAME OR SCHOOL NAME**

**c. OTHER ACCIDENT?**
YES ☐   NO ☐

**c. INSURANCE PLAN NAME OR PROGRAM NAME**

**d. INSURANCE PLAN NAME OR PROGRAM NAME**

**10d. RESERVED FOR LOCAL USE**

**d. IS THERE ANOTHER HEALTH BENEFIT PLAN?**
YES ☐   NO ☐   If yes, return to and complete item 9a–d

READ BACK OF FORM BEFRE COMPLETING & SIGNING THIS FORM.
**12. PATIENT'S OR AUTHORIZED PERSON'S SIGNATURE** I authorize the release of any medical or other information necessary to process this claim. I also request payment of government benefits either to myself or to the party who accepts assignment below.

SIGNED _____ DATE _____

**13. INSURED'S OR AUTHORIZED PERSON'S SIGNATURE**
I authorize payment of medical benefits to the undersigned physician or Supplier for services described below.

SIGNED _____

**14. DATE OF CURRENT:**  ILLNESS (First symptom) OR
MM DD YY   INJURY (Accident) OR
PREGNANCY (LMP)

**15. IF PATIENT HAS HAD SAME OR SIMILAR ILLNESS, GIVE FIRST DATE**
MM DD YY

**16. DATES PATIENT UNABLE TO WORK IN CURRENT OCCUPATION**
MM DD YY   MM DD YY
FROM             TO

**17. NAME OF REFERRING PHYSICIAN**

**17a. ID NUMBER OF REFERRING PHYSICIAN**

**18. HOSPITALIZATION DATES RELATED TO CURRENT SERVICES**
MM DD YY   MM DD YY
FROM             TO

**19. RESERVED FOR LOCAL USE**

**20. OUTSIDE LAB?**        $ CHARGES
☐ YES   ☐ NO

**21. DIAGNOSIS OR NATURE OF ILLNESS OR INJURY (RELATE ITEMS 1,2,3 OR 4 TO ITEM 24E BY LINE)**

1. _____   3. _____

2. _____   4. _____

**22. MEDICAID RESUBMISSION**
CODE            ORIGINAL REF. NO.

**23. PRIOR AUTHORIZATION NUMBER**

| 24. | A | B | C | D | | E | F | G | H | I | J | K |
|---|---|---|---|---|---|---|---|---|---|---|---|---|
| | DATE(S) OF SERVICE From To MM DD YY MM DD YY | Place of Service | Type of Service | PROCEDURES, SERVICES, OR SUPPLIES (Explain Unusual Circumstances) CPT/HCPCS | MODIFIER | DIAGNOSIS CODE | $ CHARGES | DAYS OR UNITS | EPSDT Family Plan | EMG | COB | RESVD FOR LOCAL USE |
| | | | | | | | | | | | | |
| | | | | | | | | | | | | |
| | | | | | | | | | | | | |
| | | | | | | | | | | | | |
| | | | | | | | | | | | | |

**25. FEDERAL TAX ID NUMBER   SSN EIN**
☐ ☐

**26. PATIENT'S ACCOUNT NO.**

**27. ACCEPT ASSIGNMENT?**
(For govt. claims, see back)
☐ YES   ☐ NO

**28. TOTAL CHARGE**
$

**29. AMOUNT PAID**
$

**30. BALANCE DUE**
$

**31. SIGNATURE OF PHYSICIAN OR SUPPLIER INCLUDING DEGREES OR CREDENTIALS** (I certify that the statements on the reverse apply to this bill and are made a part thereof.)

SIGNED _____ DATE _____

**32. NAME AND ADDRESS OF FACILITY WHERE SERVICES WERE RENDERED** (If other than home or office)

**33. PHYSICIAN'S, SUPPLIER'S BILLING NAME, ADDRESS, ZIP CODE & PHONE #**

PIN #            GRP #

FORM HCFA-1500

Reproduced from Centers for Medicare and Medicaid Services

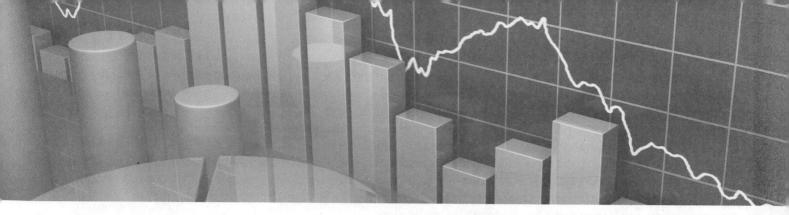

# CHAPTER 3

# Financial Environment of Healthcare Organizations

## REAL-WORLD SCENARIO

Joshua Douglas, chief financial officer at Marshall Regional Hospital, was exploring an option to convert his hospital to critical access hospital (CAH) status under the Medicare program. The CEO of the hospital, Mikaela Grace, had directed Josh to investigate this possible option at the last hospital board meeting. The hospital has been losing money for the last 4 years, and cash positions have been eroding to the point of possible default on a small debt issue.

Marshall Regional is a 13-bed acute-care hospital with a 10-bed skilled nursing facility. It is located in a rural area of a western state and is 50 miles from the nearest hospital. The current economic climate in the region is not good and is not expected to improve in the near future. Because of its low volume, Marshall's cost per unit for acute inpatient and outpatient procedures is very high. As a result the hospital has been losing large sums of money on its sizable Medicare volume. Josh has estimated that the hospital loses 45 cents for every dollar of Medicare payment. Because a high percentage of the local population is elderly, Medicare is the hospital's largest source of business. Medicare represents 50% of all outpatient revenue and 65% of inpatient revenue. Most inpatient procedures are not complex, and severely ill patients are transferred to a larger hospital 50 miles up the interstate.

Mikaela Grace had been to a recent seminar and learned that her hospital might be eligible for CAH status. If the hospital was successful in its application for CAH status, it would no longer be paid under prospective payment.

Instead, Marshall Regional would receive the cost incurred in delivering services to Medicare patients plus 1%. Josh estimated that this change in payment could result in a substantial improvement in operating margins and should help the hospital to secure its financial future.

Upon Josh's review of CAH materials, he learned that over 1,300 hospitals in the United States are designated as CAH. Although a number of criteria must be met, it seemed that the hospital would be eligible. It was under the 25-bed maximum, and it was more than 35 miles from the nearest hospital. It also maintained an acute-care length of stay less than 96 hours and had round-the-clock emergency care available. Although there were other criteria, Josh was very optimistic about Marshall's chances of receiving CAH status, and he drafted a memo to Mikaela recommending that they move forward with an application.

Almost any measure of size indicates that the healthcare industry is big business. For several decades its proportion of the gross domestic product has been steadily increasing and it now represents approximately 18%, with over 3 trillion dollars in annual expenditures. Paralleling this growth, the pressures for cost control within the system have increased tremendously, especially at the federal and state levels for control of Medicare and Medicaid. Healthcare organizations (HCOs) that are not able to deal effectively with these pressures face an uncertain future. In short, as the expected demand for health services continues to increase during the next several decades as our population ages, successful HCOs must become increasingly cost efficient.

---

### *Learning Objective 1*

Describe factors that influence the financial viability of a healthcare organization.

---

## ▶ **Financial Viability**

Not only is an HCO a basic provider of health services, it is also a business. The environment of an HCO viewed from a financial perspective is depicted in **FIGURE 3-1**.

In the long run the HCO must receive dollar payments from the community in an amount at least equal to the dollar payments it makes to its suppliers. In very simple terms, this is the essence of financial viability.

The community in Figure 3-1 is the provider of funds to the HCO. The flow of funds is either directly or indirectly related to the delivery of services by the HCO. For our purposes, the community may be categorized as follows:

1. Patients
   a. Self-payer
   b. Third-party payer
      • Blue Cross and Blue Shield
      • Commercial insurance, including managed care
      • Medicaid
      • Medicare
      • Self-insured employer
      • Other
2. Nonpatients
   a. Grants
   b. Contributions
   c. Tax support
   d. Miscellaneous

In most HCOs the greater proportion of funds is derived from patients who receive services directly. The largest percentage of these payments usually comes from third-party sources such as Blue Cross, Medicare, Medicaid, and managed-care organizations. In addition, some nonpatient funds are derived from government sources in the form of grants for research purposes or direct payments to subsidized HCOs, such as county facilities. Some HCOs also receive significant sums of money from individuals, foundations, or corporations in the form of contributions. Although these sums may be small relative to the total amounts of money received from patient services, their importance in overall viability should not be understated. In many HCOs these contributed dollars mean the difference between net income and loss.

The suppliers in Figure 3-1 provide the HCO with resources that are necessary for delivery of quality health care. The major categories of suppliers are the following:

- Employees
- Equipment suppliers
- Service contractors
- Vendors of consumable supplies
- Lenders

Payments for employees usually represent the largest single category of expenditures. For example, in many hospitals payments for employees represent about 60% of total expenditures. **TABLE 3-1** is an example of a statement of operations (similar to

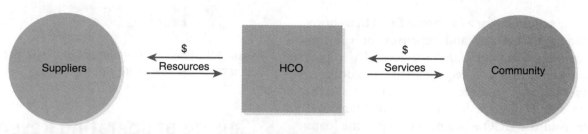

**FIGURE 3-1 Financial Environment of Healthcare Organizations**

**TABLE 3-1** Statement of Operations for Memorial Hospital, Year Ended 20X7 (in Thousands)

| | 20X7 | % |
|---|---|---|
| Unrestricted revenues, gains, and other support: | | |
| Net patient service revenue | $85,502 | 85.84 |
| Premium revenue | 11,195 | 11.24 |
| Other operating revenue | 2,913 | 2.92 |
| Total operating revenue | $99,610 | 100.0 |
| Expenses | | |
| Salaries and benefits | 40,258 | 40.41 |
| Medical supplies and drugs | 27,542 | 27.65 |
| Professional fees | 16,857 | 16.92 |
| Insurance | 5,568 | 5.59 |
| Depreciation and amortization | 3,952 | 3.97 |
| Interest | 1,456 | 1.46 |
| Provision for bad debts | 1,152 | 1.16 |
| Other | 523 | 0.53 |
| Total expenses | $97,308 | 97.69 |
| Operating income | 2,302 | 2.31 |
| Investment income | 1,846 | 1.86 |
| Excess of revenues, gains, and other support over expenses | 4,148 | 4.17 |
| Net assets released from restrictions used for purchase of property and equipment | 192 | 0.19 |
| Increase in unrestricted net assets | $4,340 | 4.36 |

an income statement for a for-profit firm) that shows percentages of revenues and expenses for a hospital. Payments for physicians' services also represent important financial requirements. In addition, lenders such as commercial banks or investment bankers supply dollars in the form of loans and receive from the HCO a promise to repay the loans with interest according to a defined repayment schedule. This financial requirement has grown steadily as HCOs have become more dependent on debt financing.

## ▶ Sources of Operating Revenue

**TABLE 3-2** provides a historical breakdown of the relative size of the healthcare industry and its individual industrial segments. The largest segment is the hospital

**TABLE 3-2**  National Healthcare Expenditures (in Descending Order of 2014 Percentage)

| Type of Expenditure (billions $) | 2009 Actual | 2014 Actual | 2025 Projected | Annualized % Change (2009–2014) | Annualized % Change (2014–2025) | % of 2014 Total NHE |
|---|---|---|---|---|---|---|
| Hospital care | 778.1 | 971.8 | 1,800.5 | 4.5% | 5.8% | 32% |
| Physician and clinical services | 500.5 | 603.7 | 1,092.8 | 3.8% | 5.5% | 20% |
| Prescription drugs | 252.7 | 297.7 | 614.5 | 3.3% | 6.8% | 10% |
| Net cost of private health insurance | 137.9 | 194.6 | 382.6 | 7.1% | 6.3% | 6% |
| Nursing care facilities and continuing care retirement communities | 136.9 | 155.6 | 276.4 | 2.6% | 5.4% | 5% |
| Other health, residential, and personal care | 123.3 | 150.4 | 264.5 | 4.1% | 5.3% | 5% |
| Dental services | 102.3 | 113.5 | 198.9 | 2.1% | 5.2% | 4% |
| Investment: structures and equipment | 93.6 | 108.3 | 198.0 | 3.0% | 5.6% | 4% |
| Other professional services | 66.6 | 84.4 | 154.9 | 4.9% | 5.7% | 3% |
| Home health care | 67.4 | 83.2 | 159.5 | 4.3% | 6.1% | 3% |
| Government public health activities | 74.1 | 79.0 | 147.8 | 1.3% | 5.9% | 3% |
| Other non-durable medical products | 50.3 | 56.9 | 96.3 | 2.5% | 4.9% | 2% |
| Durable medical equipment | 37.8 | 46.4 | 85.5 | 4.2% | 5.7% | 2% |
| Investment: research | 45.4 | 45.5 | 71.4 | 0.0% | 4.2% | 2% |
| Government administration | 29.6 | 40.2 | 87.3 | 6.3% | 7.3% | 1% |
| Total national health expenditures | $2,496.4 | $3,031.3 | $5,631.0 | 4.0% | 5.8% | 100% |

industry, which absorbs about 32% of all healthcare expenditures. This percentage has been stable over the last few years and is projected to be roughly the same percentage in 2025. The physician segment absorbs approximately 20% of total healthcare expenditures; this has also been steady in recent years but still represents a modest decrease over the prior decade when expressed as a percentage of total healthcare expenditures. Prescription drugs represent the third largest healthcare segment, reflecting the rapid rise in prescription drug use. Whereas in the past nursing homes represented the third largest healthcare segment, prescription drugs have overtaken nursing homes. Prescription drugs now constitute about 10% of all healthcare expenditures, although annualized growth rates have slowed recently.

Another area experiencing significant growth has been the administration of private health insurance, representing 7% of health expenditures. This area, which represents the overhead and profit for administering commercial health insurance, had the highest annualized growth of any health expenditure segment during the historical period. The once rapid increases in Medicare spending for skilled nursing facilities (SNFs) have been tempered by the change to prospective payment (explained later in the chapter). Annual growth rates in spending for nursing home care are two-thirds that of the overall health spending growth rates—although this is expected to change in the projected period due to the continued aging of the U.S. society.

**TABLE 3-3** depicts the sources of operating funds for the four largest healthcare segments: hospitals, physicians, prescription drugs, and nursing homes. Dramatic differences in financing among these four segments can be seen easily.

The hospital industry derives roughly half of its total funding from public sources, largely from Medicare and Medicaid. Of the two, Medicare is by far the larger, representing about 26% of all hospital revenue. This gives the federal government enormous control over hospitals and their financial positions. Few hospitals can choose to ignore the Medicare program because of its sheer size. Another 37% of total hospital funding results from private insurance, largely from Blue Cross, commercial insurance carriers, managed-care organizations, and self-insured employers. Direct payments by patients to hospitals represent approximately 3% of total revenue. The implication of this distribution for hospitals is the creation of an oligopsonistic marketplace. The buying power for hospital services is concentrated in the hands of relatively few third-party purchasers, namely the federal government, the state government, Blue Cross, a few commercial insurance carriers, and some large self-insured employers.

The physician marketplace is somewhat different from the marketplace for hospital services. A much larger percentage of physician funding is derived from direct payments by patients (approximately 9%). Compared with hospital funding, a slightly larger percentage of physician funding results from private

| **TABLE 3-3** Sources of Health Services Funding: 2014 and Projected 2025 | | | | | | | | |
|---|---|---|---|---|---|---|---|---|
| | **Hospital** | | **Physicians** | | **Prescription Drugs** | | **Nursing Homes** | |
| **Source** | **2014** | **2025** | **2014** | **2025** | **2014** | **2025** | **2014** | **2025** |
| Private health insurance | 37.3 | 35.6 | 42.2 | 39.3 | 42.8 | 39.7 | 8.4 | 9.1 |
| Out-of-pocket payments | 3.2 | 3.0 | 9.0 | 7.7 | 15.0 | 12.4 | 26.5 | 27.8 |
| Medicare | 25.8 | 27.0 | 22.9 | 25.1 | 29.0 | 35.0 | 22.9 | 28.0 |
| Medicaid | 17.3 | 18.6 | 10.6 | 13.3 | 9.2 | 9.6 | 31.9 | 25.5 |
| Other government | 6.2 | 6.2 | 4.2 | 3.9 | 3.3 | 2.7 | 3.0 | 2.6 |
| Other government and private sources | 10.3 | 9.6 | 11.2 | 10.7 | 0.7 | 0.5 | 7.3 | 7.0 |

insurance sources, largely from Blue Cross and commercial insurance carriers. Physicians derive approximately 42% of their total funds from this source; the hospital segment derives 37% of total funds from this source. Public programs, although still significant, are the smallest source of physician funding, representing 37% of total funds. This situation results because more physician services, such as routine physical examinations and many deductible and copayment services, are excluded from Medicare payment.

Similar to the market for physicians, most payments for prescription drugs (43%) come from private insurance sources. The impact of Medicare coverage can be clearly seen in Table 3-3. By 2025, projections show that Medicare will be funding 35% of all prescription drug costs. Many state Medicaid plans (which are more than 50% federally funded) do provide prescription drug benefits. Medicaid represents over 9% of prescription drug payments.

The nursing home segment receives almost no funding from private insurance sources. The major public program for nursing homes is Medicaid, not Medicare. However, the federal government pays more than 50% of all Medicaid expenditures. Medicare payments to nursing homes are largely restricted to skilled nursing care, whereas most Medicaid payments to nursing homes are for intermediate-level (custodial) care. Out-of-pocket payments are a very significant funding source for this segment, more so than any of the other three, as insurance coverage for these services can require significant patient responsibility. In addition, there are a number of individuals who may not be eligible for Medicaid and do not carry long-term care insurance that pays directly for care.

In these four segments, excluding nursing homes, one important point is seen: government programs, Medicare in particular, are projected to account for more healthcare funding, by percentage, in the future. This is an especially critical point for providers. As government programs have traditionally been less favorable payers with regard to margin, additional pressure will be placed on providers to either cut costs or backfill government payment deficiencies through commercial payment increases. And as commercial payers are increasingly being tasked with slowing the rate of healthcare expenditures, additional cost cutting could be the only viable option.

*Learning Objective 3*

Discuss the major reimbursement methods that are used in health care.

# Healthcare Payment Systems

One of the most important financial differences between healthcare firms and other businesses is the way in which their customers or patients make payment for the services they receive. Most businesses have only one basic type of payment: billed charges. Each customer is presented with a bill that represents the product of the quantity of goods or services received and their appropriate prices. Some selective discounting of the price may take place to move slow inventory during slack periods or to encourage large-volume orders. The basic payment system, however, remains the same: a fixed price per unit of service that is set by the business, not the customer.

In contrast, the typical healthcare firm may have several hundred different contractual relationships with payers, which specify different rates of payment for an identical basket of services. Although different payers may negotiate different rates of payment, the critical distinction is the unit of payment. For example, some payers pay physicians a discount from their charges, other payers pay on fee schedule, Medicare pays on a relative value scale referred to as the **resource-based relative value scale (RBRVS)**, and some health maintenance organizations may pay on an enrolled capitated or bundled basis as part of a larger agreement with other providers. Similar scenarios apply in other sectors of the healthcare industry. Alternative payment units have a different effect on the firm's financial position and might lead to different conclusions with respect to business strategy. It is thus extremely important to understand the financial implications of the various payment units used to pay healthcare firms. Five major payment units are discussed:

1. Historical cost reimbursement
2. Specific services (charge payment)
3. Fee schedules
4. Capitated rates
5. Bundled services

## Historical Cost Reimbursement

Until the early 1980s, cost reimbursement by Medicare was the predominant form of payment for most hospitals and other institutional providers. In addition to Medicare, most state Medicaid plans and a large number of Blue Cross plans paid hospitals on the basis of "reasonable" historical costs. Today, the major payers have abandoned historical cost reimbursement and substituted other payment systems. We provide some discussion of cost reimbursement for two reasons. First, it is used in some limited settings for payment. For example, Medicare still pays on a cost basis for services performed in comprehensive cancer centers, critical-access hospitals (CAHs), and at times, sole community hospitals (SCHs). Second, some policy analysts have suggested that "regulated cost reimbursement" might be a legitimate way to maintain the quality of patient care.

Two key elements in historical cost reimbursement are reasonable cost and apportionment. **Reasonable cost** is simply a qualification introduced by the payer to limit its total payment by excluding certain categories of cost or placing limits on costs that the payer deems reasonable. Examples of costs often defined as unreasonable and therefore not reimbursable are costs for charity care, patient telephones, and nursing education. *Apportionment* refers to the manner in which costs are assigned or allocated to a specific payer such as Medicare. For example, assume that a small hospital has total reasonable costs of $10 million, which represent the costs of servicing all patients. If Medicare is a historical cost reimbursement payer, an allocation or apportionment of that $10 million is necessary to determine Medicare's share of the total cost. Quite often, the apportionment is related to billed charges. For example, if charges for services to Medicare patients were $3 million and total charges to all patients were $15 million, then 3/15 or 20% of the $10 million cost would be apportioned to Medicare.

Several important financial principles of cost reimbursement should be emphasized. First, cost reimbursement can insulate management somewhat from the financial results of poor financial planning. New clinical programs that do not achieve targeted volume or exceed projected costs may still be viable because of extensive cost reimbursement. This assumes that the payer does not regard the costs as unreasonable. Second, cost reimbursement can often be increased through careful planning, just as taxes can often be reduced through tax planning. The key objective is to maximize the amount of cost apportioned to cost payers subject to any tests for reasonableness.

## Specific Services (Charge Payment)

Most healthcare firms have some master price list that identifies the appropriate charge for a defined unit of service. These master price lists are often referred to as charge description masters or CDMs. (See example in Table 2-8.) The charges that are applicable for specific services may bear no relationship to amounts actually paid. For example, a hospital may have charges for a patient categorized as Medicare severity–diagnosis-related group (MS-DRG) #292 (Heart Failure and Shock w CC) for $20,000, but Medicare could determine that the applicable rate of payment was $7,000. Although the charges for specific services of $20,000 are recorded on the patient's bill, the actual charges for specific services are not the basis for payment.

Most institutional providers, such as hospitals and nursing homes, record their charges for specific services on Centers for Medicare and Medicaid Services form CMS-1450 or Uniform Bill 2004 (UB-04). Physician bills are often submitted on a CMS-1500. A sample of both the UB-04 and the CMS-1500 are presented in Appendix 2-A. Both forms are designed by CMS, and they are the standard for claims submission that is required by most payers.

Many medical and surgical procedures often have an assigned code designated as either current procedural terminology (CPT, developed and maintained by the American Medical Association) or **Healthcare Common Procedure Coding System** (HCPCS; developed and maintained by the CMS). Supply and pharmaceutical items usually do not have CPT codes but may have specific HCPCS codes, although most have neither. The sample UB-04 consolidates individual charges for specific services by departmental or revenue code. (See Appendix 2-A.) Note that there is no listing of specific services in this bill because the services are consolidated to a revenue code level. If the patient or their insurance plan requested a detailed bill, then the specific services provided would be listed.

Payers who pay on a specific-service basis usually fall into three categories. First, they could be patients who do not have insurance coverage or lack coverage for the procedures performed. These patients are usually responsible for the total billed charges represented on the claim. Second, the patients could have coverage from an insurance firm that does not have a formal contract with the provider. In the absence of a contract, the patient and/or his or her carrier is responsible for the entire billed charges. This often happens when a provider that is out of the carrier's network treats a patient. Third, some insurance firms negotiate contracts with providers on a discounted-charge basis. The carrier agrees to make payment based on the total billed charges for the claim but at something less than 100%. While many payers negotiate terms that are "fixed" for providers—utilizing fee schedules or bundled payments, as examples—nearly all will have some elements that are sensitive to specific service charges in some form. For example, many payers with fixed payment rates will transition to charges if total patient charges are above a fixed payment amount (a stop-loss provision) or are below a fixed payment amount (a "lesser-of" provision). These provisions exist to protect providers and payers in outlier cases.

Payment for specific services has several important implications for financial management. First, revenue from specific services may represent the major source of profit for many healthcare firms. In these situations pricing or rate setting becomes an important policy. (Rate setting is addressed in Chapter 6.) Second, the firm's rate structure should be based on projected volume and cost. Any unexpected deviation from the projections may require pricing changes. If these changes are not made, there could be a significant effect on the firm's cash flow.

## Fee Schedules

Fee schedule payment is fairly simple to understand. In this situation, the payer and provider agree to some fixed payment amount for a specific service, regardless of the provider's charge (in most cases). Most of these agreements will list the negotiated payment amount by CPT or HCPCS code. As an example, a commercial payer may have a fee schedule amount of $500 for CPT 99283 (Level 3 Emergency Department Visit). When that code appears on an outpatient claim, the hospital receives that amount of payment. There are nuances to this form of payment; however, the basic understanding is important. While many hospitals have commercial payer agreements that utilize fee schedules, nearly every physician practice does. Many contracts that utilize this payment form will also have a "lesser-of" provision that pays the provider whichever is lower: the fee schedule amount or the provider's charge. Given this relationship, it is important that providers ensure their prices are at or above the fee schedule rates in order to capture the full payment amount for the service.

## Capitated Rates

Capitation is a type of payment arrangement where healthcare providers are paid a set amount for each third-party payer enrolled person assigned to them, per period of time, regardless of the amount or type of care the person requires. In some respects a capitated rate is a form of bundled service because the unit of payment is the enrollee. A medical group, hospital, or some association of providers may agree to provide some or all healthcare services for enrollees during a specified period of time. Most often the provider agrees to pay only for specific services they perform. For example, a cardiology group might agree

to provide all cardiology services to an employer or a health maintenance organization for a fixed fee per member per month. Historically, it was rare that a single healthcare provider would agree to provide all medical services to an enrolled population; however, accountable care organizations (ACOs) are changing that dynamic. When this does occur, the term *global capitation* is used to describe the nature of the contractual relationship. Capitation arrangements were more common in the mid-1990s, then experienced a significant decline, but are seeing new life in the form of ACOs. ACOs represent groups of providers that come together to deliver coordinated care to patients. The ACO can be paid on a fully capitated basis or in some modified method, but the end result for the payer is to have more control over the global costs of care for an enrolled population.

In a capitated payment environment, financial planning and control are critical—even more critical than in a bundled services payment situation. In a capitated payment arrangement the provider is responsible not only for the costs of services provided but also their utilization. Changes in either costs or utilization can have a dramatic effect on profitability. Unexpected increases in costs are not usually a basis for contract renegotiation. It is imperative therefore that management knows the cost of providing a unit of service required in the contract. For example, if the negotiated rate is to provide all hospital services to subscribers of a health maintenance organization for a fixed fee per subscriber (capitation), the hospital must know both the utilization and the cost per unit of the required services. Sometimes management may assess the financial desirability of a capitation contract on an incremental basis. This simply means that management is interested in the change in costs and change in revenue that result if the contract is signed. The firm's cost accounting system should be able to define the incremental costs likely to be incurred in a given contract so they can be compared with the incremental revenue likely to result from the contract.

## Bundled Services

Many payment plans pay healthcare providers in what in today's environment could be classified as bundled services arrangements. A bundled services payment plan has two key features. First, payments to the provider are not necessarily related to the list of specific services provided to the patient and identified in the UB-04 or the CMS-1500. Instead, payment is grouped into a mutually exclusive set of service categories. For example, hospitals are paid by some healthcare plans on a per diem (meaning per day) or per case payment rate. Both are examples of bundled service payment. Second, bundled services arrangements have a fixed fee specified per unit of service. For example, in the per diem arrangement, revenue from treating a patient is equal to the length of stay times the negotiated per diem rate.

Medicare has developed bundled services payment plans for most healthcare providers. We discuss some of these plans in detail later in this chapter. Medicare's payment methods have a profound impact on the rest of the industry because they tend to become the standard for payment by many health plans. For example, Medicare pays physicians on an RBRVS basis, and this is often used as the payment basis by many healthcare plans, with one slight wrinkle., These plans most often do not pay the Medicare rate but instead pay some greater or lesser percentage, such as 110% of RBRVS. **TABLE 3-4** presents the unit of payment used by Medicare in a variety of healthcare sectors.

Healthcare providers that are paid under bundled service arrangements need to understand and monitor their costs of production. A bundled service unit is simply a set of specific services that may be grouped or classified into a bundled unit of some kind. Total cost of producing the bundled services unit is therefore a product of two factors.

- Services provided
- Cost per unit of services provided

First, the set of specific services that comprises a bundled unit forms the basis for the cost computation. It is important to recognize, however, that the set of services may not always be fixed. For example, home health firms are paid on a 60-day episode-of-care basis. The number of specific visits per episode is not necessarily fixed. In some cases there may be 30 individual case visits to the patient in the 60-day episode, whereas in other cases 45 individual visits may be necessary. Second, the cost of producing each of the specific services that comprises the bundled unit is multiplied times the number of units required. Whether 30 or 45 visits of care are required, management must control the unit cost of individual visits by monitoring the productivity of nursing staff. Management's overall objective is to minimize the total cost of production, which means keeping total units of service provided at a minimum and producing each unit of service at an efficient level of cost. Naturally, all this must happen within a quality-of-care constraint.

Bundles of care have traditionally been contained to a single provider; however, larger bundles, across multiple providers have recently been created for payment purposes. These larger bundles are often called "episodes" because they involve a longer duration of patient care and involve more providers. For instance, a payer might create an episodic payment form for joint replacement. That episode could involve a patient's presurgical physician visits, the surgical procedure, and recovery care provided at the hospital, as well as physical therapy once the patient has been discharged. Formerly, this example would involve three separate payments to the three providers. Now, a single episode payment could be made to cover the patient's expected full course of treatment. In the end, this newer form of payment is really just a larger bundle.

## Payment Reform

Payment for healthcare services has been changing based on both the continued growth of expenditures and legislative changes. Most notably, the Affordable Care Act (ACA), which was signed into law in 2010, has prompted some significant payment changes. One of the key changes was to integrate more quality or "value" elements

**TABLE 3-4** Medicare Payment Units for Healthcare Sectors

| Healthcare Sector | Payment Unit |
| --- | --- |
| Hospital inpatient | Medicare severity–diagnosis-related groups (MS-DRGs) |
| Hospital outpatient | Ambulatory patient classifications (APCs) |
| Physicians | Resource-based relative value scale (RBRVS) |
| Skilled nursing facilities | Resource utilization groups (RUGs) |
| Home health agencies | Home health resource groups (HHRGs) |

into the healthcare payment structure. While these delivery and payment reforms have been implemented by CMS, the effects have rippled through the entire industry as many other payers have integrated similar elements. Some key areas of reform are listed here:

1. Hospital Readmissions Reduction Program (HRRP): This program reduces payments to hospitals with excessive readmissions.

2. Hospital Value-Based Purchasing (VBP): CMS reduced the base operating payment for hospitals, with the opportunity to gain back payment based on quality performance.

3. Accountable Care Organizations (ACOs): Described earlier in this chapter, these organizations were truly launched as a direct result of ACA. There have been several models, from full capitation, to structures where providers continue to receive fee-for-service payments during the year and then reconcile payment based on cost and quality performance during that period. The latter model seeks to distribute the "shared savings" of treating the population between the payer and the providers.

4. Bundled Payments: The most significant programs that CMS has launched have been the Bundled Payments for Care Improvement (BPCI) and the Comprehensive Care for Joint Replacement (CJR) initiatives. In both programs, the CMS is shifting risk to providers by determining a target price for clinical episodes and holding providers financially accountable if the provision of services within the episode is higher than the target.

5. Hospital-Acquired Condition (HAC) Reduction Program: CMS reduces payments to hospitals that rank among the lowest in prevention of patient conditions that have been linked to hospital care and should be avoidable (surgical site infections, as example).

The integration of quality and cost-efficiency related components into healthcare payment is only likely to continue. While these forms reflect changes, the fundamental elements of payment still fall into the five categories just discussed. The difference is that these five fundamental forms are being adjusted to improve value in the system by providing cost reduction and quality enhancement.

---

*Learning Objective 4*

Discuss the major aspects of Medicare benefits.

---

# ▶ Medicare Benefits

Medicare has four basic benefit programs for its beneficiaries: Part A (hospital insurance), Part B (medical insurance), Part C (Medicare Advantage plans), and Part D (prescription drug coverage). Part A, or hospital insurance, typically is provided free to all beneficiaries if they have 40 or more covered quarters of Medicare employment. Part B, or Medical insurance, usually requires a monthly payment by the beneficiary. In 2016 this payment was $121.80 per month for most beneficiaries. Part C and Part D are options for beneficiaries and can involve additional beneficiary payments depending on coverage options.

Medicare benefits are provided to three categories of individuals. Far and away the largest single group is people over 65 years of age. The second group is disabled individuals, and the third group includes people with end-stage renal disease.

There are two primary ways that Medicare beneficiaries may receive care through the system. The most popular method is the so-called traditional or original plan (Parts A and B). In this plan Medicare beneficiaries can go to any hospital, doctor, or specialist that accepts Medicare to receive care. The second method is a Medicare managed-care plan (Part C). Part C comprises plans offered by private companies that contract with Medicare to provide Part A and Part B benefits to people with Medicare who enroll in the plan. Some of these plans may also include other health provider/service coverage, including prescription drugs, which can result in additional fees for Medicare beneficiaries. Essentially, this is commercial payer coverage provided to Medicare beneficiaries where Medicare pays a portion or all of the expense. Under this method beneficiaries are enrolled in a private healthcare plan or health maintenance organization, and they are usually limited in terms of the providers that they can visit for care to those included in the plan's network. Usually, Medicare managed-care plans provide a wider range of benefits, such as routine physicals and prescription drugs, to offset their restricted networks.

Benefits under Part A include hospital stays, skilled nursing care, hospice care, and some home health services. Under Part A there is a deductible, which means the patient is responsible for this amount before any payment by Medicare. In 2016 the hospital deductible was $1,288. **Coinsurance** arrangements also exist under Part A coverage. Patients who stay beyond 60 days in a hospital were required to pay fees for each additional day, depending on the total length of stay. Patients in SNFs had no deductible but were required to pay an additional $161 per day for lengths of stay between 21 and 100 days. Generally speaking, hospice and home health are also covered with limited beneficiary exposure; however, limits do exist.

Benefits under Part B include a wide range of services, such as doctor's fees, hospital outpatient services, clinical laboratory tests, durable medical equipment, and a number of other preventive medical services. In 2016, there was a $166 deductible for medical services received under Part B. Part B benefits also require a coinsurance payment in many cases. This coinsurance is 20% of approved amounts. This coinsurance amount can be no less than 20% of the total payment due (although it can be larger) to the provider of services, which includes Medicare's payment and the coinsurance.

Part D, the Medicare drug plan, was initiated on January 1, 2006. Medicare beneficiaries have the ability to choose from a variety of plan providers that fall into two categories: a prescription drug plan (covering drugs only) or Medicare advantage plan (covering medical services and drugs). Both plan types have differing costs and benefits for beneficiaries, although the government stipulates some basic requirements.

Many Medicare beneficiaries purchase additional insurance from private insurance firms to pay for deductibles and coinsurance amounts that exist in the Medicare program. This coverage is often referred to as supplemental or Medigap coverage and may also provide limited coverage for other healthcare services. For a more complete picture of specific benefits under the Medicare program, visit Medicare's website, www.medicare.gov.

### Learning Objective 5

Describe how Medicare reimburses the major types of providers, and discuss the implications of these methods for an organization's resource management.

## ▶ Medicare Payments

### Hospital Inpatient

Medicare pays hospitals for inpatient care on a bundled services unit basis referred to as a **prospective payment system (PPS)**. Medicare officially launched PPS on October 1, 1983. All hospitals participating in the Medicare program are required to participate in PPS, except those excluded by statute:

- Children's hospitals
- Distinct psychiatric and rehabilitation units
- Hospitals outside the 50 states
- Hospitals in states with an approved waiver
- CAHs

PPS provides payment for all hospital nonphysician services provided to hospital inpatients. This payment also covers services provided by outside suppliers, such as laboratory or radiology units. Medicare makes one comprehensive all-inclusive payment to the hospital, which is then responsible for paying outside suppliers or nonphysician services.

Total payments to a hospital under Medicare can be split into the following elements (see **FIGURE 3-2**):

- Prospective payments
  - DRG operating payment
  - DRG capital payment
- Reasonable cost payments

First, let's discuss the elements of prospective payment. The basis of PPS payment is the DRG system developed by Yale University, which takes all possible diagnoses from the *International Classification of Diseases Clinical Modification* system and classifies them into 25 major diagnostic categories based on organ systems. These 25 categories are further broken down into distinct medically meaningful groupings or DRGs. Medicare contends that the resources required to treat a given DRG entity should be similar for all patients within a DRG category. However, in federal fiscal year 2016, DRGs were expanded to account for patient acuity. The number of DRGs increased significantly as a result. At the time of publication, the total number of MS-DRGs was 758. (**Appendix 3-A** lists 758 MS-DRGs.)

The MS-DRG operating payment results from the multiplication of the hospital dollar rate and the specific case weight of the MS-DRG. Appendix 3-A provides the most recent case weight for the 758 MS-DRGs. The case weight for MS-DRG 001, Heart Transplant with MCC, is 26.2466. This measure indicates that in terms of expected cost, MS-DRG 001 would cost about 26 times more than the average case. A specific value is assigned to each of the 758 MS-DRGs.

The dollar rate is broken down into labor and nonlabor components. The labor component is adjusted for cost of living. **TABLE 3-5** provides hypothetical rates that might be defined by Medicare.

Every hospital in the United States has a wage index value assigned to it. That wage index is multiplied by the labor component of the Medicare standardized payment to yield the DRG operating payment. If we assume that a hospital has a wage index of 1.2509, its DRG operating payment for DRG 001 would be calculated as follows:

$$\text{Payment} = \text{DRG weight} \times ([\text{Labor amount} \times \text{Wage index}] + \text{Nonlabor amount})$$

$$\text{Payment} = 26.2466([\$3,800 \times 1.2509] + \$1,700)$$
$$= \$169,380$$

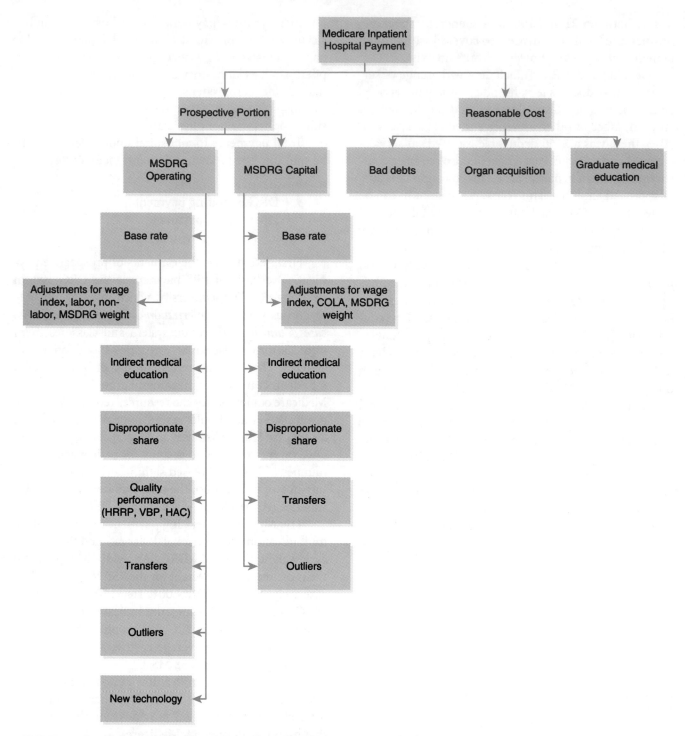

**FIGURE 3-2** **Breakdown of Medicare Inpatient Payments to a Hospital**

| **TABLE 3-5** Hypothetical Medicare Rates According to Hospital Status | |
| --- | --- |
| **Rate** | |
| Labor | Nonlabor |
| $3,800 | $1,700 |

This dollar payment may be modified to address the following areas:

■  Indirect medical education: The add-on payment for teaching hospitals related to the numbers of interns and residents at the hospital and the hospital's bed size. The allowance is over and above salaries paid to interns and residents, which are already covered as a reasonable cost. The additional payment is meant to cover the additional costs that the teaching hospital incurs in the treatment of patients.

- **Disproportionate share/uncompensated care:** Separate payment is also provided to hospitals that treat a large percentage of Medicaid, Medicaid-eligible, and uninsured patients.
- **New technology:** Cases that involve certain approved new technologies receive additional payment to reflect the additional cost of care.
- **Quality-based programs (Hospital VBP, Hospital Readmissions Reduction, and HAC Reduction Program):** Medicare adjusts payment based on quality performance, as previously described in this chapter.
- **Transfers:** Payments are reduced for cases that are transferred to another hospital or post-acute provider.
- **Outlier payments:** Additional payments for patients who use an unusually large amount of resources. We discuss their computation next.

An additional payment for a high-cost outlier is made when the actual cost of the case exceeds MS-DRG payment by $22,544, the 2016 required amount. To determine whether this threshold is met, one must define actual costs for the specific case under consideration. Costs are defined using the hospital's overall ratio of cost to charges. For example, a claim with $100,000 of charges in a hospital with a ratio of cost to charges of 0.75 would have a designated cost of $75,000. If this cost were above the threshold, Medicare would make payment at 80% of the difference. The reason that Medicare does not pay 100% of the difference relates to the concept of marginal cost. Medicare believes that additional costs incurred to treat outlier patients are not 100% of average cost.

Separate from the prospective operating payment portion, there is a national standardized federal payment rate for capital costs that is similar to the national rates for labor and nonlabor costs discussed earlier. In 2016 the federal rate for capital costs was $438.65. This rate would be adjusted for the following factors:

- Geographical adjustment, using the wage index to impute higher costs to higher wage areas
- Case mix, using the MS-DRG relative weight
- Disproportionate share adjustment
- Indirect medical education
- Outlier adjustments

As an illustration, assume that we wish to calculate capital payment for MS-DRG 001 when the federal payment rate for capital was approximately $438.65.

We also assume our hospital is in a large urban area with a geographical adjustment factor of 1.194. Note that a hospital's geographical adjustment factor and its wage index usually are not the same. We assume that no other adjustments are applicable. The amount of payment would be as follows:

$$\text{Capital payment} = \text{DRG weight} \times (\text{Standard amount} \times \text{Geographical adjustment factor})$$

$$\text{Capital payment} = 26.2466 \times (\$438.65 \times 1.194)$$
$$= \$13,747$$

There is still a portion of the total Medicare payment that is related to reasonable cost, as shown in Figure 3-2. Costs that are still paid on this basis are:

- Direct medical education costs
- Organ acquisition costs
- Bad debts for copayments and deductibles (reimbursed at 65%)

Hospitals have separate reporting for these areas to document costs and the appropriate additional reimbursement that would result. This reporting and reconciliation of payment is typically conducted through the Medicare cost report that each hospital is required to complete upon completion of its fiscal year. To give the reader some idea of payment composition for an average U.S. hospital, **TABLE 3-6** presents the median payment by category for all U.S. hospitals for a MS-DRG with a case weight of 1.00 in 2016.

**TABLE 3-6** Median Medicare Payment for U.S. Hospitals, MS-DRG Case Weight of 1.00, 2016

| Category | Median Payment |
|---|---|
| DRG operating payment | $5,836 |
| DRG capital payment | 460 |
| Indirect medical education | 169 |
| Disproportionate share | 161 |
| Coinsurance and deductible | 591 |
| Outlier payments | 226 |
| Other | 138 |
| Total | $7,581 |

Courtesy of Cleverley & Associates

There are a number of ways that a hospital can try to increase its total payment under Medicare inpatient PPS payment rules. For example, it can try to get the hospital reclassified to a higher wage index, document bad debts better on Medicare patients, change its ratio of residents to beds to increase its indirect medical education payment, and change the MS-DRG assignment. Far and away the most likely source of increased payment is MS-DRG reclassification. MS-DRGs are assigned by a software package referred to as a grouper. The grouper assigns a MS-DRG based on the patient's age, the **principal diagnosis**, procedures performed, and **secondary diagnosis**. In many cases missed secondary diagnoses can cost the hospital significant amounts of reimbursement.

MS-DRG 179 (Respiratory Infections) carries a MS-DRG weight of 0.9659, whereas MS-DRG 195 (Simple Pneumonia and Pleurisy) carries a weight of 0.7111. For a hospital with an average payment of $5,000 per case weight of 1.000, a patient erroneously assigned to MS-DRG 195 instead of MS-DRG 179 would cost the hospital $1,274: ($5,000 × [0.9659 − 0.7111]). What would cause a patient with an assignment of MS-DRG 195 to be moved to MS-DRG 179? Very simply, is there a specified cause for the pneumonia? For example, if the physician identified salmonella as the bacterial cause, the patient could be legitimately coded as MS-DRG 179. Medical record coders must be on the alert for this information in the physician's note and other documents, and physicians must be educated about the importance of accurate documentation.

There are hundreds of situations like this within a hospital. The importance of accurate coding cannot be overstated in today's payment environment. On the other hand, hospitals should seek to accurately code and not overcode to maximize reimbursement. Hospital executives who intentionally upcode may fall under the government's fraud-and-abuse regulations, which can impose severe civil and criminal penalties.

## Physicians

Beginning in January 1992 Medicare began paying for physician services using the new RBRVS. This payment system replaced the old reasonable-charge method that had been the basis for physician payment since the inception of the Medicare program in the 1960s. Medicare pays the lesser of the actual billed charge or the fee-schedule amount.

From Medicare's perspective, physicians are categorized as participating or nonparticipating physicians. A **participating physician** is one who agrees to accept Medicare's payment for a service as payment in full and will bill the patient for the copayment portion only. The copayment portion is usually 20% of the charge. As an example, assume that a patient received a service from a physician who had an approved fee schedule of $100. The participating physician receives $80 directly from Medicare and then bills the patient for $20, which represents the copayment portion of the bill. If the physician's bill for the service was only $80, Medicare would pay 80%, or $64, and the patient would be billed 20%, or $16. A participating physician agrees to accept assignment on each and every Medicare patient that he or she treats.

A **nonparticipating physician** can choose to accept assignment on a case-by-case basis. Although initially this arrangement might seem advantageous, there are several major drawbacks. First, a nonparticipating physician has a lower fee schedule. The limiting charge is equal to 95% of the approved fee schedule. If the physician in the illustration just discussed were nonparticipating, the amount of the Medicare payment would be $95, not $100. This difference may not seem so important if the physician can recover any of the difference from the patient. However, Medicare has placed some limits on the amount that a nonparticipating physician can recover from the patient. Medicare sets a maximum fee for a nonparticipating physician equal to 115% of the approved fee for nonparticipating physician, which is already only 95% of the approved fee schedule for a participating physician.

A simple illustration may help to better explain this narrative. Assume that a nonparticipating physician provides services to a patient in the amount of $200, but Medicare's approved schedule for a participating physician is only $100. How much can the physician collect? The answer depends on whether the physician accepts or rejects Medicare assignment. First, assume that the physician rejects assignment. The maximum amount that can be collected from this service is as follows:

$$\$109.25 = (0.95 \times \$100) \times 1.15$$

The entire amount will come from the patient directly. No check will be sent to the physician from Medicare. The final total payment could be allocated as follows:

| | |
|---|---|
| Medicare payment to patient (0.80 × $95.00) | $76.00 |
| Patient's copayment (0.20 × $95.00) | 19.00 |
| Additional patient payment | 14.25 |
| Total payment to physician | $109.25 |

The nonparticipating physician can also choose to accept assignment on a case-by-case basis. The advantage realized with assignment is that Medicare will now pay the physician directly for its portion of the bill. The disadvantage is that the physician is subject to the fee schedule for nonparticipating physicians, which is only 95% of the fee approved for participating physicians. In the example above, the nonparticipating physician who agreed to accept assignment on this patient would receive the following payments:

| | |
|---|---|
| Medicare payment to physician (0.80 × $95.00) | $76.00 |
| Patient's copayment (0.20 × $95.00) | <u>19.00</u> |
| Total payment to physician | $95.00 |

The participating physician, on the other hand, would receive $100.00 for this service because of the higher approved-fee schedule. Of the total $100.00 in payment, $80.00 would come directly from Medicare and $20.00 from the patient as the copayment portion.

At the present time Medicare payment rates exist for more than 10,000 physician services, usually broken out by CPT or HCPCS code. Additionally, there are specific values for those codes that vary by region, and there are distinct values for each of the Medicare carrier localities. These payment rates result from the multiplication of three relative values and regional cost indexes. For every procedure there are three components that together reflect the cost of a particular procedure:

1. Work: This factor represents not only physician time involved but also skill levels, stress, and other factors.
2. Practice expense: This factor represents nonphysician costs, excluding malpractice costs.
3. Malpractice: This factor represents the cost of malpractice insurance.

Each individual relative value is then multiplied by a region-specific set of price indexes. To illustrate this adjustment, the weighted value for excision of neck cyst (CPT #42810) for Los Angeles is presented in **TABLE 3-7**. To determine the payment rate for this procedure in Los Angeles, the index-adjusted relative value is multiplied by a conversion factor. If we assume that the conversion factor is $40.00, the approved charge for excision of neck cyst in Los Angeles is $370.80 (9.27 × $40.00).

Medicare also differentiates the payment by the setting in which the procedure was performed. If the procedure was performed in a facility setting (generally a hospital, SNF, or ambulatory surgery center), the amount allowed for practice expense is reduced from what it would be if the procedure was performed in a nonfacility setting. For example, the allowed practice expense weight for excision of neck cyst in a facility setting is 4.56, but if the procedure was performed in a nonfacility setting, the allowed weight is 7.39. The rationale for these differences is related to the additional payment that Medicare would make to the facility. A procedure performed in a hospital involves a payment to the hospital as well as to the physician.

**TABLE 3-7** Components of Price Adjustment for Excision of Neck Cyst in Los Angeles

| | RVU | Geographical Cost Index for Los Angeles | Product |
|---|---|---|---|
| Work | 3.38 | 1.047 | 3.54 |
| Practice expense | 4.56 | 1.161 | 5.29 |
| Malpractice | 0.49 | 0.908 | 0.44 |
| | | | |
| Total | | | 9.27 |

Courtesy of Cleverley & Associates

## Hospital Outpatient

The Balanced Budget Act of 1997 directed CMS to implement a prospective payment system (PPS) under Medicare for hospital outpatient services. All services paid under the new PPS are classified into groups called **ambulatory payment classifications** (APCs). Services in each APC are similar clinically and in terms of the resources they require. A payment rate is established for each APC. Depending on the services provided, hospitals may be paid for more than one APC for an encounter. Not all hospital outpatient procedures have an assigned APC code; some procedures are paid on a fee-schedule basis, such as lab tests, and others may not be paid at all because they are considered incidental services, such as some drugs and medical supply items.

The Balanced Budget Act also changed the way beneficiary coinsurance is determined for the services included under the PPS. A coinsurance amount is initially calculated for each APC based on 20% of the national median charge for services in the APC. The coinsurance amount for an APC will not change until such time as the amount becomes 20% of the total APC payment. In addition, no coinsurance amount can be greater than the hospital inpatient deductible in a given year. This is a major change for Medicare and means that the total burden of payment shifts more to Medicare in the future. A similar change for physician payment was made in 1992.

Both the total APC payment and the portion paid as coinsurance amounts are adjusted to reflect geographical wage variations using the hospital wage index. It is assumed that 60% of the total payment is labor related and thus subject to the wage-index adjustment. Each APC is assigned a relative weight and that weight is then multiplied times the current conversion factor to determine total payment. This methodology framework is used throughout most of Medicare's payment plans.

To illustrate the details discussed, assume that APC #5188 (Diagnostic Heart Catheterization) has a relative weight of 34.576 and the national conversion rate is $73.73. The total amount paid for this APC is $2,549 (34.576 × $73.73). We further assume that Medicare has set the national coinsurance for APC #5188 at $784. To adjust actual payment for a hospital with a wage index of 1.200, the following computations are made to adjust the total payment and the coinsurance payment:

$$\text{Total payment} = (0.60 \times \$2{,}549 \times 1.200) + (0.40 \times \$2{,}549) = \$2{,}855$$

$$\text{Coinsurance} = (0.60 \times \$784 \times 1.200) + (0.40 \times \$784) = \$878$$

**TABLE 3-8** illustrates the Medicare payment for a specific outpatient claim taken from a hospital-submitted UB-04 on a patient who had a left heart cardiac catheterization. The example claim shows that total payment for this claim is $2,549, with $784 coming from the patient as coinsurance. The majority of the items are coded as "N"—incidental services that are packaged

**TABLE 3-8** Example Medicare Payment for Outpatient Diagnostic Heart Catheterization: APC Reimbursement, APC #5188

| Revenue Code | Revenue Code Description | HCPCS | Units | Total Charges | Payment Status Indicator | APC Total Payment | Copayment |
|---|---|---|---|---|---|---|---|
| 300 | Laboratory | 80051 | 1 | $50 | N | $0 | $0 |
| 300 | Laboratory | 82565 | 1 | $200 | N | $0 | $0 |
| 300 | Laboratory | 84520 | 1 | $165 | N | $0 | $0 |
| 300 | Laboratory | 85027 | 1 | $180 | N | $0 | $0 |
| 300 | Laboratory | 85730 | 1 | $190 | N | $0 | $0 |
| 460 | Pulmonary function general | 94760 | 1 | $90 | N | $0 | $0 |
| 481 | Cardiology cardiac cath lab | 93458 | 1 | $12,000 | T | $2,549 | $784 |
| 481 | Cardiology cardiac cath lab | 93463 | 1 | $1,000 | N | $0 | $0 |
| 481 | Cardiology cardiac cath lab | 93464 | 1 | $1,250 | N | $0 | $0 |
| 636 | Pharmacy: drugs requiring detailed coding | J7040 | 1 | $50 | N | $0 | $0 |
| 710 | Recovery room general | | 6 | $800 | | $0 | $0 |
| | | | | $15,975 | | $2,549 | $784 |

into the APC rate. Many of these procedures are either lab or drug administration services that are considered to be a part of CPT 93458 (Left Heart Catheterization). This procedure has a "T" status indicator code, which indicates it is discounted at 50% if another "T"-coded procedure was performed. In our example, there is no other "T"-coded procedure present in the claim, so the procedure is not discounted. When multiple "T"-coded procedures are performed, the highest-value procedure is paid at 100%, but all other "T"-coded procedures are paid at 50%. It is also important to note that Medicare provides additional payments to hospitals for outliers. Outlier payments are made on an APC basis and are equal to 50% of the cost of the APC that is above 175%

of the actual APC payment. However, in addition to meeting the 175% provision, the cost must also exceed a fixed dollar threshold of $3,250 (FY 2016 amount) plus the APC payment. For example, if an APC had a total payment, including the coinsurance, of $1,000 and the estimated cost of the APC was $4,000, then Medicare would pay an additional $1,125: (0.50 × [$4,000 − $1,750]). Please recognize that the cost of the APC does include incidental services or "N"-status items, which makes it important to include these items and to charge for them even if Medicare does not recognize them as APC or fee-schedule items. A list of all status codes and corresponding Medicare OPPS payment can be found in **TABLE 3-9**.

**TABLE 3-9** Status Codes

| Status Indicator | Item/Code/Service | OPPS Payment Status |
|---|---|---|
| A | Services furnished to a hospital outpatient that are paid under a fee schedule or payment system other than OPPS, for example:<br>■ Ambulance services<br>■ Separately payable clinical diagnostic laboratory services<br>■ Separately payable nonimplantable prosthetics and orthotics<br>■ Physical, occupational, and speech therapy<br>■ Diagnostic mammography<br>■ Screening mammography | Not paid under OPPS. Paid by MACs under a fee schedule or payment system other than OPPS. Services are subject to deductible or coinsurance unless indicated otherwise.<br><br>Not subject to deductible or coinsurance.<br><br><br>Not subject to deductible or coinsurance. |
| B | Codes that are not recognized by OPPS when submitted on an outpatient hospital Part B bill type (12x and 13x). | Not paid under OPPS.<br>■ May be paid by MACs when submitted on a different bill type, for example, 75x (CORF), but not paid under OPPS.<br>■ An alternate code that is recognized by OPPS when submitted on an outpatient hospital Part B bill type (12x and 13x) may be available. |
| C | Inpatient procedures | Not paid under OPPS. Admit patient. Bill as inpatient. |
| D | Discontinued codes | Not paid under OPPS or any other Medicare payment system. |
| E | Items, codes, and services:<br>■ For which pricing information is not available<br>■ Not covered by any Medicare outpatient benefit category<br>■ Statutorily excluded by Medicare<br>■ Not reasonable and necessary | Not paid by Medicare when submitted on outpatient claims (any outpatient bill type). |

*(continues)*

**TABLE 3-9** Status Codes *(continued)*

| Status Indicator | Item/Code/Service | OPPS Payment Status |
|---|---|---|
| F | Corneal tissue acquisition; Certain CRNA services and hepatitis B vaccines | Not paid under OPPS. Paid at reasonable cost. |
| G | Pass-through drugs and biologicals | Paid under OPPS; separate APC payment. |
| H | Pass-through device categories | Separate cost-based pass-through payment; not subject to copayment. |
| J1 | Hospital Part B services paid through a comprehensive APC | Paid under OPPS; all covered Part B services on the claim are packaged with the primary "J1" service for the claim, except services with OPPS SI = F, G, H, L, and U; ambulance services; diagnostic and screening mammography; all preventive services; and certain Part B inpatient services. |
| J2 | Hospital Part B services that may be paid through a comprehensive APC | Paid under OPPS; Addendum B displays APC assignments when services are separately payable. <br>(1) Comprehensive APC payment based on OPPS comprehensive-specific payment criteria. Payment for all covered Part B services on the claim is packaged into a single payment for specific combinations of services, except services with OPPS SI = F, G, H, L, and U; ambulance services; diagnostic and screening mammography; all preventive services; and certain Part B inpatient services. <br>(2) Packaged APC payment if billed on the same claim as a HCPCS code assigned status indicator "J1." <br>(3) In other circumstances, payment is made through a separate APC payment or packaged into payment for other services. |
| K | Non-pass-through drugs and nonimplantable biologicals, including therapeutic radiopharmaceuticals | Paid under OPPS; separate APC payment. |
| L | Influenza vaccine; pneumococcal pneumonia vaccine | Not paid under OPPS. Paid at reasonable cost; not subject to deductible or coinsurance. |
| M | Items and services not billable to the MAC | Not paid under OPPS. |
| N | Items and services packaged into APC rates | Paid under OPPS; payment is packaged into payment for other services. Therefore, there is no separate APC payment. |
| P | Partial hospitalization | Paid under OPPS; per diem APC payment. |

| Q1 | STV-packaged codes | Paid under OPPS; Addendum B displays APC assignments when services are separately payable. (1) Packaged APC payment if billed on the same date of service as a HCPCS code assigned status indicator "S," "T," or "V." (2) In other circumstances, payment is made through a separate APC payment. |
|----|--------------------|----------------------------------|
| Q2 | T-packaged codes | Paid under OPPS; Addendum B displays APC assignments when services are separately payable. (1) Packaged APC payment if billed on the same date of service as a HCPCS code assigned status indicator "T." (2) In other circumstances, payment is made through a separate APC payment. |
| Q3 | Codes that may be paid through a composite APC | Paid under OPPS; Addendum B displays APC assignments when services are separately payable. Addendum M displays composite APC assignments when codes are paid through a composite APC. (1) Composite APC payment based on OPPS composite-specific payment criteria. Payment is packaged into a single payment for specific combinations of services. (2) In other circumstances, payment is made through a separate APC payment or packaged into payment for other services. |
| Q4 | Conditionally packaged laboratory tests | Paid under OPPS or CLFS. (1) Packaged APC payment if billed on the same claim as a HCPCS code assigned published status indicator "J1," "J2," "S," "T," "V," "Q1," "Q2," or "Q3." (2) In other circumstances, laboratory tests should have an SI = A and payment is made under the CLFS. |
| R | Blood and blood products | Paid under OPPS; separate APC payment. |
| S | Procedure or service, not discounted when multiple | Paid under OPPS; separate APC payment. |
| T | Procedure or service, multiple procedure reduction applies | Paid under OPPS; separate APC payment. |
| U | Brachytherapy sources | Paid under OPPS; separate APC payment. |
| V | Clinic or emergency department visit | Paid under OPPS; separate APC payment. |
| Y | Nonimplantable durable medical equipment | Not paid under OPPS. All institutional providers other than home health agencies bill to DMERC. |

Resource management under APC reimbursement is more difficult than it is under DRGs because payment is not fixed. In a DRG payment environment, once the patient is classified, cost minimization is the optimal financial strategy because payment does not increase if additional services are provided. In an APC payment situation, payments may increase when more services are provided. Management must determine from a financial perspective whether the marginal revenue of additional services is greater than the marginal cost of providing those services. Medicare is changing this dynamic, however, with the implementation of Comprehensive APCs (C-APCs). In general, C-APCs work like DRGs whereby there is a single payment for the encounter, as opposed to multiple payments for each item with a paid status. The single payment is driven by the designated primary procedure with all ancillary or secondary services provided in conjunction with the primary procedure receiving no additional payment. It is anticipated that Medicare will continue to expand the number of C-APCs in the future. As of fiscal year 2016, there are 35 C-APCs, which mostly include observation and procedures for the implantation of costly medical devices.

## Skilled Nursing Facilities

As you can see from our discussion of Medicare payments for hospital inpatient, hospital outpatient, and physician services, Medicare payment is a complex set of rules. Medicare has paid SNFs on a prospective basis since July 1, 1998. The rate is a per diem rate that is calculated to include the costs of all services, including routine, ancillary, and capital. Per diem payments for each admission are case-mix adjusted using a resident classification system known as **resource utilization groups IV** (RUG IV). As with most CMS payments, the actual payment amounts are adjusted for differences in cost of living by the hospital wage index on the labor portion of the payment.

There are 8 major categories of patients under RUG IV with 66 distinct payment categories, as shown in **TABLE 3-10**. Patients are assigned to one of the payment categories by a "RUG IV grouper" based on 6 key determinants:

- Number of minutes per week needed for rehabilitation services
- Number of different rehabilitation disciplines needed
- Specific treatments received
- Resident's ability to perform activities of daily living
- ICD-10 diagnoses
- Resident's cognitive performance

**TABLE 3-10** Number of Payment Categories for Major RUG IV

| Major RUG IV Group | Number of Payment Categories |
|---|---|
| Rehabilitation plus extensive | 9 |
| Rehabilitation | 14 |
| Extensive services | 3 |
| Special care high | 8 |
| Special care low | 8 |
| Clinically complex | 10 |
| Behavioral symptoms and cognitive performance | 4 |
| Reduced physical function | 10 |

To properly classify residents, SNFs must complete resident assessments on the 5th, 14th, 30th, 60th, and 90th days after admission. These forms are extensive and require another layer of administrative support to properly record and report to CMS.

To see how the payment system operates, let us assume that a rehabilitation patient has been categorized as "ultra high with treatment minimum of 720 minutes per week." Payment per day for this patient is computed as shown in **TABLE 3-11**. The rates used in this example are updated over time as most Medicare rates are adjusted to reflect inflation.

## Home Health Agencies

The Balanced Budget Act of 1997 called for the development and implementation of a PPS for Medicare home health services to be implemented October 1, 2000. Under prospective payment, Medicare pays home health agencies (HHAs) a predetermined base payment. The payment is adjusted for the health condition and care needs of the beneficiary. The payment is also adjusted for the geographical differences in wages for HHAs across the country. The adjustment for the health condition, or clinical characteristics, and service needs of the beneficiary is referred to as the *case-mix adjustment*. The home health PPS provides HHAs with payments for each 60-day episode of care for each beneficiary. If a beneficiary is still eligible for care after the end of the first episode, a second episode can begin; there are

**TABLE 3-11** Components of Payment under RUG IV Categorization of "Ultra High plus Extensive Services, High (RUX)"

| Category | Dollar Amount |
| --- | --- |
| Nursing care | $457.02 |
| Occupational, physical, and speech therapies | $241.12 |
| Capital and general and administrative | $87.36 |
| Total allowed per diem | $785.50 |
| x Labor % | 0.691 |
| Labor per diem | $542.78 |
| x Wage index | 0.964 |
| Labor adjusted per diem | $523.24 |
| Nonlabor per diem | $242.72 |
| Case-mix adjusted per diem | $765.96 |

no limits to the number of episodes a beneficiary who remains eligible for the home health benefit can receive. Although payment for each episode is adjusted to reflect the beneficiary's health condition and needs, a special outlier provision exists to ensure appropriate payment for those beneficiaries who need the most expensive care. Adjusting payment to reflect the HHA's cost in caring for each beneficiary, including the most ill, should ensure that all beneficiaries have access to home health services for which they are eligible.

The home health PPS is composed of five main features:

1. ***60-day episode***. The unit of payment under HHA PPS is for a 60-day episode of care. An agency receives half of the estimated base payment for the full 60 days as soon as the **fiscal intermediary** receives the initial claim. This estimate is based on the patient's condition and care needs (case-mix assignment). The agency receives the residual half of the payment at the close of the 60-day episode unless there is an applicable adjustment to that amount. The full payment is the sum of the initial and residual percentage payments, unless there is an applicable adjustment. This split-percentage payment approach provides reasonable and balanced cash flow for HHAs. Another 60-day episode can be initiated for longer-stay patients.

2. ***Case-mix adjustment***. After a physician prescribes a home health plan of care, the HHA assesses the patient's condition and likely skilled nursing care, therapy, medical, and social services and home health aide service needs at the beginning of the episode of care. The assessment must be done for each subsequent episode of care a patient receives. A nurse or therapist from the HHA uses the Outcome and Assessment Information Set (OASIS) instrument to assess the patient's condition. (All HHAs have been using OASIS since July 19, 1999.) OASIS items describing the patient's condition and the expected therapy needs (physical, speech-language pathology, or occupational) are used to determine the case-mix adjustment to the standard payment rate. This adjustment is the case-mix adjustment. There are 153 case-mix groups, or **home health resource groups**, available for patient classification using three classification criteria: clinical severity, functional severity, and service utilization severity. The Home Health Resource Grouping system in the proposed rule uses data from a large-scale case-mix research project conducted between 1997 and 1999.

3. ***Outlier payments***. Additional payments are made to the 60-day case-mix-adjusted episode payments for beneficiaries who incur unusually large costs. These outlier payments are made for episodes whose imputed cost exceeds a threshold amount for each case-mix group. The amount of the outlier payment is a proportion of the amount of imputed costs beyond the threshold. Outlier costs are imputed for each episode by applying standard per visit amounts to the number of visits by discipline (skilled nursing visits; physical, speech-language pathology, and occupational therapy; or home health aide services) reported on the claims. Total national outlier payments for home health services annually are no more than 2.5% of estimated total payments under home health PPS.

**TABLE 3-12** National HHA Payments Unadjusted for Wage Index

| Discipline | Per Visit Rate |
|---|---|
| Home health aide | $60.87 |
| Medical social service | 215.47 |
| Occupational therapy | 147.95 |
| Physical therapy | 146.95 |
| Skilled nursing | 134.42 |
| Speech pathology | 159.71 |

4. ***Adjustments for beneficiaries who require only a few visits during the 60-day episode.*** The proposed home health PPS has a low-utilization payment adjustment for beneficiaries whose episodes consist of four or fewer visits. These episodes are paid the standardized, service-specific, per visit amount multiplied by the number of visits actually provided during the episode. **TABLE 3-12** shows the national payments unadjusted for wage index for HHAs that submit quality data for 2016.

5. ***Adjustments for beneficiaries who change HHAs.*** The home health PPS includes a partial episode payment adjustment. A new episode clock is triggered when a beneficiary elects to transfer to another HHA or when a beneficiary is discharged and readmitted to the same HHA during the 60-day episode. The partial episode payment provides a simplified approach to the episode definition that takes into account key intervening health events in a patient's care. The partial episode payment allows the 60-day episode clock to end and a new clock to begin if a beneficiary transfers to another HHA or is discharged but returns because of a decline in his or her condition to the same HHA within the 60-day episode. When a new 60-day episode begins, a new plan of care and a new assessment are necessary. The original 60-day episode payment is proportionally adjusted to reflect the length of time the beneficiary remained under the agency's care before the intervening event. The new episode is paid an initial episode payment of one-half of the new case-mix group, and the 60-day clock is restarted.

To illustrate the actual payment determination for an episode of care under the HHA PPS program, assume that a patient has been classified as 1 severity for clinical, 1 severity for functional, and 2 severity for services utilization (C1F1S2). Payment for this patient under the PPS program is calculated as follows:

| | |
|---|---|
| National standardized payment rate | $2,965.12 |
| Case weight | $\times$ 0.7197 |
| Case-mix adjusted payment | $2,134.00 |

This amount is then adjusted for the actual wage index of the provider. Under the HHA PPS program, 77.5% of the payment is assumed to be labor related, whereas the remaining 21.5% is assumed to be nonlabor. Actual payment for a provider with a wage index of 1.2000 is $2,341.15:

$$(\$2{,}134 \times 0.73535 \times 1.2000) + (\$2{,}134 \times 0.21465) = \$2{,}341.15$$

## ▶ SUMMARY

Compared with most businesses, HCOs are financially complex. Not only do they provide a large number of specific services, but their individual services often also have different effective price structures. Services may be bundled in different ways to determine prices, according to the agreements in place with each specific payer. One customer may choose to pay on the basis of cost, whereas another may pay full charges. Prices may be determined prospectively or may be capitated for broad scopes of care. This variation in payment patterns creates problems in the establishment of prices for products and services. Indeed, the revenue function of a typical healthcare entity is usually much more complex than that of a comparably sized nonhealthcare business. Furthermore, organizations within different segments of the healthcare industry are affected by changes in payment arrangements in different ways.

Healthcare entities also depend quite heavily on a very limited number of key clients for most of their operating funding. Their largest client is often the federal government or the state government. Doing business with the government involves a significant amount of reporting to ensure compliance and adherence to governmental regulations. Moreover, because the federal government is such a large purchaser of services, a thorough understanding of the nature and implications of the Medicare payment system's rules and regulations is a must for effective management of an HCO. Important differences exist in setting rates and **bundling** services between hospital inpatient and outpatient care, physician services, SNFs, and home health care. Each system has differing implications for the management of resources by the HCO.

The revenue function of a typical healthcare entity is usually much more complex than that of a comparably sized nonhealthcare business. Organizations can have vastly different revenue structures, depending on the segments of the healthcare industry in which they are active. Government commands enormous influence as a purchaser of healthcare services and maintains complex payment systems. Because payment arrangements are determined primarily by the payer, an effective healthcare administrator must have a firm understanding of the various systems, both public and private, that exist. Yet, although HCOs may be complex from a financial perspective, they are still businesses. Their financial viability requires the receipt of funds in amounts sufficient to meet their financial requirements.

## ASSIGNMENTS

**TABLE 3-13**  Revenue to Meet Hospital Financial Requirements

| Volume | |
|---|---|
| Medicare cases | 1,000 |
| Cost-paying cases | 400 |
| Charity care and bad-debt cases | 100 |
| Charge-paying cases | 500 |
| Total cases | 2,000 |
| Financial data | |
| Budgeted expenses | $6,000,000 |
| Debt principal payment | 200,000 |
| Working capital increase | 250,000 |
| Capital expenditures | 400,000 |
| Present payment structure | |
| Medicare pays only $2,800 per case, or a total of $2,800,000. | |
| All other cost payers pay their share of existing expenses. | |

1. From the data in **TABLE 3-13**, determine the amount of revenue that needs to be generated to meet hospital financial requirements.
2. Why is the accumulation of funded reserves for capital replacement more critical for nonprofit healthcare entities than for investor-owned healthcare facilities?
3. Teaching hospitals receive an additional payment to recognize the indirect costs of medical education. What rationale might be used to justify this extra payment?
4. Depreciation expense is recognized as a reimbursable cost by a number of payers who pay prospective rates for operating costs. Would you prefer accelerated depreciation (sum of the year's digits) or price-level depreciation for a 5-year life asset with a $150,000 cost? Assume that inflation is projected to be 6% per year.

**TABLE 3-14**  Repair of Mitral Valve

| Product | Relative Value | Chicago Index | Units |
|---|---|---|---|
| Work | 26.07 | 1.028 | 26.80 |
| Practice expense | 31.96 | 1.080 | 34.52 |
| Malpractice | 5.80 | 1.382 | 8.02 |
|  |  |  | 69.34 |

5. Using the data from Problem 1, calculate the impact of a 10% reduction in operating expenses, that is, down to $5,400,000, on the required revenue and rate structure. Discuss the implications of your findings.
6. Calculate the RBRVS rate for CPT 33426, repair of mitral valve for a physician in Chicago, Illinois. Assume the conversion factor is 40.7986. **TABLE 3-14** provides relevant values to complete this calculation.
7. Medicare currently reimburses hospitals for 65% of bad debts written off on Medicare patients, copayments, and deductibles. If a hospital had $1,000,000 in Medicare deductibles and copayments, what amount might Medicare pay for its bad debts if 15% of the total will remain uncollectable?
8. Discussions with a group of physicians regarding employment status of your hospital are taking place. If the physicians were employed by your hospital, they would be performing all surgical procedures at your hospital instead of in their current offices. This could mean a sizable change in total revenue, especially from Medicare patients. To see the effect of this change, assume the example in Table 3-7 for CPT #42810, excision of a neck cyst. If Medicare pays the hospital $1,600 for the facility fee and the physicians receive $370.80, calculate the amount the physicians would lose if the procedure were paid in a nonfacility setting. Assume the nonfacility practice expense weight is 7.39.
9. Your hospital is reviewing its DRG coding patterns for Medicare. It has focused on two DRGs: 640 (Misc disorders of nutrition, metabolism, fluids/electrolytes w MCC) and 641 (Misc disorders of nutrition, metabolism, fluids/electrolytes w/o MCC). There were 100 patients assigned to these two DRGs: 50 to 640 and 50 to 641. National averages suggest that 85 should have been assigned to DRG 640 and 15 to DRG 641. Assuming an average payment of $6,000 per DRG with a case weight of 1.0, how much lost payment from Medicare may be resulting from poor coding and documentation? Use case weight values from Appendix 3-A.

## SOLUTIONS AND ANSWERS

1. The relevant calculation is as follows:

$$\text{Revenue} = \frac{\text{Budgeted expense} + \text{Desired net income} - \text{Noncharge-paying payments}}{\text{Proportion of charge-paying patients}}$$

$$\text{Revenue} = \frac{\$6,000,000 + \$850,000 - \$4,000,000}{0.25} = \$11,400,00 \text{ or } \$5,700 \text{ per case}$$

Desired net income = $850,000 = $200,000 + $250,000 + $400,000

Noncharge-paying patient payments = Medicare payments + Cost-paying patient payments = $4,000,000

$$\text{Propotion of charge-paying patient} = \frac{500}{2,000} = 0.25$$

**TABLE 3-15** Price Level and Sum-of-the-Years Digits Depreciation

| | Price Level Sum-of-the-Years Digits | |
| --- | --- | --- |
| | Depreciation* | Depreciation† |
| Year 1 | $31,800 | $50,000 |
| Year 2 | 33,708 | 40,000 |
| Year 3 | 35,730 | 30,000 |
| Year 4 | 37,874 | 20,000 |
| Year 5 | 40,147 | 10,000 |
| | $179,259 | $150,000 |

*Depreciation in year $t = 150,000/5 \, (1.06)^t$. This term reflects compounding of straight-line depreciation at 6% per year.

†Depreciation in year $t$ of an $N$-year life asset is equal to the historical cost times: $2(N + 1 - t)/N(N + 1)$.

2. A nonprofit entity does not have the same opportunities for capital formation that an investor-owned organization does. Specifically, the nonprofit entity cannot sell new shares or ownership interests. Its sources of capital are limited to its accumulated funded reserves and new debt. In some special situations, nonprofit organizations may receive contributions, but these amounts are usually not significant.

3. Part of the rationale used is related to severity of patients. It is widely believed that teaching hospitals treat more severely ill patients. The currently used DRG classification system does not incorporate severity adjustments.

4. The relevant comparative data are provided in **TABLE 3-15**.
   In year 1, the depreciation is $150,000 \times 10 \div 30$, or $50,000. In most cases price-level-adjusted depreciation would be better. However, for short-lived assets accelerated depreciation may provide greater levels of reimbursement in earlier years to offset lower returns in later years. The lower the rate of asset inflation, the more desirable accelerated depreciation becomes.

5. The relevant calculation would be as follows:

$$\text{Revenue} = \frac{\$5,400,000 + \$850,000 - \$3,880,000}{0.25} = \$9,480,000, \text{ or } \$4,740 \text{ per case}$$

   A 10% reduction in operating expenses permitted a 17% reduction in rates ($5,700 to $4,740 per case). Cost control is critical in healthcare entities, especially in those with relatively low levels of cost payers. A reduction in rates is especially important when competing for major contracts in which price is a predominant determinant.

6. The RBRVS rate for this procedure is

$$\$2,829 = \$40.7986 \times 69.34$$

7. Although the total Medicare deductible and copayment amount is $1,000,000, a small percentage will most likely remain unpaid. Many Medicare beneficiaries have supplemental insurance that pays for deductibles and copayments. In addition, many Medicare patients do pay for their deductibles and copayments. In our example, 15% of the total will remain uncollectable, so, this means $150,000 of reported bad debts. Medicare would then pay 65% ($97,500).

8. The current practice expense weight in a facility setting is 4.56, per Table 3-7. The weight in a nonfacility setting is 7.39, per discussion in the text. The lost payment the doctors would experience is as follows:

Payments if hospital based

$1,600 (Hospital payment) + 370.80 (Physician payment) = $1,970.80

Physician payment

$370.80 (Payment if hospital based) = $131.43

(Additional payment if nonhospital based) = $502.23

$131.43 = (7.39 − 4.56) × 1.161 × $40

Net loss in payment = $1,468.57

9. If the hospital had the same coding percentages as the national average, it would have had 35 more cases coded as 640 and 35 fewer cases coded as 641. Using the case weights in Appendix 3-A and the $6,000 payment per case weight of 1.0, the additional payment is as follows:

35 cases × (1.1318 − 0.7221) × $6,000 = $86,037

# Appendix 3-A

## List of MS-DRGs and Relative Weights for Fiscal Year 2016

| MS-DRG | MDC | Type | MS-DRG Title | Weights | Geometric Mean LOS |
|--------|-----|------|--------------|---------|--------------------|
| 001 | PRE | SURG | HEART TRANSPLANT OR IMPLANT OF HEART ASSIST SYSTEM W MCC | 26.2166 | 29.4 |
| 002 | PRE | SURG | HEART TRANSPLANT OR IMPLANT OF HEART ASSIST SYSTEM W/O MCC | 14.6448 | 16.6 |
| 003 | PRE | SURG | ECMO OR TRACH W MV >96 HRS OR PDX EXC FACE, MOUTH & NECK W MAJ O.R. | 17.6569 | 25.5 |
| 004 | PRE | SURG | TRACH W MV >96 HRS OR PDX EXC FACE, MOUTH & NECK W/O MAJ O.R. | 10.9458 | 20.0 |
| 005 | PRE | SURG | LIVER TRANSPLANT W MCC OR INTESTINAL TRANSPLANT | 10.7263 | 15.3 |
| 006 | PRE | SURG | LIVER TRANSPLANT W/O MCC | 4.8330 | 7.9 |
| 007 | PRE | SURG | LUNG TRANSPLANT | 9.7007 | 15.8 |
| 008 | PRE | SURG | SIMULTANEOUS PANCREAS/KIDNEY TRANSPLANT | 5.4338 | 9.8 |
| 010 | PRE | SURG | PANCREAS TRANSPLANT | 4.3039 | 8.1 |
| 011 | PRE | SURG | TRACHEOSTOMY FOR FACE, MOUTH & NECK DIAGNOSES W MCC | 4.7501 | 11.3 |
| 012 | PRE | SURG | TRACHEOSTOMY FOR FACE, MOUTH & NECK DIAGNOSES W CC | 3.4047 | 8.4 |
| 013 | PRE | SURG | TRACHEOSTOMY FOR FACE, MOUTH & NECK DIAGNOSES W/O CC/MCC | 2.1906 | 5.8 |
| 014 | PRE | SURG | ALLOGENEIC BONE MARROW TRANSPLANT | 11.5928 | 22.7 |
| 016 | PRE | SURG | AUTOLOGOUS BONE MARROW TRANSPLANT W CC/MCC | 6.1746 | 17.8 |

(continues)

| MS-DRG | MDC | Type | MS-DRG Title | Weights | Geometric Mean LOS |
|--------|-----|------|--------------|---------|--------------------|
| 017 | PRE | SURG | AUTOLOGOUS BONE MARROW TRANSPLANT W/O CC/MCC | 4.3721 | 10.0 |
| 020 | 01 | SURG | INTRACRANIAL VASCULAR PROCEDURES W PDX HEMORRHAGE W MCC | 9.7571 | 13.6 |
| 021 | 01 | SURG | INTRACRANIAL VASCULAR PROCEDURES W PDX HEMORRHAGE W CC | 7.1549 | 12.3 |
| 022 | 01 | SURG | INTRACRANIAL VASCULAR PROCEDURES W PDX HEMORRHAGE W/O CC/MCC | 4.9977 | 6.7 |
| 023 | 01 | SURG | CRANIO W MAJOR DEV IMPL/ACUTE COMPLEX CNS PDX W MCC OR CHEMO IMPLANT | 5.3486 | 7.9 |
| 024 | 01 | SURG | CRANIO W MAJOR DEV IMPL/ACUTE COMPLEX CNS PDX W/O MCC | 3.7976 | 4.2 |
| 025 | 01 | SURG | CRANIOTOMY & ENDOVASCULAR INTRACRANIAL PROCEDURES W MCC | 4.2965 | 7.2 |
| 026 | 01 | SURG | CRANIOTOMY & ENDOVASCULAR INTRACRANIAL PROCEDURES W CC | 2.9958 | 4.6 |
| 027 | 01 | SURG | CRANIOTOMY & ENDOVASCULAR INTRACRANIAL PROCEDURES W/O CC/MCC | 2.2835 | 2.4 |
| 028 | 01 | SURG | SPINAL PROCEDURES W MCC | 5.3695 | 9.3 |
| 029 | 01 | SURG | SPINAL PROCEDURES W CC OR SPINAL NEUROSTIMULATORS | 3.0548 | 4.8 |
| 030 | 01 | SURG | SPINAL PROCEDURES W/O CC/MCC | 1.7982 | 2.6 |
| 031 | 01 | SURG | VENTRICULAR SHUNT PROCEDURES W MCC | 3.7834 | 7.4 |
| 032 | 01 | SURG | VENTRICULAR SHUNT PROCEDURES W CC | 2.0352 | 3.3 |
| 033 | 01 | SURG | VENTRICULAR SHUNT PROCEDURES W/O CC/MCC | 1.5734 | 2.0 |
| 034 | 01 | SURG | CAROTID ARTERY STENT PROCEDURE W MCC | 3.6851 | 4.8 |
| 035 | 01 | SURG | CAROTID ARTERY STENT PROCEDURE W CC | 2.3048 | 2.1 |
| 036 | 01 | SURG | CAROTID ARTERY STENT PROCEDURE W/O CC/MCC | 1.7180 | 1.3 |
| 037 | 01 | SURG | EXTRACRANIAL PROCEDURES W MCC | 3.0888 | 5.3 |
| 038 | 01 | SURG | EXTRACRANIAL PROCEDURES W CC | 1.5560 | 2.3 |

| MS-DRG | MDC | Type | MS-DRG Title | Weights | Geometric Mean LOS |
|--------|-----|------|--------------|---------|--------------------|
| 039 | 01 | SURG | EXTRACRANIAL PROCEDURES W/O CC/MCC | 1.0609 | 1.3 |
| 040 | 01 | SURG | PERIPH/CRANIAL NERVE & OTHER NERV SYST PROC W MCC | 3.8044 | 8.2 |
| 041 | 01 | SURG | PERIPH/CRANIAL NERVE & OTHER NERV SYST PROC W CC OR PERIPH NEUROSTIM | 2.1354 | 4.7 |
| 042 | 01 | SURG | PERIPH/CRANIAL NERVE & OTHER NERV SYST PROC W/O CC/MCC | 1.9242 | 2.7 |
| 052 | 01 | MED | SPINAL DISORDERS & INJURIES W CC/MCC | 1.4915 | 4.1 |
| 053 | 01 | MED | SPINAL DISORDERS & INJURIES W/O CC/MCC | 0.8625 | 2.8 |
| 054 | 01 | MED | NERVOUS SYSTEM NEOPLASMS W MCC | 1.3570 | 4.0 |
| 055 | 01 | MED | NERVOUS SYSTEM NEOPLASMS W/O MCC | 1.0401 | 3.0 |
| 056 | 01 | MED | DEGENERATIVE NERVOUS SYSTEM DISORDERS W MCC | 1.8513 | 5.2 |
| 057 | 01 | MED | DEGENERATIVE NERVOUS SYSTEM DISORDERS W/O MCC | 1.0716 | 3.7 |
| 058 | 01 | MED | MULTIPLE SCLEROSIS & CEREBELLAR ATAXIA W MCC | 1.7198 | 5.5 |
| 059 | 01 | MED | MULTIPLE SCLEROSIS & CEREBELLAR ATAXIA W CC | 1.0134 | 3.7 |
| 060 | 01 | MED | MULTIPLE SCLEROSIS & CEREBELLAR ATAXIA W/O CC/MCC | 0.8130 | 3.1 |
| 061 | 01 | MED | ACUTE ISCHEMIC STROKE W USE OF THROMBOLYTIC AGENT W MCC | 2.6843 | 5.4 |
| 062 | 01 | MED | ACUTE ISCHEMIC STROKE W USE OF THROMBOLYTIC AGENT W CC | 1.8918 | 3.9 |
| 063 | 01 | MED | ACUTE ISCHEMIC STROKE W USE OF THROMBOLYTIC AGENT W/O CC/MCC | 1.5238 | 2.9 |
| 064 | 01 | MED | INTRACRANIAL HEMORRHAGE OR CEREBRAL INFARCTION W MCC | 1.7326 | 4.5 |
| 065 | 01 | MED | INTRACRANIAL HEMORRHAGE OR CEREBRAL INFARCTION W CC OR TPA IN 24 HRS | 1.0593 | 3.3 |
| 066 | 01 | MED | INTRACRANIAL HEMORRHAGE OR CEREBRAL INFARCTION W/O CC/MCC | 0.7574 | 2.4 |

*(continues)*

| MS-DRG | MDC | Type | MS-DRG Title | Weights | Geometric Mean LOS |
|--------|-----|------|--------------|---------|--------------------|
| 067 | 01 | MED | NONSPECIFIC CVA & PRECEREBRAL OCCLUSION W/O INFARCT W MCC | 1.4338 | 4.0 |
| 068 | 01 | MED | NONSPECIFIC CVA & PRECEREBRAL OCCLUSION W/O INFARCT W/O MCC | 0.8731 | 2.4 |
| 069 | 01 | MED | TRANSIENT ISCHEMIA | 0.7227 | 2.1 |
| 070 | 01 | MED | NONSPECIFIC CEREBROVASCULAR DISORDERS W MCC | 1.6283 | 4.7 |
| 071 | 01 | MED | NONSPECIFIC CEREBROVASCULAR DISORDERS W CC | 1.0079 | 3.5 |
| 072 | 01 | MED | NONSPECIFIC CEREBROVASCULAR DISORDERS W/O CC/MCC | 0.7329 | 2.4 |
| 073 | 01 | MED | CRANIAL & PERIPHERAL NERVE DISORDERS W MCC | 1.3359 | 3.8 |
| 074 | 01 | MED | CRANIAL & PERIPHERAL NERVE DISORDERS W/O MCC | 0.9063 | 3.0 |
| 075 | 01 | MED | VIRAL MENINGITIS W CC/MCC | 1.6917 | 5.3 |
| 076 | 01 | MED | VIRAL MENINGITIS W/O CC/MCC | 0.8302 | 2.9 |
| 077 | 01 | MED | HYPERTENSIVE ENCEPHALOPATHY W MCC | 1.5448 | 4.4 |
| 078 | 01 | MED | HYPERTENSIVE ENCEPHALOPATHY W CC | 0.9676 | 3.1 |
| 079 | 01 | MED | HYPERTENSIVE ENCEPHALOPATHY W/O CC/MCC | 0.6862 | 2.3 |
| 080 | 01 | MED | NONTRAUMATIC STUPOR & COMA W MCC | 1.2159 | 3.7 |
| 081 | 01 | MED | NONTRAUMATIC STUPOR & COMA W/O MCC | 0.7651 | 2.7 |
| 082 | 01 | MED | TRAUMATIC STUPOR & COMA, COMA >1 HR W MCC | 2.0170 | 3.4 |
| 083 | 01 | MED | TRAUMATIC STUPOR & COMA, COMA >1 HR W CC | 1.3006 | 3.3 |
| 084 | 01 | MED | TRAUMATIC STUPOR & COMA, COMA >1 HR W/O CC/MCC | 0.8469 | 2.1 |
| 085 | 01 | MED | TRAUMATIC STUPOR & COMA, COMA <1 HR W MCC | 2.0357 | 4.7 |

| MS-DRG | MDC | Type | MS-DRG Title | Weights | Geometric Mean LOS |
|--------|-----|------|--------------|---------|--------------------|
| 086 | 01 | MED | TRAUMATIC STUPOR & COMA, COMA <1 HR W CC | 1.1394 | 3.3 |
| 087 | 01 | MED | TRAUMATIC STUPOR & COMA, COMA <1 HR W/O CC/MCC | 0.7918 | 2.2 |
| 088 | 01 | MED | CONCUSSION W MCC | 1.3653 | 3.7 |
| 089 | 01 | MED | CONCUSSION W CC | 0.9759 | 2.8 |
| 090 | 01 | MED | CONCUSSION W/O CC/MCC | 0.7394 | 1.9 |
| 091 | 01 | MED | OTHER DISORDERS OF NERVOUS SYSTEM W MCC | 1.5880 | 4.2 |
| 092 | 01 | MED | OTHER DISORDERS OF NERVOUS SYSTEM W CC | 0.9075 | 3.1 |
| 093 | 01 | MED | OTHER DISORDERS OF NERVOUS SYSTEM W/O CC/MCC | 0.6981 | 2.2 |
| 094 | 01 | MED | BACTERIAL & TUBERCULOUS INFECTIONS OF NERVOUS SYSTEM W MCC | 3.4429 | 8.2 |
| 095 | 01 | MED | BACTERIAL & TUBERCULOUS INFECTIONS OF NERVOUS SYSTEM W CC | 2.3282 | 5.7 |
| 096 | 01 | MED | BACTERIAL & TUBERCULOUS INFECTIONS OF NERVOUS SYSTEM W/O CC/MCC | 2.1855 | 4.8 |
| 097 | 01 | MED | NON-BACTERIAL INFECT OF NERVOUS SYS EXC VIRAL MENINGITIS W MCC | 3.1221 | 8.1 |
| 098 | 01 | MED | NON-BACTERIAL INFECT OF NERVOUS SYS EXC VIRAL MENINGITIS W CC | 1.8410 | 5.7 |
| 099 | 01 | MED | NON-BACTERIAL INFECT OF NERVOUS SYS EXC VIRAL MENINGITIS W/O CC/MCC | 1.2570 | 4.1 |
| 100 | 01 | MED | SEIZURES W MCC | 1.5639 | 4.2 |
| 101 | 01 | MED | SEIZURES W/O MCC | 0.7942 | 2.6 |
| 102 | 01 | MED | HEADACHES W MCC | 1.0685 | 3.1 |
| 103 | 01 | MED | HEADACHES W/O MCC | 0.7199 | 2.3 |
| 113 | 02 | SURG | ORBITAL PROCEDURES W CC/MCC | 2.0118 | 4.0 |
| 114 | 02 | SURG | ORBITAL PROCEDURES W/O CC/MCC | 1.2094 | 2.4 |

*(continues)*

| MS-DRG | MDC | Type | MS-DRG Title | Weights | Geometric Mean LOS |
|--------|-----|------|--------------|---------|--------------------|
| 115 | 02 | SURG | EXTRAOCULAR PROCEDURES EXCEPT ORBIT | 1.3151 | 3.5 |
| 116 | 02 | SURG | INTRAOCULAR PROCEDURES W CC/MCC | 1.5015 | 3.5 |
| 117 | 02 | SURG | INTRAOCULAR PROCEDURES W/O CC/MCC | 0.8340 | 2.0 |
| 121 | 02 | MED | ACUTE MAJOR EYE INFECTIONS W CC/MCC | 0.9934 | 3.8 |
| 122 | 02 | MED | ACUTE MAJOR EYE INFECTIONS W/O CC/MCC | 0.5850 | 3.0 |
| 123 | 02 | MED | NEUROLOGICAL EYE DISORDERS | 0.7171 | 2.1 |
| 124 | 02 | MED | OTHER DISORDERS OF THE EYE W MCC | 1.2163 | 3.8 |
| 125 | 02 | MED | OTHER DISORDERS OF THE EYE W/O MCC | 0.7256 | 2.5 |
| 129 | 03 | SURG | MAJOR HEAD & NECK PROCEDURES W CC/MCC OR MAJOR DEVICE | 2.2292 | 3.7 |
| 130 | 03 | SURG | MAJOR HEAD & NECK PROCEDURES W/O CC/MCC | 1.3596 | 2.3 |
| 131 | 03 | SURG | CRANIAL/FACIAL PROCEDURES W CC/MCC | 2.4094 | 4.3 |
| 132 | 03 | SURG | CRANIAL/FACIAL PROCEDURES W/O CC/MCC | 1.4401 | 2.2 |
| 133 | 03 | SURG | OTHER EAR, NOSE, MOUTH & THROAT O.R. PROCEDURES W CC/MCC | 1.8573 | 3.8 |
| 134 | 03 | SURG | OTHER EAR, NOSE, MOUTH & THROAT O.R. PROCEDURES W/O CC/MCC | 1.0635 | 1.9 |
| 135 | 03 | SURG | SINUS & MASTOID PROCEDURES W CC/MCC | 1.9100 | 4.1 |
| 136 | 03 | SURG | SINUS & MASTOID PROCEDURES W/O CC/MCC | 1.1905 | 1.9 |
| 137 | 03 | SURG | MOUTH PROCEDURES W CC/MCC | 1.4261 | 3.8 |
| 138 | 03 | SURG | MOUTH PROCEDURES W/O CC/MCC | 0.8272 | 2.0 |
| 139 | 03 | SURG | SALIVARY GLAND PROCEDURES | 0.9828 | 1.6 |
| 146 | 03 | MED | EAR, NOSE, MOUTH & THROAT MALIGNANCY W MCC | 1.8740 | 5.7 |
| 147 | 03 | MED | EAR, NOSE, MOUTH & THROAT MALIGNANCY W CC | 1.2419 | 3.9 |
| 148 | 03 | MED | EAR, NOSE, MOUTH & THROAT MALIGNANCY W/O CC/MCC | 0.8094 | 2.2 |

| MS-DRG | MDC | Type | MS-DRG Title | Weights | Geometric Mean LOS |
|--------|-----|------|--------------|---------|--------------------|
| 149 | 03 | MED | DYSEQUILIBRIUM | 0.6707 | 2.1 |
| 150 | 03 | MED | EPISTAXIS W MCC | 1.2560 | 3.6 |
| 151 | 03 | MED | EPISTAXIS W/O MCC | 0.7033 | 2.3 |
| 152 | 03 | MED | OTITIS MEDIA & URI W MCC | 1.0612 | 3.4 |
| 153 | 03 | MED | OTITIS MEDIA & URI W/O MCC | 0.7042 | 2.5 |
| 154 | 03 | MED | OTHER EAR, NOSE, MOUTH & THROAT DIAGNOSES W MCC | 1.4090 | 4.0 |
| 155 | 03 | MED | OTHER EAR, NOSE, MOUTH & THROAT DIAGNOSES W CC | 0.8733 | 3.1 |
| 156 | 03 | MED | OTHER EAR, NOSE, MOUTH & THROAT DIAGNOSES W/O CC/MCC | 0.6662 | 2.3 |
| 157 | 03 | MED | DENTAL & ORAL DISEASES W MCC | 1.4949 | 4.5 |
| 158 | 03 | MED | DENTAL & ORAL DISEASES W CC | 0.8582 | 3.0 |
| 159 | 03 | MED | DENTAL & ORAL DISEASES W/O CC/MCC | 0.6176 | 2.1 |
| 163 | 04 | SURG | MAJOR CHEST PROCEDURES W MCC | 5.0016 | 10.5 |
| 164 | 04 | SURG | MAJOR CHEST PROCEDURES W CC | 2.5822 | 5.3 |
| 165 | 04 | SURG | MAJOR CHEST PROCEDURES W/O CC/MCC | 1.8148 | 3.1 |
| 166 | 04 | SURG | OTHER RESP SYSTEM O.R. PROCEDURES W MCC | 3.6796 | 8.5 |
| 167 | 04 | SURG | OTHER RESP SYSTEM O.R. PROCEDURES W CC | 1.9367 | 5.0 |
| 168 | 04 | SURG | OTHER RESP SYSTEM O.R. PROCEDURES W/O CC/MCC | 1.2950 | 2.9 |
| 175 | 04 | MED | PULMONARY EMBOLISM W MCC | 1.4839 | 4.9 |
| 176 | 04 | MED | PULMONARY EMBOLISM W/O MCC | 0.9375 | 3.3 |
| 177 | 04 | MED | RESPIRATORY INFECTIONS & INFLAMMATIONS W MCC | 1.9033 | 6.0 |
| 178 | 04 | MED | RESPIRATORY INFECTIONS & INFLAMMATIONS W CC | 1.3575 | 4.8 |
| 179 | 04 | MED | RESPIRATORY INFECTIONS & INFLAMMATIONS W/O CC/MCC | 0.9659 | 3.6 |

*(continues)*

| MS-DRG | MDC | Type | MS-DRG Title | Weights | Geometric Mean LOS |
|--------|-----|------|--------------|---------|--------------------|
| 180 | 04 | MED | RESPIRATORY NEOPLASMS W MCC | 1.6767 | 5.2 |
| 181 | 04 | MED | RESPIRATORY NEOPLASMS W CC | 1.1775 | 3.7 |
| 182 | 04 | MED | RESPIRATORY NEOPLASMS W/O CC/MCC | 0.8553 | 2.6 |
| 183 | 04 | MED | MAJOR CHEST TRAUMA W MCC | 1.4723 | 4.7 |
| 184 | 04 | MED | MAJOR CHEST TRAUMA W CC | 1.0125 | 3.4 |
| 185 | 04 | MED | MAJOR CHEST TRAUMA W/O CC/MCC | 0.7182 | 2.5 |
| 186 | 04 | MED | PLEURAL EFFUSION W MCC | 1.5734 | 4.7 |
| 187 | 04 | MED | PLEURAL EFFUSION W CC | 1.0835 | 3.5 |
| 188 | 04 | MED | PLEURAL EFFUSION W/O CC/MCC | 0.7860 | 2.7 |
| 189 | 04 | MED | PULMONARY EDEMA & RESPIRATORY FAILURE | 1.2265 | 3.9 |
| 190 | 04 | MED | CHRONIC OBSTRUCTIVE PULMONARY DISEASE W MCC | 1.1578 | 4.0 |
| 191 | 04 | MED | CHRONIC OBSTRUCTIVE PULMONARY DISEASE W CC | 0.9321 | 3.3 |
| 192 | 04 | MED | CHRONIC OBSTRUCTIVE PULMONARY DISEASE W/O CC/MCC | 0.7313 | 2.7 |
| 193 | 04 | MED | SIMPLE PNEUMONIA & PLEURISY W MCC | 1.4261 | 4.8 |
| 194 | 04 | MED | SIMPLE PNEUMONIA & PLEURISY W CC | 0.9695 | 3.7 |
| 195 | 04 | MED | SIMPLE PNEUMONIA & PLEURISY W/O CC/MCC | 0.7111 | 2.8 |
| 196 | 04 | MED | INTERSTITIAL LUNG DISEASE W MCC | 1.6315 | 5.2 |
| 197 | 04 | MED | INTERSTITIAL LUNG DISEASE W CC | 1.0406 | 3.6 |
| 198 | 04 | MED | INTERSTITIAL LUNG DISEASE W/O CC/MCC | 0.7775 | 2.8 |
| 199 | 04 | MED | PNEUMOTHORAX W MCC | 1.7503 | 5.7 |
| 200 | 04 | MED | PNEUMOTHORAX W CC | 1.0443 | 3.5 |
| 201 | 04 | MED | PNEUMOTHORAX W/O CC/MCC | 0.7354 | 2.7 |
| 202 | 04 | MED | BRONCHITIS & ASTHMA W CC/MCC | 0.8980 | 3.1 |
| 203 | 04 | MED | BRONCHITIS & ASTHMA W/O CC/MCC | 0.6697 | 2.5 |

| MS-DRG | MDC | Type | MS-DRG Title | Weights | Geometric Mean LOS |
|---|---|---|---|---|---|
| 204 | 04 | MED | RESPIRATORY SIGNS & SYMPTOMS | 0.7291 | 2.2 |
| 205 | 04 | MED | OTHER RESPIRATORY SYSTEM DIAGNOSES W MCC | 1.4478 | 4.1 |
| 206 | 04 | MED | OTHER RESPIRATORY SYSTEM DIAGNOSES W/O MCC | 0.8164 | 2.5 |
| 207 | 04 | MED | RESPIRATORY SYSTEM DIAGNOSIS W VENTILATOR SUPPORT >96 HOURS | 5.3498 | 12.2 |
| 208 | 04 | MED | RESPIRATORY SYSTEM DIAGNOSIS W VENTILATOR SUPPORT <96 HOURS | 2.3055 | 4.9 |
| 215 | 05 | SURG | OTHER HEART ASSIST SYSTEM IMPLANT | 15.8738 | 12.0 |
| 216 | 05 | SURG | CARDIAC VALVE & OTH MAJ CARDIOTHORACIC PROC W CARD CATH W MCC | 9.4642 | 12.7 |
| 217 | 05 | SURG | CARDIAC VALVE & OTH MAJ CARDIOTHORACIC PROC W CARD CATH W CC | 6.2576 | 8.5 |
| 218 | 05 | SURG | CARDIAC VALVE & OTH MAJ CARDIOTHORACIC PROC W CARD CATH W/O CC/MCC | 5.4815 | 6.5 |
| 219 | 05 | SURG | CARDIAC VALVE & OTH MAJ CARDIOTHORACIC PROC W/O CARD CATH W MCC | 7.5590 | 9.6 |
| 220 | 05 | SURG | CARDIAC VALVE & OTH MAJ CARDIOTHORACIC PROC W/O CARD CATH W CC | 5.1074 | 6.5 |
| 221 | 05 | SURG | CARDIAC VALVE & OTH MAJ CARDIOTHORACIC PROC W/O CARD CATH W/O CC/MCC | 4.5406 | 4.8 |
| 222 | 05 | SURG | CARDIAC DEFIB IMPLANT W CARDIAC CATH W AMI/HF/SHOCK W MCC | 8.5188 | 10.2 |
| 223 | 05 | SURG | CARDIAC DEFIB IMPLANT W CARDIAC CATH W AMI/HF/SHOCK W/O MCC | 6.4026 | 5.4 |
| 224 | 05 | SURG | CARDIAC DEFIB IMPLANT W CARDIAC CATH W/O AMI/HF/SHOCK W MCC | 7.6140 | 8.0 |
| 225 | 05 | SURG | CARDIAC DEFIB IMPLANT W CARDIAC CATH W/O AMI/HF/SHOCK W/O MCC | 5.8561 | 4.1 |
| 226 | 05 | SURG | CARDIAC DEFIBRILLATOR IMPLANT W/O CARDIAC CATH W MCC | 6.9737 | 6.8 |
| 227 | 05 | SURG | CARDIAC DEFIBRILLATOR IMPLANT W/O CARDIAC CATH W/O MCC | 5.4816 | 3.1 |

*(continues)*

| MS-DRG | MDC | Type | MS-DRG Title | Weights | Geometric Mean LOS |
|---|---|---|---|---|---|
| 228 | 05 | SURG | OTHER CARDIOTHORACIC PROCEDURES W MCC | 6.9512 | 10.8 |
| 229 | 05 | SURG | OTHER CARDIOTHORACIC PROCEDURES W CC | 4.5589 | 6.5 |
| 230 | 05 | SURG | OTHER CARDIOTHORACIC PROCEDURES W/O CC/MCC | 4.3018 | 4.3 |
| 231 | 05 | SURG | CORONARY BYPASS W PTCA W MCC | 7.8056 | 9.9 |
| 232 | 05 | SURG | CORONARY BYPASS W PTCA W/O MCC | 5.7779 | 7.9 |
| 233 | 05 | SURG | CORONARY BYPASS W CARDIAC CATH W MCC | 7.3581 | 11.6 |
| 234 | 05 | SURG | CORONARY BYPASS W CARDIAC CATH W/O MCC | 4.9076 | 8.0 |
| 235 | 05 | SURG | CORONARY BYPASS W/O CARDIAC CATH W MCC | 5.8103 | 8.9 |
| 236 | 05 | SURG | CORONARY BYPASS W/O CARDIAC CATH W/O MCC | 3.8013 | 6.0 |
| 239 | 05 | SURG | AMPUTATION FOR CIRC SYS DISORDERS EXC UPPER LIMB & TOE W MCC | 4.8380 | 10.5 |
| 240 | 05 | SURG | AMPUTATION FOR CIRC SYS DISORDERS EXC UPPER LIMB & TOE W CC | 2.6835 | 7.0 |
| 241 | 05 | SURG | AMPUTATION FOR CIRC SYS DISORDERS EXC UPPER LIMB & TOE W/O CC/MCC | 1.4476 | 4.5 |
| 242 | 05 | SURG | PERMANENT CARDIAC PACEMAKER IMPLANT W MCC | 3.7836 | 5.7 |
| 243 | 05 | SURG | PERMANENT CARDIAC PACEMAKER IMPLANT W CC | 2.6444 | 3.6 |
| 244 | 05 | SURG | PERMANENT CARDIAC PACEMAKER IMPLANT W/O CC/MCC | 2.1394 | 2.5 |
| 245 | 05 | SURG | AICD GENERATOR PROCEDURES | 4.6864 | 4.0 |
| 246 | 05 | SURG | PERC CARDIOVASC PROC W DRUG-ELUTING STENT W MCC OR 4+ VESSELS/STENTS | 3.2494 | 4.1 |
| 247 | 05 | SURG | PERC CARDIOVASC PROC W DRUG-ELUTING STENT W/O MCC | 2.1307 | 2.2 |
| 248 | 05 | SURG | PERC CARDIOVASC PROC W NON-DRUG-ELUTING STENT W MCC OR 4+ VES/STENTS | 3.0696 | 4.8 |

| MS-DRG | MDC | Type | MS-DRG Title | Weights | Geometric Mean LOS |
|---|---|---|---|---|---|
| 249 | 05 | SURG | PERC CARDIOVASC PROC W NON-DRUG-ELUTING STENT W/O MCC | 1.9140 | 2.5 |
| 250 | 05 | SURG | PERC CARDIOVASC PROC W/O CORONARY ARTERY STENT W MCC | 2.6975 | 4.2 |
| 251 | 05 | SURG | PERC CARDIOVASC PROC W/O CORONARY ARTERY STENT W/O MCC | 1.6863 | 2.4 |
| 252 | 05 | SURG | OTHER VASCULAR PROCEDURES W MCC | 3.2872 | 5.5 |
| 253 | 05 | SURG | OTHER VASCULAR PROCEDURES W CC | 2.6028 | 4.3 |
| 254 | 05 | SURG | OTHER VASCULAR PROCEDURES W/O CC/MCC | 1.7232 | 2.4 |
| 255 | 05 | SURG | UPPER LIMB & TOE AMPUTATION FOR CIRC SYSTEM DISORDERS W MCC | 2.6202 | 6.8 |
| 256 | 05 | SURG | UPPER LIMB & TOE AMPUTATION FOR CIRC SYSTEM DISORDERS W CC | 1.6241 | 5.3 |
| 257 | 05 | SURG | UPPER LIMB & TOE AMPUTATION FOR CIRC SYSTEM DISORDERS W/O CC/MCC | 1.0844 | 3.4 |
| 258 | 05 | SURG | CARDIAC PACEMAKER DEVICE REPLACEMENT W MCC | 2.8590 | 4.9 |
| 259 | 05 | SURG | CARDIAC PACEMAKER DEVICE REPLACEMENT W/O MCC | 1.9456 | 2.9 |
| 260 | 05 | SURG | CARDIAC PACEMAKER REVISION EXCEPT DEVICE REPLACEMENT W MCC | 3.7299 | 7.6 |
| 261 | 05 | SURG | CARDIAC PACEMAKER REVISION EXCEPT DEVICE REPLACEMENT W CC | 1.8639 | 3.5 |
| 262 | 05 | SURG | CARDIAC PACEMAKER REVISION EXCEPT DEVICE REPLACEMENT W/O CC/MCC | 1.5125 | 2.5 |
| 263 | 05 | SURG | VEIN LIGATION & STRIPPING | 2.0854 | 4.1 |
| 264 | 05 | SURG | OTHER CIRCULATORY SYSTEM O.R. PROCEDURES | 2.8080 | 5.8 |
| 265 | 05 | SURG | AICD LEAD PROCEDURES | 2.9681 | 3.1 |
| 266 | 05 | SURG | ENDOVASCULAR CARDIAC VALVE REPLACEMENT W MCC | 8.5986 | 7.3 |
| 267 | 05 | SURG | ENDOVASCULAR CARDIAC VALVE REPLACEMENT W/O MCC | 6.5575 | 4.4 |

*(continues)*

| MS-DRG | MDC | Type | MS-DRG Title | Weights | Geometric Mean LOS |
|--------|-----|------|--------------|---------|--------------------|
| 268 | 05 | SURG | AORTIC AND HEART ASSIST PROCEDURES EXCEPT PULSATION BALLOON W MCC | 6.2807 | 6.9 |
| 269 | 05 | SURG | AORTIC AND HEART ASSIST PROCEDURES EXCEPT PULSATION BALLOON W/O MCC | 3.9041 | 1.9 |
| 270 | 05 | SURG | OTHER MAJOR CARDIOVASCULAR PROCEDURES W MCC | 4.7349 | 6.5 |
| 271 | 05 | SURG | OTHER MAJOR CARDIOVASCULAR PROCEDURES W CC | 3.1426 | 4.5 |
| 272 | 05 | SURG | OTHER MAJOR CARDIOVASCULAR PROCEDURES W/O CC/MCC | 2.2508 | 2.3 |
| 273 | 05 | SURG | PERCUTANEOUS INTRACARDIAC PROCEDURES W MCC | 3.5499 | 6.0 |
| 274 | 05 | SURG | PERCUTANEOUS INTRACARDIAC PROCEDURES W/O MCC | 2.4197 | 2.7 |
| 280 | 05 | MED | ACUTE MYOCARDIAL INFARCTION, DISCHARGED ALIVE W MCC | 1.6971 | 4.5 |
| 281 | 05 | MED | ACUTE MYOCARDIAL INFARCTION, DISCHARGED ALIVE W CC | 1.0232 | 2.9 |
| 282 | 05 | MED | ACUTE MYOCARDIAL INFARCTION, DISCHARGED ALIVE W/O CC/MCC | 0.7557 | 2.0 |
| 283 | 05 | MED | ACUTE MYOCARDIAL INFARCTION, EXPIRED W MCC | 1.6613 | 2.9 |
| 284 | 05 | MED | ACUTE MYOCARDIAL INFARCTION, EXPIRED W CC | 0.7827 | 1.8 |
| 285 | 05 | MED | ACUTE MYOCARDIAL INFARCTION, EXPIRED W/O CC/MCC | 0.5473 | 1.4 |
| 286 | 05 | MED | CIRCULATORY DISORDERS EXCEPT AMI, W CARD CATH W MCC | 2.1775 | 5.1 |
| 287 | 05 | MED | CIRCULATORY DISORDERS EXCEPT AMI, W CARD CATH W/O MCC | 1.1562 | 2.5 |
| 288 | 05 | MED | ACUTE & SUBACUTE ENDOCARDITIS W MCC | 2.7933 | 7.5 |
| 289 | 05 | MED | ACUTE & SUBACUTE ENDOCARDITIS W CC | 1.6969 | 5.6 |
| 290 | 05 | MED | ACUTE & SUBACUTE ENDOCARDITIS W/O CC/MCC | 1.0546 | 3.7 |

| MS-DRG | MDC | Type | MS-DRG Title | Weights | Geometric Mean LOS |
|--------|-----|------|--------------|---------|--------------------|
| 291 | 05 | MED | HEART FAILURE & SHOCK W MCC | 1.4809 | 4.6 |
| 292 | 05 | MED | HEART FAILURE & SHOCK W CC | 0.9707 | 3.6 |
| 293 | 05 | MED | HEART FAILURE & SHOCK W/O CC/MCC | 0.6737 | 2.6 |
| 294 | 05 | MED | DEEP VEIN THROMBOPHLEBITIS W CC/MCC | 0.9826 | 3.8 |
| 295 | 05 | MED | DEEP VEIN THROMBOPHLEBITIS W/O CC/MCC | 0.7427 | 3.2 |
| 296 | 05 | MED | CARDIAC ARREST, UNEXPLAINED W MCC | 1.2864 | 1.9 |
| 297 | 05 | MED | CARDIAC ARREST, UNEXPLAINED W CC | 0.6488 | 1.3 |
| 298 | 05 | MED | CARDIAC ARREST, UNEXPLAINED W/O CC/MCC | 0.4477 | 1.1 |
| 299 | 05 | MED | PERIPHERAL VASCULAR DISORDERS W MCC | 1.4216 | 4.3 |
| 300 | 05 | MED | PERIPHERAL VASCULAR DISORDERS W CC | 0.9994 | 3.5 |
| 301 | 05 | MED | PERIPHERAL VASCULAR DISORDERS W/O CC/MCC | 0.7023 | 2.6 |
| 302 | 05 | MED | ATHEROSCLEROSIS W MCC | 1.0590 | 2.9 |
| 303 | 05 | MED | ATHEROSCLEROSIS W/O MCC | 0.6427 | 2.0 |
| 304 | 05 | MED | HYPERTENSION W MCC | 1.0109 | 3.3 |
| 305 | 05 | MED | HYPERTENSION W/O MCC | 0.6626 | 2.2 |
| 306 | 05 | MED | CARDIAC CONGENITAL & VALVULAR DISORDERS W MCC | 1.4029 | 4.0 |
| 307 | 05 | MED | CARDIAC CONGENITAL & VALVULAR DISORDERS W/O MCC | 0.8044 | 2.5 |
| 308 | 05 | MED | CARDIAC ARRHYTHMIA & CONDUCTION DISORDERS W MCC | 1.2150 | 3.8 |
| 309 | 05 | MED | CARDIAC ARRHYTHMIA & CONDUCTION DISORDERS W CC | 0.7851 | 2.6 |
| 310 | 05 | MED | CARDIAC ARRHYTHMIA & CONDUCTION DISORDERS W/O CC/MCC | 0.5608 | 2.0 |
| 311 | 05 | MED | ANGINA PECTORIS | 0.6091 | 1.8 |
| 312 | 05 | MED | SYNCOPE & COLLAPSE | 0.7630 | 2.4 |

*(continues)*

| MS-DRG | MDC | Type | MS-DRG Title | Weights | Geometric Mean LOS |
|--------|-----|------|--------------|---------|--------------------|
| 313 | 05 | MED | CHEST PAIN | 0.6621 | 1.8 |
| 314 | 05 | MED | OTHER CIRCULATORY SYSTEM DIAGNOSES W MCC | 1.9334 | 4.9 |
| 315 | 05 | MED | OTHER CIRCULATORY SYSTEM DIAGNOSES W CC | 0.9722 | 3.1 |
| 316 | 05 | MED | OTHER CIRCULATORY SYSTEM DIAGNOSES W/O CC/MCC | 0.6498 | 2.0 |
| 326 | 06 | SURG | STOMACH, ESOPHAGEAL & DUODENAL PROC W MCC | 5.4452 | 11.0 |
| 327 | 06 | SURG | STOMACH, ESOPHAGEAL & DUODENAL PROC W CC | 2.6399 | 5.7 |
| 328 | 06 | SURG | STOMACH, ESOPHAGEAL & DUODENAL PROC W/O CC/MCC | 1.5154 | 2.5 |
| 329 | 06 | SURG | MAJOR SMALL & LARGE BOWEL PROCEDURES W MCC | 5.0709 | 11.5 |
| 330 | 06 | SURG | MAJOR SMALL & LARGE BOWEL PROCEDURES W CC | 2.5511 | 7.0 |
| 331 | 06 | SURG | MAJOR SMALL & LARGE BOWEL PROCEDURES W/O CC/MCC | 1.6491 | 4.1 |
| 332 | 06 | SURG | RECTAL RESECTION W MCC | 4.5570 | 10.2 |
| 333 | 06 | SURG | RECTAL RESECTION W CC | 2.4254 | 6.0 |
| 334 | 06 | SURG | RECTAL RESECTION W/O CC/MCC | 1.6480 | 3.5 |
| 335 | 06 | SURG | PERITONEAL ADHESIOLYSIS W MCC | 4.1261 | 10.4 |
| 336 | 06 | SURG | PERITONEAL ADHESIOLYSIS W CC | 2.3340 | 6.7 |
| 337 | 06 | SURG | PERITONEAL ADHESIOLYSIS W/O CC/MCC | 1.5675 | 4.0 |
| 338 | 06 | SURG | APPENDECTOMY W COMPLICATED PRINCIPAL DIAG W MCC | 2.9719 | 7.5 |
| 339 | 06 | SURG | APPENDECTOMY W COMPLICATED PRINCIPAL DIAG W CC | 1.7693 | 4.8 |
| 340 | 06 | SURG | APPENDECTOMY W COMPLICATED PRINCIPAL DIAG W/O CC/MCC | 1.1773 | 2.9 |
| 341 | 06 | SURG | APPENDECTOMY W/O COMPLICATED PRINCIPAL DIAG W MCC | 2.1523 | 4.5 |

| MS-DRG | MDC | Type | MS-DRG Title | Weights | Geometric Mean LOS |
|--------|-----|------|--------------|---------|--------------------|
| 342 | 06 | SURG | APPENDECTOMY W/O COMPLICATED PRINCIPAL DIAG W CC | 1.3275 | 2.7 |
| 343 | 06 | SURG | APPENDECTOMY W/O COMPLICATED PRINCIPAL DIAG W/O CC/MCC | 1.0099 | 1.7 |
| 344 | 06 | SURG | MINOR SMALL & LARGE BOWEL PROCEDURES W MCC | 3.1029 | 8.0 |
| 345 | 06 | SURG | MINOR SMALL & LARGE BOWEL PROCEDURES W CC | 1.6268 | 5.2 |
| 346 | 06 | SURG | MINOR SMALL & LARGE BOWEL PROCEDURES W/O CC/MCC | 1.2143 | 3.7 |
| 347 | 06 | SURG | ANAL & STOMAL PROCEDURES W MCC | 2.4457 | 6.1 |
| 348 | 06 | SURG | ANAL & STOMAL PROCEDURES W CC | 1.4486 | 4.0 |
| 349 | 06 | SURG | ANAL & STOMAL PROCEDURES W/O CC/MCC | 0.9265 | 2.4 |
| 350 | 06 | SURG | INGUINAL & FEMORAL HERNIA PROCEDURES W MCC | 2.4982 | 5.6 |
| 351 | 06 | SURG | INGUINAL & FEMORAL HERNIA PROCEDURES W CC | 1.4110 | 3.4 |
| 352 | 06 | SURG | INGUINAL & FEMORAL HERNIA PROCEDURES W/O CC/MCC | 0.9764 | 2.1 |
| 353 | 06 | SURG | HERNIA PROCEDURES EXCEPT INGUINAL & FEMORAL W MCC | 2.9142 | 6.2 |
| 354 | 06 | SURG | HERNIA PROCEDURES EXCEPT INGUINAL & FEMORAL W CC | 1.6640 | 3.9 |
| 355 | 06 | SURG | HERNIA PROCEDURES EXCEPT INGUINAL & FEMORAL W/O CC/MCC | 1.2366 | 2.5 |
| 356 | 06 | SURG | OTHER DIGESTIVE SYSTEM O.R. PROCEDURES W MCC | 3.7588 | 8.2 |
| 357 | 06 | SURG | OTHER DIGESTIVE SYSTEM O.R. PROCEDURES W CC | 2.0801 | 5.1 |
| 358 | 06 | SURG | OTHER DIGESTIVE SYSTEM O.R. PROCEDURES W/O CC/MCC | 1.3515 | 3.1 |
| 368 | 06 | MED | MAJOR ESOPHAGEAL DISORDERS W MCC | 1.7848 | 4.8 |

*(continues)*

| MS-DRG | MDC | Type | MS-DRG Title | Weights | Geometric Mean LOS |
|--------|-----|------|--------------|---------|--------------------|
| 369 | 06 | MED | MAJOR ESOPHAGEAL DISORDERS W CC | 1.0630 | 3.4 |
| 370 | 06 | MED | MAJOR ESOPHAGEAL DISORDERS W/O CC/MCC | 0.7355 | 2.4 |
| 371 | 06 | MED | MAJOR GASTROINTESTINAL DISORDERS & PERITONEAL INFECTIONS W MCC | 1.7854 | 5.8 |
| 372 | 06 | MED | MAJOR GASTROINTESTINAL DISORDERS & PERITONEAL INFECTIONS W CC | 1.1090 | 4.4 |
| 373 | 06 | MED | MAJOR GASTROINTESTINAL DISORDERS & PERITONEAL INFECTIONS W/O CC/MCC | 0.7817 | 3.3 |
| 374 | 06 | MED | DIGESTIVE MALIGNANCY W MCC | 2.0345 | 5.9 |
| 375 | 06 | MED | DIGESTIVE MALIGNANCY W CC | 1.2302 | 4.0 |
| 376 | 06 | MED | DIGESTIVE MALIGNANCY W/O CC/MCC | 0.9093 | 2.8 |
| 377 | 06 | MED | G.I. HEMORRHAGE W MCC | 1.7509 | 4.7 |
| 378 | 06 | MED | G.I. HEMORRHAGE W CC | 0.9949 | 3.2 |
| 379 | 06 | MED | G.I. HEMORRHAGE W/O CC/MCC | 0.6712 | 2.3 |
| 380 | 06 | MED | COMPLICATED PEPTIC ULCER W MCC | 1.9549 | 5.3 |
| 381 | 06 | MED | COMPLICATED PEPTIC ULCER W CC | 1.0690 | 3.5 |
| 382 | 06 | MED | COMPLICATED PEPTIC ULCER W/O CC/MCC | 0.8238 | 2.7 |
| 383 | 06 | MED | UNCOMPLICATED PEPTIC ULCER W MCC | 1.3545 | 4.2 |
| 384 | 06 | MED | UNCOMPLICATED PEPTIC ULCER W/O MCC | 0.8481 | 2.8 |
| 385 | 06 | MED | INFLAMMATORY BOWEL DISEASE W MCC | 1.7195 | 5.7 |
| 386 | 06 | MED | INFLAMMATORY BOWEL DISEASE W CC | 0.9996 | 3.8 |
| 387 | 06 | MED | INFLAMMATORY BOWEL DISEASE W/O CC/MCC | 0.7379 | 3.0 |
| 388 | 06 | MED | G.I. OBSTRUCTION W MCC | 1.5813 | 5.2 |
| 389 | 06 | MED | G.I. OBSTRUCTION W CC | 0.8707 | 3.5 |
| 390 | 06 | MED | G.I. OBSTRUCTION W/O CC/MCC | 0.6067 | 2.7 |
| 391 | 06 | MED | ESOPHAGITIS, GASTROENT & MISC DIGEST DISORDERS W MCC | 1.1925 | 3.8 |

| MS-DRG | MDC | Type | MS-DRG Title | Weights | Geometric Mean LOS |
|--------|-----|------|--------------|---------|--------------------|
| 392 | 06 | MED | ESOPHAGITIS, GASTROENT & MISC DIGEST DISORDERS W/O MCC | 0.7400 | 2.7 |
| 393 | 06 | MED | OTHER DIGESTIVE SYSTEM DIAGNOSES W MCC | 1.6335 | 4.6 |
| 394 | 06 | MED | OTHER DIGESTIVE SYSTEM DIAGNOSES W CC | 0.9502 | 3.3 |
| 395 | 06 | MED | OTHER DIGESTIVE SYSTEM DIAGNOSES W/O CC/MCC | 0.6756 | 2.4 |
| 405 | 07 | SURG | PANCREAS, LIVER & SHUNT PROCEDURES W MCC | 5.5888 | 10.5 |
| 406 | 07 | SURG | PANCREAS, LIVER & SHUNT PROCEDURES W CC | 2.8075 | 5.9 |
| 407 | 07 | SURG | PANCREAS, LIVER & SHUNT PROCEDURES W/O CC/MCC | 2.0026 | 4.1 |
| 408 | 07 | SURG | BILIARY TRACT PROC EXCEPT ONLY CHOLECYST W OR W/O C.D.E. W MCC | 3.6476 | 9.6 |
| 409 | 07 | SURG | BILIARY TRACT PROC EXCEPT ONLY CHOLECYST W OR W/O C.D.E. W CC | 2.4648 | 6.6 |
| 410 | 07 | SURG | BILIARY TRACT PROC EXCEPT ONLY CHOLECYST W OR W/O C.D.E. W/O CC/MCC | 1.5576 | 4.5 |
| 411 | 07 | SURG | CHOLECYSTECTOMY W C.D.E. W MCC | 3.5782 | 8.9 |
| 412 | 07 | SURG | CHOLECYSTECTOMY W C.D.E. W CC | 2.4981 | 6.6 |
| 413 | 07 | SURG | CHOLECYSTECTOMY W C.D.E. W/O CC/MCC | 1.7996 | 4.1 |
| 414 | 07 | SURG | CHOLECYSTECTOMY EXCEPT BY LAPAROSCOPE W/O C.D.E. W MCC | 3.5283 | 8.5 |
| 415 | 07 | SURG | CHOLECYSTECTOMY EXCEPT BY LAPAROSCOPE W/O C.D.E. W CC | 2.0071 | 5.5 |
| 416 | 07 | SURG | CHOLECYSTECTOMY EXCEPT BY LAPAROSCOPE W/O C.D.E. W/O CC/MCC | 1.3342 | 3.4 |
| 417 | 07 | SURG | LAPAROSCOPIC CHOLECYSTECTOMY W/O C.D.E. W MCC | 2.4734 | 5.8 |
| 418 | 07 | SURG | LAPAROSCOPIC CHOLECYSTECTOMY W/O C.D.E. W CC | 1.6584 | 3.9 |
| 419 | 07 | SURG | LAPAROSCOPIC CHOLECYSTECTOMY W/O C.D.E. W/O CC/MCC | 1.2540 | 2.5 |

*(continues)*

| MS-DRG | MDC | Type | MS-DRG Title | Weights | Geometric Mean LOS |
|--------|-----|------|--------------|---------|--------------------|
| 420 | 07 | SURG | HEPATOBILIARY DIAGNOSTIC PROCEDURES W MCC | 3.6609 | 8.1 |
| 421 | 07 | SURG | HEPATOBILIARY DIAGNOSTIC PROCEDURES W CC | 1.7451 | 4.1 |
| 422 | 07 | SURG | HEPATOBILIARY DIAGNOSTIC PROCEDURES W/O CC/MCC | 1.2941 | 2.8 |
| 423 | 07 | SURG | OTHER HEPATOBILIARY OR PANCREAS O.R. PROCEDURES W MCC | 4.2650 | 9.8 |
| 424 | 07 | SURG | OTHER HEPATOBILIARY OR PANCREAS O.R. PROCEDURES W CC | 2.3049 | 6.0 |
| 425 | 07 | SURG | OTHER HEPATOBILIARY OR PANCREAS O.R. PROCEDURES W/O CC/MCC | 1.6000 | 3.6 |
| 432 | 07 | MED | CIRRHOSIS & ALCOHOLIC HEPATITIS W MCC | 1.6567 | 4.7 |
| 433 | 07 | MED | CIRRHOSIS & ALCOHOLIC HEPATITIS W CC | 0.9164 | 3.2 |
| 434 | 07 | MED | CIRRHOSIS & ALCOHOLIC HEPATITIS W/O CC/MCC | 0.6235 | 2.3 |
| 435 | 07 | MED | MALIGNANCY OF HEPATOBILIARY SYSTEM OR PANCREAS W MCC | 1.7476 | 5.1 |
| 436 | 07 | MED | MALIGNANCY OF HEPATOBILIARY SYSTEM OR PANCREAS W CC | 1.1686 | 3.8 |
| 437 | 07 | MED | MALIGNANCY OF HEPATOBILIARY SYSTEM OR PANCREAS W/O CC/MCC | 0.9051 | 2.7 |
| 438 | 07 | MED | DISORDERS OF PANCREAS EXCEPT MALIGNANCY W MCC | 1.6612 | 4.9 |
| 439 | 07 | MED | DISORDERS OF PANCREAS EXCEPT MALIGNANCY W CC | 0.8823 | 3.5 |
| 440 | 07 | MED | DISORDERS OF PANCREAS EXCEPT MALIGNANCY W/O CC/MCC | 0.6368 | 2.6 |
| 441 | 07 | MED | DISORDERS OF LIVER EXCEPT MALIG, CIRR, ALC HEPA W MCC | 1.8767 | 5.0 |
| 442 | 07 | MED | DISORDERS OF LIVER EXCEPT MALIG, CIRR, ALC HEPA W CC | 0.9371 | 3.4 |
| 443 | 07 | MED | DISORDERS OF LIVER EXCEPT MALIG, CIRR, ALC HEPA W/O CC/MCC | 0.6545 | 2.5 |

| MS-DRG | MDC | Type | MS-DRG Title | Weights | Geometric Mean LOS |
|--------|-----|------|--------------|---------|--------------------|
| 444 | 07 | MED | DISORDERS OF THE BILIARY TRACT W MCC | 1.5895 | 4.5 |
| 445 | 07 | MED | DISORDERS OF THE BILIARY TRACT W CC | 1.0553 | 3.3 |
| 446 | 07 | MED | DISORDERS OF THE BILIARY TRACT W/O CC/MCC | 0.7633 | 2.4 |
| 453 | 08 | SURG | COMBINED ANTERIOR/POSTERIOR SPINAL FUSION W MCC | 11.4304 | 9.2 |
| 454 | 08 | SURG | COMBINED ANTERIOR/POSTERIOR SPINAL FUSION W CC | 8.0698 | 4.9 |
| 455 | 08 | SURG | COMBINED ANTERIOR/POSTERIOR SPINAL FUSION W/O CC/MCC | 6.1934 | 3.0 |
| 456 | 08 | SURG | SPINAL FUS EXC CERV W SPINAL CURV/MALIG/ INFEC OR EXT FUS W MCC | 9.4061 | 9.8 |
| 457 | 08 | SURG | SPINAL FUS EXC CERV W SPINAL CURV/MALIG/ INFEC OR EXT FUS W CC | 7.0741 | 5.5 |
| 458 | 08 | SURG | SPINAL FUS EXC CERV W SPINAL CURV/MALIG/ INFEC OR EXT FUS W/O CC/MCC | 5.2986 | 3.3 |
| 459 | 08 | SURG | SPINAL FUSION EXCEPT CERVICAL W MCC | 6.5455 | 6.7 |
| 460 | 08 | SURG | SPINAL FUSION EXCEPT CERVICAL W/O MCC | 3.9717 | 2.9 |
| 461 | 08 | SURG | BILATERAL OR MULTIPLE MAJOR JOINT PROCS OF LOWER EXTREMITY W MCC | 5.0977 | 6.3 |
| 462 | 08 | SURG | BILATERAL OR MULTIPLE MAJOR JOINT PROCS OF LOWER EXTREMITY W/O MCC | 3.2145 | 3.2 |
| 463 | 08 | SURG | WND DEBRID & SKN GRFT EXC HAND, FOR MUSCULO-CONN TISS DIS W MCC | 5.1028 | 10.2 |
| 464 | 08 | SURG | WND DEBRID & SKN GRFT EXC HAND, FOR MUSCULO-CONN TISS DIS W CC | 3.0937 | 6.2 |
| 465 | 08 | SURG | WND DEBRID & SKN GRFT EXC HAND, FOR MUSCULO-CONN TISS DIS W/O CC/MCC | 1.9349 | 3.8 |
| 466 | 08 | SURG | REVISION OF HIP OR KNEE REPLACEMENT W MCC | 5.0394 | 6.6 |
| 467 | 08 | SURG | REVISION OF HIP OR KNEE REPLACEMENT W CC | 3.4376 | 3.7 |
| 468 | 08 | SURG | REVISION OF HIP OR KNEE REPLACEMENT W/O CC/MCC | 2.7513 | 2.7 |

*(continues)*

| MS-DRG | MDC | Type | MS-DRG Title | Weights | Geometric Mean LOS |
|--------|-----|------|--------------|---------|--------------------|
| 469 | 08 | SURG | MAJOR JOINT REPLACEMENT OR REATTACHMENT OF LOWER EXTREMITY W MCC | 3.2962 | 5.9 |
| 470 | 08 | SURG | MAJOR JOINT REPLACEMENT OR REATTACHMENT OF LOWER EXTREMITY W/O MCC | 2.0816 | 2.8 |
| 471 | 08 | SURG | CERVICAL SPINAL FUSION W MCC | 4.9033 | 6.2 |
| 472 | 08 | SURG | CERVICAL SPINAL FUSION W CC | 2.9051 | 2.4 |
| 473 | 08 | SURG | CERVICAL SPINAL FUSION W/O CC/MCC | 2.2650 | 1.5 |
| 474 | 08 | SURG | AMPUTATION FOR MUSCULOSKELETAL SYS & CONN TISSUE DIS W MCC | 3.6260 | 8.7 |
| 475 | 08 | SURG | AMPUTATION FOR MUSCULOSKELETAL SYS & CONN TISSUE DIS W CC | 2.1001 | 5.7 |
| 476 | 08 | SURG | AMPUTATION FOR MUSCULOSKELETAL SYS & CONN TISSUE DIS W/O CC/MCC | 1.1427 | 3.1 |
| 477 | 08 | SURG | BIOPSIES OF MUSCULOSKELETAL SYSTEM & CONNECTIVE TISSUE W MCC | 3.1211 | 8.3 |
| 478 | 08 | SURG | BIOPSIES OF MUSCULOSKELETAL SYSTEM & CONNECTIVE TISSUE W CC | 2.1992 | 5.4 |
| 479 | 08 | SURG | BIOPSIES OF MUSCULOSKELETAL SYSTEM & CONNECTIVE TISSUE W/O CC/MCC | 1.7158 | 3.5 |
| 480 | 08 | SURG | HIP & FEMUR PROCEDURES EXCEPT MAJOR JOINT W MCC | 2.9990 | 6.7 |
| 481 | 08 | SURG | HIP & FEMUR PROCEDURES EXCEPT MAJOR JOINT W CC | 1.9790 | 4.6 |
| 482 | 08 | SURG | HIP & FEMUR PROCEDURES EXCEPT MAJOR JOINT W/O CC/MCC | 1.6228 | 3.7 |
| 483 | 08 | SURG | MAJOR JOINT/LIMB REATTACHMENT PROCEDURE OF UPPER EXTREMITIES | 2.4127 | 1.9 |
| 485 | 08 | SURG | KNEE PROCEDURES W PDX OF INFECTION W MCC | 3.2132 | 8.1 |
| 486 | 08 | SURG | KNEE PROCEDURES W PDX OF INFECTION W CC | 2.0690 | 5.4 |
| 487 | 08 | SURG | KNEE PROCEDURES W PDX OF INFECTION W/O CC/MCC | 1.5484 | 3.9 |

| MS-DRG | MDC | Type | MS-DRG Title | Weights | Geometric Mean LOS |
|--------|-----|------|--------------|---------|--------------------|
| 488 | 08 | SURG | KNEE PROCEDURES W/O PDX OF INFECTION W CC/MCC | 1.7591 | 3.4 |
| 489 | 08 | SURG | KNEE PROCEDURES W/O PDX OF INFECTION W/O CC/MCC | 1.2991 | 2.3 |
| 492 | 08 | SURG | LOWER EXTREM & HUMER PROC EXCEPT HIP, FOOT, FEMUR W MCC | 3.1585 | 6.2 |
| 493 | 08 | SURG | LOWER EXTREM & HUMER PROC EXCEPT HIP, FOOT, FEMUR W CC | 2.0557 | 3.9 |
| 494 | 08 | SURG | LOWER EXTREM & HUMER PROC EXCEPT HIP, FOOT, FEMUR W/O CC/MCC | 1.5796 | 2.7 |
| 495 | 08 | SURG | LOCAL EXCISION & REMOVAL INT FIX DEVICES EXC HIP & FEMUR W MCC | 3.0151 | 7.3 |
| 496 | 08 | SURG | LOCAL EXCISION & REMOVAL INT FIX DEVICES EXC HIP & FEMUR W CC | 1.7451 | 4.0 |
| 497 | 08 | SURG | LOCAL EXCISION & REMOVAL INT FIX DEVICES EXC HIP & FEMUR W/O CC/MCC | 1.2436 | 2.1 |
| 498 | 08 | SURG | LOCAL EXCISION & REMOVAL INT FIX DEVICES OF HIP & FEMUR W CC/MCC | 2.2492 | 5.4 |
| 499 | 08 | SURG | LOCAL EXCISION & REMOVAL INT FIX DEVICES OF HIP & FEMUR W/O CC/MCC | 1.0512 | 2.2 |
| 500 | 08 | SURG | SOFT TISSUE PROCEDURES W MCC | 3.2024 | 7.4 |
| 501 | 08 | SURG | SOFT TISSUE PROCEDURES W CC | 1.6064 | 4.3 |
| 502 | 08 | SURG | SOFT TISSUE PROCEDURES W/O CC/MCC | 1.1752 | 2.4 |
| 503 | 08 | SURG | FOOT PROCEDURES W MCC | 2.2679 | 6.7 |
| 504 | 08 | SURG | FOOT PROCEDURES W CC | 1.5941 | 5.0 |
| 505 | 08 | SURG | FOOT PROCEDURES W/O CC/MCC | 1.2590 | 2.9 |
| 506 | 08 | SURG | MAJOR THUMB OR JOINT PROCEDURES | 1.3490 | 3.4 |
| 507 | 08 | SURG | MAJOR SHOULDER OR ELBOW JOINT PROCEDURES W CC/MCC | 1.8698 | 4.3 |
| 508 | 08 | SURG | MAJOR SHOULDER OR ELBOW JOINT PROCEDURES W/O CC/MCC | 1.6134 | 2.2 |

*(continues)*

| MS-DRG | MDC | Type | MS-DRG Title | Weights | Geometric Mean LOS |
|--------|-----|------|--------------|---------|--------------------|
| 509 | 08 | SURG | ARTHROSCOPY | 1.6562 | 3.4 |
| 510 | 08 | SURG | SHOULDER, ELBOW OR FOREARM PROC, EXC MAJOR JOINT PROC W MCC | 2.4420 | 4.8 |
| 511 | 08 | SURG | SHOULDER, ELBOW OR FOREARM PROC, EXC MAJOR JOINT PROC W CC | 1.7018 | 3.3 |
| 512 | 08 | SURG | SHOULDER, ELBOW OR FOREARM PROC, EXC MAJOR JOINT PROC W/O CC/MCC | 1.3531 | 2.1 |
| 513 | 08 | SURG | HAND OR WRIST PROC, EXCEPT MAJOR THUMB OR JOINT PROC W CC/MCC | 1.5025 | 3.8 |
| 514 | 08 | SURG | HAND OR WRIST PROC, EXCEPT MAJOR THUMB OR JOINT PROC W/O CC/MCC | 0.9055 | 2.3 |
| 515 | 08 | SURG | OTHER MUSCULOSKELET SYS & CONN TISS O.R. PROC W MCC | 3.1862 | 7.0 |
| 516 | 08 | SURG | OTHER MUSCULOSKELET SYS & CONN TISS O.R. PROC W CC | 2.0670 | 4.3 |
| 517 | 08 | SURG | OTHER MUSCULOSKELET SYS & CONN TISS O.R. PROC W/O CC/MCC | 1.7716 | 2.6 |
| 518 | 08 | SURG | BACK & NECK PROC EXC SPINAL FUSION W MCC OR DISC DEVICE/NEUROSTIM | 2.9249 | 3.8 |
| 519 | 08 | SURG | BACK & NECK PROC EXC SPINAL FUSION W CC | 1.6805 | 3.1 |
| 520 | 08 | SURG | BACK & NECK PROC EXC SPINAL FUSION W/O CC/MCC | 1.1812 | 1.9 |
| 533 | 08 | MED | FRACTURES OF FEMUR W MCC | 1.4430 | 4.5 |
| 534 | 08 | MED | FRACTURES OF FEMUR W/O MCC | 0.7353 | 2.9 |
| 535 | 08 | MED | FRACTURES OF HIP & PELVIS W MCC | 1.2235 | 4.0 |
| 536 | 08 | MED | FRACTURES OF HIP & PELVIS W/O MCC | 0.7241 | 3.0 |
| 537 | 08 | MED | SPRAINS, STRAINS, & DISLOCATIONS OF HIP, PELVIS & THIGH W CC/MCC | 0.9046 | 3.3 |
| 538 | 08 | MED | SPRAINS, STRAINS, & DISLOCATIONS OF HIP, PELVIS & THIGH W/O CC/MCC | 0.6282 | 2.5 |
| 539 | 08 | MED | OSTEOMYELITIS W MCC | 1.8365 | 6.0 |

| MS-DRG | MDC | Type | MS-DRG Title | Weights | Geometric Mean LOS |
|--------|-----|------|--------------|---------|--------------------|
| 540 | 08 | MED | OSTEOMYELITIS W CC | 1.2832 | 4.7 |
| 541 | 08 | MED | OSTEOMYELITIS W/O CC/MCC | 0.9098 | 3.4 |
| 542 | 08 | MED | PATHOLOGICAL FRACTURES & MUSCULOSKELET & CONN TISS MALIG W MCC | 1.9100 | 5.7 |
| 543 | 08 | MED | PATHOLOGICAL FRACTURES & MUSCULOSKELET & CONN TISS MALIG W CC | 1.1171 | 4.0 |
| 544 | 08 | MED | PATHOLOGICAL FRACTURES & MUSCULOSKELET & CONN TISS MALIG W/O CC/MCC | 0.7805 | 3.1 |
| 545 | 08 | MED | CONNECTIVE TISSUE DISORDERS W MCC | 2.4409 | 5.9 |
| 546 | 08 | MED | CONNECTIVE TISSUE DISORDERS W CC | 1.1645 | 3.8 |
| 547 | 08 | MED | CONNECTIVE TISSUE DISORDERS W/O CC/MCC | 0.7882 | 2.7 |
| 548 | 08 | MED | SEPTIC ARTHRITIS W MCC | 1.8733 | 6.0 |
| 549 | 08 | MED | SEPTIC ARTHRITIS W CC | 1.1824 | 4.2 |
| 550 | 08 | MED | SEPTIC ARTHRITIS W/O CC/MCC | 0.8129 | 2.9 |
| 551 | 08 | MED | MEDICAL BACK PROBLEMS W MCC | 1.5573 | 4.6 |
| 552 | 08 | MED | MEDICAL BACK PROBLEMS W/O MCC | 0.8648 | 3.1 |
| 553 | 08 | MED | BONE DISEASES & ARTHROPATHIES W MCC | 1.2287 | 4.1 |
| 554 | 08 | MED | BONE DISEASES & ARTHROPATHIES W/O MCC | 0.7337 | 2.8 |
| 555 | 08 | MED | SIGNS & SYMPTOMS OF MUSCULOSKELETAL SYSTEM & CONN TISSUE W MCC | 1.2656 | 3.7 |
| 556 | 08 | MED | SIGNS & SYMPTOMS OF MUSCULOSKELETAL SYSTEM & CONN TISSUE W/O MCC | 0.7440 | 2.6 |
| 557 | 08 | MED | TENDONITIS, MYOSITIS & BURSITIS W MCC | 1.4295 | 4.8 |
| 558 | 08 | MED | TENDONITIS, MYOSITIS & BURSITIS W/O MCC | 0.8457 | 3.3 |
| 559 | 08 | MED | AFTERCARE, MUSCULOSKELETAL SYSTEM & CONNECTIVE TISSUE W MCC | 1.9202 | 5.0 |
| 560 | 08 | MED | AFTERCARE, MUSCULOSKELETAL SYSTEM & CONNECTIVE TISSUE W CC | 1.0814 | 3.5 |

*(continues)*

| MS-DRG | MDC | Type | MS-DRG Title | Weights | Geometric Mean LOS |
|--------|-----|------|--------------|---------|--------------------|
| 561 | 08 | MED | AFTERCARE, MUSCULOSKELETAL SYSTEM & CONNECTIVE TISSUE W/O CC/MCC | 0.6842 | 2.1 |
| 562 | 08 | MED | FX, SPRN, STRN & DISL EXCEPT FEMUR, HIP, PELVIS & THIGH W MCC | 1.3662 | 4.2 |
| 563 | 08 | MED | FX, SPRN, STRN & DISL EXCEPT FEMUR, HIP, PELVIS & THIGH W/O MCC | 0.7870 | 3.0 |
| 564 | 08 | MED | OTHER MUSCULOSKELETAL SYS & CONNECTIVE TISSUE DIAGNOSES W MCC | 1.5225 | 4.7 |
| 565 | 08 | MED | OTHER MUSCULOSKELETAL SYS & CONNECTIVE TISSUE DIAGNOSES W CC | 0.9598 | 3.5 |
| 566 | 08 | MED | OTHER MUSCULOSKELETAL SYS & CONNECTIVE TISSUE DIAGNOSES W/O CC/MCC | 0.7159 | 2.5 |
| 570 | 09 | SURG | SKIN DEBRIDEMENT W MCC | 2.4504 | 7.0 |
| 571 | 09 | SURG | SKIN DEBRIDEMENT W CC | 1.4569 | 5.2 |
| 572 | 09 | SURG | SKIN DEBRIDEMENT W/O CC/MCC | 1.0391 | 3.7 |
| 573 | 09 | SURG | SKIN GRAFT FOR SKIN ULCER OR CELLULITIS W MCC | 3.9130 | 8.6 |
| 574 | 09 | SURG | SKIN GRAFT FOR SKIN ULCER OR CELLULITIS W CC | 2.8430 | 7.4 |
| 575 | 09 | SURG | SKIN GRAFT FOR SKIN ULCER OR CELLULITIS W/O CC/MCC | 1.6141 | 4.4 |
| 576 | 09 | SURG | SKIN GRAFT EXC FOR SKIN ULCER OR CELLULITIS W MCC | 5.3493 | 8.9 |
| 577 | 09 | SURG | SKIN GRAFT EXC FOR SKIN ULCER OR CELLULITIS W CC | 2.2579 | 4.4 |
| 578 | 09 | SURG | SKIN GRAFT EXC FOR SKIN ULCER OR CELLULITIS W/O CC/MCC | 1.3812 | 2.6 |
| 579 | 09 | SURG | OTHER SKIN, SUBCUT TISS & BREAST PROC W MCC | 2.6848 | 7.0 |
| 580 | 09 | SURG | OTHER SKIN, SUBCUT TISS & BREAST PROC W CC | 1.6155 | 4.0 |
| 581 | 09 | SURG | OTHER SKIN, SUBCUT TISS & BREAST PROC W/O CC/MCC | 1.1834 | 2.2 |

| MS-DRG | MDC | Type | MS-DRG Title | Weights | Geometric Mean LOS |
|--------|-----|------|--------------|---------|--------------------|
| 582 | 09 | SURG | MASTECTOMY FOR MALIGNANCY W CC/MCC | 1.3370 | 2.2 |
| 583 | 09 | SURG | MASTECTOMY FOR MALIGNANCY W/O CC/MCC | 1.1856 | 1.6 |
| 584 | 09 | SURG | BREAST BIOPSY, LOCAL EXCISION & OTHER BREAST PROCEDURES W CC/MCC | 1.6794 | 3.7 |
| 585 | 09 | SURG | BREAST BIOPSY, LOCAL EXCISION & OTHER BREAST PROCEDURES W/O CC/MCC | 1.5184 | 2.1 |
| 592 | 09 | MED | SKIN ULCERS W MCC | 1.4255 | 5.0 |
| 593 | 09 | MED | SKIN ULCERS W CC | 1.0198 | 4.2 |
| 594 | 09 | MED | SKIN ULCERS W/O CC/MCC | 0.7049 | 3.1 |
| 595 | 09 | MED | MAJOR SKIN DISORDERS W MCC | 1.8480 | 5.4 |
| 596 | 09 | MED | MAJOR SKIN DISORDERS W/O MCC | 0.9375 | 3.6 |
| 597 | 09 | MED | MALIGNANT BREAST DISORDERS W MCC | 1.7397 | 5.3 |
| 598 | 09 | MED | MALIGNANT BREAST DISORDERS W CC | 1.0617 | 3.7 |
| 599 | 09 | MED | MALIGNANT BREAST DISORDERS W/O CC/MCC | 0.7211 | 2.3 |
| 600 | 09 | MED | NON-MALIGNANT BREAST DISORDERS W CC/MCC | 0.9843 | 3.7 |
| 601 | 09 | MED | NON-MALIGNANT BREAST DISORDERS W/O CC/MCC | 0.6799 | 2.8 |
| 602 | 09 | MED | CELLULITIS W MCC | 1.4371 | 4.9 |
| 603 | 09 | MED | CELLULITIS W/O MCC | 0.8429 | 3.5 |
| 604 | 09 | MED | TRAUMA TO THE SKIN, SUBCUT TISS & BREAST W MCC | 1.3527 | 3.9 |
| 605 | 09 | MED | TRAUMA TO THE SKIN, SUBCUT TISS & BREAST W/O MCC | 0.8019 | 2.6 |
| 606 | 09 | MED | MINOR SKIN DISORDERS W MCC | 1.3708 | 4.3 |
| 607 | 09 | MED | MINOR SKIN DISORDERS W/O MCC | 0.7258 | 2.8 |
| 614 | 10 | SURG | ADRENAL & PITUITARY PROCEDURES W CC/MCC | 2.3916 | 3.9 |
| 615 | 10 | SURG | ADRENAL & PITUITARY PROCEDURES W/O CC/MCC | 1.4254 | 2.1 |

*(continues)*

| MS-DRG | MDC | Type | MS-DRG Title | Weights | Geometric Mean LOS |
|---|---|---|---|---|---|
| 616 | 10 | SURG | AMPUTAT OF LOWER LIMB FOR ENDOCRINE, NUTRIT, & METABOL DIS W MCC | 4.0054 | 10.3 |
| 617 | 10 | SURG | AMPUTAT OF LOWER LIMB FOR ENDOCRINE, NUTRIT, & METABOL DIS W CC | 2.0064 | 6.0 |
| 618 | 10 | SURG | AMPUTAT OF LOWER LIMB FOR ENDOCRINE, NUTRIT, & METABOL DIS W/O CC/MCC | 1.1804 | 4.3 |
| 619 | 10 | SURG | O.R. PROCEDURES FOR OBESITY W MCC | 2.9418 | 3.8 |
| 620 | 10 | SURG | O.R. PROCEDURES FOR OBESITY W CC | 1.8407 | 2.5 |
| 621 | 10 | SURG | O.R. PROCEDURES FOR OBESITY W/O CC/MCC | 1.5484 | 1.8 |
| 622 | 10 | SURG | SKIN GRAFTS & WOUND DEBRID FOR ENDOC, NUTRIT & METAB DIS W MCC | 3.5239 | 8.6 |
| 623 | 10 | SURG | SKIN GRAFTS & WOUND DEBRID FOR ENDOC, NUTRIT & METAB DIS W CC | 1.8623 | 5.6 |
| 624 | 10 | SURG | SKIN GRAFTS & WOUND DEBRID FOR ENDOC, NUTRIT & METAB DIS W/O CC/MCC | 1.1292 | 3.7 |
| 625 | 10 | SURG | THYROID, PARATHYROID & THYROGLOSSAL PROCEDURES W MCC | 2.6133 | 4.9 |
| 626 | 10 | SURG | THYROID, PARATHYROID & THYROGLOSSAL PROCEDURES W CC | 1.3936 | 2.2 |
| 627 | 10 | SURG | THYROID, PARATHYROID & THYROGLOSSAL PROCEDURES W/O CC/MCC | 0.9108 | 1.3 |
| 628 | 10 | SURG | OTHER ENDOCRINE, NUTRIT & METAB O.R. PROC W MCC | 3.4413 | 7.0 |
| 629 | 10 | SURG | OTHER ENDOCRINE, NUTRIT & METAB O.R. PROC W CC | 2.1952 | 6.1 |
| 630 | 10 | SURG | OTHER ENDOCRINE, NUTRIT & METAB O.R. PROC W/O CC/MCC | 1.3601 | 3.0 |
| 637 | 10 | MED | DIABETES W MCC | 1.3823 | 4.1 |
| 638 | 10 | MED | DIABETES W CC | 0.8463 | 3.0 |
| 639 | 10 | MED | DIABETES W/O CC/MCC | 0.6007 | 2.2 |
| 640 | 10 | MED | MISC DISORDERS OF NUTRITION, METABOLISM, FLUIDS/ELECTROLYTES W MCC | 1.1318 | 3.3 |

| MS-DRG | MDC | Type | MS-DRG Title | Weights | Geometric Mean LOS |
|--------|-----|------|--------------|---------|--------------------|
| 641 | 10 | MED | MISC DISORDERS OF NUTRITION, METABOLISM, FLUIDS/ELECTROLYTES W/O MCC | 0.7221 | 2.7 |
| 642 | 10 | MED | INBORN AND OTHER DISORDERS OF METABOLISM | 1.2246 | 3.4 |
| 643 | 10 | MED | ENDOCRINE DISORDERS W MCC | 1.6249 | 5.3 |
| 644 | 10 | MED | ENDOCRINE DISORDERS W CC | 1.0123 | 3.7 |
| 645 | 10 | MED | ENDOCRINE DISORDERS W/O CC/MCC | 0.7255 | 2.8 |
| 652 | 11 | SURG | KIDNEY TRANSPLANT | 3.1540 | 5.5 |
| 653 | 11 | SURG | MAJOR BLADDER PROCEDURES W MCC | 6.0456 | 11.9 |
| 654 | 11 | SURG | MAJOR BLADDER PROCEDURES W CC | 3.0267 | 7.2 |
| 655 | 11 | SURG | MAJOR BLADDER PROCEDURES W/O CC/MCC | 2.2796 | 4.8 |
| 656 | 11 | SURG | KIDNEY & URETER PROCEDURES FOR NEOPLASM W MCC | 3.4617 | 6.8 |
| 657 | 11 | SURG | KIDNEY & URETER PROCEDURES FOR NEOPLASM W CC | 2.0091 | 4.2 |
| 658 | 11 | SURG | KIDNEY & URETER PROCEDURES FOR NEOPLASM W/O CC/MCC | 1.5337 | 2.6 |
| 659 | 11 | SURG | KIDNEY & URETER PROCEDURES FOR NON-NEOPLASM W MCC | 3.4848 | 7.5 |
| 660 | 11 | SURG | KIDNEY & URETER PROCEDURES FOR NON-NEOPLASM W CC | 1.9030 | 4.1 |
| 661 | 11 | SURG | KIDNEY & URETER PROCEDURES FOR NON-NEOPLASM W/O CC/MCC | 1.3981 | 2.3 |
| 662 | 11 | SURG | MINOR BLADDER PROCEDURES W MCC | 2.8897 | 7.6 |
| 663 | 11 | SURG | MINOR BLADDER PROCEDURES W CC | 1.6652 | 4.1 |
| 664 | 11 | SURG | MINOR BLADDER PROCEDURES W/O CC/MCC | 1.2987 | 2.0 |
| 665 | 11 | SURG | PROSTATECTOMY W MCC | 3.1132 | 8.9 |
| 666 | 11 | SURG | PROSTATECTOMY W CC | 1.7878 | 4.6 |
| 667 | 11 | SURG | PROSTATECTOMY W/O CC/MCC | 0.9964 | 2.3 |

*(continues)*

| MS-DRG | MDC | Type | MS-DRG Title | Weights | Geometric Mean LOS |
|--------|-----|------|--------------|---------|--------------------|
| 668 | 11 | SURG | TRANSURETHRAL PROCEDURES W MCC | 2.4521 | 6.3 |
| 669 | 11 | SURG | TRANSURETHRAL PROCEDURES W CC | 1.3111 | 3.1 |
| 670 | 11 | SURG | TRANSURETHRAL PROCEDURES W/O CC/MCC | 0.9207 | 2.1 |
| 671 | 11 | SURG | URETHRAL PROCEDURES W CC/MCC | 1.5705 | 4.1 |
| 672 | 11 | SURG | URETHRAL PROCEDURES W/O CC/MCC | 0.8742 | 1.9 |
| 673 | 11 | SURG | OTHER KIDNEY & URINARY TRACT PROCEDURES W MCC | 3.3559 | 7.3 |
| 674 | 11 | SURG | OTHER KIDNEY & URINARY TRACT PROCEDURES W CC | 2.3148 | 5.4 |
| 675 | 11 | SURG | OTHER KIDNEY & URINARY TRACT PROCEDURES W/O CC/MCC | 1.5595 | 2.4 |
| 682 | 11 | MED | RENAL FAILURE W MCC | 1.5085 | 4.6 |
| 683 | 11 | MED | RENAL FAILURE W CC | 0.9406 | 3.5 |
| 684 | 11 | MED | RENAL FAILURE W/O CC/MCC | 0.6272 | 2.5 |
| 685 | 11 | MED | ADMIT FOR RENAL DIALYSIS | 1.0369 | 2.9 |
| 686 | 11 | MED | KIDNEY & URINARY TRACT NEOPLASMS W MCC | 1.6670 | 5.3 |
| 687 | 11 | MED | KIDNEY & URINARY TRACT NEOPLASMS W CC | 1.0161 | 3.5 |
| 688 | 11 | MED | KIDNEY & URINARY TRACT NEOPLASMS W/O CC/MCC | 0.6607 | 2.2 |
| 689 | 11 | MED | KIDNEY & URINARY TRACT INFECTIONS W MCC | 1.0821 | 4.0 |
| 690 | 11 | MED | KIDNEY & URINARY TRACT INFECTIONS W/O MCC | 0.7828 | 3.1 |
| 691 | 11 | MED | URINARY STONES W ESW LITHOTRIPSY W CC/MCC | 1.5470 | 2.8 |
| 692 | 11 | MED | URINARY STONES W ESW LITHOTRIPSY W/O CC/MCC | 1.2566 | 1.9 |
| 693 | 11 | MED | URINARY STONES W/O ESW LITHOTRIPSY W MCC | 1.3323 | 3.8 |
| 694 | 11 | MED | URINARY STONES W/O ESW LITHOTRIPSY W/O MCC | 0.7294 | 2.0 |
| 695 | 11 | MED | KIDNEY & URINARY TRACT SIGNS & SYMPTOMS W MCC | 1.2494 | 4.1 |

| MS-DRG | MDC | Type | MS-DRG Title | Weights | Geometric Mean LOS |
|---|---|---|---|---|---|
| 696 | 11 | MED | KIDNEY & URINARY TRACT SIGNS & SYMPTOMS W/O MCC | 0.6934 | 2.6 |
| 697 | 11 | MED | URETHRAL STRICTURE | 0.9417 | 2.8 |
| 698 | 11 | MED | OTHER KIDNEY & URINARY TRACT DIAGNOSES W MCC | 1.5524 | 5.0 |
| 699 | 11 | MED | OTHER KIDNEY & URINARY TRACT DIAGNOSES W CC | 1.0246 | 3.5 |
| 700 | 11 | MED | OTHER KIDNEY & URINARY TRACT DIAGNOSES W/O CC/MCC | 0.7163 | 2.6 |
| 707 | 12 | SURG | MAJOR MALE PELVIC PROCEDURES W CC/MCC | 1.7753 | 2.8 |
| 708 | 12 | SURG | MAJOR MALE PELVIC PROCEDURES W/O CC/MCC | 1.3146 | 1.4 |
| 709 | 12 | SURG | PENIS PROCEDURES W CC/MCC | 1.9721 | 4.0 |
| 710 | 12 | SURG | PENIS PROCEDURES W/O CC/MCC | 1.4170 | 1.8 |
| 711 | 12 | SURG | TESTES PROCEDURES W CC/MCC | 1.9959 | 5.2 |
| 712 | 12 | SURG | TESTES PROCEDURES W/O CC/MCC | 0.9475 | 2.3 |
| 713 | 12 | SURG | TRANSURETHRAL PROSTATECTOMY W CC/MCC | 1.5077 | 3.4 |
| 714 | 12 | SURG | TRANSURETHRAL PROSTATECTOMY W/O CC/MCC | 0.8072 | 1.7 |
| 715 | 12 | SURG | OTHER MALE REPRODUCTIVE SYSTEM O.R. PROC FOR MALIGNANCY W CC/MCC | 1.8793 | 5.2 |
| 716 | 12 | SURG | OTHER MALE REPRODUCTIVE SYSTEM O.R. PROC FOR MALIGNANCY W/O CC/MCC | 1.1508 | 1.6 |
| 717 | 12 | SURG | OTHER MALE REPRODUCTIVE SYSTEM O.R. PROC EXC MALIGNANCY W CC/MCC | 1.7645 | 4.7 |
| 718 | 12 | SURG | OTHER MALE REPRODUCTIVE SYSTEM O.R. PROC EXC MALIGNANCY W/O CC/MCC | 0.9069 | 2.1 |
| 722 | 12 | MED | MALIGNANCY, MALE REPRODUCTIVE SYSTEM W MCC | 1.7370 | 5.5 |
| 723 | 12 | MED | MALIGNANCY, MALE REPRODUCTIVE SYSTEM W CC | 1.0979 | 3.8 |

*(continues)*

| MS-DRG | MDC | Type | MS-DRG Title | Weights | Geometric Mean LOS |
|--------|-----|------|--------------|---------|--------------------|
| 724 | 12 | MED | MALIGNANCY, MALE REPRODUCTIVE SYSTEM W/O CC/MCC | 0.6545 | 2.0 |
| 725 | 12 | MED | BENIGN PROSTATIC HYPERTROPHY W MCC | 1.3198 | 4.5 |
| 726 | 12 | MED | BENIGN PROSTATIC HYPERTROPHY W/O MCC | 0.7406 | 2.7 |
| 727 | 12 | MED | INFLAMMATION OF THE MALE REPRODUCTIVE SYSTEM W MCC | 1.4461 | 4.9 |
| 728 | 12 | MED | INFLAMMATION OF THE MALE REPRODUCTIVE SYSTEM W/O MCC | 0.7838 | 3.1 |
| 729 | 12 | MED | OTHER MALE REPRODUCTIVE SYSTEM DIAGNOSES W CC/MCC | 1.1169 | 3.5 |
| 730 | 12 | MED | OTHER MALE REPRODUCTIVE SYSTEM DIAGNOSES W/O CC/MCC | 0.6036 | 2.3 |
| 734 | 13 | SURG | PELVIC EVISCERATION, RAD HYSTERECTOMY & RAD VULVECTOMY W CC/MCC | 2.5255 | 4.5 |
| 735 | 13 | SURG | PELVIC EVISCERATION, RAD HYSTERECTOMY & RAD VULVECTOMY W/O CC/MCC | 1.2207 | 1.8 |
| 736 | 13 | SURG | UTERINE & ADNEXA PROC FOR OVARIAN OR ADNEXAL MALIGNANCY W MCC | 4.3286 | 9.9 |
| 737 | 13 | SURG | UTERINE & ADNEXA PROC FOR OVARIAN OR ADNEXAL MALIGNANCY W CC | 2.0037 | 5.1 |
| 738 | 13 | SURG | UTERINE & ADNEXA PROC FOR OVARIAN OR ADNEXAL MALIGNANCY W/O CC/MCC | 1.3498 | 3.0 |
| 739 | 13 | SURG | UTERINE, ADNEXA PROC FOR NON-OVARIAN/ADNEXAL MALIG W MCC | 3.4082 | 6.6 |
| 740 | 13 | SURG | UTERINE, ADNEXA PROC FOR NON-OVARIAN/ADNEXAL MALIG W CC | 1.6920 | 3.3 |
| 741 | 13 | SURG | UTERINE, ADNEXA PROC FOR NON-OVARIAN/ADNEXAL MALIG W/O CC/MCC | 1.1973 | 1.8 |
| 742 | 13 | SURG | UTERINE & ADNEXA PROC FOR NON-MALIGNANCY W CC/MCC | 1.5586 | 3.0 |
| 743 | 13 | SURG | UTERINE & ADNEXA PROC FOR NON-MALIGNANCY W/O CC/MCC | 1.0090 | 1.8 |
| 744 | 13 | SURG | D&C, CONIZATION, LAPAROSCOPY & TUBAL INTERRUPTION W CC/MCC | 1.6851 | 4.1 |

| MS-DRG | MDC | Type | MS-DRG Title | Weights | Geometric Mean LOS |
|--------|-----|------|--------------|---------|--------------------|
| 745 | 13 | SURG | D&C, CONIZATION, LAPAROSCOPY & TUBAL INTERRUPTION W/O CC/MCC | 0.9719 | 2.0 |
| 746 | 13 | SURG | VAGINA, CERVIX & VULVA PROCEDURES W CC/MCC | 1.4628 | 3.3 |
| 747 | 13 | SURG | VAGINA, CERVIX & VULVA PROCEDURES W/O CC/MCC | 0.9099 | 1.6 |
| 748 | 13 | SURG | FEMALE REPRODUCTIVE SYSTEM RECONSTRUCTIVE PROCEDURES | 1.1241 | 1.6 |
| 749 | 13 | SURG | OTHER FEMALE REPRODUCTIVE SYSTEM O.R. PROCEDURES W CC/MCC | 2.6452 | 6.1 |
| 750 | 13 | SURG | OTHER FEMALE REPRODUCTIVE SYSTEM O.R. PROCEDURES W/O CC/MCC | 1.3346 | 2.4 |
| 754 | 13 | MED | MALIGNANCY, FEMALE REPRODUCTIVE SYSTEM W MCC | 1.9204 | 5.8 |
| 755 | 13 | MED | MALIGNANCY, FEMALE REPRODUCTIVE SYSTEM W CC | 1.1325 | 3.7 |
| 756 | 13 | MED | MALIGNANCY, FEMALE REPRODUCTIVE SYSTEM W/O CC/MCC | 0.5908 | 2.2 |
| 757 | 13 | MED | INFECTIONS, FEMALE REPRODUCTIVE SYSTEM W MCC | 1.3717 | 5.2 |
| 758 | 13 | MED | INFECTIONS, FEMALE REPRODUCTIVE SYSTEM W CC | 1.0090 | 4.1 |
| 759 | 13 | MED | INFECTIONS, FEMALE REPRODUCTIVE SYSTEM W/O CC/MCC | 0.7595 | 3.2 |
| 760 | 13 | MED | MENSTRUAL & OTHER FEMALE REPRODUCTIVE SYSTEM DISORDERS W CC/MCC | 0.8524 | 2.8 |
| 761 | 13 | MED | MENSTRUAL & OTHER FEMALE REPRODUCTIVE SYSTEM DISORDERS W/O CC/MCC | 0.5355 | 1.9 |
| 765 | 14 | SURG | CESAREAN SECTION W CC/MCC | 1.1442 | 3.7 |
| 766 | 14 | SURG | CESAREAN SECTION W/O CC/MCC | 0.7807 | 2.8 |
| 767 | 14 | SURG | VAGINAL DELIVERY W STERILIZATION &/OR D&C | 1.2965 | 2.7 |
| 768 | 14 | SURG | VAGINAL DELIVERY W O.R. PROC EXCEPT STERIL &/OR D&C | 1.2618 | 3.6 |

*(continues)*

| MS-DRG | MDC | Type | MS-DRG Title | Weights | Geometric Mean LOS |
|---|---|---|---|---|---|
| 769 | 14 | SURG | POSTPARTUM & POST ABORTION DIAGNOSES W O.R. PROCEDURE | 2.1737 | 4.4 |
| 770 | 14 | SURG | ABORTION W D&C, ASPIRATION CURETTAGE OR HYSTEROTOMY | 0.8272 | 1.9 |
| 774 | 14 | MED | VAGINAL DELIVERY W COMPLICATING DIAGNOSES | 0.7509 | 2.6 |
| 775 | 14 | MED | VAGINAL DELIVERY W/O COMPLICATING DIAGNOSES | 0.5865 | 2.1 |
| 776 | 14 | MED | POSTPARTUM & POST ABORTION DIAGNOSES W/O O.R. PROCEDURE | 0.6766 | 2.4 |
| 777 | 14 | MED | ECTOPIC PREGNANCY | 0.9386 | 1.9 |
| 778 | 14 | MED | THREATENED ABORTION | 0.5332 | 2.0 |
| 779 | 14 | MED | ABORTION W/O D&C | 0.6850 | 1.7 |
| 780 | 14 | MED | FALSE LABOR | 0.2062 | 1.1 |
| 781 | 14 | MED | OTHER ANTEPARTUM DIAGNOSES W MEDICAL COMPLICATIONS | 0.8182 | 2.7 |
| 782 | 14 | MED | OTHER ANTEPARTUM DIAGNOSES W/O MEDICAL COMPLICATIONS | 0.5454 | 1.7 |
| 789 | 15 | MED | NEONATES, DIED OR TRANSFERRED TO ANOTHER ACUTE CARE FACILITY | 1.5860 | 1.8 |
| 790 | 15 | MED | EXTREME IMMATURITY OR RESPIRATORY DISTRESS SYNDROME, NEONATE | 5.2300 | 17.9 |
| 791 | 15 | MED | PREMATURITY W MAJOR PROBLEMS | 3.5719 | 13.3 |
| 792 | 15 | MED | PREMATURITY W/O MAJOR PROBLEMS | 2.1552 | 8.6 |
| 793 | 15 | MED | FULL TERM NEONATE W MAJOR PROBLEMS | 3.6692 | 4.7 |
| 794 | 15 | MED | NEONATE W OTHER SIGNIFICANT PROBLEMS | 1.2987 | 3.4 |
| 795 | 15 | MED | NORMAL NEWBORN | 0.1758 | 3.1 |
| 799 | 16 | SURG | SPLENECTOMY W MCC | 4.7569 | 9.2 |
| 800 | 16 | SURG | SPLENECTOMY W CC | 2.7364 | 5.3 |
| 801 | 16 | SURG | SPLENECTOMY W/O CC/MCC | 1.7458 | 2.8 |

| MS-DRG | MDC | Type | MS-DRG Title | Weights | Geometric Mean LOS |
|--------|-----|------|--------------|---------|--------------------|
| 802 | 16 | SURG | OTHER O.R. PROC OF THE BLOOD & BLOOD FORMING ORGANS W MCC | 3.3880 | 8.1 |
| 803 | 16 | SURG | OTHER O.R. PROC OF THE BLOOD & BLOOD FORMING ORGANS W CC | 1.8719 | 4.7 |
| 804 | 16 | SURG | OTHER O.R. PROC OF THE BLOOD & BLOOD FORMING ORGANS W/O CC/MCC | 1.1715 | 2.3 |
| 808 | 16 | MED | MAJOR HEMATOL/IMMUN DIAG EXC SICKLE CELL CRISIS & COAGUL W MCC | 2.2346 | 6.0 |
| 809 | 16 | MED | MAJOR HEMATOL/IMMUN DIAG EXC SICKLE CELL CRISIS & COAGUL W CC | 1.2235 | 3.8 |
| 810 | 16 | MED | MAJOR HEMATOL/IMMUN DIAG EXC SICKLE CELL CRISIS & COAGUL W/O CC/MCC | 0.8644 | 2.7 |
| 811 | 16 | MED | RED BLOOD CELL DISORDERS W MCC | 1.2992 | 3.7 |
| 812 | 16 | MED | RED BLOOD CELL DISORDERS W/O MCC | 0.8572 | 2.8 |
| 813 | 16 | MED | COAGULATION DISORDERS | 1.7350 | 3.7 |
| 814 | 16 | MED | RETICULOENDOTHELIAL & IMMUNITY DISORDERS W MCC | 1.6622 | 4.7 |
| 815 | 16 | MED | RETICULOENDOTHELIAL & IMMUNITY DISORDERS W CC | 0.9803 | 3.2 |
| 816 | 16 | MED | RETICULOENDOTHELIAL & IMMUNITY DISORDERS W/O CC/MCC | 0.6962 | 2.4 |
| 820 | 17 | SURG | LYMPHOMA & LEUKEMIA W MAJOR O.R. PROCEDURE W MCC | 5.9153 | 12.1 |
| 821 | 17 | SURG | LYMPHOMA & LEUKEMIA W MAJOR O.R. PROCEDURE W CC | 2.3113 | 4.7 |
| 822 | 17 | SURG | LYMPHOMA & LEUKEMIA W MAJOR O.R. PROCEDURE W/O CC/MCC | 1.2851 | 2.1 |
| 823 | 17 | SURG | LYMPHOMA & NON-ACUTE LEUKEMIA W OTHER O.R. PROC W MCC | 4.4536 | 11.1 |
| 824 | 17 | SURG | LYMPHOMA & NON-ACUTE LEUKEMIA W OTHER O.R. PROC W CC | 2.3467 | 6.0 |
| 825 | 17 | SURG | LYMPHOMA & NON-ACUTE LEUKEMIA W OTHER O.R. PROC W/O CC/MCC | 1.3967 | 2.9 |

*(continues)*

| MS-DRG | MDC | Type | MS-DRG Title | Weights | Geometric Mean LOS |
|--------|-----|------|--------------|---------|--------------------|
| 826 | 17 | SURG | MYELOPROLIF DISORD OR POORLY DIFF NEOPL W MAJ O.R. PROC W MCC | 5.1814 | 10.8 |
| 827 | 17 | SURG | MYELOPROLIF DISORD OR POORLY DIFF NEOPL W MAJ O.R. PROC W CC | 2.3141 | 5.0 |
| 828 | 17 | SURG | MYELOPROLIF DISORD OR POORLY DIFF NEOPL W MAJ O.R. PROC W/O CC/MCC | 1.5139 | 2.8 |
| 829 | 17 | SURG | MYELOPROLIF DISORD OR POORLY DIFF NEOPL W OTHER O.R. PROC W CC/MCC | 3.3241 | 6.8 |
| 830 | 17 | SURG | MYELOPROLIF DISORD OR POORLY DIFF NEOPL W OTHER O.R. PROC W/O CC/MCC | 1.3670 | 2.6 |
| 834 | 17 | MED | ACUTE LEUKEMIA W/O MAJOR O.R. PROCEDURE W MCC | 5.5990 | 10.4 |
| 835 | 17 | MED | ACUTE LEUKEMIA W/O MAJOR O.R. PROCEDURE W CC | 2.3024 | 4.9 |
| 836 | 17 | MED | ACUTE LEUKEMIA W/O MAJOR O.R. PROCEDURE W/O CC/MCC | 1.1381 | 2.9 |
| 837 | 17 | MED | CHEMO W ACUTE LEUKEMIA AS SDX OR W HIGH DOSE CHEMO AGENT W MCC | 6.1348 | 15.7 |
| 838 | 17 | MED | CHEMO W ACUTE LEUKEMIA AS SDX W CC OR HIGH DOSE CHEMO AGENT | 2.7707 | 7.0 |
| 839 | 17 | MED | CHEMO W ACUTE LEUKEMIA AS SDX W/O CC/MCC | 1.3190 | 4.9 |
| 840 | 17 | MED | LYMPHOMA & NON-ACUTE LEUKEMIA W MCC | 3.1449 | 7.6 |
| 841 | 17 | MED | LYMPHOMA & NON-ACUTE LEUKEMIA W CC | 1.6118 | 4.7 |
| 842 | 17 | MED | LYMPHOMA & NON-ACUTE LEUKEMIA W/O CC/MCC | 1.1167 | 3.1 |
| 843 | 17 | MED | OTHER MYELOPROLIF DIS OR POORLY DIFF NEOPL DIAG W MCC | 1.8464 | 5.6 |
| 844 | 17 | MED | OTHER MYELOPROLIF DIS OR POORLY DIFF NEOPL DIAG W CC | 1.1233 | 4.0 |
| 845 | 17 | MED | OTHER MYELOPROLIF DIS OR POORLY DIFF NEOPL DIAG W/O CC/MCC | 0.8261 | 2.8 |
| 846 | 17 | MED | CHEMOTHERAPY W/O ACUTE LEUKEMIA AS SECONDARY DIAGNOSIS W MCC | 2.4618 | 5.9 |

| MS-DRG | MDC | Type | MS-DRG Title | Weights | Geometric Mean LOS |
|--------|-----|------|--------------|---------|--------------------|
| 847 | 17 | MED | CHEMOTHERAPY W/O ACUTE LEUKEMIA AS SECONDARY DIAGNOSIS W CC | 1.1883 | 3.4 |
| 848 | 17 | MED | CHEMOTHERAPY W/O ACUTE LEUKEMIA AS SECONDARY DIAGNOSIS W/O CC/MCC | 0.9352 | 2.8 |
| 849 | 17 | MED | RADIOTHERAPY | 1.6745 | 4.9 |
| 853 | 18 | SURG | INFECTIOUS & PARASITIC DISEASES W O.R. PROCEDURE W MCC | 5.1334 | 10.7 |
| 854 | 18 | SURG | INFECTIOUS & PARASITIC DISEASES W O.R. PROCEDURE W CC | 2.3804 | 6.6 |
| 855 | 18 | SURG | INFECTIOUS & PARASITIC DISEASES W O.R. PROCEDURE W/O CC/MCC | 1.5124 | 3.5 |
| 856 | 18 | SURG | POSTOPERATIVE OR POST-TRAUMATIC INFECTIONS W O.R. PROC W MCC | 4.6569 | 9.8 |
| 857 | 18 | SURG | POSTOPERATIVE OR POST-TRAUMATIC INFECTIONS W O.R. PROC W CC | 2.0516 | 5.6 |
| 858 | 18 | SURG | POSTOPERATIVE OR POST-TRAUMATIC INFECTIONS W O.R. PROC W/O CC/MCC | 1.3300 | 3.8 |
| 862 | 18 | MED | POSTOPERATIVE & POST-TRAUMATIC INFECTIONS W MCC | 1.8550 | 5.5 |
| 863 | 18 | MED | POSTOPERATIVE & POST-TRAUMATIC INFECTIONS W/O MCC | 1.0089 | 3.7 |
| 864 | 18 | MED | FEVER | 0.8481 | 2.8 |
| 865 | 18 | MED | VIRAL ILLNESS W MCC | 1.5273 | 4.2 |
| 866 | 18 | MED | VIRAL ILLNESS W/O MCC | 0.7739 | 2.8 |
| 867 | 18 | MED | OTHER INFECTIOUS & PARASITIC DISEASES DIAGNOSES W MCC | 2.6068 | 6.7 |
| 868 | 18 | MED | OTHER INFECTIOUS & PARASITIC DISEASES DIAGNOSES W CC | 1.0292 | 3.8 |
| 869 | 18 | MED | OTHER INFECTIOUS & PARASITIC DISEASES DIAGNOSES W/O CC/MCC | 0.7091 | 2.8 |
| 870 | 18 | MED | SEPTICEMIA OR SEVERE SEPSIS W MV >96 HOURS | 5.8782 | 12.6 |

*(continues)*

| MS-DRG | MDC | Type | MS-DRG Title | Weights | Geometric Mean LOS |
|--------|-----|------|--------------|---------|--------------------|
| 871 | 18 | MED | SEPTICEMIA OR SEVERE SEPSIS W/O MV >96 HOURS W MCC | 1.7926 | 5.0 |
| 872 | 18 | MED | SEPTICEMIA OR SEVERE SEPSIS W/O MV >96 HOURS W/O MCC | 1.0427 | 3.9 |
| 876 | 19 | SURG | O.R. PROCEDURE W PRINCIPAL DIAGNOSES OF MENTAL ILLNESS | 3.0841 | 7.8 |
| 880 | 19 | MED | ACUTE ADJUSTMENT REACTION & PSYCHOSOCIAL DYSFUNCTION | 0.7227 | 2.4 |
| 881 | 19 | MED | DEPRESSIVE NEUROSES | 0.6618 | 3.4 |
| 882 | 19 | MED | NEUROSES EXCEPT DEPRESSIVE | 0.6924 | 3.3 |
| 883 | 19 | MED | DISORDERS OF PERSONALITY & IMPULSE CONTROL | 1.3737 | 4.6 |
| 884 | 19 | MED | ORGANIC DISTURBANCES & MENTAL RETARDATION | 1.1483 | 4.3 |
| 885 | 19 | MED | PSYCHOSES | 1.0575 | 5.6 |
| 886 | 19 | MED | BEHAVIORAL & DEVELOPMENTAL DISORDERS | 0.8718 | 3.9 |
| 887 | 19 | MED | OTHER MENTAL DISORDER DIAGNOSES | 0.9939 | 3.0 |
| 894 | 20 | MED | ALCOHOL/DRUG ABUSE OR DEPENDENCE, LEFT AMA | 0.4859 | 2.1 |
| 895 | 20 | MED | ALCOHOL/DRUG ABUSE OR DEPENDENCE W REHABILITATION THERAPY | 1.2435 | 9.3 |
| 896 | 20 | MED | ALCOHOL/DRUG ABUSE OR DEPENDENCE W/O REHABILITATION THERAPY W MCC | 1.5678 | 4.8 |
| 897 | 20 | MED | ALCOHOL/DRUG ABUSE OR DEPENDENCE W/O REHABILITATION THERAPY W/O MCC | 0.7231 | 3.3 |
| 901 | 21 | SURG | WOUND DEBRIDEMENTS FOR INJURIES W MCC | 3.9370 | 9.2 |
| 902 | 21 | SURG | WOUND DEBRIDEMENTS FOR INJURIES W CC | 1.8265 | 5.3 |
| 903 | 21 | SURG | WOUND DEBRIDEMENTS FOR INJURIES W/O CC/MCC | 1.1723 | 3.3 |
| 904 | 21 | SURG | SKIN GRAFTS FOR INJURIES W CC/MCC | 3.2140 | 7.1 |
| 905 | 21 | SURG | SKIN GRAFTS FOR INJURIES W/O CC/MCC | 1.4233 | 3.6 |

| MS-DRG | MDC | Type | MS-DRG Title | Weights | Geometric Mean LOS |
|--------|-----|------|--------------|---------|--------------------|
| 906 | 21 | SURG | HAND PROCEDURES FOR INJURIES | 1.5670 | 2.8 |
| 907 | 21 | SURG | OTHER O.R. PROCEDURES FOR INJURIES W MCC | 3.8073 | 7.5 |
| 908 | 21 | SURG | OTHER O.R. PROCEDURES FOR INJURIES W CC | 1.9904 | 4.3 |
| 909 | 21 | SURG | OTHER O.R. PROCEDURES FOR INJURIES W/O CC/MCC | 1.2992 | 2.6 |
| 913 | 21 | MED | TRAUMATIC INJURY W MCC | 1.3561 | 3.8 |
| 914 | 21 | MED | TRAUMATIC INJURY W/O MCC | 0.7317 | 2.5 |
| 915 | 21 | MED | ALLERGIC REACTIONS W MCC | 1.6040 | 3.7 |
| 916 | 21 | MED | ALLERGIC REACTIONS W/O MCC | 0.5582 | 1.8 |
| 917 | 21 | MED | POISONING & TOXIC EFFECTS OF DRUGS W MCC | 1.4065 | 3.5 |
| 918 | 21 | MED | POISONING & TOXIC EFFECTS OF DRUGS W/O MCC | 0.6859 | 2.2 |
| 919 | 21 | MED | COMPLICATIONS OF TREATMENT W MCC | 1.7611 | 4.5 |
| 920 | 21 | MED | COMPLICATIONS OF TREATMENT W CC | 0.9991 | 3.1 |
| 921 | 21 | MED | COMPLICATIONS OF TREATMENT W/O CC/MCC | 0.6960 | 2.3 |
| 922 | 21 | MED | OTHER INJURY, POISONING & TOXIC EFFECT DIAG W MCC | 1.5833 | 4.0 |
| 923 | 21 | MED | OTHER INJURY, POISONING & TOXIC EFFECT DIAG W/O MCC | 0.8117 | 2.5 |
| 927 | 22 | SURG | EXTENSIVE BURNS OR FULL THICKNESS BURNS W MV >96 HRS W SKIN GRAFT | 15.9672 | 23.5 |
| 928 | 22 | SURG | FULL THICKNESS BURN W SKIN GRAFT OR INHAL INJ W CC/MCC | 5.7399 | 11.3 |
| 929 | 22 | SURG | FULL THICKNESS BURN W SKIN GRAFT OR INHAL INJ W/O CC/MCC | 2.4661 | 5.5 |
| 933 | 22 | MED | EXTENSIVE BURNS OR FULL THICKNESS BURNS W MV >96 HRS W/O SKIN GRAFT | 2.8685 | 2.6 |
| 934 | 22 | MED | FULL THICKNESS BURN W/O SKIN GRFT OR INHAL INJ | 1.6716 | 4.2 |

*(continues)*

| MS-DRG | MDC | Type | MS-DRG Title | Weights | Geometric Mean LOS |
|--------|-----|------|--------------|---------|--------------------|
| 935 | 22 | MED | NON-EXTENSIVE BURNS | 1.5141 | 3.4 |
| 939 | 23 | SURG | O.R. PROC W DIAGNOSES OF OTHER CONTACT W HEALTH SERVICES W MCC | 2.9866 | 6.2 |
| 940 | 23 | SURG | O.R. PROC W DIAGNOSES OF OTHER CONTACT W HEALTH SERVICES W CC | 1.9107 | 3.7 |
| 941 | 23 | SURG | O.R. PROC W DIAGNOSES OF OTHER CONTACT W HEALTH SERVICES W/O CC/MCC | 1.3589 | 2.1 |
| 945 | 23 | MED | REHABILITATION W CC/MCC | 1.2781 | 8.8 |
| 946 | 23 | MED | REHABILITATION W/O CC/MCC | 1.0151 | 6.8 |
| 947 | 23 | MED | SIGNS & SYMPTOMS W MCC | 1.1323 | 3.5 |
| 948 | 23 | MED | SIGNS & SYMPTOMS W/O MCC | 0.7356 | 2.7 |
| 949 | 23 | MED | AFTERCARE W CC/MCC | 1.1197 | 3.3 |
| 950 | 23 | MED | AFTERCARE W/O CC/MCC | 0.5798 | 2.3 |
| 951 | 23 | MED | OTHER FACTORS INFLUENCING HEALTH STATUS | 0.9885 | 2.7 |
| 955 | 24 | SURG | CRANIOTOMY FOR MULTIPLE SIGNIFICANT TRAUMA | 5.6773 | 8.4 |
| 956 | 24 | SURG | LIMB REATTACHMENT, HIP & FEMUR PROC FOR MULTIPLE SIGNIFICANT TRAUMA | 3.7116 | 6.4 |
| 957 | 24 | SURG | OTHER O.R. PROCEDURES FOR MULTIPLE SIGNIFICANT TRAUMA W MCC | 6.5504 | 9.4 |
| 958 | 24 | SURG | OTHER O.R. PROCEDURES FOR MULTIPLE SIGNIFICANT TRAUMA W CC | 3.8565 | 6.9 |
| 959 | 24 | SURG | OTHER O.R. PROCEDURES FOR MULTIPLE SIGNIFICANT TRAUMA W/O CC/MCC | 2.1705 | 4.2 |
| 963 | 24 | MED | OTHER MULTIPLE SIGNIFICANT TRAUMA W MCC | 2.6295 | 5.4 |
| 964 | 24 | MED | OTHER MULTIPLE SIGNIFICANT TRAUMA W CC | 1.4205 | 4.1 |
| 965 | 24 | MED | OTHER MULTIPLE SIGNIFICANT TRAUMA W/O CC/MCC | 0.9217 | 3.0 |
| 969 | 25 | SURG | HIV W EXTENSIVE O.R. PROCEDURE W MCC | 5.0291 | 11.2 |
| 970 | 25 | SURG | HIV W EXTENSIVE O.R. PROCEDURE W/O MCC | 2.7871 | 5.1 |

| MS-DRG | MDC | Type | MS-DRG Title | Weights | Geometric Mean LOS |
|--------|-----|------|--------------|---------|--------------------|
| 974 | 25 | MED | HIV W MAJOR RELATED CONDITION W MCC | 2.6531 | 6.6 |
| 975 | 25 | MED | HIV W MAJOR RELATED CONDITION W CC | 1.3589 | 4.5 |
| 976 | 25 | MED | HIV W MAJOR RELATED CONDITION W/O CC/MCC | 0.9073 | 3.3 |
| 977 | 25 | MED | HIV W OR W/O OTHER RELATED CONDITION | 1.1577 | 3.5 |
| 981 | PRE | SURG | EXTENSIVE O.R. PROCEDURE UNRELATED TO PRINCIPAL DIAGNOSIS W MCC | 4.8532 | 9.5 |
| 982 | PRE | SURG | EXTENSIVE O.R. PROCEDURE UNRELATED TO PRINCIPAL DIAGNOSIS W CC | 2.7416 | 5.4 |
| 983 | PRE | SURG | EXTENSIVE O.R. PROCEDURE UNRELATED TO PRINCIPAL DIAGNOSIS W/O CC/MCC | 1.7615 | 2.8 |
| 984 | PRE | SURG | PROSTATIC O.R. PROCEDURE UNRELATED TO PRINCIPAL DIAGNOSIS W MCC | 3.3844 | 9.3 |
| 985 | PRE | SURG | PROSTATIC O.R. PROCEDURE UNRELATED TO PRINCIPAL DIAGNOSIS W CC | 1.9339 | 4.8 |
| 986 | PRE | SURG | PROSTATIC O.R. PROCEDURE UNRELATED TO PRINCIPAL DIAGNOSIS W/O CC/MCC | 1.2079 | 2.4 |
| 987 | PRE | SURG | NON-EXTENSIVE O.R. PROC UNRELATED TO PRINCIPAL DIAGNOSIS W MCC | 3.2123 | 8.0 |
| 988 | PRE | SURG | NON-EXTENSIVE O.R. PROC UNRELATED TO PRINCIPAL DIAGNOSIS W CC | 1.7533 | 4.6 |
| 989 | PRE | SURG | NON-EXTENSIVE O.R. PROC UNRELATED TO PRINCIPAL DIAGNOSIS W/O CC/MCC | 1.0425 | 2.2 |
| 998 | | ** | PRINCIPAL DIAGNOSIS INVALID AS DISCHARGE DIAGNOSIS | | |
| 999 | | ** | UNGROUPABLE | | |

MS-DRGs 998 and 999 contain cases that could not be assigned to valid DRGs.

Note: If there is no value in either the geometric mean length of stay or the arithmetic mean length of stay columns, the volume of cases is insufficient to determine a meaningful computation of these statistics.

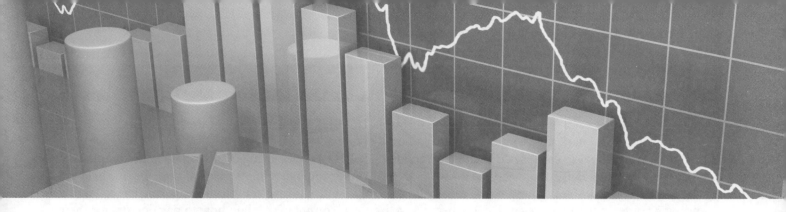

# CHAPTER 4

# Legal and Regulatory Environment

**Peter A. Pavarini**, Esq.

## LEARNING OBJECTIVES

After studying this chapter, you should be able to do the following:

1. Understand how legal and regulatory issues shape and define good financial management of an HCO.
2. Appreciate the consequences of failing to manage the finances of an HCO with regard for the complex and ever-changing array of laws and regulations that are unique to this industry.
3. Identify the major components of a corporate compliance plan, including the establishment of internal controls relating to the finances of an organization.
4. Recognize when and how to involve legal counsel on a Medicare or Medicaid reimbursement issue or other financial matter that has regulatory compliance implications or would otherwise require you to seek legal advice before making a decision.
5. Be aware of the most important aspects of the Patient Protection and Affordable Care Act of 2010 (Affordable Care Act, or ACA)[1] as it relates to financial management in the post-reform environment. Describe how the ACA's three pillars—insurance reforms, care delivery system reforms, and financial savings reforms—are changing the American healthcare system.
6. Identify the most common federal regulatory issues, such as fraud and abuse, Stark Law, HIPAA, EMTALA, and IRS requirements for tax-exempt organizations, as well as less common concerns that arise under the antitrust laws and federal and state laws regulating third-party payers.
7. Be prepared to respond to a compliance audit or investigation, particularly when the subject of that inquiry includes financial records.

---

[1]Patient Protection and Affordable Care Act, Pub. Law No. 111-148 (2010).

Opener image: © A1Stock/Shutterstock

## REAL-WORLD SCENARIO

Claudio Bravo, the CFO of Sinking Springs Regional Hospital (SSRH), has been asked by the hospital's CEO, Doris Devine, to help her prepare a presentation to SSRH's board of directors seeking approval for a major restructuring of the hospital's cardiovascular service line. For several years SSRH has been losing market share to its competitors because of perceived quality issues and the growing disloyalty of cardiologists on its medical staff. Devine believes that SSRH needs to do "something bold" to reverse this trend and improve the hospital's performance. While attending a conference in Las Vegas, Devine heard a well-known consultant explain how to pay doctors for their exclusive use of a hospital as long as it is done in the context of a quality improvement program.

To his credit, Bravo is skeptical of any arrangement that pays doctors for their referrals, but he was told by Devine that this "concept" had already been approved by the U.S. Department of Health and Human Services Office of Inspector General so he does not need to run it by SSRH's legal counsel. Devine has given Bravo an outline of a service line management program that would do the following: (1) Cardiology Care, Inc. (CCI), a group of nine cardiologists, would be paid a base fee of $1.5 million annually to improve the quality of cardiovascular care at SSRH, plus various incentive payments for increased volumes in the operating room and catheterization lab, increased revenues from diagnostic tests, and improved public opinion of the SSRH; (2) CVS Associates, P.C. (CVS), the primary cardiovascular surgery group in the region, would be paid $500,000 for each additional surgeon it recruits to handle the expected increase in inpatient volumes; (3) all of SSRH's employed primary care physicians would be required, as a condition of their employment, to refer their patients to CCI as the service line manager; and (4) up to $4.5 million in funds from a refinancing of SSRH's tax-exempt debt would be used to purchase new technology for the heart program.

Bravo decides to do some due diligence on CCI and CVS before beginning work on the board presentation. He learns from Sidney Slade, the business manager of CCI, that her company has been under a corporate integrity agreement with the Office of Inspector General for 3 years due to Medicare billing problems at another hospital. Slade also tells Bravo she believes a closer relationship with SSRH would be a "good idea" because the cardiologists' incomes have declined dramatically since she was hired. Slade is worried that her job is at risk and that CCI doesn't have the staff to manage its practice, let alone a department of the hospital.

Bravo also contacts Dr. Emil Sikorsky, the lead surgeon at CVS, to see what he knows about Devine's proposal. Sikorsky tells Bravo there's very little SSRH can do to increase its market share because heart surgery volumes are down everywhere. Sikorsky himself would like to be retrained in vascular procedures because he believes "that's the next gold mine." He asks Bravo whether the hospital would be willing to pay for him to enroll in a 6-month fellowship in advanced vascular procedures as long as he promises to come back to SSRH. Bravo says that he will inquire of Devine. Before their conversation ends, Sikorsky asks whether Bravo had heard that the hospital's cardiovascular program is going to be audited next week. Supposedly, SSRH has been found to have (1) a readmission rate on Medicare heart failure patients that is "off the chart" and (2) poor documentation to support why patients are being readmitted with such frequency.

Armed with this new information, Bravo begins developing financial projections for how SSRH would pay for these additional expenditures in its cardiovascular program. The only scenario that would justify this investment in SSRH's heart program is one that achieves market dominance within 3 to 5 years (over 80% of heart patients in SSRH's primary and secondary service areas). Although Bravo believes that is highly unlikely, he prepares a spreadsheet and a PowerPoint presentation that shows how Devine's proposal will work. He also assumes that with the increased bargaining power of having physicians on board he will be able to negotiate substantially higher rates from managed care payers.

Also included in Bravo's proposal is a description of two potential new health information technology (HIT) initiatives he received from SSRH's Chief Information Officer Tiffany Technophile. The first proposal is a telemedicine initiative that would enable select SSRH-affiliated providers to conduct remote appointments with their patients via telemedicine. The provider–patient interaction would be housed on the platform of a third-party telemedicine company.

Technophile's second proposal is for the creation of a software application that would allow patients to upload certain physical fitness data that is collected through "wearable" devices (e.g., smartwatches, step monitors, and other activity trackers). Using this data (which would be accessible via the hospital's internal network), SSRH-affiliated providers could develop individualized wellness plans tailored to each patient's needs and desires. In addition, SSRH plans on selling this data to reputable buyers (e.g., insurance companies and pharmaceutical researchers), enabling SSRH to fund several badly needed construction projects.

Because Bravo is about to leave for a 2-week vacation, he does not have enough time to have the presentation reviewed by legal counsel before it goes out with the board packet. One of the board members, an attorney in a downtown law firm, receives the presentation and immediately calls his health law partner to ask whether anything in the document could expose the hospital's senior management or directors to civil or criminal penalties.

# ▶ Part I. Knowledge of the Law and Regulations Is an Essential Part of Healthcare Financial Management

## Learning Objective 1

Understand how legal and regulatory issues shape and define good financial management of a healthcare organization.

## Developing an Awareness of the Rapidly Changing Legal and Regulatory Environment Is Critical to the Successful Financial Management of a Healthcare Organization

The enactment of the ACA in March 2010 represented a landmark change in the federal law that shapes virtually every financial aspect of the nation's healthcare delivery system. The ACA's most significant provisions were designed to address long-standing problems with the availability and affordability of health insurance. Most importantly, as discussed later, the ACA imposes important new requirements on insurance plans, particularly individual and small group markets, as well as imposes a tax on certain individuals who fail to purchase some form of health insurance.

The ACA also sets the stage for systemic changes in how health care is delivered by moving away from a fee-for-service payment to a model that rewards healthcare providers who can achieve superior outcomes for their patients. Since the enactment of the ACA, the federal government has signaled its intention to make value-based payment its dominant form of reimbursement. In response to this emphasis on quality, cost-effective care, providers have begun to accept the concept of delivering care via accountable care organizations (ACOs)—networks of providers

sharing financial and medical responsibility for select populations of patients. ACO participants are eligible to share in savings realized as a result of delivering cost-effective care. As of early 2016, ACOs covered more than 23 million lives in the United States, a number that is expected to grow to 105 million by 2020.

While the effectiveness of certain ACA reforms remains uncertain, the number of Americans with health insurance has continued to climb, especially in states that expanded Medicaid coverage using ACA incentives. Nationally, the percentage of uninsured persons is the lowest it has been in years. This has been especially true among young adults (ages 19–25) whose uninsured rate fell 52% between the ACA's first open enrollment and the end of the third quarter of 2015. The participation of young adults who generally impose a lesser claims burden on the insurance system is critical to the ACA's overall success.

Despite continued political debate over the ACA, many of its payment reforms have rapidly become permanent fixtures of the American health system. Consequently, those entrusted with the financial management of healthcare organizations (HCOs) must continue to remain attentive to ongoing efforts to implement and refine the provisions of this law.

## Learning Objective 2

Appreciate the consequences of managing the finances of a healthcare organization without regard for the complex and ever-changing array of laws and regulations that are unique to this industry.

## Understanding Regulatory Compliance in a Healthcare Organization
### Corporate Compliance Plans

The U.S. Department of Health and Human Services (DHHS) Office of Inspector General (OIG) was established as an independent and objective oversight unit of the DHHS to carry out the mission of promoting economy, efficiency, and effectiveness through the elimination of waste, abuse, and fraud. The OIG strongly recommends adopting a corporate compliance plan because it helps reduce the risk of compliance errors and can limit the liability of directors and management. An effective plan can also reduce liability under the Federal Sentencing Guidelines.

A well-written corporate compliance plan helps an organization's employees understand how laws and regulations relate to their jobs and enables management to know that these legal requirements are being followed.

The OIG has said that an effective corporate compliance plan should contain the following elements:

- Adoption of reasonable compliance standards of conduct and procedures. The provider must organize its compliance materials, learn what laws and regulations govern its practices, and put in writing the steps necessary for a high-level compliance officer to be certain that it obeys the law.
- Appointment of a high-level compliance officer. For the plan to be effective, this officer must be someone who can insist on compliance from anyone in the organization, so the compliance officer should be someone at the highest level of management.
- Employee education and systematic compliance training.
- Development of effective lines of communication. There must be easy access to the compliance officer so that problems can be reported and corrected. There must also be a guarantee that employees can report compliance issues without fear of retaliation. In larger organizations experts suggest a 24-hour hotline so employees can report problems anonymously.
- Consistent and continuous enforcement of compliance standards through well-publicized disciplinary standards. OIG suggests that every plan contain disciplinary standards so there are consequences for serious deviations from the organization's standards of conduct. Disciplinary standards should apply not just for the employee who erred, but also for the supervisor who failed to detect the problem. OIG also suggests that employers use background checks for new employees to ensure they have not been involved in healthcare fraud. OIG maintains a national databank that lists people who have been sanctioned for healthcare fraud.
- Development of auditing and monitoring programs. A monitoring program should include regular reports to the compliance officer and to senior management. For larger organizations this program will probably include compliance audits by internal or outside auditors who are experts in federal billing regulations.

- Development of a mechanism for reporting detected violations to the appropriate agency and for correcting the problem prospectively.
- Information about the guidelines for compliance can be found at the OIG website (http://oig.hhs.gov/fraud/complianceguidance.asp).

In addition, an organization should routinely assess the areas of compliance risk it can reasonably be expected to encounter. For example, almost every healthcare provider should consider the applicability of laws and regulations pertaining to tax, antitrust, environmental, employment, intellectual property, confidentiality, licensing, and controlled substances.

The greatest risk for most organizations is erroneous or fraudulent billing. In these cases the first phase of plan development should be to get a snapshot of the organization's billing practices. The risk analysis should usually be made under the supervision of the organization's lawyers.

An HCO is particularly vulnerable to fraudulent activities that are taken on its behalf by employees or agents. Many of these are commonplace but can result in considerable economic and reputational harm to the institution. For example, billing for services provided by inadequately supervised medical residents could result in liability under the False Claims Act. Without a properly enforced compliance plan, relatively minor infractions left unchecked can result in multimillion-dollar penalties to the organization.

Developing a plan can take anywhere from several months for a small medical practice to a year or longer for a large hospital. However, the protection afforded by such a plan makes the investment of time and resources well worth the effort.

---

*Learning Objective 3*

---

Identify the major components of a corporate compliance plan, including the establishment of internal controls relating to the finances of an organization.

---

## Internal Control as a Part of Corporate Compliance

As described by the American Institute of Certified Public Accountants (AICPA), "internal control is a process effected by an entity's board of directors, management, and other personnel designed to provide reasonable assurance regarding the achievement of objectives in the following categories: reliability of financial reporting, effectiveness and efficiency of operations, and compliance with applicable laws and regulations."[2] This definition emphasizes the fact that internal control is a function of the board, management, and other personnel within the organization. The responsibility for internal control rests squarely on the shoulders of management.

The AICPA identifies the five interrelated components of internal control as follows:

- *Control environment* sets the tone of an organization, influencing the control consciousness of its people. It is the foundation for all other components of internal control, providing discipline and structure.
- *Risk assessment* is the entity's identification and analysis of relevant risks to achievement of its objectives, forming a basis for determining how the risks should be managed.
- *Control activities* are the policies and procedures that help ensure management directives are carried out.
- *Information and communication* are the identification, capture, and exchange of information in a form and time frame that enable people to carry out their responsibilities.
- *Monitoring* is a process that assesses the quality of internal control performance over time.

Internal control is not the equivalent of corporate compliance, but it should be a key component of a corporate compliance plan. The two programs should function together to ensure that an organization is soundly managed from both a financial and legal perspective.

# ▶ Part II. Primary Regulatory Issues Confronting Healthcare Organizations Today

---

## *Learning Objective 4*

Recognize when and how to involve legal counsel on a Medicare or Medicaid reimbursement issue or other financial matter that has regulatory compliance implications or would otherwise require you to seek legal advice before making a decision.

---

[2]Thomas A. Ratcliffe & Charles E. Landes, *Understanding Internal Control and Internal Control Services 2* (New York: American Institute of Certified Public Accountants, Inc., 2009).

## Medicare Reimbursement

In 1965 Medicare was established as a social insurance program, like Social Security, to provide health insurance coverage for individuals aged 65 and older and for younger people with permanent disabilities. Before 1965 about half of all seniors lacked medical insurance; today, almost all seniors have health insurance coverage under Medicare. Medicare covers approximately 55 million people: 46.3 million people aged 65 and older and another 9 million people with permanent disabilities who are under age 65. Medicare helps pay for many healthcare services, including hospitalizations, physician services, and prescription drugs. Individuals contribute to Medicare through payroll taxes throughout their working lives and generally become eligible for Medicare when they reach age 65, regardless of their income or health status.

Encompassing approximately 15% of the federal budget in 2015 and 23% of national personal health spending in 2014, Medicare is a significant part of both federal spending and healthcare spending in the United States. Medicare is administered by the DHHS Centers for Medicare and Medicaid Services (CMS).

Medicare offers a number of programs for its beneficiaries, including health facility coverage, reimbursement of doctor's fees, and prescription coverage. Additionally, Medicare offers a managed care plan, Medicare Advantage, that bundles a number of these offerings.

- *Part A. Hospital Insurance*: Most people do not pay a premium for Part A because they or a spouse already paid for it through their payroll taxes while working. Medicare Part A helps cover inpatient care in hospitals, including critical access hospitals and skilled nursing facilities, but not custodial or long-term care. It also helps cover hospice care and some home health care. Beneficiaries must meet certain conditions to get these benefits.
- *Part B. Medical Insurance*: Most people pay a monthly premium for Part B. Medicare Part B helps cover doctors' services and outpatient care. It also covers some other medical services that Part A does not cover, such as some of the services of physical and occupational therapists and some home health care. Part B helps pay for these covered services and supplies when they are medically necessary.
- *Medicare Supplemental Insurance ("Medigap" Policies)*: Medicare Parts A and B are commonly referred to as the "original Medicare plan." A Medigap policy is health insurance sold by private insurance companies to fill the "gaps" in original Medicare plan coverage. Medigap policies help

pay some of the healthcare costs that the original Medicare plan does not cover. Insurance companies are permitted to sell only "standardized" Medigap policies. Generally, an eligible beneficiary with a Medigap policy will have Medicare Part A and Part B. The beneficiary will have to pay the monthly Medicare Part B premium and a premium to the Medigap insurance provider.

- *Part C. Medicare Advantage*: Medicare Advantage Plans are managed care health plan options that are part of the Medicare program. Eligible beneficiaries who join one of these plans generally get all their Medicare-covered health care through that plan. Coverage can include prescription drug coverage. Medicare Advantage Plans include one of the following:
  - Medicare health maintenance organization
  - Preferred provider organizations
  - Private fee-for-service plans
  - Medicare special needs plans
- Eligible beneficiaries who join a Medicare Advantage Plan use the health insurance card they receive from the plan for their health care. In most of these plans, generally there are extra benefits and lower copayments than in the original Medicare plan. However, beneficiaries may have to see doctors or go to hospitals that participate in the plan.
- To join a Medicare Advantage Plan, a beneficiary must have Medicare Part A and Part B and pay a monthly Medicare Part B premium to Medicare. Additionally, a beneficiary may also pay a monthly premium to a Medicare Advantage Plan for the extra benefits offered through the plan. A beneficiary who joins a Medicare Advantage Plan will not have any deductibles, copayments, or other cost sharing under their Medicare Health Plan. Accordingly, a beneficiary would not need a Medigap policy.
- *Part D. Prescription Drug Coverage*: Beginning on January 1, 2006, the Medicare prescription drug coverage was available to everyone with Medicare. Part D coverage may help lower prescription drug costs and help protect against higher costs in the future. Medicare Prescription Drug Coverage is insurance offered through private companies. Beneficiaries choose a drug plan and pay a monthly premium.

## Certification of Provider of Item or Service

Institutional providers, physicians, nonphysician practitioners, and other healthcare suppliers must enroll in the Medicare program to be eligible to receive Medicare payment for covered services provided to Medicare beneficiaries. The Medicare enrollment application is used to collect information about the institutions and other providers and suppliers and to secure the necessary documentation to ensure the organization is qualified and eligible to enroll in the Medicare program.

The usual process for becoming a certified Part A institutional **Medicare provider** is as follows:

1. The applicant completes and submits the Medicare enrollment application to its designated Medicare fee-for-service contractor.
2. The fee-for-service contractor reviews the application and makes a recommendation for approval or denial to the applicable CMS Regional Office.
3. Once the fee-for-service contractor makes a recommendation to approve enrollment, the state agency or, if applicable, a CMS-recognized accrediting organization conducts a survey. Based on the survey results the state agency makes a recommendation for approval or denial (a certification of compliance or noncompliance) to the CMS Regional Office.
4. The CMS Regional Office makes the final decision regarding program eligibility. The CMS Regional Office also works with the Office of Civil Rights to obtain the necessary Civil Rights clearances. If approved, the provider must typically sign a provider agreement.

In Part B, "participation" means a Part B noninstitutional provider agrees to always accept assignment of claims for all services furnished to Medicare beneficiaries. By agreeing to always accept assignment, the provider accepts Medicare-allowed amounts as payment in full and does not collect more than the Medicare deductible and coinsurance from the beneficiary. Unlike many private insurance plans, the Social Security Act requires providers to submit claims for Medicare beneficiaries whether they participate or not.

The participating provider application should be submitted simultaneously with the Medicare enrollment form. Providers that choose to participate receive 5% higher reimbursement than those who do not participate. Medicare payments are issued directly to the physician/supplier because the claims are always assigned, and claim information is forwarded to Medigap insurers.

## Payment for the Item or Service

For Part A inpatient institutional care, such as hospital and nursing home care, Medicare uses the "inpatient prospective payment system." A prospective payment system is one in which the healthcare institution receives a certain payment for each episode of care provided to a patient, regardless of the actual amount of care used. The amount of the payment is based on the value of a certain diagnosis as determined by CMS in the form of **diagnosis-related groups (DRGs)**. DRGs make up a classification system that groups similar clinical conditions (diagnoses) and the procedures furnished by the hospital during the stay. Related therapeutic outpatient department services provided within 3 days before admission are included in the payment for the inpatient stay and may not be separately billed. Since October 1, 2007, a new DRG system, called Medicare Severity-DRG, has been used to better account for severity of illness and resource consumption for Medicare beneficiaries.

In addition to the base-rate per DRG payments, hospitals can receive additional outlier payments for extremely costly procedures, for the cost of graduate medical education if the hospital has an approved program, and for treating a disproportionate share of low-income patients, as well as for the use of certain new technology. Payments may be reduced if a patient has a short length of stay and is transferred to another hospital.

For several decades, hospitals were reimbursed under Part B for most outpatient hospital services in accordance with the outpatient prospective payment system (OPPS). However, as a result of the enactment of the Balanced Budget Act of 2015 (BBA), most services administered in a hospital outpatient department (HOPD) will be reimbursed under the Medicare physician fee schedule (MPFS) or the ambulatory surgical center fee schedule (ASCFS), both of which are less generous than OPPS. The BBA's HOPD reforms are an important first step in what many expect will be a wave of site-neutral payment reforms, which seek to reimburse providers according to the service provided, rather than the setting in which the service is provided.

Most services are paid separately, including, but not limited to, most surgical, diagnostic, and nonsurgical therapeutic procedures; blood and blood products; most clinic and emergency department visits; and some drugs and biologicals. Within each ambulatory patient classification (APC), payment for ancillary and supportive items and services is packaged into payment for the primary independent service. Separate payments are not made for a packaged service, which is considered an integral part of another service that is paid under the OPPS. Some examples of usual packaged services are routine supplies, anesthesia, operating and recovery room use, implantable medical devices, inexpensive drugs under a per day drug threshold

packaging amount ($100 in 2016), guidance services, and imaging supervision and interpretation services.

Medicare Part B pays for physician services based on the MPFS, which lists the more than 7,000 covered services and their payment rates. Physician services include office visits, surgical procedures, and a range of other diagnostic and therapeutic services.

The fee schedule assigns relative value units to each outpatient healthcare service. The Medicare reimbursement for a physician calculation includes the relative value unit for the procedure, relative value units for the practice expense, a geographical adjustment factor for geographical variations in payments, and a conversion factor. Indicative of federal policy supporting value-based payment, the Medicare Access and CHIP Reauthorization Act of 2015 authorized the payment of providers based on two models that factor in the quality of care, the amount of resources consumed, clinical practice improvement activities, and the meaningful use of certified electronic health record (EHR) technology.

## Medicare Appeals

### Appeal Rights: Medicare Beneficiaries

A **Medicare beneficiary** has the right to appeal any decision about the beneficiary's Medicare services regardless of the coverage plan. If Medicare does not pay for an item or service provided to the beneficiary or if the beneficiary is not given an item or service the beneficiary believes he or she should receive, they can appeal.

**Original Medicare** An enrollee in original Medicare can appeal a Medicare denial of payment or underpayment for an item or service received. Appeal rights are printed on the back of the Explanation of Medicare Benefits or Medicare Summary Notice that is mailed to the beneficiary. The notice also explains why the bill was not paid and the appeal steps.

**Medicare Part C** An enrollee in a Medicare managed care plan can appeal a denial of payment or a disallowance of service that should be covered or provided. If a fast decision is requested, the plan must answer the appeal within 72 hours. The Medicare managed care plan must describe the appeal process in writing. If a plan does not decide in favor of the beneficiary, the appeal is reviewed by an independent organization that works for Medicare, not for the plan.

**Medicare Part D** A Medicare prescription drug plan enrollee can appeal a plan sponsor's decision not to provide or pay for a Part D prescription drug that the enrollee believes the plan sponsor should provide or pay for. The word *provide* includes such things as authorizing prescription drugs, paying for prescription drugs, or continuing to provide a Part D prescription drug that the enrollee has been receiving. The Medicare prescription drug plan must inform the enrollee in writing how to request an appeal.

A standard appeal must be answered by the plan sponsor within 7 calendar days after receiving the request. An enrollee or the enrollee's physician can request an expedited 72-hour appeal if the enrollee's health could be seriously harmed by waiting up to 7 calendar days for a decision. If the plan sponsor does not decide in favor of the enrollee, that decision can be appealed to an independent organization that works for Medicare, not for the plan sponsor.

## Appeal Rights: Medicare Providers, Physicians, and Other Suppliers

Once an initial claim determination is made there are five levels of appeal to protect providers, physicians, and other suppliers. Physicians and other suppliers who do not take assignment on claims have limited appeal rights. Beneficiaries may transfer their appeal rights to nonparticipating physicians or other suppliers who provide the items or services and do not otherwise have appeal rights. All appeal requests must be made in writing.

Medicare offers five levels in the Part A and Part B appeals process. The levels, listed in order, are as follows:

1. *Redetermination by a financial institution, carrier, or Medicare Administrative Contractor (MAC)*: A redetermination is an examination of a claim by the financial institution, carrier, or MAC personnel who are different from the personnel who made the initial determination. The appellant (the individual filing the appeal) has 120 days from the date of receipt of the initial claim determination to file an appeal. A minimum monetary threshold is not required to request a redetermination.
2. *Reconsideration by a qualified independent contractor (QICs)*: A party to the redetermination may request a reconsideration if dissatisfied with the redetermination. A QIC conducts the reconsideration. The QIC reconsideration process allows for an independent review of medical necessity issues by a panel of physicians or other healthcare professionals. A minimum monetary threshold is not required to request a reconsideration.
3. *Hearing by an administrative law judge (ALJ)*: If at least $150 remains in controversy after the QIC's decision, a party to the reconsideration may request an ALJ hearing within 60 days of receipt of the reconsideration. Appellants must also send notice of the ALJ hearing request to all parties to the QIC reconsideration and verify this on the hearing request form or in the written request.
4. *Review by the Medicare Appeals Council within the Departmental Appeals Board ("the Appeals Council")*: If a party to the ALJ hearing is dissatisfied with the ALJ's decision, the party may request a review by the Appeals Council. There are no requirements regarding the amount of money in controversy. The request for Appeals Council review must be submitted in writing within 60 days of receipt of the ALJ's decision and must specify the issues and findings that are being contested.
5. *Judicial review in U.S. District Court*: If at least $1,500 is still in controversy after the Appeals Council's decision, a party to the decision may request judicial review before a U.S. District Court judge. The appellant must file the request for review within 60 days of receipt of the Appeals Council's decision. The Appeals Council's decision contains information about the procedures for requesting judicial review.

## Medicaid Reimbursement

The Medicaid program was established by Congress in 1965 and covers health and long-term care services for many of the sickest and poorest Americans. The Medicaid program is a federal-state partnership in which the federal government provides matching grants to states to finance care for certain "mandatory" groups of people. So long as they cover these "mandatory" groups to the extent required by federal law, states have broad discretion to vary the terms of their Medicaid programs. Since there is no funding cap on the Medicaid dollars a state can receive, federal funds are permitted to flow to states based on actual need.

Federal law provides that the state must ensure adequate funding for the nonfederal share of expenditures from state or local sources for the amount, duration, scope, or quality of care and services available under the state plan. Recognized sources of the state share of Medicaid payments include legislative **appropriations** to the single state agency, intergovernmental transfers, certified public expenditures, and permissible taxes and provider donations. Before approval of a state plan amendment, CMS must verify that the source of the state share meets applicable statutory and regulatory requirements to authorize federal financial participation for the covered services.

Federal law directs payment of federal financial participation at different matching rates, for amounts "found necessary by the Secretary for the proper and efficient administration of the State plan."[3] The Secretary of the DHHS is the final arbiter of which activities fall under this definition. Claims held under this authority must be directly related to the administration of the Medicaid program. In addition, payment may only be made for the percentage of time spent actually attributable to Medicaid-eligible individuals.

CMS has approved cost allocation plans from states that include the following types of administrative costs necessary for the proper and efficient administration of the State plan:

- Medicaid eligibility determinations
- Medicaid outreach
- Prior authorization for Medicaid services
- Medicaid Management Information System development and operation
- Early and periodic screening, diagnostic and treatment administration
- Third-party liability activities
- Utilization review
- Medicaid financial operations and reporting

In part due to the ACA, Medicaid has been dramatically expanded. In 2013, nearly 72.5 million people, including one-fourth of all children, received Medicaid coverage for at least some portion of the year. Without Medicaid, most of its beneficiaries would remain uninsured.

Like Medicare, Medicaid is a major source of funding for the U.S. healthcare system. It is the main source of financing for long-term care, paying 40% of the nation's bill for both nursing home care and long-term care. Additionally, Medicaid is the largest source of public funding for mental health care. Safety-net hospitals and health centers that care for the uninsured and much of the low-income population also depend on Medicaid.

## Eligibility Determinations

Agencies in each state administer Medicaid under the oversight of CMS. Although participation is voluntary, all states participate in Medicaid. States have broad authority to define eligibility, benefits, provider payment, and other aspects of their programs subject to basic minimum requirements required under federal law. Consequently, Medicaid operates as a distinct program in each state, the District of Columbia, and the U.S. territories. These variations and the demographic differences among the states result in variations of covered populations from state to state.

As noted previously, federal law requires each state to cover certain "mandatory" groups to receive the federal match. Traditionally, such mandatory groups included only pregnant women, children under age 6 with family income below 133% of the federal poverty level, children ages 6 to 18 below 100% federal poverty level, parents below states' July 1996 welfare eligibility levels (often below 50% federal poverty level), and most elderly and persons with disabilities receiving Supplemental Security Income, for which income eligibility equates to 74% federal poverty level for an individual.

With the passage of the ACA, states were required to expand Medicaid to all nonelderly individuals with income up to 138% of the federal poverty level, or risk losing federal Medicaid payments. In *NFIB v. Sebelius*, however, the United States Supreme Court ruled that Congress could not condition all of a state's Medicaid funding on its willingness to expand Medicaid to these poor, childless adults. The result of this ruling is that if a state chooses to cover childless adults in the way the ACA contemplates, it receives additional funding from the federal government.

Accordingly, in the 32 states and territories that have adopted the Medicaid expansion as of April 2016, adults with an income below 138% of the poverty level are guaranteed coverage through Medicaid. The income thresholds adults must meet to qualify for Medicaid vary by state.[4] The ACA's Medicaid expansion provisions are estimated to result in 18.3 million new Medicaid enrollees by 2021.

## Coverage of Item or Service

Medicaid covers the health services typically covered by private insurance to address the many different healthcare needs of its diverse enrollees and their

---

[3]42 U.S.C. § 1396b.

[4]http://kff.org/health-reform/state-indicator/medicaid-income-eligibility-limits-for-adults-as-a-percent-of-the-federal-poverty-level/

limited ability to afford care out of pocket. Medicaid also covers many additional services, such as dental and vision care, transportation, and long-term care services. Some covered benefits, such as services provided by federally qualified health centers, reflect the unique role certain institutions play in furnishing healthcare services to the low-income population. To control costs, states use numerous tools to manage utilization, such as prior authorization and case management.

As with eligibility, state Medicaid programs must cover certain "**mandatory services**" specified under federal law to receive any federal matching funds.

Medicaid services are covered subject to medical necessity, as determined by the state Medicaid program or a managed care plan that is under contract to the state. Federal law also permits states to cover many services that are designated as "optional services," such as prescription drugs, which all states cover, and personal care services.

## Waivers of Medicaid Requirements

In general, states are required to comply with certain requirements in order to receive federal matching funds under the Medicaid program. However, the Social Security Act gives the Secretary of DHHS authority to waive certain requirements to allow an experimental, pilot, or demonstration project that promotes the objectives of the Medicaid and Children's Health Insurance programs.[5] Projects eligible for such "section 1115 waivers" include those that expand eligibility to individuals who are not otherwise Medicaid or CHIP eligible, provide services not typically covered by Medicaid, or use innovative service delivery systems that improve care, increase efficiency, and reduce costs. Section 1115 waivers must be budget neutral and generally are for an initial 5-year period followed by an additional 3-year period if the state obtains an extension from DHHS. The ACA requires opportunity for public comment and greater transparency of the section 1115 waiver process.

## Provider Payment Rates

Each state has its own Medicaid reimbursement methodology. CMS reviews state plan reimbursement methodologies for services provided under the state plan for consistency with federal statutes and regulations. These laws require that states "assure that payments are consistent with efficiency, economy, and quality of care and are sufficient to enlist enough providers so

that care and services are available under the plan at least to the extent that such care and services are available to the general population in the geographic area."[6]

In general, CMS reviews state payment methodologies and supporting documentation to ensure that the state plan methodology may be audited and is comprehensively described and that payment rates are economic, efficient, and sufficient to attract willing and qualified providers. In addition, the law requires that Medicaid payments to qualified hospitals, nursing facilities, intermediate care facilities for the mentally retarded (ICF/MRs), and clinics not exceed a reasonable estimate of the amount that Medicare would pay for equivalent services in the aggregate within state-owned or operated, non-state-owned or operated, and private facilities.

Together with the ACA, the Health Care and Education Reconciliation Act of 2010 (HCERA) alters Medicaid payment methodology for certain physicians. In 2013 and 2014, HCERA required that physicians practicing in pediatrics, family medicine, or general internal medicine receive reimbursement equal to at least 100% of the Medicare Part B physician fee, meaning that these physicians could not be paid a smaller fee for seeing Medicaid patients than they would be for seeing Medicare patients. In light of the shortage of practitioners in these areas, it is likely that Congress and agencies will consider exploring ways to attract and retain providers by devising generous reimbursement models.

## Disproportionate Share Hospital Payments

Medicaid makes special payments to hospitals that serve a disproportionate share of low-income and uninsured patients. Approximately 6% of Medicaid spending is attributable to supplemental payments to hospitals that serve a disproportionate share of low-income and uninsured patients. Known as "DSH" payments, they help support the safety-net hospitals that provide substantial uncompensated care to this population.

Because Congress expected the ACA to expand coverage (reducing uncompensated care), it included a provision in that law that phases out DSH payments over time. These phase-outs have had a significant impact on safety-net hospitals, especially in states where Medicaid has not been expanded. Unless Congress acts to correct this unintended consequence of the ACA, it is likely that hospitals in states

---

[5]42 U.S.C. §1315(a).

[6]42 U.S.C. § 1396(a)(30)(A).

where Medicaid has not been expanded will see their uncompensated care costs continue to increase.

---

### Learning Objective 5

Be aware of the most important aspects of the ACA as it relates to financial management in the post-reform environment.

---

## Effect of Healthcare Reform

Among the ACA's most sweeping reforms are those in the area of payment for healthcare services administered to Medicare beneficiaries. This section discusses several ACA-implemented reforms that share a common theme: financially rewarding providers who participate in the Medicare program in models that promote cost-efficient, quality patient outcomes.

The first ACA-contained payment reform is the Medicare Shared Savings Program (MSSP).[7] The MSSP rewards providers who deliver high-quality care to Medicare beneficiaries via ACOs by allowing them to share in any cost savings realized by the federal government. An ACO is a group of providers or suppliers (or a network of such groups) that is jointly responsible for the cost and quality of health care provided to Medicare beneficiaries.

An ACO must apply and be approved for participation in the MSSP by CMS. In order to participate, the ACA requires that ACOs (among other things) (1) be accountable for the overall care of a defined group of not less than 5,000 Medicare beneficiaries; (2) have sufficient participation of primary care physicians; (3) have processes that promote evidence-based medicine, report on quality and costs, and be capable of coordinating care; and (4) consist of a group of providers and suppliers who have an established mechanism for joint decision making.

ACOs participate in the MSSP in either a one-sided model (in which the ACO receives a lower share of savings enjoyed by the federal government, but is not responsible for any cost increases) or a two-sided model (in which the ACO receives a higher share of savings enjoyed by the federal government, but is also liable for any increased care costs associated with its Medicare beneficiary pool). While the ACA's ACO reforms only have a direct impact on government payers, private payers are increasingly encouraging provider participation in accountable care models, with 2015 estimates indicating that more than 50% of accountable care payment arrangements involve commercial payers. From a compliance perspective, there is an inherent tension between collaborative care models (especially ACOs) and the key thrust of the fraud and abuse laws, namely to target certain cooperative relationships among otherwise unaffiliated healthcare providers. As discussed below, CMS has taken steps to alleviate providers' concerns relating to antitrust compliance by issuing "fraud and abuse waivers" that allow ACO participants to deliver high-quality, cost-effective care in collaborative arrangements without running afoul of the fraud and abuse laws.[8] These waivers are discussed more thoroughly in the fraud and abuse section.

The second ACA-contained payment reform is the National Pilot Program on Payment Bundling.[9] Under bundled payment methodologies, providers (e.g., hospitals and physicians) receive a single payment for all care provided for an episode of illness, rather than a separate fee for each service rendered in the course of treating a patient. For example, if a patient has knee replacement surgery, rather than making one payment to the hospital, a second payment to the surgeon, and a third payment to the anesthesiologist, the payer would combine these payments for the specific episode of care (i.e., knee replacement surgery). By requiring each provider in the continuum of care to share one payment "pool," this payment model seeks to encourage cost-effective, quality care by allowing collaborating providers to share in any savings realized by the payer for treatment delivered through the bundled payment model.

To promote the use of bundled payments, the ACA created the Center for Medicare and Medicaid Innovation (Innovation Center). The Innovation Center was charged with testing innovative payment and service delivery models that have the potential to reduce Medicare, Medicaid, or CHIP expenditures while preserving or enhancing the quality of care for beneficiaries. In exercising this duty, the Innovation Center created the Bundled Payments for Care Improvement (BPCI) initiative,[10] which consists of four broadly defined models of care that link payments for the multiple services that beneficiaries receive during an episode of care. While the ACA has ensured that public payers will remain active promotors of bundled care payment models, private payers—including large employers such as Lowe's[11]—have likewise been eager to engage providers in bundled payment arrangements.

---

[7]ACA § 3022; 42 U.S.C. 1395jjj.

[8]https://www.cms.gov/Medicare/Fraud-and-Abuse/PhysicianSelfReferral/Fraud-and-Abuse-Waivers.html

[9]ACA § 3023; 42 U.S.C. 1395cc-4.

[10]https://innovation.cms.gov/initiatives/bundled-payments/

[11]http://www.npr.org/sections/health-shots/2016/04/20/474413496/some-firms-save-money-by-offering-employees-free-surgery

A third ACA-contained payment reform is the payment adjustment for conditions acquired in hospitals.[12] Specifically, the ACA penalizes hospitals whose patients are plagued by a high number of hospital-acquired conditions (HACs) by reducing their Medicare payments. Since fiscal year 2015, hospitals have been ranked based on their number of HACs, with the 25% of "worst-offender" hospitals in the top quarter experiencing overall inpatient payment reductions of 1% (in addition to current payment penalties for HACs).

A fourth ACA-contained payment reform is the Hospital Readmissions Reduction Program (HRRP).[13] The HRRP requires CMS to reduce payments to hospitals paid under the inpatient prospective payment systems (IPPS) for excess readmissions. More information on the HRRP program can be found on CMS's website.[14]

A fifth and final ACA-contained payment reform involves the treatment of Patient-Centered Medical Homes (PCMHs). Similar to the ACO model, the PCMH model is based on a vision of primary care practice in which a "team" of health professionals provides comprehensive and timely care to patients who are more actively involved in receiving care. The PCMH model finds support in several ACA provisions,[15] and generally seeks to promote a cooperative, ongoing relationship between primary care physician and patient, including by incentivizing the early discovery and management of chronic conditions.

As these and other ACA payment reforms become increasingly widespread, relationships among institutional providers, physicians, outpatient clinics, and post–acute care providers such as skilled nursing and home health care will require a much higher level of integration and cooperation than exists in the current system.

### Learning Objective 6

Identify the most common federal regulatory issues, such as fraud and abuse, Stark Law, HIPAA, EMTALA, and IRS requirements for tax-exempt organizations, as well as less common concerns that arise under the antitrust laws and federal and state laws regulating third-party payers.

[12]ACA § 3008; 42 U.S.C. § 1395ww(p).

[13]ACA, §§ 3025, 10309; 42 U.S.C. § 1395ww(p).

[14]https://www.cms.gov/medicare/medicare-fee-for-service-payment/acuteinpatientpps/readmissions-reduction-program.html

[15]ACA, §§ 3021, 3502, 5301, 5405.

## Fraud, Abuse, and Penalties

Fraud consists of intentional acts of deception, whereas abuse involves improper acts that are inconsistent with standard practice and may result in overpayment or overutilization. Fraud and abuse can take many forms. Providers may bill for services not delivered or not medically necessary. Double billing for a single procedure can occur, as can improper "upcoding" to receive a higher reimbursement rate. Kickbacks for referrals or medical procedures are another frequently cited form of fraud.

The Medicare program involves claims for services submitted by thousands of providers on behalf of more than 55 million beneficiaries. The cumulative effect of even small overpayments can translate to significant program losses because of the number of claims and providers involved. The Health Care Fraud and Abuse Control Program, under the joint direction of the U.S. Attorney General and the Secretary of the DHHS, acting through the OIG, was designed to coordinate federal, state, and local law enforcement activities with respect to enforcing laws to minimize healthcare fraud and abuse.

## Criminal Statutes

A number of criminal statutes address false or fraudulent representations made to, and false claims filed with, Medicare or other federally funded healthcare programs. The Medicare and Medicaid Anti-Fraud and Abuse Amendments provide criminal penalties for making false statements of material fact in a claim made for Medicare or Medicaid payment and for failing to disclose or conceal an event affecting the right to receive a benefit or payment. In addition, these amendments provide criminal penalties for improper use of Medicare or Medicaid benefits, presenting claims by unlicensed physicians, and advising a person to transfer assets to gain Medicaid eligibility.

In addition to the direct criminal statutes, criminal mail or wire fraud also apply to the use of mail or wire for the purpose of a scheme or plan to defraud or for obtaining money or property by means of false or fraudulent representations. The Racketeer Influenced and Corrupt Organizations Act (RICO Act) prohibits a person from receiving income from a pattern of activity including committing an enumerated act (such as mail or wire fraud) at least twice in 10 years. Furthermore, criminal money laundering is the act of knowingly engaging in a monetary transaction in criminally derived property of a value greater than $10,000 and derived from specific unlawful activity (such as mail or wire fraud or any act or activity constituting an offense involving a federal healthcare offense).

Finally, a person may not knowingly and willfully falsify, conceal, or cover up by trick, scheme, or device a material fact, or make any materially false, fictitious, or fraudulent statements or representations, or make or use a materially false writing or document knowing the same to contain any materially false, fictitious, or fraudulent statement or entry. Such false statements are also criminal acts. These various criminal laws illustrate that Medicare fraud can result in a variety of criminal charges. In addition, the Anti-Kickback Statute includes criminal penalties and is discussed in more detail next.

## Self-Referrals and Kickbacks

The Anti-Kickback Statute (AKS) and the Stark Physician Self-Referral Law (Stark Law) are two important fraud and abuse authorities. They are among the most important regulatory restrictions and must be considered when structuring business relationships between healthcare entities. Violations of these laws can result in nonpayment of Medicare claims, civil monetary penalties, exclusion from the Medicare program, and liability under the False Claims Act, discussed later. Under current law, submitting a claim to Medicare when the provider has violated AKS or the Stark Law may be a false claim, because claims include a certification that the provider is in compliance with Medicare laws and regulations. In addition, violation of AKS can result in criminal penalties, including imprisonment and fines.

Unfortunately, AKS and the Stark Law include much uncertainty, in part because the regulations governing their implementation change so frequently. Both AKS and the Stark Law have relatively short statutory language, there are significant regulations adding safe harbors and exceptions, and specifying details are left unclear in the statute. Therefore, following rule-making procedures, the OIG can change the AKS regulations, and the CMS can change the Stark Law regulations, without any action of Congress.

Implementation of AKS and the Stark Law is difficult because the requirements often conflict with the economic interests of the parties structuring the relationship. In addition, both AKS and the Stark Law have a complex web of exceptions, safe harbors, and interpretation from the OIG and CMS in the form of commentary to the rules, advisory opinions, and other published guidance.

For example, AKS and the Stark Law often frustrate parties' efforts to enter into collaborative arrangements (especially ACOs) that are both encouraged by

the ACA and widely viewed as integral to decreasing the cost of health care while simultaneously improving outcomes. This is so because AKS and Stark, broadly speaking, are primarily concerned with discouraging certain collaborative relationships among healthcare providers, based on the theory that such relationships frequently result in "sweetheart" deals that are at odds with the government's interest in cost-efficient care and patients' interest in neutral medical advice that is not shaded by a provider's financial bias. Unfortunately, this silo-based conception of healthcare delivery is at odds with the growing recognition—especially among government and private payers—that provider integration and cooperation leads to increasingly efficient care and better outcomes.

In response to provider concerns over the intersection between the fraud and abuse laws and MSSP ACOs, CMS issued an October 2015 final rule[16] aimed at "adequately protecting beneficiaries and federal healthcare programs while promoting innovative structures within the [MSSP]." While legal counsel must be engaged to determine whether an arrangement satisfies one or more of the final rule's five waivers, a brief description of each follows:

- *The ACO Pre-Participation Waiver* waives the requirements of the Stark Law and AKS with respect to start-up arrangements that predate an ACO's agreement to participate in the MSSP.
- *The ACO Participation Waiver* waives the requirements of the Stark Law and AKS with respect to any arrangement of (1) an ACO, (2) one or more of its ACO participants or its ACO providers/suppliers, or (3) a combination thereof, provided that ACO's governing body has determined that the arrangement is reasonably related to the purposes of the MSSP.
- *The Shared Savings Distribution Waiver* waives the requirements of the Stark Law and AKS with respect to shared savings paid by CMS to the ACO and then distributed either (1) to ACO participants, providers, and suppliers during the year shared savings were earned or (2) outside the ACO for activities necessary for (or directly related to) the ACO's participation in and operations under the MSSP.
- *The Compliance with the Stark Law Waiver* provides that with respect to any financial relationship between or among the ACO, its participants, or its provider/suppliers that implicates the Stark Law but falls within an exception, AKS's requirements are

---

[16]80 Fed. Reg. 66,726 (Oct. 29, 2015).

waived. This waiver obviates the need for duplicate legal review under the AKS where an arrangement qualifies for an exception under the Stark Law.

■ *The Patient Incentives Waiver* waives the requirements of AKS (and the Beneficiary Inducements CMP[17]) with respect to items or services provided to beneficiaries for free or below market value by an ACO, its participants, or its providers/suppliers.

While the Waivers have alleviated some fraud and abuse concerns, their detailed requirements and the steep penalties associated with noncompliance have discouraged many providers from organizing into models that have the potential to deliver the quality, cost-efficient outcomes that stakeholders universally agree are sorely needed.

While AKS and the Stark Law are important federal statutory and regulatory schemes addressing entities with relationships to Medicare and Medicaid, many states also have their own versions of anti-kickback and physician self-referral prohibitions. These state laws vary in complexity and coverage, addressing relationships between healthcare entities either reimbursed by Medicaid, other state-payers, or in some cases, limit relationships regardless of payment source. Because of length constraints, state law is not addressed in this chapter.

**Stark Law** The Stark Law prohibits a physician from referring a patient for certain "designated health services" to an entity with which the physician has a "financial relationship."[18] In addition, a provider may not bill Medicare for a claim based on a prohibited referral. Unlike AKS, the Stark Law is a strict liability statute and may be violated irrespective of intent. In addition, the Stark Law only applies to referrals made by physicians.

The Stark Law was premised on the assumption that a physician may not make the best medical decision for a patient when the physician has economic ties to a related for-profit business. If the physician's self-interest impacts decision making, care may be compromised. In addition, healthcare costs may be increased by referring for services that may not be medically necessary as well as by a prearranged referral source.

To understand the Stark Law, a clear understanding of the definitions in the basic rule is needed. A "financial relationship" is defined to include investment or ownership interests and compensation relationships.

In addition, the definition of financial relationship includes both direct and indirect relationships. Therefore, referrals may be prohibited between a physician and a hospital where a physician has an impermissible contractual relationship with a physician group that shares a parent entity with the hospital.

"Designated health services" is specifically defined to include the following:

■ Clinical laboratory services
■ Physical therapy, occupational therapy, and speech-language pathology services
■ Radiology and certain other imaging services
■ Radiation therapy services and supplies
■ Durable medical equipment and supplies
■ Parenteral and enteral nutrients, equipment, and supplies
■ Prosthetics, orthotics, and prosthetic devices
■ Home health services and supplies
■ Outpatient prescription drugs
■ Inpatient and outpatient hospital services

Excluded from "designated health services" are those services reimbursed as part of a composite rate, unless the service itself is reimbursed as a composite rate above (e.g., home health and inpatient hospital services).

Violation of the Stark Law can result in denial of payment of Medicare claims, refunds of amounts collected in violation of the Stark Law, civil monetary penalties of up to $15,000 for each claim that a person knows or should know was made in violation of the Stark Law, and three times the amount of the improper collection. Finally, where a claim is submitted in violation of the Stark Law, the FCA may also be implicated, as discussed previously.

Although the Stark Law prohibition is broad, there are a number of statutory and regulatory exceptions.[19] Some of these exceptions apply to ownership arrangements only, compensation arrangements only, or both ownership and compensation arrangements.

For physicians practicing as part of a group practice, there are "in-office ancillary services" and "physician services" exceptions that allow a physician to refer for services within the group practice. However, the group practice must meet the Stark Law's complicated definition of "group practice," the physician or another member of the group practice must personally furnish or directly supervise the furnishing of the services, the services must be provided in a space meeting the exception's location requirements, and the services must be billed by the performing or

---

[17]42 U.S.C. § 1320a–7a(a)(5).
[18]42 U.S.C. § 1395nn.

[19]42 C.F.R. §§ 411.350 *et seq.*

supervising physician, his/her group, an entity wholly owned by any of the above, or a third-party billing company as agent for any of the above.

Compensation-related exceptions generally focus on ensuring relationships are consistent with fair market value and commercially reasonable and require that compensation does not vary with or take into account the volume or value of referrals. For example, in *United States ex rel. Drakeford v. Toumey*,[20] the court concluded that the Stark Law was violated by a hospital's part-time employment of 19 physicians for outpatient surgeries. Specifically, the court noted that the physicians—who were paid a base salary based on past production with a substantial productivity bonus equal to nearly 80% of compensation—had a compensation package on which Toumey stood to lose $1.5 to 2 million per year on the physician's compensation when compared to their collections. In addition, the physicians' compensation was deemed to vary based on the volume or value of referrals because every case involved compensation via technical and facility fees, which were earned from professional procedures that had to be delivered at the hospital's outpatient facilities. Accordingly, the physicians did not qualify for a Stark Law exception for bona fide employment arrangements, and the agreement was otherwise non-compliant with Stark. As a result of submitting claims for payment in violation of the Stark Law, Toumey was found to be in violation of the False Claims Act, and ordered to pay damages and civil penalties totaling $237,454,000 (which was reduced to $72.4 million in a final settlement agreement reached with regulators). There are also exceptions to Stark liability for renting office space and renting equipment, each with a number of specific requirements. Importantly, both the equipment and space rental exceptions forbid "perclick" and percentage-based compensation. Therefore, an equipment rental relationship may not be compensated on a per use basis but must be used for certain prearranged blocks of time to meet the Stark exception.

Other major Stark exceptions include those for personal services and bona fide employment, and both exceptions have a number of requirements. Unlike AKS, which only requires bona fide employment to meet an exception, the Stark Law employment exception requires that the employment be for identifiable services, compensation be consistent with fair market value and commercially reasonable, and not take into account the volume or value of referrals. Such limitation does not prohibit productivity bonuses if the bonuses are based on services performed personally by the employee.

Like AKS, Stark has a process by which providers may self-disclose actual or potential violations in an effort to reduce penalties, avoid exclusion, and provide protection from *qui tam* suits. Known as the self-referral disclosure protocol, this process—though by no means effortless—can help providers avoid the ruinous liability that sometimes accompanies violations of the Stark Law.

**Anti-Kickback Statute** AKS states that no person may offer or request, give, or receive remuneration in exchange for a referral for a good or service that may be reimbursed under a federal healthcare program (e.g., Medicare).[21] Note that at least one district court has held that a referral does not need to actually be made: "the Government need only prove that the money was paid in exchange for the promise of referrals."[22] In addition, AKS prohibits both the payment and the receipt of such kickbacks. AKS applies to all healthcare providers and any other person that may fall under its prohibition, as compared with the Stark Law, which is limited to physicians.

"Remuneration" under AKS is interpreted broadly. It is clear when, for example, an imaging provider hands cash to a physician in exchange for a promise to refer patients for magnetic resonance imaging that remuneration has been given in exchange for referrals. However, remuneration can also be given or received in the form of free or discounted goods or services. For example, a hospital providing office space to a physician for below-market rent in exchange for referrals from that physician is also considered remuneration in exchange for referrals. As a result, healthcare providers should take care to ensure that all financial arrangements are consistent with fair market value. The concept of fair market value arises in most AKS safe harbors to ensure that improper remuneration is not given either by above-market compensation (i.e., extra cash) or below-market compensation (i.e., improper discount).

AKS is intent based, so to violate the statute a person must have the intent to give or receive remuneration for referrals. However, even if the physician performs some service for the money received, the potential for unnecessary drain on Medicare remains. If the payments were intended to induce a provider to refer for services, the statute was violated, even if the payments were also intended to compensate for professional services.[23] AKS is violated if *one purpose* of

---

[20]792 F.3d 364 (4th Cir. 2015).

[21]42 U.S.C. § 1320a-7b(b).
[22]*United States v. Picciotti*, 40 F.Supp.2d 242, 248 (D.N.J. 1999).
[23]*United States v. Greber*, 760 F.2d 68 (3d Cir. 1985).

the payment is to induce referrals.[24] The one purpose does not even need to be the main purpose; one court found that "the issue of sole versus primary reason for payments is irrelevant since any amount of inducement is illegal."[25] Therefore, any intent to induce referrals would fulfill the requirements under AKS.[26]

AKS includes a few statutory exceptions, including bona fide employment. It is indicative of the breadth of AKS that an exception for employment was made. According to the statutory language, a bona fide employee may be compensated in any otherwise-legal manner. It is important to note that the Stark Law is not so liberal in exceptions to employment and places some requirements on physician employment (discussed later).

The OIG has identified various payment practices that, although potentially capable of inducing referrals of business under Medicare and Medicaid, are essentially harmless or efficient and therefore should not be viewed as kickbacks for purposes of criminal prosecution or civil remedies. The resulting regulations, often referred to as the "safe harbor rules," are intended to give guidance and comfort to providers who engage in certain narrowly prescribed business practices that Congress did not intend to prohibit by AKS and, in some instances, should be encouraged by the federal government.

There are 25 safe harbors identified by the OIG. Some commonly used safe harbors are for space rental, equipment rental, and personal services agreements between healthcare entities and/or providers. For each of these arrangements, the safe harbor requires that the arrangement be in writing, for a term of at least 1 year, that the compensation be set in advance, and that the compensation be consistent with fair market value and be commercially reasonable. As discussed earlier, the OIG wants to make sure that, for example, a hospital is leasing a magnetic resonance imaging facility to a physician practice for its fair market value and not leasing it for "bargain basement" prices in exchange for referrals from the physicians to the hospital. In addition, there are safe harbors for investment in healthcare entities, for certain discounts for products, and for waiver of coinsurance or deductibles, among others. These safe harbors each contain a number of requirements that must be met before an arrangement is protected.

If an arrangement fully complies with a safe harbor, AKS is not violated. Failure of an arrangement to comply with a safe harbor can mean one of three things: (1) the arrangement is not intended to induce the referral of business reimbursable under Medicare or Medicaid, so there is no violation of AKS or need for a safe harbor; (2) the arrangement could be a clear statutory violation and also not qualify for safe harbor protection and therefore at high risk for prosecution; or (3) the arrangement may violate the statute in a less serious manner although not be in compliance with a safe harbor provision. The degree of the risk depends on an evaluation of the many factors that are part of the decision-making process regarding case selection for investigation and prosecution.

The OIG has the primary responsibility for enforcing AKS. In addition to its audit function, the OIG issues advisory opinions at the request of various parties, which lend guidance to the statutes and regulations that make up AKS. The OIG also implements a self-disclosure protocol, under which a party who has violated AKS (or other Medicare law) can report the wrongdoing in exchange for lenient treatment. However, there is no guarantee of leniency, and the Department of Justice is informed of all self-disclosures made to the OIG.

## False Claims Act

The False Claims Act (FCA) is the federal government's primary civil remedy for improper or fraudulent claims.[27] Although the FCA applies to all federal programs, not just to public healthcare benefits, it increasingly has been applied in health care, due in part to the large dollar amounts involved. Under the FCA healthcare providers who knowingly make false or fraudulent claims to the government are fined $5,500 to $11,000 per claim plus up to three times the amount of the damages caused to the federal program. Large fines can quickly accrue, because providers routinely submit thousands of claims to the government each year. For example, on March 10, 2000, the Department of Justice filed claims under the FCA seeking recovery of over $1 billion from Vencor Inc., a long-term healthcare provider, for its alleged knowing submission of false claims. The Department of Justice alleged that Vencor was engaged in improper billing practices, claims for services not rendered, provision of medically unnecessary services, misrepresenting eligibility or credentials, and substandard quality of care.

---

[24]*United States v. Kats*, 871 F.2d 105 (9th Cir. 1989).

[25]*U.S. ex rel. Pogue v. Diabetes Treatment Centers*, 565 F.Supp.2d 153, 162 (D.D.C. 2008).

[26]42 C.F.R. § 1001.952.

[27]31 U.S.C. §§ 3729 *et seq.*

Specific intent to defraud the government is not required to violate the FCA; the government need only establish that the claim submitted is false and that it was submitted knowingly. Thus, the FCA prohibits activity that does not fall under the traditional definition of fraud, which requires actual knowledge and the intent to defraud. In addition, an amendment to the FCA was passed in 2009 that defines a claim under the FCA as a claim for payment made either directly to the government or to a government contractor. As a result, where, for example, a physician group bills a hospital for services provided, if those services are ultimately paid for by Medicare, such a bill is available for prosecution under the FCA. As with most other civil actions, the government must establish its case by presenting a preponderance of the evidence rather than by meeting the higher burden of proof that applies in criminal cases.

To prove that a healthcare provider has knowingly submitted a false claim, the government must establish that the person submitted the claim with actual knowledge, in deliberate ignorance, or with reckless disregard for the claim's truth or falsity. The FCA is not intended to apply to honest mistakes and negligence. Yet, those doing business with the government are obligated to make at least limited inquiries as to the accuracy of the claims they submit.

## Qui Tam *Actions*

FCA claims may be brought against an entity not only by the Department of Justice or other governmental organization, but also by an individual. When such an action is brought by an individual, it is referred to as a "*qui tam*" action, and the individual is referred to as a "relator." *Qui tam* actions are also known as "whistleblower" suits. In a *qui tam* action, a relator with personal knowledge of a fraud brings the suit against a defendant on behalf of the government. The knowledge with which the relator brings a *qui tam* action must not be public knowledge, but information that would not otherwise be available without the *qui tam* suit.

The relator in a *qui tam* action does not need to have been personally harmed by the alleged false claim. However, the relator receives a certain percentage of any award or settlement amount. Once a relator files a *qui tam* action, the government has the option of joining the action as a plaintiff. If the government joins, the relator is entitled to between 15% and 25% of any award or settlement, depending on the assistance provided. If the government decides not to join, the relator is entitled to between 25% and 30% of any award or settlement. By granting a relator a percentage

of a successful *qui tam* action, the FCA provides individuals with incentive to assist the government in identifying fraud, especially where insider knowledge is required to identify such acts.

## Privacy of Healthcare Information under HIPAA

The Health Insurance Portability and Accountability Act of 1996 (HIPAA) was enacted to improve the Medicare and Medicaid programs and the efficiency and effectiveness of the healthcare system by encouraging the development of a health information system through the establishment of standards and requirements for the electronic transmission of certain health information.[28]

The American Recovery and Reinvestment Act of 2009 contains the Health Information Technology for Economic and Clinical Health Act (HITECH Act), which amends HIPAA.[29] The 2013 Omnibus Rule was issued to implement certain provisions of the HITECH Act.

By law, DHHS is required to issue HIPAA regulations regarding standards for privacy of individually identifiable health information (the "Privacy Standards"); security standards for the protection of electronic protected health information (PHI; the "Security Standards"); standards for notification in case of a breach of unsecured PHI (the "Breach Notification Standards"); and rules for compliance and investigations, impositions of civil monetary penalties, and procedures for hearings (the "Enforcement Rule"). After a brief overview of HIPAA's structure, this section examines the four HIPAA rules and standards in detail.

## Overview of HIPAA

HIPAA rules and regulations apply to "covered entities." Covered entities by statutory definition include healthcare providers, health plans, and healthcare clearinghouses. "Healthcare provider" refers to any provider of healthcare services as defined in relevant Medicare provisions and to any other person or organization that furnishes, bills, or is paid for healthcare services or supplies in the normal course of business. "Health plan" is defined broadly to include any individual or group plan that provides or pays the cost of medical care. "Healthcare clearinghouse" is defined as

---

[28]Pub. Law No. 104-191, 110 Stat. 1936 (1996).
[29]Pub. Law No. 111–5, 123 Stat. 115 §§ 13400 *et seq.* (2009).

a public or private entity that processes or facilitates the processing of nonstandard data elements of health information into standard data elements. Billing companies are an example of a healthcare clearinghouse.

The regulations also affect "business associates" of covered entities. A business associate is a "person who performs functions or activities on behalf of, or certain services for, a covered entity or another business associate that involve the use or disclosure of protected health information." Examples of business associates include independent contractors or other persons or entities receiving information for the purposes noted above, including lawyers, accountants, auditors, consultants, and billing firms. The Omnibus Rule specified that the following types of service providers are considered business associates: providers of certain data transmission services, a person that offers a personal health record, and a subcontractor who handles PHI on behalf of the business associate.

While a covered entity is generally liable for compliance with all HIPAA rules and standards, business associate liability is narrower. Specifically, in addition to liability for impermissible uses and disclosures of PHI, a business associate is directly liable under the HIPAA rules for a failure to (1) provide breach notification to the covered entity; (2) provide access to a copy of electronic PHI to either the covered entity, the individual, or the individual's designee, as specified in the parties' contract; (3) disclose PHI where required by DHHS to investigate or determine the business associate's compliance with HIPAA; (4) provide an accounting of disclosures; and (5) comply with the requirements of the Security Standards.

**Privacy Standards** In general, the Privacy Standards were designed to accomplish three broad objectives:

- Define and limit the circumstances in which entities use and disclose PHI.
- Establish certain individual rights regarding PHI.
- Require covered entities to adopt administrative safeguards to protect the confidentiality and privacy of PHI.

Although the law does not require the collection or electronic transmission of any health information, it does require that the standards be followed any time transactions are conducted electronically.

PHI is defined as health information used or disclosed by a covered entity in any form (electronic, paper records, oral communications) that identifies an individual and relates to the individual's past, present, or future physical or mental health or condition; the provision of health care to the individual; or the past,

present, or future payment for the provision of health care to the individual.

The HIPAA Privacy Standards prohibit covered entities from using or disclosing individually identifiable health information that is or has been transmitted or maintained electronically, except in certain circumstances. Unlike many medical records statutes, this requirement is not limited to the record in which the information appears but rather applies to the information itself. Thus, any information that has been transmitted by fax, telephone, computer, electronic handheld device, or any other electronic means is protected by the HIPAA standards thereafter in whatever form it might appear, including oral communications.

Under the Privacy Standards, an individual has rights over his or her health information, including the right to request restrictions on certain uses and disclosures of PHI, the right to receive confidential communications of PHI, the right to inspect and copy PHI, the right to amend PHI, and the right to receive an accounting of disclosures of PHI. An individual also has a right to adequate notice of the covered entity's legal duties with respect to PHI. This notice is provided through the ubiquitous "Notice of Privacy Practices" one receives from healthcare providers. This notice contains a statement of the individual's rights with respect to PHI and a brief description of how the individual may exercise these rights.

A covered entity may not use or disclose PHI, unless permitted or required by the HIPAA standards. A covered entity is permitted to use or disclose PHI to the individual; for treatment, payment, or healthcare operations, including disclosures to business associates, pursuant to and in compliance with a valid patient authorization, as required by law; or, under certain circumstances, if the PHI is stripped of information that may identify the patient. Furthermore, a covered entity is required to disclose PHI to an individual by request and when required by the Secretary of DHHS to conduct certain investigations. With few exceptions, when using or disclosing PHI or when requesting PHI from another covered entity, a covered entity must make reasonable efforts to limit PHI to the minimum necessary to accomplish the intended purpose of the use, disclosure, or request.

The Privacy Standards specify that covered entities may not disclose PHI to business associates without "satisfactory assurances" that the business associate complies with relevant standards. Satisfactory assurances include certain contractual language that must be included in all contracts between the covered entities and the business associates. Accordingly, covered entities would need to consider HIPAA provisions when drafting contracts with independent contractors.

**Security Standards** Covered entities must comply with the Security Standards with respect to electronic PHI (e-PHI). Compliance requires the covered entity to meet the following standards:

- Ensure the confidentiality, integrity, and availability of all e-PHI the covered entity creates, receives, maintains, or transmits.
- Protect against any reasonably anticipated threats or hazards to the security or integrity of such information.
- Protect against any reasonably anticipated uses or disclosures of such information that are not permitted or required under the Privacy Standards.
- Ensure compliance with HIPAA by its workforce.

The Security Standards require a covered entity to comply with specific administrative safeguards, physical safeguards, technical safeguards, and organizational requirements, and to implement reasonable and appropriate policies and procedures to comply with the standards, implementation specifications, or other requirements of the Security Standards. Under the HITECH Act business associates must also comply with all but the organizational requirements of these provisions. Although compliance with each element is important, the technical safeguards deserve particular attention.

Technical safeguards refer to the technology, and the policies and procedures regarding the technology, that protect e-PHI and control access. The technical safeguards include mandatory standards for access controls, audit controls, data integrity, person or entity authentication, and transmission security.

The access controls standard requires implementation of technical policies and procedures for electronic information systems that maintain e-PHI to allow access only to those persons or software programs that have been granted access rights. The required implementation specifications include assignment of a unique name and/or number for identifying and tracking user identity and the establishment (and implementation as needed) of procedures for obtaining necessary e-PHI during an emergency. The addressable implementation specifications include implementation of electronic procedures that terminate an electronic session after a predetermined time of inactivity and implementation of a mechanism to encrypt and decrypt e-PHI.

The audit controls standard requires implementation of hardware, software, and/or procedural mechanisms that record and examine activity in information systems that contain or use e-PHI. The data integrity standard requires implementation of policies and procedures to protect e-PHI from improper alteration or destruction. The addressable implementation specification requires assessing the implementation of electronic mechanisms to corroborate that e-PHI has not been altered or destroyed in an unauthorized manner.

The person or entity authentication standard requires implementation of procedures to verify that a person or entity seeking access to e-PHI is the one claimed. The transmission security standard requires implementation of technical security measures to guard against unauthorized access to e-PHI that is being transmitted over an electronic communications network. The addressable implementation specifications include implementation of security measures to ensure that electronically transmitted e-PHI is not improperly modified without detection until disposed of and implementation of a mechanism to encrypt e-PHI whenever deemed appropriate.

**Breach Notification Standards** The Breach Notification Rule was issued as part of the 2013 Omnibus Rule and sheds significant light on when a breach involving patient information occurs, what entities can be held liable for such a breach, and what obligations are triggered in the event of a breach.

A "breach" is the "acquisition, access, use, or disclosure" of PHI "in a manner not permitted" under the Privacy Rule, which "compromises the security or privacy" of the PHI. Breaches do not include instances in which (1) a workforce member—acting in good faith, unintentionally, and within the scope of employment—acquires or accesses PHI in a way that does not result in further use or disclosure, (2) a person authorized to access PHI inadvertently discloses PHI to another authorized person within the same organization, so long as the PHI is not further used or disclosed, or (3) the covered entity makes a disclosure to a person the entity reasonably believes would not have been able to retain the PHI.

Unless a covered entity or business associate can satisfy one of these three exceptions, any activity meeting the definition is presumptively a breach unless a party can show "low probability" that the PHI has been compromised. Based on agency commentary, it seems unlikely that a low probability of compromise will be found in most situations.

Once a covered entity or business associate discovers (or, if it had exercised reasonable diligence, would have discovered) a breach, certain notification requirements are implicated. First, when a business associate discovers it has committed a breach, it is required to notify the covered entity "without unreasonable delay" (which in no case can exceed 60 days).

Second, and more importantly, both covered entities and providers are required to notify each individual whose PHI has been compromised by a breach. This notification must be made "without unreasonable delay," and in no case later than 60 days after discovery of the breach, unless a law enforcement exception applies. The required notification must be written in plain language and include, to the extent possible: (1) a brief description of what happened, including the date of the breach and the date of the discovery of the breach, if known; (2) a description of the types of unsecured PHI that were involved in the breach; (3) any steps individuals should take to protect themselves from potential harm resulting from the breach; (4) a brief description of what the covered entity or business associate is doing to investigate the breach, to mitigate harm to individuals, and to protect against any further breaches; and (5) contact procedures for individuals to ask questions or learn additional information.

Third, if the breach involves more than 500 residents of a state, the covered entity must—within the time frame described earlier—notify prominent media outlets serving the state. Fourth, a covered entity must also notify DHHS following the discovery of a breach of unsecured PHI. For breaches involving 500 or more individuals, a covered entity must provide notification to DHHS contemporaneously with the notice to the individual. For breaches involving less than 500 individuals, a covered entity must maintain a log or other documentation of such breaches and, not later than 60 days after the end of each calendar year, provide notification to the DHHS for such breaches in the manner specified on the DHHS website.

**Enforcement Rule**  The HIPAA Enforcement Rule contains several important provisions relating to compliance and investigations, the imposition of civil money penalties for violations of HIPAA, and procedures for related hearings. The HITECH Act revised the HIPAA Enforcement Rule in the following ways:

- Establishing four categories of violations with increasing levels of liability
- Establishing four corresponding tiers of civil money penalties that significantly increase the minimum penalty amount for each violation
- Establishing a maximum civil money penalty amount of $1.5 million for all violations of an identical provision in a calendar year

- Eliminating the previous bar on the imposition of civil money penalties where there was no knowledge of the violation
- Prohibiting imposition of penalties for any violation that is not due to willful neglect and is corrected within a 30-day time period

Subject to a number of affirmative defenses, a civil money penalty may be imposed on a covered entity (or business associate) if DHHS determines that the covered entity (or business associate) has violated a provision of HIPAA. It is important to note that if the Secretary determines that more than one covered entity or business associate was responsible for a violation, the Secretary will impose a civil money penalty against each such covered entity or business associate. Additionally, a covered entity is liable for certain acts of an agent, including a workforce member or business associate, acting within the scope of the agency.

Civil money penalties range from $100 to $50,000 per violation, up to a maximum of $1.5 million per calendar year for violating the same requirement of the HIPAA rules. Criminal penalties are $50,000 and/or 1 year in prison for wrongful disclosure and up to $250,000 and/or 10 years in prison for an offense committed with intent to sell, transfer, or use PHI for commercial advantage. These penalties apply to both covered entities and business associates. Furthermore, the attorney general of any state may bring civil action for damages and may recover court costs and attorney fees.

## Emergency Medical Transfer and Active Labor Act

The Emergency Medical Treatment and Active Labor Act (EMTALA) requires all Medicare or Medicaid-participating hospitals with an emergency department to provide appropriate medical screening to each patient requesting emergency care to determine whether the patient requires such care.[30] Originally passed by Congress in 1985 as part of the Consolidated Omnibus Budget Reconciliation Act of 1985, EMTALA often is referred to as the "antidumping law" because it prohibits hospitals from transferring an emergency patient to another hospital simply because of the patient's inability to pay.

If emergency care is needed, the statute requires the hospital to medically stabilize the patient (assuming the hospital has the medical capabilities to do so),

---

[30]42 U.S.C. § 1395dd.

irrespective of the patient's ability to pay. Hospitals are prohibited from posting payment information in their emergency rooms. Patients who have medical conditions that the hospital is incapable of stabilizing (as certified by a physician) or who ask to be transferred to another facility before the hospital can stabilize their condition must be transferred to another facility in accordance with specific requirements of EMTALA. If after evaluation the patient is found not to have a medical emergency, the hospital's obligation to the patient under EMTALA ends.

EMTALA also requires that a Medicare- or Medicaid-participating hospital ensures that emergency department staff does not engage the patient in discussion regarding his or her financial or insurance information before conducting the medical screening examination and stabilization of the emergency condition. Hospitals may, however, commence normal registration procedures, which may include asking whether the patient carries insurance, as long as such procedures do not delay screening and stabilization.

To avoid EMTALA violations, hospitals should perform the following:

- Require all clinical, administrative, and contract staff to review and understand the EMTALA requirements.
- Ensure that all patients who decide to leave the hospital without receiving treatment or withdraw their request for emergency treatment are offered a medical examination and treatment within the hospital facilities before they leave, and that staff who can identify and stabilize a patient's medical condition always are available in the hospital to provide these services within the limits of the hospital staff's medical capabilities.
- Ensure that all reasonable steps are taken to obtain the patient's written informed consent to refuse any examination or treatment services, and that the patient's medical record contains a description of the examination, treatment, or both as well as documentation of the patient's refusal to receive emergency care.
- Ensure that emergency department staff have reviewed and understand all statutory requirements regarding transfer of patients to another facility.
- Instruct hospital staff to refrain from asking patients to complete financial forms or inquiring about patients' financial or insurance status, even if the patient engages the staff in conversation, until the medical screening examination has been conducted and the patient's emergency medical condition has been stabilized.

## Tax Exemption Issues for Healthcare Organizations

Nonprofit HCOs are a significant part of the healthcare industry. At the state level, the traditional rule has historically been that state exemption usually follows from federal tax exemption. While that still remains mostly true, a noteworthy trend seems to indicate that states will no longer uniformly follow federal determinations with respect to tax-exempt status.[31]

The most common way for an HCO to achieve tax-exempt status is via § 501(c)(3) of the Internal Revenue Code. The Internal Revenue Service (IRS) not only enforces the code, but also provides guidance to assist in understanding the rules surrounding tax-exempt organizations.

### Qualification as a § 501(c)(3) Organization

There are two advantages to qualifying as a tax-exempt organization under § 501(c)(3) rather than a different section of the code. First, § 501(c)(3) organizations are eligible for tax-exempt financing. Second, donors who make contributions to § 501(c)(3) organizations can deduct the donation to the fullest extent permitted under the code.

Organizations may qualify as § 501(c)(3) if they are charitable, religious, educational, or scientific in nature. The IRS has found that the "promotion of health" is a charitable purpose.[32] Therefore, most § 501(c)(3) HCOs qualify as organizations by being both organized and operated for charitable purposes.

To be organized for charitable purposes, an organization must include limits in its articles of incorporation by enumerating the charitable purposes and disallowing all but an insubstantial part of its activities any activities that are (1) not in furtherance of the charitable purposes, (2) attempting to influence legislation, (3) influencing or participating in a political campaign of a candidate for public office, or (4) have objectives that characterize it as an action organization. Furthermore, the organization must be required to distribute its assets upon dissolution to one or more exempt purposes.

A § 501(c)(3) organization must also comply with the operational requirements of § 501(c)(3). The organization must meet four requirements:

1. *Primary purpose*: An organization must engage "primarily" in activities that accomplish one or more exempt purposes, and no

---

[31]http://www.modernhealthcare.com/article/20151111/NEWS/151119974

[32]Rev. Rul. 69-545, 1969-2 C.B. 117.

more than an insubstantial part of its activities can be toward a nonexempt purpose.

2. *Private inurement*: The net earnings of an organization may not "inure" to the benefit of private shareholders or individuals.

3. *Public benefit*: The organization must serve a public rather than a private interest and may not be operated for the benefit of private interests, such as individuals, the creator, shareholders, or other persons controlled by such private interests.

4. *Lobbying or political activities*: No substantial part of an organization's activities may constitute the carrying on of propaganda or attempting to influence legislation or participate in a political campaign on behalf of any candidate for public office.

## Public Charity Versus Private Foundation

Organizations with § 501(c)(3) status are either public charity or private foundation organizations. Being a private foundation has a number of disadvantages. For example, private foundations are taxed on investment income and have certain restrictions on how their funds may be spent and invested. In addition, tax deductions on individual contributions to private foundations are more limited than those to public charities. Finally, private foundations must file additional reports not required of public charities.

Every § 501(c)(3) organization is considered a "private foundation" unless it fits within one of the specific forms of "public charity."[33] A § 501(c)(3) organization may meet public charity requirements as a result of its status if the organization is a church, a hospital, an educational organization, or a governmental unit. In addition, an organization qualifies as a public charity if it is "publicly supported"—that is, if it normally receives at least one-third of its total support from the government and/or public donations. Finally, if a § 501(c)(3) organization is not publicly supported and does not meet a status requirement, it may be a public charity only where it is operated exclusively for the benefit of one or more organizations that independently qualify as a public charity and is operated, supervised, or controlled by such organization.

As noted above, hospitals with § 501(c)(3) status automatically qualify as public charities. In regulations, the IRS has defined "hospital" to include not only traditional inpatient hospitals but also rehabilitation institutions, outpatient clinics, or community mental health or drug treatment centers if the principal purpose or function is the providing of hospital care or the treatment of any physical or mental disability or condition, whether on an inpatient or outpatient basis, provided that the cost of such treatment is deductible to the patient. However, a hospital in this context does not include long-term care facilities that do not provide medical services or healthcare management companies.[34]

## Charity Care

As stated above, the IRS has found that the "promotion of health" is a charitable purpose. In addition, the tax-exempt organization does not need to provide a direct benefit to all members of the community, but the organization must ensure that the group of potential beneficiaries of the organization is not so small that there is no benefit to the community. This "community benefit" standard is further defined by the IRS to include a hospital that operates an emergency room open to everyone regardless of means or healthcare coverage and that provides nonemergency hospital care to everyone in the community able to pay for such care.

The IRS has not historically required nonemergency charity care as a requirement for a hospital's tax-exempt status. However, for other healthcare entities or a hospital without an emergency department, the IRS has indicated that a charity care policy is an important factor in determination of the organization's tax-exempt status.

In addition, the community benefit standard also includes who controls the operations of the organization. Specifically, who sits on the organization's board of directors, whether the hospital has an open medical staff policy, whether it accepts and treats Medicare and Medicaid patients, and whether it uses surplus funds to improve facilities, equipment, and patient care and to provide health-related education, training, and research are fundamental to the community benefit analysis.

The ACA imposes new requirements on nonprofit hospitals related to charity care requirements. Specifically, nonprofit hospitals will be required to (1) engage in a mandated triennial community health needs assessment and related plan to address the community's needs, (2) maintain written financial assistance and emergency care policies, (3) charge uninsured patients only the lowest rate charged to insured

[33]26 U.S.C. § 509.

[34]Treas. Reg. § 1.170A-9(c)(1).

patients for emergency or other medically necessary care, and (4) make reasonable efforts to determine whether a patient is eligible for the previously mentioned financial assistance policy before engaging in extraordinary measures for collection.

The new rules apply to any "hospital organization," defined as any organization that operates a facility that is required to be licensed or registered as a hospital under state law, as well as any organization that the Secretary of the Treasury Department determines provides hospital care as the principal basis for its tax exemption. For a hospital organization that operates more than one hospital facility, the organization must meet the new requirements separately for each facility and will lose § 501(c)(3) status with respect to any facility that does not separately meet the new requirements.

## Unrelated Business Income Tax

If a § 501(c)(3) organization realizes income from activities outside of its specific exempt functions, it may have to pay tax on that amount, referred to as unrelated business income tax (UBIT). UBIT prevents tax-exempt organizations from unfairly competing with for-profit entities in the marketplace.

UBIT is imposed on income to a tax-exempt organization from an unrelated trade or business.[35] An unrelated trade or business exists where three factors are met:

1. The activity constitutes a trade or business, generally meaning the sale of goods or services in exchange for income.
2. The activity is regularly carried on, meaning that it is conducted in a manner comparable with competing for-profit taxable entities. An activity is not regularly carried on if it only occurs once per year.
3. The activity is not substantially related to the exempt purposes of the organization. An activity is substantially related where there is a substantial causal relationship between the activity and the exempt purpose. The IRS has found that just because an activity is a source of funding for an exempt purpose does not make it substantially related.

Certain activities are specifically excluded from the definition of "unrelated trade or business" under the code. Specifically, a trade or business in which substantially all work is performed by volunteers,

carried on for the convenience of an organization's members, students, patients, officers or employees; the sale of goods, substantially all of which are **donations**; certain entertainment or trade show activities; and a few other very narrow exceptions.

A tax-exempt HCO's income is not subject to UBIT if the income is in the form of **dividends**, interest, royalties, certain rent of real property, gain from the sale of noninventory property, or research income. Tax-exempt organizations must report UBIT on their annual Form 990 filings with the IRS, discussed later. In addition, excessive UBIT could lead to loss of tax-exempt status. Generally, an organization should be concerned where more than one-fourth of its total revenues are derived from unrelated trade or business activities.

The IRS has specifically commented on a number of business activities in which HCOs commonly participate. For example, the IRS has found that both pharmacy sales and laboratory tests performed by a tax-exempt HCO are substantially related to exempt purposes and therefore income is exempt from taxes, where sales are to, or tests are performed for, patients. However, sales to nonpatients are subject to UBIT. The IRS defined patients as people who are (1) admitted as inpatients, (2) treated at the entity's outpatient facilities, (3) referred to an outpatient facility for diagnosis or treatment, (4) refilling prescriptions received during treatment as a patient, (5) receiving medical services as part of a hospital-administered home care program, or (6) receiving medical services in a hospital-affiliated extended care facility.

In addition, the IRS generally has found that cafeterias, gift shops, and parking facilities at tax-exempt hospitals are substantially related to the hospital's exempt purpose. However, management or consulting to unrelated entities generally results in unrelated taxable income. Income from billing services may or may not be taxable, based on the facts.

## Form 990

Tax-exempt § 501(c)(3) HCOs are required to file an annual disclosure form with the IRS called Form 990. Information provided to the IRS on the Form 990 is open for public inspection, with the exception of the organization's contributors. The organization must make available its three most recent Form 990s for inspection and copying at certain offices of the organization. In addition, Form 990-T, the annual return form for UBIT, is subject to the same public disclosure requirements as the Form 990 information return.[36]

[35]26 U.S.C. §§ 511–14.

[36]26 U.S.C. §§ 6033 & 6104.

The Form 990 has evolved over the years, through statutory changes, input through public comment, and based on information gathered by the IRS when auditing tax-exempt organizations. In December 2007 the IRS issued a significantly redesigned Form 990, which has individualized schedules depending on the type of tax-exempt organization. The new Schedule H, specific to HCOs, requires more detail regarding how the organization is satisfying the community benefit standard, discussed previously.

An organization that is required to file a Form 990 but fails to do so is penalized $20 per day or $100 per day if the organization has annual gross receipts exceeding $1 million. In addition, if the IRS makes a written demand for filing a Form 990 on a reasonable, future date after one failure to file, the individuals responsible for the failure to meet the second deadline will be personally liable for $10 per day of continued failure.[37]

## Antitrust in Health Care

The purpose of the antitrust laws is to promote a competitive, free marketplace; these laws are intended to protect the public from the adverse effects of monopoly power and business practices that unreasonably restrain trade. The federal government and all state governments have antitrust laws, which reflect a public policy principle that a competitive marketplace protects consumers, restrains private economic power, and generally produces the best allocation of quality goods and services at the lowest prices.

The three main sources of federal antitrust law are the Sherman Act, the Clayton Act, and the Federal Trade Commission Act. Section 1 of the Sherman Act prohibits all conspiracies or agreements that restrain trade. Section 2 of the Sherman Act prohibits monopolization. Section 7 of the Clayton Act prohibits all mergers and acquisitions of stock or assets that may substantially lessen competition or that tend to create a monopoly. Section 5 of the Federal Trade Commission Act prohibits unfair methods of competition.

## Sherman Act

As interpreted by the courts, Section 1 of the Sherman Act applies to agreements that unreasonably restrain trade, which may include agreements or conspiracies to fix prices, divide market territories or groups of customers, boycott other firms, or use coercive tactics with the intent and effect of injuring competition. Some types of conduct, such as agreements among firms to fix prices or divide markets, are on their face antitrust violations and are called "per se" violations. Actions not considered per se violations are evaluated under the more lenient "rule of reason."

The Sherman Act penalizes conduct that is likely to result in higher prices or lower quality of services to the ultimate consumer. Many business practices that are penalized under the Sherman Act may have a business justification but are deemed illegal because they "unreasonably" restrain trade (i.e., the anticompetitive effect of the business practices outweigh their pro-business justifications). An example of such a practice would be a "noncompete" clause prohibiting the seller of a business from ever engaging in a similar business activity. Although such a noncompete clause might be justified on business grounds to protect the value of the business acquired by the buyer, the clause's provision could nevertheless unreasonably restrain trade if it is not geographically and temporally reasonable. Some practices, however, are penalized because there are no acceptable justifications for the conduct. An example of such a practice is an agreement among competitors to fix prices.

Price-fixing concerns arise in the healthcare setting where physician organizations (POs), physician hospital organizations (PHOs), or other networks of otherwise unaffiliated healthcare providers negotiate with payers as a group. Keep in mind, where healthcare providers are all owned by the same parent, sharing price information is always acceptable. However, otherwise independent providers negotiating as a unit without meeting certain requirements is considered price fixing and violates antitrust law. From an antitrust perspective, these providers may be viewed as competitors that are jointly setting the price they will charge for their services. However, there are a number of contexts in which POs and PHOs can legally assist providers with negotiating payer agreements. These are discussed further later in this chapter.

Enforcement of antitrust laws is jointly shared by the Department of Justice (DOJ) and the Federal Trade Commission (FTC), and the agencies have largely overlapping jurisdiction. Over the years the agencies have developed expertise in particular industries or markets. For example, the FTC devotes most of its resources to certain segments of the economy, including those where consumer spending is high: health care, pharmaceuticals, professional services, food, energy, and certain high-tech industries like computer technology and Internet services. When issuing guidance the agencies have historically come to an agreement on how to enforce a certain area of antitrust law.

---

[37]26 U.S.C. § 6652.

In August 1996 the Department of Justice and FTC issued their current guidelines, *Statements of Antitrust Enforcement Policy in Health Care*, outlining general enforcement policies regarding certain types of practices of healthcare providers. The 1996 *Statements* specify how agencies will apply the antitrust laws to nine types of conduct of hospitals, physicians, nursing homes, and other providers, such as joint purchasing, information exchange, and formation of PHOs.

The ninth policy statement applies to any organization composed of various types of providers that combine to jointly offer healthcare services, including POs and PHOs. According to the statement, if members of the network offer only complementary or unrelated services, they do not compete and there are no antitrust concerns. If a group of competing providers forms the network, however, the antitrust agencies are concerned that the network may interfere with competition and with the market efficiencies that competition protects. To address these concerns, the antitrust agencies identified ways in which PHOs and others may be structured to create incentives for providers to operate efficiently even in the absence of competition.

One way in which provider networks can minimize the antitrust risks associated with joint conduct is by sharing "substantial" financial risk, referred to as "financial integration." Financial integration can be achieved, for example, if the compensation each provider receives through the network depends on the overall performance of the network as a whole. For example, a network may negotiate capitated payer agreements with health maintenance organizations because the network is provided a flat amount per beneficiary and as a result bears the financial risk when providing services. Alternatively, a PHO could receive a fixed amount for a "package" of complex or extended services delivered by its participating providers, even though services may require numerous providers and the aggregate cost of furnishing services might vary significantly from patient to patient. For example, a system consisting of a hospital, obstetricians/gynecologists, pediatricians, and anesthesiologists could collectively agree to furnish all necessary prenatal, delivery, and post-delivery services to enrollees for a fixed fee.

As an alternative, the antitrust agencies suggest that a network may be able to adopt and strictly enforce clinical standards that guarantee the efficient delivery of care even in the absence of risk sharing or competition, referred to as "clinical integration." The FTC has approved a number of existing clinically integrated networks through a series of advisory opinions, which have provided guidance regarding exactly what is required to jointly negotiate with payers. The lessons learned from these opinions include the importance of evidence-based clinical practice guidelines, including data collection mechanisms for measuring performance; participation and buy-in from all physicians, including primary care and specialists; and that the network not be exclusive and not have market power in the community. With the increased incentives for adopting electronic health records, some PHOs and POs have used the opportunity to begin adopting the data collection systems to implement the required systems for analyzing network participant performance against clinical standards toward implementing a fully clinically integrated panel.

Where there is neither financial integration nor clinical integration, a network may not jointly contract for its providers, for example, for a general fee-for-service payer agreement. However, the "messenger model" is a means of allowing networks to assist their providers in contracting without joint negotiation. An acceptable messenger model exists where there are significant safeguards against providers sharing rate information with one another. When the network and payer want to enter into an agreement for provider services, the payer suggests a certain compensation level, which the network "messengers" to its providers. Each provider then either accepts the offer or counters with its own offer. In this way the network assists providers with payer contracting, but rate information is not shared in violation of antitrust law.

As previously explained, healthcare reform has encouraged a variety of collaborative relationships between payers and providers in the interest of reducing cost and improving quality. One such initiative is the MSSP, which establishes provider-controlled contracting networks known as ACOs. If the ACOs' participants include otherwise independent providers who join together to provide an array of services and contract with payers, the Sherman Act's prohibition on agreements that restrain trade is logically implicated.

Accordingly, in response to concerns by providers interested in forming ACOs, the FTC and DOJ released the 2011 *Statement of Antitrust Enforcement Policy Regarding Accountable Care Organizations Participating in the Medicare Shared Savings Program* (the "Policy Statement"). Despite the Policy Statement's reference to the MSSP only, the Agencies have made clear that it is intended to ensure that "health care providers have the antitrust clarity and guidance needed to form procompetitive ACOs that participate in both Medicare and commercial markets." Consistent with earlier pronouncements in similar contexts, the Policy

Statement indicates that the permissibility of an ACO arrangement will turn, in large measure, on whether its participants are either financially or clinically integrated. Financial integration is analyzed using the approach outlined above, while clinical integration exists where the ACO meets CMS's eligibility conditions for participation in the MSSP program (which concern establishing a formal legal structure, a leadership and management structure that includes clinical and administrative processes, and other factors). In other words, so long as an ACO meets CMS's eligibility requirements, it will be subject to antitrust review under a deferential "rule-of-reason" approach.

In order to further insulate itself from antitrust scrutiny, an ACO may attempt to operate in a way that would bring it within an antitrust "safety zone." The Policy Statement explains that an ACO is within the "safety zone" where—among other requirements—its participants neither (1) demonstrate an impermissible control of a given market for services, as measured by the ACO's percentage of the market share, nor (2) require participants to exclusively contract with payers via the ACO. The Policy Statement explains that even if an ACO does not fall within the "safety zone," its conduct "may be pro-competitive and legal," but its participants should take care to ensure that certain safeguards are implemented (such as prohibitions on sharing competitively sensitive information and tying arrangements).

## Clayton Act

Section 7 of the Clayton Act prohibits mergers and acquisitions that may substantially lessen competition "in any line of commerce … in any section of the country."[38] Enacted in 1914 the Clayton Act made price discrimination, tying and exclusive dealing contracts, mergers of competing companies, and interlocking directorates illegal but not criminal.

Under the Clayton Act either the DOJ or FTC may investigate a merger or joint venture between two or more hospitals, although the FTC has tended to handle most hospital merger investigations. These agencies have established a procedure for deciding, on the basis of staff expertise, prior dealings with the parties involved, and caseload, which agency investigates a particular merger or joint venture. Although either agency may investigate a merger or joint venture for civil violations, once criminal conduct is suspected, the case is referred to DOJ. Private parties and state attorneys general may also sue to block

mergers or joint ventures under either the Sherman or Clayton Act.

The Hart-Scott-Rodino Antitrust Improvements Act of 1976 requires that parties notify both the FTC and DOJ of certain mergers, acquisitions, joint ventures, or tender offers before consummation of the agreements.[39] Parties satisfying the HSR filing thresholds (currently, transactions where assets or voting securities valued in excess of $78.2 million are being acquired) are required to file HSR forms with the agencies and then wait 30 days before consummating the transaction. Based on information provided in the HSR forms, the DOJ and FTC decide whether to allow the proposed merger to proceed or, if the transaction raises potential competition concerns, to extend the HSR waiting period and investigate the transaction more thoroughly. The investigation may involve issuance of a "Second Request" for additional information, after which the agencies will decide whether to challenge the proposed merger or collaboration as a potential violation of antitrust laws.

Reviews of potentially problematic mergers often include interviews of customers and competitors, as well as an in-depth analysis of the marketplace. The views of customers are particularly important to the merger analysis and have proven to be a source of valuable evidence in cases where the agencies have sought to challenge a transaction.

The DOJ/FTC *Horizontal Merger Guidelines*, issued in 1992 and subsequently revised in 2010, outline the general analytical methodology used by the agencies in deciding if they will challenge a merger. In most cases, the agencies will first determine the relevant market(s) impacted by the transaction and whether the merger will result in market concentration levels that indicate a likelihood of anticompetitive effects. If not, then the analysis generally will typically not proceed any further. However, if so, then the agencies will assess the significance of the anticompetitive concerns, taking into account whether another competitor can make a timely market entry to deter or counteract the competitive concern. Then, the agencies will assess any merger-specific efficiencies resulting from the transaction, and may also consider ancillary issues, such as whether either party to the merger would fail absent the merger, resulting in the failing party's assets exiting the market.

Since the ACA's enactment in 2010, the agencies have shown an increased willingness to challenge mergers and acquisitions by both hospitals and physician practices. In the hospital context, the FTC

---

[38]15 U.S.C. § 18.

[39]15 U.S.C. § 18a.

challenged a merger agreement between ProMedica and St. Luke's, the largest and fourth largest hospital providers in the Toledo, Ohio area. After a 5-year legal battle with the FTC, ProMedica was forced to divest St. Luke's. Other FTC challenges to hospital mergers include the 2015 merger of two large Chicago-area health systems (Advocate Health Care and North-Shore University Health System), as well as the 2015 merger of a large medical center and health system in Pennsylvania (Penn State Hershey Medical Center and Pinnacle Health System).

In the physician acquisition context, the FTC has been similarly eager to challenge what it views as anti-competitive conduct by hospitals and health systems. In 2012, the FTC challenged Renown Health's successive acquisitions of 15 and 16 physician cardiology practices in Reno, Nevada, claiming that the acquisition would result in Renown controlling 88% of the market for adult cardiology services. To resolve the allegations, Renown entered into a consent decree requiring a rare "structural" remedy: divestiture. Specifically, Renown agreed to release 10 cardiologists from their contractual noncompete provisions, allowing them to work at competing practices without penalty.

## Third-Party Payer Contracts

Patients generally do not pay out of pocket for their healthcare services and supplies. Therefore, every healthcare provider needs to be able to seek reimbursement from the **third-party payer** that is responsible for the patient's healthcare costs. There is a variety of payers, as well as a variety of products payers offer, that healthcare providers may encounter. It is important to understand the differences and regulatory structures through which payer agreements are regulated.

Payers may be public or private. The most significant public payers are Medicare and Medicaid, which were discussed earlier. In addition, the State Children's Health Insurance Program, the armed services health plan, and Federal Employees Health Benefits Program are all examples of public payers.

Private payers offer products in the form of insurance, in which the payer collects premiums to finance health benefits. The insurance plan then bears the risk and pays the provider for a beneficiary's healthcare services based on the rules of the plan. Other times, an insurance company or other third-party administrator may administrate a program for a self-funded employer or other organization. Self-funded plans are employers or other organizations that collect the premiums, bear the risk, and are liable for the cost of beneficiaries' healthcare services to the providers but pay the administrator to process claims.

Payers often have any number of products available to employers and beneficiaries. The products fall into one of the following four categories.

## Traditional Indemnity or Fee-for-Service

Early hospital and medical plans offered by insurance companies paid either a fixed amount for specific diseases or medical procedures (schedule benefits) or a percentage of the provider's fee. The patient received medical care and was responsible for paying the provider. If the service was covered by the policy, the insurance company was responsible for reimbursing the patient based on the provisions of the insurance contract. Health insurance plans that are not based on a network of contracted providers or that base payments on a percentage of provider charges are still described as indemnity or fee-for-service plans. These plans are less common.

## Managed Care

**Managed care** products are based on a panel or network of contracted healthcare providers. **Preferred provider organizations** contract with providers to secure certain rates but also reimburse a certain smaller percentage of healthcare services provided by out-of-network providers. Exclusive provider organizations only reimburse providers within the network. Both preferred provider and exclusive provider organizations reimburse providers on a fee-for-service basis, either as a percentage of costs or pursuant to a negotiated fee schedule. Managed care network plans often include:

- A set of selected providers that furnish a comprehensive array of healthcare services to enrollees
- Explicit standards for selecting providers
- Formal utilization review and quality improvement programs

## Health Maintenance Organizations

A **health maintenance organization** (HMO) is a type of **managed care organization** that provides healthcare coverage that is fulfilled through a specific closed network. An HMO covers only care rendered by those doctors and other professionals who have agreed to treat patients in accordance with the HMO's guidelines and restrictions. Providers may be employees of the HMO ("staff model"), employees of a provider group that has contracted with the HMO ("group model"), or members of an independent practice association ("IPA model"). HMOs may also use a combination of these approaches. HMOs reimburse providers on a capitated basis, meaning that the **provider network** receives a fixed fee for each patient, and the risk that the patient will use more or fewer resources is therefore shifted to the providers.

## Self-Insured Plans

Self-insured plans are health plans sponsored by an employer or organization and offered to employees or members through which the employer or organization retains the risk associated with the plan. Self-insured plans often enter into an administrative services only arrangement for administration of the plan with an insurance company or third-party administrators. The administrative services only arrangement ensures that the risk stays with the self-insured group; the insurance company or third-party administrator merely provides certain claims, billing, medical management, and/or other administrative services. Self-insured plans may include any of a variety of products described above, including indemnity plans, preferred provider organizations, or HMOs.

## State Law

In general, insurance is regulated primarily at the state level. Each state has its own specific laws regulating health insurance plans. The activities of the organization determine the different licensure requirements. For example, private payers that are risk-bearing entities are subject to the licensure requirements of the state insurance department. In addition, selling a specific insurance product in a state likely requires state licensure for that product by the insurance department. Finally, states often require specific third-party administrator licensure where entities provide administrative services only.

States may have a variety of laws regulating payer plans and payer–provider agreements. For example, "any willing provider" laws require a managed care organization to enter into an agreement with any provider who meets the requirements of that network or product. Some states require continuity of care provisions, which require providers to treat a patient either for a fixed period of time or for the duration of an illness, regardless of whether benefits through the managed care organization have been terminated. States may also require a managed care organization or HMO to cover emergency services, even if those services are provided out of network under a closed-network policy. Another important state insurance regulation concerns a practice known as "balance billing." Balance billing occurs when a provider bills a patient for all charges not paid for by the patient's insurance plan (e.g., where an out-of-network emergency room seeks

to bill a patient for nonemergency services that the insurer refuses to pay). While most states allow some measure of balance billing, many regulate the types of services and patients that can be balance billed. Especially in states with restrictive balance billing laws (e.g., New York's "Surprise Bill" Law), a provider's uncompensated care costs can be affected by balance billing restrictions.

Certain state laws enforce protections for providers against certain acts of managed care organizations. For example, a payer may be required to disclose medical review criteria and other policies and procedures to providers. Payers may be subject to "prompt pay" laws, requiring that "clean claims," or claims made consistent with payer requirements, are paid within a certain period of time. States may also disallow managed care organizations from requiring providers from participating in all plans rather than just those plans in which the provider chooses to participate.

## Federal Law

Self-insurance plans are regulated by the Employee Retirement Income Security Act of 1974 (ERISA).[40] Plans subject to ERISA must include certain mandated benefits and other requirements that protect members of the self-funded plan. ERISA preemption (areas where the federal ERISA law preempts state insurance law) is subject to complex rules that have been evolving over time through court cases. ERISA provides three standards used to determine the extent of preemption:

1. If a state law "relates to" a self-funded plan governed by ERISA, then the federal ERISA preempts state law.
2. State laws "regulating insurance" avoid ERISA preemption.
3. Self-funded employee benefit plans are not considered insurance companies by states, so state insurance laws do not apply to such plans.

With the enactment of the ACA in 2010, the federal government now heavily regulates many aspects of insurance in a way that traditionally was the province of state government. While an in-depth exploration of the ACA's impact on insurers is beyond the scope of this chapter, a few of the most important ACA provisions are detailed here. It should be noted that several ACA reforms apply only to individual and small group insurance plans, while others also apply to large group insurance plans.

---

[40]29 U.S.C. § 1001 *et seq.*

First, insurers are required to spend a certain portion of premiums received (between 80 and 85%, depending on the type of insurer) on care and quality improvement. If an insurer fails to meet these requirements, it must issue a rebate to either the group policyholder or to individual participants.

Second, insurers are responsible for paying several annual fees, which are used in part to fund research to improve healthcare delivery and outcomes. These fees vary depending on number of covered lives, type of insurer, rate of premium growth, and other factors.

Third, insurers are required to sell plans containing coverage for "essential health benefits," a category that includes ambulatory patient services, emergency services, hospitalization, maternity and newborn care, mental health and substance use disorder services, prescription drugs, rehabilitative and habilitative services and devices, laboratory services, preventive and wellness services and chronic disease management, and pediatric services, including oral and vision care.

Fourth, insurers must provide coverage for preexisting conditions (i.e., medical conditions that existed when benefits under a plan commenced).

Fifth, when determining premium rates for certain plans, insurers may consider only whether the plan is for individual or family coverage, geographic rating area, age, and tobacco use. This requirement effectively disallows consideration of many factors that were once central to premium rate determinations (e.g., health status, gender, industry, and use of an intermediary to obtain health coverage).

Sixth, the ACA imposes a 40% excise tax on any "excess benefit" provided through certain types of employer-sponsored, high cost health coverage. Commonly referred to as the "Cadillac Tax," this controversial measure has been delayed until 2020, but will likely be the target of repeal efforts before then. Should it go into effect, the Cadillac Tax seeks to lower healthcare expenditures by limiting overutilization of care, which proponents argue frequently accompanies plans that allow covered individuals to seek care with little regard for out-of-pocket expenses.

Seventh, the ACA created the reinsurance, risk corridor, and risk adjustment programs (3Rs), which will likely have a profound impact on how risk is redistributed among carriers in certain markets.

## Clinical Integration

Since the 1980s, the American healthcare system has experienced an increase in clinical integration (CI). CI occurs where a network of otherwise independent physicians collectively commit to deliver high-quality, cost-effective care to patients by working closely with one another. While participants in a clinically integrated network (CIN) often remain organized in separate legal structures, their combined bargaining power gives them leverage in negotiations with—and the ability to extract more favorable reimbursement rates from—commercial payers. While they have enjoyed a resurgence, CI models are not new. Previous decades have seen competing physicians organizing in both independent practice associations (IPAs) and physician hospital organizations (PHOs) to negotiate jointly with payers.

Generally speaking, CINs are multispecialty in nature and involve some or all of the following attributes:

- A set of clinical and administrative metrics defining the CIN's performance improvement goals
- Membership limited to those physicians able to advance those goals
- A system to monitor physician attainment of these goals
- A physician-led governance structure—supported by administrative staff—to oversee program operations
- A health information technology (HIT) infrastructure to identify improvement opportunities and facilitate the exchange of patient information among participants
- Performance-based payment incentives to incentivize physician productivity
- Joint contracting with commercial payers for physician services

While CINs and ACOs both seek to encourage collaborative relationships among HCOs in the interest of quality, cost-efficient care, there are two distinctions worth emphasizing. First, while CI efforts are focused on improving care by physician practices across specialty types, ACOs focus on care improvement for an entire patient population across the entire care continuum (including, in addition to physicians, hospitals, post-acute care providers, and others). Second, while a CIN can serve as the basis for an ACO, not every CIN takes the additional steps required to become an ACO. For example, a CIN might choose to focus primarily on basic quality and efficiency improvement metrics without taking on the full spectrum of care coordination and population health management functions needed to succeed in the reimbursement risk–heavy ACO model.

## Payer–Provider Convergence

Payer–provider convergence is defined as the joining of disparate subsectors within the healthcare industry that previously operated separately.

Payers have been acquiring provider groups, allowing them to realize several benefits, including (1) market share gains, as patients change plans to maintain their current providers, (2) increased customer satisfaction through expanded provider networks, and (3) improved coordination between the financial and clinical aspects of the care continuum.

While payers are increasingly performing many of the functions traditionally associated with providers, the same can also be said of providers who have taken steps to form health plans of their own. According to 2015 data, roughly 13% of health systems currently offer a health plan. Collectively, these 107 systems operate health plans covering 18 million members, approximately 8% of all insured lives. Benefits to a health system of offering a health plan include the potential for increased volume, the opportunity to leverage economies of scale and skill, the creation of strategic option value for the future (e.g., through revamped utilization management efforts), lower barriers to entry in many markets, and preserving market competition in areas dominated by a few payers.

While the distinction between traditional payer and provider functions is unlikely to collapse entirely, ACA-driven payment reforms will eventually require most providers and payers to achieve a level of clinical integration that promotes the delivery of quality, cost-efficient care. While the appropriate level of clinical integration for a given organization must be determined on a case-by-case basis, an ability to appreciate the challenges and opportunities presented by post-reform payment models is essential for successful navigation of this ever-changing landscape.

### *Learning Objective 7*

Be prepared to respond to a compliance audit or investigation, particularly when the subject of that inquiry includes financial records.

## ▶ Legal Audits and Investigations

A legal audit or investigation is a complete review of an organization's legal obligations where violation of the obligations could result in the imposition of civil or criminal sanctions. An HCO is exposed to many areas of risk where legal audits and investigations, as part of a robust and comprehensive compliance program, should occur on a routine and ongoing basis. Some of the more notable areas of the law under which audits and investigations may occur include the FCA, Medicare and Medicaid laws, HIPAA, ERISA, and federal and state self-referral and anti-kickback laws.

Legal audits and investigations are formalized and structured processes that result in reliable reports that an organization and/or an outside investigational agency can rely on to determine whether any laws or regulations have been violated and if so, the extent of liability and potential harm. Only if an investigation or audit is conducted by or under the direction of an attorney, will the attorney–client privilege or work product doctrine apply to the interviews, records, and reports produced by the investigation or audit. Accordingly, it is essential to structure the audit or investigation to meet the elements of the attorney–client privilege and work product doctrine. Engaging outside counsel, as opposed to inside counsel, to direct or conduct the audit or investigation enhances the claim of attorney–client privilege and work product doctrine.

From the beginning of the audit or investigation it should be expressly documented, preferably by the governing body, that the purpose of the audit or investigation is to secure legal advice for the organization. Counsel should be empowered to direct all aspects of the audit or investigation, and all employees should be directed to cooperate fully and exclusively with counsel. Furthermore, all reports and records should be marked "private and confidential," "attorney–client privilege," and "attorney work product" as appropriate and maintained in a segregated and secure file system. Finally, all audit and investigation reports issued by counsel should reflect counsel's legal advice and risk assessment to improve the likelihood of maintaining protections of the attorney–client privilege and work product doctrine.

The audit and investigation team, led by or conducted by counsel, should include members who are independent of physicians and line management; have access to existing audit and healthcare resources, relevant personnel, and all relevant areas of operation; can present written evaluative reports on compliance activities to the CEO, governing body, and members of the compliance committee on a regular basis; and specifically identify areas where corrective actions are needed. Although it is important that the team include employees of the organization, those team members should not be involved with a review of an area over which they are responsible. Additionally, the team may include consultants with specific content knowledge of clinical areas, accounting, or billing and coding. For purposes of retaining attorney–client privilege, any outside consultants preparing reports or records should be engaged by counsel.

Once chartered by the governing body or senior management and counsel is engaged, an audit or investigation begins with the preparation of a detailed audit plan. The audit plan identifies all areas and subject matter to be reviewed and the specific areas of interest to the audit team.

An audit or investigation may use a variety of techniques, including site visits, interviews with management operations, coding, claims processing, patient care, and other related reviews; questionnaires developed to solicit impressions of a broad cross section of the organization's employees and staff; reviews of related medical and financial records and other source documents; reviews of written materials and documentation prepared by the different divisions of the organization; and **trend analysis**, or longitudinal studies, that seeks deviations, positive or negative, in specific areas over a given period.

Violations of an organization's compliance program or failures to comply with applicable federal or state law may threaten an organization's status as a reliable, honest, and trustworthy provider capable of participating in federal healthcare programs. Detected but uncorrected misconduct can seriously endanger the mission, reputation, and legal status of the organization. Accordingly, if an audit or investigation identifies areas of suspected noncompliance, counsel should advise the governing body or senior management of the legal risks and an appropriate course of action that may include further investigation, specific remedies to mitigate harm, and perhaps an immediate referral to criminal and/or civil law enforcement authorities.

## Hospital Employment of Physicians

### Physician Employment Models

In the post-reform environment, hospitals and physicians are increasingly seeking to affiliate via employer–employee relationships, which better reflect the continued emergence of shared-risk models. Although physicians historically have resisted efforts to sacrifice a measure of autonomy by becoming hospital employees, this trend has begun to reverse itself, with approximately 43% of physicians working as employees in 2014. Given the expected increase in hospital employment of physicians, the remainder of this section focuses on two issues, compensation and billing, that frequently concern hospitals with physician employees.

### Physician Compensation

When determining the method by which to compensate its employed physicians, a hospital should begin by asking what behavior it seeks to incentivize. For example, under the (increasingly outdated) fee-for-service model a hospital would be reimbursed for the volume of services delivered by an employed physician, which incentivized hospitals to increase a physician's compensation in a way that would reward high-volume producers.

In the post-reform environment, however, reimbursement for physician services is increasingly tied not to the quantity of procedures performed, but to the quality of outcomes experienced by patients. For example, DHHS has announced an initiative designed to tie 90% of traditional payments for healthcare services to quality or value by the year 2018. Additionally, in 2015 Congress passed the Medicare Access and CHIP Reauthorization Act of 2015 (MACRA), which repealed the so-called "Doc Fix" in favor of a system that reimburses Medicare-participating physicians under one of two models, both of which are designed to expand pay-for-performance incentives.

### Physician Billing Issues

When a hospital bills for services rendered by employed physicians, it should be mindful of several issues, including billing/coding and cash management. For a thorough exploration of the billing issues that confront HCOs, refer to Chapters 2 and 22 of this text.

## ▶ SUMMARY

This chapter has provided a general overview of the laws and regulations that govern the healthcare industry. A financial manager can expect to be confronted by these types of legal issues and should plan to address them on a regular basis. The ACA has ushered in a period of even greater regulatory oversight as access to health care has been expanded and payment methods have been dramatically altered. The failure to understand the importance of these legal requirements can put an organization at significant financial risk and expose individuals to personal liability. Corporate compliance should be considered an essential element of every HCO's culture and the foundation of its financial security.

## ▶ ACKNOWLEDGMENTS

Peter A. Pavarini, Esq. is a partner in the Columbus, Ohio, office of Squire Patton Boggs (US) LLP (www. squirepattonboggs.com) and has focused his practice on the representation of healthcare providers in transactional and regulatory matters for over 30 years. He wishes to express his sincere appreciation for the capable assistance of James M. Hafner, Jr., Esq., an associate based in the Columbus, Ohio office of Squire Patton Boggs, in the preparation of this chapter.

## ASSIGNMENTS

1. Identify at least three federal statutes that may be implicated by the proposed restructuring of SSRH's cardiovascular service line.
2. How much reliance should a CFO place upon a CEO's assertion that a novel physician–hospital relationship has been approved by DHHS-OIG? How can a CFO be sure that a particular proposal is legally acceptable?
3. How has the ACA reshaped financial arrangements among hospitals, physicians, and other providers if Medicare makes a single payment for all care received by a beneficiary from 72 hours before admission to 30 days after discharge from an inpatient facility?
4. If Bravo wanted to see for himself whether SSRH's cardiovascular program was in fact at risk of being found out of compliance with Medicare's conditions of participation, how should he go about getting relevant patient documentation without violating the privacy requirements of HIPAA?
5. Based on his legal concerns about the proposed restructuring, Bravo believes that SSRH would be on firmer legal ground if the relationship with CCI was limited to private pay patients only and if HMO, Inc., a major managed care payer in the market, was also involved in the quality improvement program. Is he right, and why?
6. What suggestions would you have to improve SSRH's corporate compliance program given that Devine's proposal may never have been reviewed by legal counsel before going to the SSRH board?
7. If SSRH implemented a policy that the hospital's emergency department could not receive heart failure patients unless the patient had first contacted a CCI cardiologist, would EMTALA be implicated? How would you confirm that the hospital is not at risk of an EMTALA violation?
8. What federal law would be most implicated by CIO Tiffany Technophile's proposal? Are there safeguards available to ensure that one or both of the proposals remain compliant with this federal law?
9. Describe how new payment models are blurring the distinction between payers and providers.
10. Compare and contrast Medicare and Medicaid.
11. Discuss the various types of third-party payers.
12. What are the four operational requirements for a § 501(c)(3) tax-exempt organization?

## SOLUTIONS AND ANSWERS

1. A number of federal statutes may be implicated by the proposed restructuring of SSRH's cardiovascular service line, including (1) the Anti-Kickback Statute, (2) the Stark Law, (3) the False Claims Act, (4) the Internal Revenue Code, and (5) Patient Protection and Affordable Care Act.
2. The CFO should have a novel physician–hospital relationship reviewed by counsel. It is likely that the CEO is referring to an advisory opinion in which the OIG has reviewed a specific arrangement and indicated that the arrangement has a low risk for violating the Anti-Kickback Statute based on a certain set of facts. To ensure that SSRH's proposed arrangement has the same low risk as the arrangement approved by the OIG, the SSRH proposed arrangement must meet all of the requirements and have all of the safeguards indicated in the advisory opinion. All such arrangements should be reviewed by counsel to minimize risk of the significant civil and criminal penalties possible for any such violation.
3. Under the current Medicare reimbursement system, hospitals are reimbursed one amount for each inpatient admission at a given rate based on the characteristics and diagnosis of the patient. Once the patient is discharged,

Medicare reimburses outpatient providers for services to the patient directly per procedure or office visit. Therefore, hospitals and outpatient providers will need to determine how to divide one payment for all services provided throughout the 33-day period for services provided, regardless of provider or location. It is likely that as the ACA continues to be implemented, hospitals and outpatient providers will merge not only for ease of distribution of reimbursement, but also to more efficiently negotiate how a bundled payment is divided. Finally, post–acute care providers, such as nursing homes and home health providers, will have to work with hospitals and other outpatient providers to negotiate how they will be reimbursed for services provided within the 33-day period for which a bundled payment is provided.

4. Bravo is the CFO of a hospital, which is a covered entity under HIPAA. A covered entity is permitted to use protected health information for healthcare operations. Ensuring that a healthcare service line is in compliance with Medicare's conditions of participation is a part of the healthcare operations of the hospital. If Bravo requires outside assistance of a consultant or attorney to determine whether the Medicare conditions of participation are being met, such consultant or attorney would be a business associate under HIPAA. Therefore, before any patient information could be transferred, the consultant and SSRH must execute a business associate agreement ensuring that the protected health information is properly secured in compliance with HIPAA requirements.

5. Although Bravo is technically correct that the Anti-Kickback Statute and the Stark Law apply only where Medicare or another federal health care program is paying for healthcare services or items, such a plan is difficult and risky in practice. If CCI is truly limited to private pay patients, the arrangement need not meet the requirements of the Stark Law. The Anti-Kickback Statute need only be considered in the context of whether the arrangement could be used as remuneration in exchange for other referrals of Medicare or Medicaid beneficiaries.

   However, there is always a risk that patients may have Medicare as a secondary payer and the hospital would mistakenly bill Medicare or other government payer for services provided under the CCI arrangement. In addition, if the relationship with CCI includes HMO, Inc. as a third-party payer, it is very likely that HMO, Inc. includes a Medicare Advantage plan and/or a Medicaid managed care plan, both of which would implicate the Stark Law and the Anti-Kickback Statute. Therefore, limiting a service line to private payers in order to avoid the requirements of the Stark Law and the Anti-Kickback Statute is not the safest way to try to comply with the laws.

6. SSRH's corporate compliance program should require all new arrangements or affiliations with independent physicians or physician groups to be reviewed by counsel, especially when the relationship or affiliation is novel, and when the physicians are in a position to refer to the hospital.

7. EMTALA requires that if emergency care is needed, a hospital with an emergency department must medically stabilize the patient. Therefore, to limit the hospital's risk of an EMTALA violation, the emergency department should ensure that a patient is stable before inquiring whether the patient contacted a CCI cardiologist. SSRH is free to transfer the patient once the patient's condition has been stabilized.

8. HIPAA is the federal law most implicated by Technophile's proposal. In order to remain HIPAA compliant, the proposal—depending on its precise details once implemented—may benefit from one or more of the following safeguards: (1) obtain individual authorization that meets the requirements of the Privacy Standard, (2) de-identify data using an expert in statistical analysis, and/or (3) obtain approval from a Privacy Board or IRB in accordance with 45 C.F.R. § 164.512(i).

9. New payment models are blurring the distinction between payers and providers in several ways. First, a growing number of provider organizations (e.g., physician practices) are owned by health plans, which may seek to tie physician reimbursement to the quality and value of outcomes they produce. Second, sophisticated risk-sharing arrangements such as ACOs are encouraging providers to shoulder some of the risks previously borne (and realize some of the rewards previously limited to) payers. Third, providers who are especially well-positioned to deliver high-quality, cost-efficient care are forming their own health plans, eliminating the need to involve a separate payer in the care continuum.

10. Medicare is a social insurance program that provides health insurance coverage for individuals aged 65 and over and individuals with permanent disabilities. Benefits include hospital insurance, doctor's services, and prescription drug coverage. Medicaid is a safety net insurance program that provides health insurance coverage to poor and very sick individuals. The single largest expenditure under Medicaid is for nursing home care. While Medicare is funded and administered through the federal government, Medicaid is funded by the federal and state governments and is administered by state government.

11. Generally, third-party payers are either public or private. Public payers include Medicare, Medicaid, the Federal Employees Health Benefit Program, and the State Children's Health Insurance Program. There are specific eligibility

requirements for each program and some degree of cost sharing between the government and the individual beneficiary. Private payers are nongovernmental entities, regulated by state law, that offer packages of health insurance benefits to businesses and individuals. The types of plans include traditional indemnity fee-for-service plans, managed care plans, health maintenance organizations, and self-insured plans.

12. The four operational requirements for a § 501(c)(3) tax-exempt organization are (1) the organization must engage "primarily" in activities that accomplish one or more exempt purposes, and no more than an insubstantial part of its activities can be toward a nonexempt purpose; (2) the net earnings of an organization may not "inure" to the benefit of private shareholders or individuals; (3) the organization must serve a public rather than a private interest and may not be operated for the benefit of private interests, such as individuals, the creator, shareholders, or other persons controlled by such private interests; and (4) no substantial part of an organization's activities may constitute the carrying on of propaganda or attempting to influence legislation or participate in a political campaign on behalf of any candidate for public office.

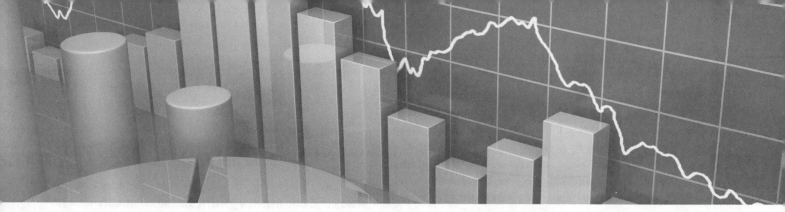

# CHAPTER 5
# Measuring Community Benefit

## LEARNING OBJECTIVES

After studying this chapter, you should be able to do the following:

1. Describe the current basis for tax exemption of not-for-profit healthcare firms.
2. Describe the elements of community benefit listed by key policy groups.
3. Assess the relative community benefits provided by proprietary and not-for-profit hospitals.
4. Develop a methodology for estimating financial benefits received by not-for-profit healthcare firms.
5. Develop a methodology for estimating financial benefits provided by not-for-profit healthcare firms.

## REAL-WORLD SCENARIO

Putnam Memorial Hospital has been the recipient of negative press coverage in their local paper. The negative publicity was precipitated by questions regarding the community benefit provided by the tax-exempt hospital in relationship to the taxes that the community has forgone, such as property taxes and local income tax. The paper has highlighted several key pieces of information regarding Putnam's recent performance. First, the newspaper documented the $1.6 million total compensation earned last year by the hospital's CEO, Douglas Marshall. Many of the paper's readers quickly identified with this point and questioned why any executive in a nonprofit setting should receive compensation at such lofty levels. The paper also noted that the hospital earned more than $40 million in profit last year and did not pay any tax on that profit nor did the hospital pay any property tax on their extensive real estate holdings. Furthermore, the paper cited huge cash reserves being held by the hospital—more than $100 million. The paper questioned why this money was not being used to pay the costs of uninsured patients. Levels of charity care provided by the hospital in the most recent year were less than 2% of revenue.

Mr. Marshall has been speaking with his financial staff about possible responses to the series of negative newspaper articles. Specifically, he wants to document the actual benefits that the hospital receives as a result of its tax-exempt status. He then wants to measure what benefits the hospital provides to the community that might not be provided if the hospital was not a charitable tax-exempt facility. Mr. Marshall believes that the benefits his hospital provides will far exceed the tax benefits received. He wants the computations done quickly and presented in a manner that a nonfinancial audience can understand so that he can diffuse the rising anger in the community against the hospital.

Most of the current interest in **community benefit** is related to nonprofit hospitals. The term *community benefit* is generally used to describe the scope of services and support (financial assistance or other) that a hospital provides to its community in return for its tax-exempt status. While not-for-profit healthcare firms exist in other healthcare sectors, the sheer size of hospitals as healthcare businesses makes them a more visible target for public scrutiny. According to the American Hospital Association (AHA), in 2014 about 78% of the 4,974 U.S. community hospitals were non-profit entities (58% private nonprofit and 20% operated by state or local governments). The remaining 22% are for-profit, investor-owned institutions. Tax exemption is the lightning rod that has attracted public attention. In addition to federal income tax exemptions, most not-for-profits receive taxation benefits in many other areas. For example, not-for-profits often do not pay any state or local income taxes; they usually do not pay property or sales taxes, and they can issue tax-exempt **bonds**.

Investor-owned hospitals have long argued that not-for-profit hospitals have received unfair tax advantages that make it harder for them to compete in markets where not-for-profit hospitals have large market share. More recently, federal and state governments have become interested in not-for-profit hospitals as a potential source of revenue. Most likely there will be significant changes in the tax profiles of not-for-profit hospitals and other not-for-profit firms in the decade ahead as demands for government funding accelerate.

---

### *Learning Objective 1*

Describe the current basis for tax exemption of not-for-profit healthcare firms.

---

## ▶ Tax Exemption Status

At the present time the Internal Revenue Service requires five factors to be present to support a hospital's tax-exempt status:

1. Operation of an emergency room open to all members of the community without regard to ability to pay
2. Governance board composed of community members
3. Use of surplus revenue for facilities improvement, patient care, medical training, education, and research
4. Provision of inpatient hospital care for all persons in the community able to pay, including those covered by Medicare and Medicaid
5. Open medical staff with privileges available to all qualifying physicians.

There is nothing in this list that references charitable care, but **not-for-profit** hospitals qualify for tax exemption under a provision of the Internal Revenue Code that relates to charitable purpose, **501(c)(3)**. Not-for-profit hospitals must accept all patients in their emergency rooms without regard to ability to pay, however they do not have to follow-up with additional care to those who are indigent unless they choose to do so. Still, **charity care**, which refers to the dollar value of services provided to patients at no cost or reduced cost has become a significant measurement area for not-for-profit hospitals in the community benefit discussion.

All not-for-profit firms with annual revenues greater than $25,000 and who are exempt from federal income tax are required to file **IRS Form 990** on an annual basis. That form contains a variety of financial information, including balance sheet and income statement data. The forms also contain information on compensation for the highest paid executives.

Since 2010 all not-for-profit hospitals must file **Schedule H** with their annual IRS 990 forms for filing year 2009. Schedule H is presented at the end of this chapter. The primary purpose of this form is to collect information regarding the provision of charity care by not-for-profit hospitals. At this point it is unclear how the data will be used, but most believe the federal government will implement specific standards for the provision of charity care and other community benefits. Not-for-profit hospitals that fail to meet these standards may then have their tax-exempt status removed. Schedule H has six sections:

1. Part I: Financial Assistance and Certain Other Community Benefits at Cost
2. Part II: Community Building Activities
3. Part III: Bad Debt, Medicare, and Collection Practices
4. Part IV: Management Companies and Joint Ventures
5. Part V: Facility Information
6. Part VI: Supplemental Information

There is little doubt that the areas identified in Part I will make the inclusion list for determining IRS community benefit. The other areas are less clear.

The Patient Protection and Affordable Care Act (ACA) of 2010 added Section 501(r) to the Internal Revenue Code, which contains four new requirements related to community benefits that nonprofit hospitals must meet to qualify for 501(c)(3) tax-exempt status. They are as follows:

- Conduct a community health needs assessment with an accompanying implementation strategy at least once every 3 years.
- Establish a written financial assistance policy for medically necessary and emergency care.
- Comply with specified limitations on hospital charges for those eligible for financial assistance.
- Comply with specified billing and collections requirements.

The new ACA requirements do not include a specific minimum value of charity care that a hospital must provide to qualify for tax-exempt status.

## State Efforts

There is significant variation among the states regarding the regulation and taxation of not-for-profit healthcare firms. The General Accounting Office (GAO) published a study in February 2009 titled "Nonprofit Hospitals Variation in Standards and Guidance Limits: Comparison of How Hospitals Meet Community Benefit Requirements." In this study they found 15 states with some form of community benefit reporting standards and or regulation. While these 15 states did have some form of community benefit standard, the GAO found that there was great variation among the states and their respective plans. All 15 of the states had some form of reporting—although in one state the reporting was voluntary. The two key elements of state regulatory plan were these questions:

- How are community benefits defined?
- Is there a penalty for violation of a community benefit standard?

The GAO defined community benefit as "a legal standard that expressly obligates a hospital to provide healthcare services or benefits to the community served by the hospital as a condition of maintaining tax-exempt status or qualifying as a not-for-profit hospital. It is generally something that hospitals are required to do beyond their role of providing care for the sick and injured in exchange for remuneration or compensation. Most of the 15 states did not define the composition of community benefit in a manner that was consistent across all hospitals. In fact, of the 15 states, only 10 of them defined community benefit in a detailed manner that would enable measurement.

Of the 15 states with community benefit requirements, 4 had explicit penalties for failure to comply and 11 states did not specify a penalty. States with explicit penalties often imposed a civil penalty for failure to submit their annual reports in a timely fashion. Some states may also retain the right to remove tax exemption, most notably property tax exemption. For example, the Illinois department of revenue ruled that a Catholic hospital did not qualify for a local property tax exemption because they provided only "the illusion of charity." Free care represented only 0.7% of the hospital's revenues. This case has been watched closely in the United States as other states eye not-for-profit hospitals as a possible revenue target.

The Hilltop Institute published a comprehensive review of state community benefit legislation in November 2015, "Hospital Community Benefits after the ACA: Trends in State Community Benefit Legislation, January–October 2015." At the point of publication there were five states (Illinois, Utah, Nevada, Pennsylvania, and Texas) that had enacted specific minimum community benefit standards to be present in order to qualify for tax exemption.

---

### *Learning Objective 2*

Describe the elements of community benefit listed by key policy groups.

---

## ▶ Community Benefit Areas

We have just seen that there is some significant variation among the 15 states that have attempted to define community benefit for not-for-profit hospitals. In this section we will identify the specific areas of community benefit that have been mentioned by specific policy groups. The policy groups reviewed include the following:

- American Hospital Association (AHA)
- Healthcare Financial Management Association (HFMA)
- Internal Revenue Service (IRS)
- Voluntary Hospitals of America (VHA)
- Catholic Healthcare Association (CHA)

While all five groups are of interest, it is the IRS that we believe is the most important. Ultimately, they will determine what community benefit standards will be employed. In this regard, we pay especially close attention to Schedule H of the IRS 990 form that is presented in the appendix to this chapter.

## Charity Care

All five of the policy groups recognize charity care as a legitimate community benefit. Furthermore, all five seem to be in agreement on the measurement of charity care. Charity care is usually defined as the unreimbursed cost of providing the care. There are several critical areas to understand given this uniform definition. First, these are patients who have been specifically defined as charity care. This is different from a patient who is uninsured and is billed for a hospital visit but does not pay. This is a bad debt and will be discussed shortly. Second, only the costs of providing the services are recognized—not the charges. In order to estimate the costs of charity care some system of cost accounting must exist to define the actual production cost of services provided.

The IRS has asked 990 filers to specify the method of estimating cost. There are generally two specific methods:

- Cost accounting system
- Cost-to-charge ratio

Many hospitals will most likely use a ratio of cost to charge (RCC) methodology. This is the easiest method to use and is widely understood and accepted at this point in time. **TABLE 5-1** illustrates the RCC methodology.

In the simple example of Table 5-1, the hospital has charges of $10,000,000 to charity patients. The actual cost of these services is defined as the RCC (35%) times the total charges. This produces an estimated cost of charity care of $3,500,000.

## Unreimbursed Cost of Means Tested Government Health Programs

All five of the policy groups also agree that the unreimbursed costs of means tested programs such as Medicaid should be included as a community benefit. A **means tested program** is one in which government sponsorship is present and beneficiaries become eligible through specific means testing. Medicaid is of course the largest and best known example. There is an implicit assumption in their inclusion that most of these programs will make payment at levels well below the actual cost of providing services. Schedule H of the IRS 990 makes it clear that the actual cost of providing services to these programs must be offset against any revenues

**TABLE 5-2** Estimation of Unreimbursed Medicaid Costs

| | |
|---|---|
| Medicaid charges | $100,000,000 |
| Ratio of cost to charges | 35% |
| Estimated cost of Medicaid services | $35,000,000 |
| Less Medicaid reimbursement | $22,000,000 |
| Unreimbursed cost of Medicaid services | $13,000,000 |

received from them. **TABLE 5-2** shows an example of a hospital that incurred $35,000,000 in cost to treat Medicaid beneficiaries, but it also received $22,000,000 in payments, which produced the $13,000,000 net cost that would be reported as an element of charity care.

## Unreimbursed Cost of Medicare

Only the AHA and HFMA include this element as a legitimate element of community benefit. The IRS has not taken a position in the area to date, but does include it in Part III of Schedule H. However, to date the elements in Schedule H are not being designated as the primary areas of community benefit. The major rationale for exclusion has been the historical relationship between Medicare and payment of costs. Initially, Medicare set payments to hospitals that matched expected costs. While Medicare still pays substantially more than Medicaid, the vast majority of hospitals do lose money on Medicare beneficiaries. In 2014, CMS estimated the average loss on inpatient and outpatient services to be 5.8%.

## Bad Debts

Only the AHA includes bad debts as an element of community benefit. The IRS includes bad debts in Part III of Schedule H along with unreimbursed Medicare costs. Most parties refuse to recognize bad debts because they believe that it is not true charity care. Historically, hospitals were required to determine charity care at the time of service provision. This has become quite difficult in today's economic climate. The HFMA Principles and Practices Board, which establishes reporting guidelines for hospitals, recently revised the long-standing guideline that eligibility for charity care must be decided based on the patient's financial status at the time of service. While appropriate for other business sectors, the complexities of healthcare delivery and coverage, compounded by federal regulations,

**TABLE 5-1** Estimation of Charitable Care Costs

| | |
|---|---|
| Charity care charges | $10,000,000 |
| Ratio of cost to charges | 35% |
| Estimated cost of charity services | $3,500,000 |

make this narrow interpretation of generally accepted accounting principles (GAAP) untenable for providers. The Principles and Practices Board has updated its guidelines to state that the timing period for determining eligibility should be addressed in the charity care policy. The IRS references HFMA's Statement number 15 in Part III of Schedule H.

**FIGURE 5-1** illustrates the four major areas of charity care as reported in four states with community benefit reporting. The data show very clearly that in these states unreimbursed Medicare costs typically represent the largest area of charity care. The second largest area is usually bad debt. It is interesting to note that the two largest areas of potential charity care are areas that most policy groups have excluded.

## Other Benefits

The IRS identifies five other areas that they refer to as "other benefits" in Part I of Schedule H. These areas include the following:

- Community health improvement
- Health profession education
- Subsidized health services
- Research
- Cash and in-kind contributions to community groups

All of these areas are netted against any revenue that may be realized.

## Community Building Activities

The IRS also identifies a series of "community-building activities" in Part II of Schedule H. At this point, these areas are information only and are not defined as charity care or community benefit services that are listed in Part I.

> *Learning Objective 3*

Assess the relative community benefits provided by proprietary and not-for-profit hospitals.

## ▶ The Community Value Index®

Investor-owned hospitals have long contended that not-for-profit hospitals provide little community benefit in relation to the tax benefits that they receive. Our objective in this section is to assess whether there is a difference in community value provided by not-for-profit hospitals versus that of proprietary hospitals. We will adopt a national metric and scoring methodology that has been used since 2004 to assess community value.

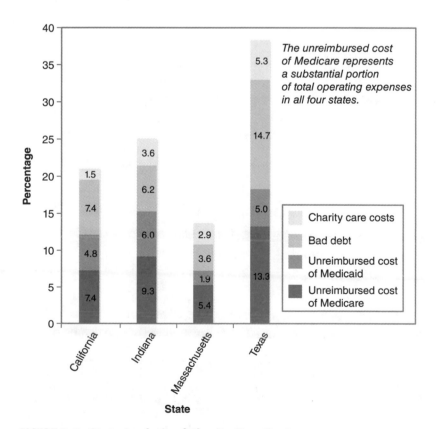

**FIGURE 5-1  State Analysis of Charity Care Costs**

The **Community Value Index® (CVI)** was created to provide a measure of the value that a hospital provides to its community. The CVI is composed of 10 measures that assess a hospital's performance in 4 areas:

1. Financial viability and plant reinvestment
2. Hospital cost structure
3. Hospital charge structure
4. Hospital quality performance

Fundamentally, the CVI suggests that a hospital provides value to the community when it is financially viable, is appropriately reinvesting back into the facility, maintains a low cost structure, has reasonable charges, and provides high-quality care to patients.

Within the 4 core areas, 10 measures (**TABLE 5-3**) were selected to determine hospital performance. A discussion of the core areas and individual measures follows.

## Core Area One: Financial Viability and Plant Reinvestment

The first core area of the CVI examines a hospital's financial viability and facility reinvestment. A hospital must be financially viable in order to be a valuable asset in the community. Perhaps there is no greater disservice than to have a facility purport to be a leading care provider to citizens and then close due to poor financial management. Certainly, a strong financial position must be achieved in order for a hospital to continue its mission of care provision while at the same time, survive in the turbulent health services market. Of course, a hospital must also continue reinvestment back into the facility in order to provide for current and emerging health needs in the community. This does not imply that hospitals should spend money just for the sake of spending it, but rather making wise investments into capital equipment that will be used efficiently.

**TABLE 5-3** Community Value Components

| Measure | Purpose |
| --- | --- |
| *Core Area One: Financial Viability and Plant Reinvestment* | |
| Total margin | Assess profitability at hospital |
| Growth in net fixed assets (2 years) | Assess level of hospital reinvestment |
| Fixed asset turnover | Assess efficiency of plant use |
| Debt financing percentage | Assess how hospital is financed |
| *Core Area Two: Hospital Cost Structure* | |
| Medicare cost per discharge (CMI/WI adj.) | Assess inpatient cost structure |
| Medicare cost per visit (RW/WI adj.) | Assess outpatient cost structure |
| *Core Area Three: Hospital Charge Structure* | |
| Medicare charge per discharge (CMI/WI adj.) | Assess level of inpatient charges |
| Medicare charge per visit (RW/WI adj.) | Assess level of outpatient charges |
| Medicaid days percentage | Assess level of low-income patients |
| *Core Area Four: Hospital Quality Performance* | |
| Hospital Quality Index | Assess process and outcomes of patient care |

*CMI, case mix index; WI, wage index; RW, relative weight*

Appropriately combining these two concepts of financial strength and reinvestment enhances a hospital's value in the community. This core area of the CVI suggests that hospitals in both for-profit and nonprofit settings should be generating a return on operations; however, they should be using those resources to continue to improve the level of care provided to the communities they serve. The four measures used to determine a hospital's performance in this core area are total margin, growth in net fixed assets, fixed asset turnover, and debt financing percentage.

**Total margin**, which is the ratio of net income to total revenue, provides information on the level of profitability at a hospital. Without appropriate returns, a hospital will be unable to continue serving the community's health needs. Perhaps this concept is confused in the nonprofit setting. At times, there seems to be a perception that because a hospital is "not-for-profit" it should not be making a profit. This could not be further from the truth. Just as individuals and for-profit businesses need resources in excess of expenses in order to meet current and future obligations, so too do nonprofit organizations require similar returns in order to ensure survival.

As suggested previously, however, providing value to the community also involves reinvestment back into the facility. To measure this concept, a growth rate in net fixed assets was determined for a 2-year period for each hospital in our study. This was balanced with an examination of how efficiently hospitals use their plant and equipment, as measured by the **fixed asset turnover ratio**. The combination of these two fixed asset measures balances any extreme results that may occur. For example, let us imagine that a hospital embarked on a major capital project that was not needed to fulfill a community health need. Of course, the hospital would have a high growth rate in net fixed assets, implying significant investment in the facility, However, the fixed asset turnover ratio would be low, suggesting that the project may not have been needed. The offsetting scores would reduce the hospital's final ranking.

Finally, **debt financing** measures how the hospital is financing its capital investments. While debt is not a negative thing, too much debt certainly will cripple a hospital, putting it into jeopardy and compromising its ability to continue to meet the needs of the community it serves.

## Core Area Two: Hospital Cost Structure

The next core area of the CVI involves a hospital's cost structure. Keeping costs low allows a hospital to provide efficient care that can result in lower costs for community members and third-party payers. Allowing for an appropriate margin on care provided to community members will be less costly to them if the hospital's underlying cost structure is lower. In the end, this efficient care also promotes value to the community.

In order to assess a hospital's performance in this area two measures were used: Medicare cost per discharge (adjusted for case mix and wage index) and Medicare cost per visit (adjusted for relative weight and wage index).

The CVI does not employ adjusted day/discharge measures to calculate cost positions or charge positions (as will be seen), because information based on these measures can often be misleading. Adjusted day/discharge measures were started in order to try and convert outpatient activity into a common inpatient unit (day or discharge). However, the methodology to do this can lead to flawed results. This issue will be further explored in Chapter 11.

Although the CVI cost measures are restricted to the Medicare population, this does not present a particularly strong case against applying the results to the rest of the hospital's patient population for two reasons. First, Medicare represents the largest patient population for almost every U.S. hospital. Second, because Medicare pays on a fixed, prospective payment methodology, hospitals have an incentive to keep costs low with these patients. If a hospital has high costs in treating Medicare patients, it can be reasonably assumed that it would also have high costs in treating other patients as well.

## Core Area Three: Hospital Charge Structure

The third core area of the CVI examines a hospital's charges. Certainly, this area has received great attention in the past few years as health expenses, in general, have been rising. Obviously, consumers and third-party payers desire health care that is reasonably priced. However, hospitals are often in a difficult position because their pricing does not reflect actual payment that will be recovered for provided care. A patient's bill may appear less shocking if the individual knew what discounted price was actually compensated by the third-party payer. In the end, however, hospitals should strive for pricing that is reasonable and competitive with peer facilities. The CVI examines this by comparing hospital charges among hospitals in similar size/geographic classes.

Similar in methodology to assessing a hospital's cost structure, the CVI determines a hospital's charges based primarily on two measures: Medicare charge per discharge (adjusted for case mix and wage index) and Medicare charge per visit (adjusted for relative weight and wage index). As stated in the cost discussion, the CVI's charge measures can be reasonably applied to the rest of the hospital's non-Medicare business because Medicare represents such a significant proportion of total business for most U.S. hospitals. Also, gross charges for Medicare patients should be applicable to gross charges for other payers as well, because prices for specific billable services do not vary by payer.

The *Medicaid days percentage* is the ratio of Medicaid and Medicaid HMO days to total patient days at the hospital. The purpose of this measure is to provide greater parity to relative charge structures at U.S. hospitals. Our belief, which is well documented, is that hospitals with higher levels of low-income patients have higher overall charge structures. The suggestion is clear: hospitals with high levels of low-income patients must set higher prices to cover financial deficiencies incurred in treating low-income patients. Including this measure does not totally erase a hospital's high charges; however, it does bring more balance to the overall charge score of the CVI.

## Core Area Four: Hospital Quality Performance

The final core area of the CVI includes the quality dimension. Quality has always been a central component of value; however, until recently there were only a limited number of metrics that were publicly available for a large number of hospitals. In addition, some metrics that were available were not consistently reported across organizations or did not adequately address a larger breadth of quality areas. As standards and number of facilities reporting have improved, the comparison of quality data has become more meaningful. For these reasons, the quality dimension is now included in the CVI calculation.

To assess this area of performance, we have analyzed Medicare's process of care and outcome of care quality measures for the most current periods. Process of care measures are reported for the period April 2014 through March 2015 and outcome of care measures are reported for the period July 2011 through June 2014.

There were 25 process of care metrics that were used in our analysis in the areas of heart attack, heart failure, pneumonia, and surgical infection prevention. These process of care areas refer to medical standards for treatment protocols (e.g., heart attack patients given aspirin on arrival). Hospitals report the percentage of time standards were met in each of the 25 areas. From this data, we determined the percentage the

hospital was above or below the U.S. average and the frequency at which the hospital performed at or above the highest performing hospitals in the country. In sum, hospitals received high process of care composite scores when a higher number of areas were reported and when performance in those areas exceeded the U.S. average and high-performance levels.

Outcome quality measurement is conducted through risk-adjusted mortality rates established for each facility by Medicare. These rates are provided for hospitals in three areas: heart attack, heart failure, and pneumonia patients. The mortality rates estimate the risk-adjusted frequency of death within 30 days of patient discharge. From the data in these areas, we created a composite score to evaluate the percentage a hospital was above or below U.S. average levels. Hospitals that had lower levels of mortality had better composite scores.

The final step in our quality analysis was to create a *hospital quality index* (HQI) based on the review of data in the process of care and outcomes areas. Combining the composite scores of these two areas created the overall HQI score. The HQI served as the overall quality score for each hospital in the CVI study.

## Comparative CVI Scores by Hospital Sector

**TABLE 5-4** provides comparative 2016 CVI scores for alternative hospital sectors categorized by ownership. Higher scores indicate better relative performance. Proprietary hospitals show the worst overall CVI scores (59.6) compared to the U.S. median (62.8).

The primary reason for the relatively low proprietary scores is related to two areas. Proprietary hospitals have very low charge scores because their prices are significantly higher than other hospitals and their Medicaid patient mix is usually low relative to other hospitals. They also have lower financial scores that are the result of higher levels of debt and lower reinvestment rates in plant and equipment.

It should be expected that proprietary hospitals would have lower CVI scores than voluntary hospitals. Voluntary hospitals have an obligation to provide services back to their communities in return for the favorable tax benefits that they receive. We next try to establish a methodology for directly estimating tax benefits received and the actual cost of benefits provided to the community in a specific case example.

---

*Learning Objective 4*

Develop a methodology for estimating financial benefits received by not-for-profit healthcare firms.

**TABLE 5-4** CVI Scores by Hospital Ownership

| Hospital Sectors | CVI Scores | | | | |
| --- | --- | --- | --- | --- | --- |
| | Financial | Cost | Charges | Quality | Overall |
| Proprietary | 47.8 | 52.7 | 34.9 | 100.3 | 59.6 |
| VNP Church | 53.2 | 57.1 | 48.5 | 100.7 | 64.5 |
| VNP Other | 51.2 | 50.7 | 52.9 | 100.9 | 63.8 |
| Government | 47.4 | 38.6 | 58.9 | 99.4 | 60.9 |
| All United States | 50.5 | 50.5 | 50.2 | 100.5 | 62.8 |

VNP, Voluntary nonprofit

## ▶ Estimating Financial Benefits in Not-for-Profit Healthcare Firms

There are a number of specific financial benefits that not-for-profit healthcare firms receive that have been cited by policy analysts over the years. In this section we will discuss the areas that are believed to be the largest in terms of financial magnitude and discuss a methodology for estimating the benefits in each area via a hypothetical example. The specific areas that will be discussed include the following:

- Property tax exemption
- Postal rate reduction
- Interest savings from tax-exempt bonds
- Sales tax exemption
- Federal unemployment tax exemption
- Income taxes
    - Local/city
    - State
    - Federal

### Property Tax Exemption

Local communities often criticize the exemption from property tax that many not-for-profit and governmental entities enjoy. Proprietary healthcare firms must pay property taxes on their real estate investments and most agree that property taxes should be accounted for as one of the financial benefits received by not-for-profit healthcare firms.

Most property taxes are based on assessed valuations. There is usually an appraisal of the property, and that appraised value is often uniformly reduced by applying an assessment percentage. **TABLE 5-5** illustrates

**TABLE 5-5** Estimation of Property Tax

| Values reported in audit | |
| --- | --- |
| Land and land improvements | $36,000,000 |
| Buildings and fixed equipment | 450,000,000 |
| Equipment | 280,000,000 |
| Construction in progress | 14,000,000 |
| Total gross property and equipment | 780,000,000 |
| Less allowance for depreciation | 400,000,000 |
| Net property plant and equipment | 380,000,000 |
| Property under assessment | |
| Land and land improvements | 36,000,000 |
| Buildings and fixed equipment | 450,000,000 |
| Construction in progress | 14,000,000 |
| Total | 500,000,000 |
| Assessment percentage | 35% |
| Assessed value | 175,000,000 |
| Estimated tax rate | 7% |
| **Real estate tax liability** | **12,250,000** |

the estimation of property tax for our hypothetical example.

In Table 5-5 we started with information in the audited financial statements. Most likely, it would be possible to get specific property tax appraisals from the taxing **authority**—most likely the county. Note that only land and land improvements, combined with the building cost and the cost of fixed equipment such as boilers, are included. Other equipment would be exempt from real estate property tax. In our example we have taken the undepreciated cost from the property, plant, and equipment section of the balance sheet for a total of $500 million. In the county where our hospital is located, only 35% of the appraised value would be assessed. This creates an assessed value base of $175 million to which we apply tax rate of 7% (the estimated property tax rate for the geographical area of the hospital). Our estimated property tax then becomes $12,250,000.

## Postal Rate Reduction

To some it may come as a surprise that not-for-profit firms are eligible for lower U.S. postal rates. Hospitals may during the course of a year send large volumes of mail, and the savings can be quite large. **TABLE 5-6** summarizes the savings for our hypothetical hospital.

## Interest Savings from Tax-exempt Bonds

Proprietary healthcare firms have long cited the ability of not-for-profit healthcare firms to issue **tax-exempt bonds** as a decisive cost advantage. Without the availability of tax-exempt financing most not-for-profit healthcare firms would find their relative cost of capital increased. **TABLE 5-7** summarizes the savings from issuance of tax-exempt bonds at the hypothetical hospital.

**TABLE 5-6**  Estimate of Postal Rate Savings

| | |
|---|---|
| Postage rate first class (for-profit) | $0.47 |
| Postage rate first class (nonprofit) | $0.23 |
| Difference | $0.24 |
| Number of first class pieces mailed | 3,500,000 |
| Savings in postage | $840,000 |

**TABLE 5-7**  Estimate of Savings from Issuance of Tax-Exempt Bonds

| | |
|---|---|
| Tax-exempt bonds audited statements | 300,000,000 |
| Expected taxable interest rate | 6.75% |
| Current tax-exempt interest rate | 5.00% |
| Difference | 1.75% |
| Estimate of interest saved | 5,250,000 |

In the example of Table 5-7, it is fairly easy to estimate the potential savings realized from tax-exempt bonds. The only real difficult part is the determination of "expected taxable interest rate." We know with certainty the effective interest rate on the bonds currently, but it may be hard to define what the equivalent taxable rate would be for several reasons. First, what time period should be used? Using the current taxable rate would give a valid value if the taxable financing were done today; however, it is being compared to a tax-exempt interest rate of a prior period. Second, can we really create an equivalent taxable financing package that mimics the tax-exempt issue in terms of maturity, interest rate swaps, and other financing features? In our example we have assumed that the current spread between a taxable and a tax-exempt issue is 175 basis points or 1.75%. Because we have $300 million of outstanding tax-exempt bonds, our expected savings is $5,250,000.

## Sales Tax Exemption

Not-for-profit firms are also exempt from state sales taxes. This can also become a sizable benefit to a not-for-profit healthcare firm. One issue that becomes important is what areas would be subject to the sales tax. Salaries and fringe benefits are not subject to state sales tax, which leaves supplies and drugs as the two biggest areas for healthcare firms. In many states drugs may be exempt from sales tax, which leaves supplies. **TABLE 5-8** summarizes the sales tax computation for our hypothetical hospital.

**TABLE 5-8**  Estimation of Sales Tax

| | |
|---|---|
| Annual purchase of supplies | 125,000,000 |
| State sales tax rate | 7.00% |
| Estimated sales tax | 8,750,000 |

## Federal Unemployment Tax Exemption

The federal government exempts not-for-profit firms from paying federal unemployment tax assessments (FUTA). States may still assess unemployment taxes, but the not-for-profit firm can choose among several alternative ways to finance its state unemployment liability. For our sample hospital, there is no FUTA tax for not-for-profits in their state. **TABLE 5-9** summarizes the computations for the FUTA.

## Income Taxes

Exemption from income taxes is the area where most people associate an advantage with not-for-profit healthcare firms. As described earlier there are three areas of income taxes for most not-for-profit healthcare firms:

- Local/city income taxes
- State income taxes
- Federal income taxes

Usually, there is a hierarchy of income taxation that proceeds as follows. Taxable income at the city level is not adjusted for state or federal income taxes. State income taxable income is reduced by city income taxes. Finally, federal taxable income is reduced by both city and state taxes. **TABLE 5-10** summarizes the estimation of income taxes at all three levels for our hypothetical hospital.

Notice that we have started with unadjusted net income as reported in the audited financial statements. To the reported level of net income we must start by adding some items that may be recognized as expenses in computing net income but are not recognized as legitimate expenses for computing income taxes. These are the so-called "disallowed items" represented in Table 5-9. The following two areas are shown in Table 5-9:

1. 50% of meals and entertainment
2. Officer life insurance premiums

| **TABLE 5-9** Federal Unemployment Tax Assessment Benefit | |
|---|---|
| Federal unemployment wage base | $ 7,000 |
| Number of FTEs | 6,000 |
| Salary base subject to FUTA | $ 42,000,000 |
| FUTA rate | 6.00% |
| FUTA liability | $ 2,520,000 |

FTEs, full-time equivalents; FUTA, federal unemployment tax assessments

| **TABLE 5-10** Income Tax Estimation | |
|---|---|
| Net income from audited | $ 72,000,000 |
| Add disallowed items | |
| 50% of meals and entertainment | $ 1,800,000 |
| Officer life insurance premiums | $ 1,200,000 |
| Total disallowed | $ 3,000,000 |
| Revised net income | $ 75,000,000 |
| Less additional deductions | |
| Sales tax | $ 8,750,000 |
| Property tax | $ 12,250,000 |
| Federal unemployment tax | $ 2,520,000 |
| Postage expense increase | $ 840,000 |
| Additional interest expense | $ 5,250,000 |
| Total additional expenses | $ 29,610,000 |
| Net income subject to local income tax | $ 45,390,000 |
| City income tax rate | 2.00% |
| **City income tax** | **$ 907,800** |
| Net income subject to state income tax | $ 44,482,200 |
| State income tax rate | 8.50% |
| **State income tax** | **$ 3,780,987** |
| Net income subject to federal tax | $ 40,701,213 |
| Federal tax rate | 35.0% |
| **Federal income tax** | **$ 14,245,425** |

For taxable corporations only 50% of the expense associated with business meals and entertainment are deductible. We have therefore added back 50% of the cost of expenses in this area to our net income. The life insurance premiums paid on behalf of an officer of a corporation are also not deductible for tax return purposes. We have also added back these expenditures to our original net income figure. This meant that our revised net income would be increased from $72 million to $ 75 million. From that $75 million we subtract all of those expenses that we would have incurred if the hospital had been taxable. For example, we would have paid $12,250,000 of property taxes if we were a taxable entity. These reductions reduced our city income taxable basis to $45,390,000. The tax then due the city at 2% was $907,800. This amount was then subtracted to determine the state income tax basis of $44,482,200. The state income tax of $3,780,987 is then subtracted to determine the federal income taxable basis of $40,701,213.

We can now summarize the total amount of financial benefits realized by our hypothetical not-for-profit hospital in **TABLE 5-11**.

In this case example, our not-for-profit hospital received $48,544,212 in taxation benefits that resulted from its not-for-profit status. The question becomes very simple. Did this hospital provide more than $48,544,212 in benefits to the community? This is the simple relationship that many are seeking to document. Do not-for-profit healthcare firms provide more benefits than they receive?

---

### Learning Objective 5

Develop a methodology for estimating financial benefits provided by not-for-profit healthcare firms.

---

## ▶ Estimating Financial Benefits Provided by Not-for-Profit Healthcare Firms

In the last section of this chapter we will identify the amount of benefits provided by our hypothetical hospital to its community. The areas to be included will match those described earlier. Specifically, the benefits to be included are the following:

- Traditional charity care
- Unpaid cost of Medicaid
- Medical education
- Other benefits
  - Subsidized health services
  - Community health services
  - Cash and in-kind donations to the community
  - Research

## Traditional Charity Care

Charity care is defined as the free or discounted health services provided to persons who cannot afford to pay, as defined by the hospital's charity care policies and procedures. Most hospitals have enacted specific discount policies in relationship to Federal Poverty Guidelines. **TABLE 5-12** provides the 2016 Federal Poverty Guideline levels. In our hypothetical hospital we will assume that all patients with income less than

---

**TABLE 5-11** Summary of Taxation Benefits

| | |
|---|---|
| Federal income tax | $ 14,245,425 |
| State income tax | $ 3,780,987 |
| City income tax | $ 907,800 |
| Forgone FUTA tax | $ 2,520,000 |
| Sales tax | $ 8,750,000 |
| Property tax | $ 12,250,000 |
| Additional postage expense | $ 840,000 |
| Interest savings on tax-exempt bonds | $ 5,250,000 |
| Total value of tax exemption | $ 48,544,212 |

---

**TABLE 5-12** 2016 Federal Poverty Guidelines

| Household Size | Poverty Level |
|---|---|
| 1 | $11,880 |
| 2 | 16,020 |
| 3 | 20,160 |
| 4 | 24,300 |
| 5 | 28,440 |
| 6 | 32,580 |
| 7 | 36,730 |
| 8 | 40,890 |

| TABLE 5-13　Estimation of Charity Care Benefit | |
|---|---|
| Charity care charge write-offs | $ 120,000,000 |
| Times cost-to-charge ratio | 38.0% |
| Cost of charity care provided | $ 45,600,000 |
| Less state disproportionate share payments | $ 9,000,000 |
| Net cost of charity care | $ 36,600,000 |

200% of the Federal Poverty Guideline will receive a 100% discount.

**TABLE 5-13** summarizes the computation of charity care benefits for the hospital. Note that in this example the state has made a $9,000,000 disproportionate payment to help cover the costs of indigent care. This payment is netted against the cost to produce the net cost of charity care of $36,600,000.

## Unpaid Cost of Medicaid and Other Means Tested Programs

The hospital has only included Medicaid and Medicaid managed-care patients. There are no other means tested programs that have been identified. **TABLE 5-14** summarizes the net cost to the hospital.

## Medical Education Programs

The hospital has defined this area to include the education and training of health professionals above and beyond the requirements mandated by the employer

| TABLE 5-14　Net Cost of Medicaid Programs | |
|---|---|
| Medicaid and Medicaid managed-care total charges | $ 100,000,000 |
| Times cost-to-charge ratio | 38.0% |
| Cost of Medicaid and Medicaid managed-care programs | $ 38,000,000 |
| Less payments | $ 31,000,000 |
| Unpaid cost of Medicaid programs | $ 7,000,000 |

| TABLE 5-15　Medical Education Benefits Provided | |
|---|---|
| Direct costs of medical education | $ 20,000,000 |
| Less payments | $ 10,000,000 |
| Net cost of medical education | $ 10,000,000 |

and for certification and licensure. This would typically include interns, residents, and nursing student training. Any offsetting payments that were received are deducted from the cost of program delivery. Medicare payments for direct medical education costs would be included as payments. **TABLE 5-15** summarizes the benefits.

## Other Benefits

There are a variety of different categories of benefits included here. **TABLE 5-16** summarizes the costs of these areas.

## Comparison of Benefits Provided to Benefits Received

We have now completed the computation of both benefits received and benefits provided by the hospital. **TABLE 5-17** summarizes the analysis.

In this example, our hypothetical hospital has received tax benefits of $48,544,212 and it has provided community benefits of $56,800,000 for a net contribution to the community of $8,255,788. This excess benefit was derived without including unreimbursed costs of Medicare or bad debt. The key remaining question is whether this level of excess community

| TABLE 5-16　Other Benefits | |
|---|---|
| Subsidized health services | $ 1,800,000 |
| Community health services | $ 1,000,000 |
| Cash and in-kind donations to the community | $ 300,000 |
| Unsubsidized research costs | $ 100,000 |
| Total | $ 3,200,000 |

**TABLE 5-17** Summary of Community Benefit Analysis

| | |
|---|---|
| Charity care (net cost) | $ 36,600,000 |
| Net cost of Medicaid programs | $ 7,000,000 |
| Net cost of medical education | $ 10,000,000 |
| Subsidized health services | $ 1,800,000 |
| Community health services | $ 1,000,000 |
| Cash and in-kind contributions | $ 300,000 |
| Research | $ 100,000 |
| **Total benefits provided** | **$ 56,800,000** |
| Federal income tax | $ 14,245,425 |
| State income tax | $ 3,780,987 |
| City income tax | $ 907,800 |
| Forgone FUTA tax | $ 2,520,000 |
| Sales tax | $ 8,750,000 |
| Property tax | $ 12,250,000 |
| Additional postage expense | $ 840,000 |
| Interest savings on tax-exempt bonds | $ 5,250,000 |
| **Total value of tax exemption** | **$ 48,544,212** |
| **Excess community benefit** | **$ 8,255,788** |

benefit justifies the tax exemptions. Many would argue the two largest areas—charity care and Medicaid—are merely costs of doing business. Others point out that proprietary hospitals provide similar benefits and are not accorded tax-exempt status.

# ▶ SUMMARY

The majority of hospitals in the United States are not-for-profit firms that are exempt from federal income tax and also many other state and local taxes. Increasingly, communities are asking a very simple question. Do these hospitals provide benefits to the community in an amount greater that the taxation benefits that they receive? This is not an easy question to answer but one that the federal government seems intent on addressing. The IRS has required not-for-profit hospitals to file Schedule H as part of their annual IRS Form 990 submissions. Schedule H will collect detailed information in a number of areas regarding the provision of charity and other community benefits. At some point the data will be fully analyzed and decisions will be made regarding the future of tax exemption for not-for-profit hospitals and other not-for-profit healthcare firms. It seems that many, perhaps most, not-for-profit hospitals will be required to pay some taxes either in the form of property taxes or income taxes. This decision to tax will then force these same not-for-profit hospitals to assess the continued advantages and disadvantages of their current ownership structure. Some not-for-profits will no doubt migrate to a proprietary ownership basis to take advantage of easier access to capital. The long-term effects of these possible changes are not clear at this point, but they could be monumental.

# ASSIGNMENTS

**TABLE 5-18** is a footnote from an actual audited financial statement of a major healthcare system. From the information in that footnote, please answer the following questions:

1. What is the single largest area of community benefit provided by Dignity Health and what dollar amount of benefit was provided?
2. What is the total dollar amount of community benefit provided by Dignity Health?
3. Why is Medicare not listed as a community benefit?
4. If Medicare were to be included as a legitimate area of community benefit, what percentage of Dignity's total expenses would be allocated to community benefit activities?

Summary of Dignity Health's community benefits for 2015, in terms of services to the poor and benefits for the broader community, which has been prepared in accordance with Internal Revenue Service Form 990, Schedule H, and the CHA publication, *A Guide for Planning and Reporting Community Benefit* (dollars in thousands).

**TABLE 5-18**  Community Benefit Footnote

| | Unaudited | | | | |
| --- | --- | --- | --- | --- | --- |
| | Persons Served | Total Benefit Expense | Direct Offsetting Revenue | Net Community Benefit | % of Total Expense |
| Benefits for the poor | | | | | |
| Traditional charity care | 155,869 | 145,519 | (1,476) | 144,043 | 1.2% |
| Unpaid costs of Medicaid | 1,529,842 | 3,541,533 | (2,958,545) | 582,988 | 4.9% |
| Other means tested programs | 269,823 | 12,299 | (3,098) | 9,201 | 0.1% |
| Community services | | | | | |
| Community health services | 376,686 | 46,687 | (4,931) | 41,756 | 0.3% |
| Health professions education | 79 | 3 | – | 3 | 0.0% |
| Subsidized health services | 96,294 | 28,890 | (4,018) | 28,872 | 0.2% |
| Donations | 123,504 | 37,313 | (780) | 36,533 | 0.3% |
| Community building activities | 7,795 | 2,658 | (840) | 1,818 | 0.0% |
| Community benefit operations | 143 | 7,347 | (223) | 7,124 | 0.1% |
| Total community services for the poor | 604,501 | 122,898 | (10,792) | 112,106 | 0.9% |
| Total benefits for the poor | 2,560,035 | 3,822,249 | (2,973,911) | 848,338 | 7.1% |
| Benefits for the broader community | | | | | |
| Community services | | | | | |
| Community health services | 278,419 | 13,225 | (1,179) | 12,046 | 0.1% |
| Health professions education | 27,306 | 77,257 | (9,342) | 67,915 | 0.6% |

*(continues)*

**TABLE 5-18** Community Benefit Footnote    *(continued)*

| | Unaudited | | | | |
| --- | --- | --- | --- | --- | --- |
| | Persons Served | Total Benefit Expense | Direct Offsetting Revenue | Net Community Benefit | % of Total Expense |
| Subsidized health services | 3,641 | 2,704 | (1,263) | 1,441 | 0.0% |
| Research | 14,806 | 31,768 | (20,858) | 10,910 | 0.1% |
| Donations | 31,341 | 8,688 | (26) | 8,662 | 0.1% |
| Community building activities | 7,583 | 3,966 | (144) | 3,822 | 0.0% |
| Community benefit operations | 31 | 1,333 | - | 1,333 | 0.0% |
| Total benefits for the broader community | 363,127 | 138,941 | (32,812) | 106,129 | .9% |
| Total community benefits | 2,923,162 | $3,961,190 | ($3,006,723) | $954,467 | 8.0% |
| Unpaid costs of Medicare | 1,042,065 | 3,003,473 | (2,247,364) | 756,109 | 6.3% |
| Total community benefits including unpaid costs of Medicare | 3,965,227 | $6,964,663 | ($5,254,087) | $1,710,576 | 14.3% |

## SOLUTIONS

CHW responses:

1. Unpaid costs of Medicaid programs amounted to $582,988,000 at Dignity and accounted for 4.9% of total expenses.
2. Dignity provided $954,467,000 of community benefit, which represented 8.0% of total expenses.
3. Dignity is a part of the Catholic Healthcare Association, which does not recognize unpaid costs of Medicare as a community benefit. The dollar amount of $756,109 is reported but not included in the community benefit total.
4. If unpaid Medicare costs were included in community benefit totals, CHW would be providing $1,710,576,000 or 14.3% of their total expenses in community benefits.

# Appendix 5-A

## Schedule H Form

| SCHEDULE H (Form 990) | **Hospitals** | OMB No. 1545-0047 |
|---|---|---|
| | ▶ Complete if the organization answered "Yes" to Form 990, Part IV, question 20. | **20**09 |
| Department of the Treasury Internal Revenue Service | ▶ Attach to Form 990.<br>▶ See separate instructions. | **Open to Public Inspection** |

| Name of the organization | Employer identification number |
|---|---|
| | |

### Part I — Charity Care and Certain Other Community Benefits at Cost

| | | Yes | No |
|---|---|---|---|
| **1a** | Does the organization have a charity care policy? If "No," skip to question 6a . . . . . . . . | **1a** | |
| **b** | If "Yes," is it a written policy? . . . . . . . . . . . . . . . . . . . . . | **1b** | |

**2** If the organization has multiple hospitals, indicate which of the following best describes application of the charity care policy to the various hospitals.

☐ Applied uniformly to all hospitals  ☐ Applied uniformly to most hospitals

☐ Generally tailored to individual hospitals

**3** Answer the following based on the charity care eligibility criteria that applies to the largest number of the organization's patients.

| | | Yes | No |
|---|---|---|---|
| **a** | Does the organization use Federal Poverty Guidelines (FPG) to determine eligibility for providing *free* care to low income individuals? If "Yes," indicate which of the following is the family income limit for eligibility for free care: . . . . <br> ☐ 100%  ☐ 150%  ☐ 200%  ☐ Other _____ % | **3a** | |
| **b** | Does the organization use FPG to determine eligibility for providing *discounted* care to low income individuals? If "Yes," indicate which of the following is the family income limit for eligibility for discounted care: . . . . . . . <br> ☐ 200%  ☐ 250%  ☐ 300%  ☐ 350%  ☐ 400%  ☐ Other _____ % | **3b** | |

**c** If the organization does not use FPG to determine eligibility, describe in Part VI the income based criteria for determining eligibility for free or discounted care. Include in the description whether the organization uses an asset test or other threshold, regardless of income, to determine eligibility for free or discounted care.

| | | Yes | No |
|---|---|---|---|
| **4** | Does the organization's policy provide free or discounted care to the "medically indigent"? . . . . . | **4** | |
| **5a** | Does the organization budget amounts for free or discounted care provided under its charity care policy? | **5a** | |
| **b** | If "Yes," did the organization's charity care expenses exceed the budgeted amount? . . . . . . . | **5b** | |
| **c** | If "Yes" to line 5b, as a result of budget considerations, was the organization unable to provide free or discounted care to a patient who was eligible for free or discounted care? . . . . . . . . . . . | **5c** | |
| **6a** | Does the organization prepare an annual community benefit report? . . . . . . . . . . . . | **6a** | |
| **b** | If "Yes," does the organization make it available to the public? . . . . . . . . . . . . . . | **6b** | |

Complete the following table using the worksheets provided in the Schedule H instructions. Do not submit these worksheets with the Schedule H.

**7** Charity Care and Certain Other Community Benefits at Cost

| Charity Care and Means-Tested Government Programs | (a) Number of activities or programs (optional) | (b) Persons served (optional) | (c) Total community benefit expense | (d) Direct offsetting revenue | (e) Net community benefit expense | (f) Percent of total expense |
|---|---|---|---|---|---|---|
| **a** Charity care at cost (from Worksheets 1 and 2) . . . . | | | | | | |
| **b** Unreimbursed Medicaid (from Worksheet 3, column a) . . | | | | | | |
| **c** Unreimbursed costs—other means-tested government programs (from Worksheet 3, column b) . . . . | | | | | | |
| **d** **Total** Charity Care and Means-Tested Government Programs . . . . . . . . | | | | | | |
| **Other Benefits** | | | | | | |
| **e** Community health improvement services and community benefit operations (from Worksheet 4) . | | | | | | |
| **f** Health professions education (from Worksheet 5) . . . | | | | | | |
| **g** Subsidized health services (from Worksheet 6) . . . . . | | | | | | |
| **h** Research (from Worksheet 7) . . | | | | | | |
| **i** Cash and in-kind contributions to community groups (from Worksheet 8) . . . . . . | | | | | | |
| **j** **Total.** Other Benefits . . . . | | | | | | |
| **k** **Total.** Add lines 7d and 7j . . | | | | | | |

For Privacy Act and Paperwork Reduction Act Notice, see the Instructions for Form 990.  Cat. No. 50192T  Schedule H (Form 990) 2009

Schedule H (Form 990) 2009
Page **2**

| **Part II** | **Community Building Activities** Complete this table if the organization conducted any community building activities. |

| | **(a)** Number of activities or programs (optional) | **(b)** Persons served (optional) | **(c)** Total community building expense | **(d)** Direct offsetting revenue | **(e)** Net community building expense | **(f)** Percent of total expense |
|---|---|---|---|---|---|---|
| 1 Physical improvements and housing | | | | | | |
| 2 Economic development | | | | | | |
| 3 Community support | | | | | | |
| 4 Environmental improvements | | | | | | |
| 5 Leadership development and training for community members | | | | | | |
| 6 Coalition building | | | | | | |
| 7 Community health improvement advocacy | | | | | | |
| 8 Workforce development | | | | | | |
| 9 Other | | | | | | |
| 10 Total | | | | | | |

| **Part III** | **Bad Debt, Medicare, & Collection Practices** |

**Section A. Bad Debt Expense**

|  |  | Yes | No |
|---|---|---|---|
| 1 | Does the organization report bad debt expense in accordance with Healthcare Financial Management Association Statement No. 15? . . . . . . . . . . . . . . . . . . . . . . . . . **1** | | |
| 2 | Enter the amount of the organization's bad debt expense (at cost) . . . . . . **2** | | |
| 3 | Enter the estimated amount of the organization's bad debt expense (at cost) attributable to patients eligible under the organization's charity care policy. . . . . . . . . **3** | | |
| 4 | Provide in Part VI the text of the footnote to the organization's financial statements that describes bad debt expense. In addition, describe the costing methodology used in determining the amounts reported on lines 2 and 3, and rationale for including other bad debt amounts in community benefit. | | |

**Section B. Medicare**

| 5 | Enter total revenue received from Medicare (including DSH and IME) . . . . . . **5** |
| 6 | Enter Medicare allowable costs of care relating to payments on line 5 . . . . . . **6** |
| 7 | Subtract line 6 from line 5. This is the surplus or (shortfall) . . . . . . . . . **7** |
| 8 | Describe in Part VI the extent to which any shortfall reported in line 7 should be treated as community benefit. Also describe in Part VI the costing methodology or source used to determine the amount reported on line 6. Check the box that describes the method used: |

    ☐ Cost accounting system    ☐ Cost to charge ratio        ☐ Other

**Section C. Collection Practices**

| 9a | Does the organization have a written debt collection policy? . . . . . . . . . . . . . . . . . . . . . **9a** | | |
| b | If "Yes," does the organization's collection policy contain provisions on the collection practices to be followed for patients who are known to qualify for charity care or financial assistance? Describe in Part VI . . . **9b** | | |

| **Part IV** | **Management Companies and Joint Ventures** |

| **(a)** Name of entity | **(b)** Description of primary activity of entity | **(c)** Organization's profit % or stock ownership % | **(d)** Officers, directors, trustees, or key employees' profit % or stock ownership % | **(e)** Physicians' profit % or stock ownership % |
|---|---|---|---|---|
| 1 | | | | |
| 2 | | | | |
| 3 | | | | |
| 4 | | | | |
| 5 | | | | |
| 6 | | | | |
| 7 | | | | |
| 8 | | | | |
| 9 | | | | |
| 10 | | | | |
| 11 | | | | |
| 12 | | | | |
| 13 | | | | |
| 14 | | | | |

Schedule H (Form 990) 2009

| Part V | Facility Information |
|---|---|

| Name and address | Licensed hospital | General medical & surgical | Children's hospital | Teaching hospital | Critical access hospital | Research facility | ER-24 hours | ER-other | Other (Describe) |
|---|---|---|---|---|---|---|---|---|---|
| | | | | | | | | | |
| | | | | | | | | | |
| | | | | | | | | | |
| | | | | | | | | | |
| | | | | | | | | | |
| | | | | | | | | | |
| | | | | | | | | | |
| | | | | | | | | | |
| | | | | | | | | | |
| | | | | | | | | | |
| | | | | | | | | | |
| | | | | | | | | | |
| | | | | | | | | | |
| | | | | | | | | | |
| | | | | | | | | | |
| | | | | | | | | | |
| | | | | | | | | | |

| Part VI | Supplemental Information |
|---------|--------------------------|

Complete this part to provide the following information.

**1** Provide the description required for Part I, line 3c; Part I, line 6a; Part I, line 7g; Part I, line 7, column (f); Part I, line 7; Part III, line 4; Part III, line 8; Part III, line 9b, and Part V. See Instructions.

**2** **Needs assessment.** Describe how the organization assesses the health care needs of the communities it serves.

**3** **Patient education of eligibility for assistance.** Describe how the organization informs and educates patients and persons who may be billed for patient care about their eligibility for assistance under federal, state, or local government programs or under the organization's charity care policy.

**4** **Community information.** Describe the community the organization serves, taking into account the geographic area and demographic constituents it serves.

**5** **Community building activities.** Describe how the organization's community building activities, as reported in Part II, promote the health of the communities the organization serves.

**6** Provide any other information important to describing how the organization's hospitals or other health care facilities further its exempt purpose by promoting the health of the community (e.g., open medical staff, community board, use of surplus funds, etc.).

**7** If the organization is part of an affiliated health care system, describe the respective roles of the organization and its affiliates in promoting the health of the communities served.

**8** If applicable, identify all states with which the organization, or a related organization, files a community benefit report.

-------------------------------------------------------------------------------

-------------------------------------------------------------------------------

-------------------------------------------------------------------------------

-------------------------------------------------------------------------------

-------------------------------------------------------------------------------

-------------------------------------------------------------------------------

-------------------------------------------------------------------------------

-------------------------------------------------------------------------------

-------------------------------------------------------------------------------

-------------------------------------------------------------------------------

-------------------------------------------------------------------------------

-------------------------------------------------------------------------------

-------------------------------------------------------------------------------

-------------------------------------------------------------------------------

-------------------------------------------------------------------------------

-------------------------------------------------------------------------------

-------------------------------------------------------------------------------

-------------------------------------------------------------------------------

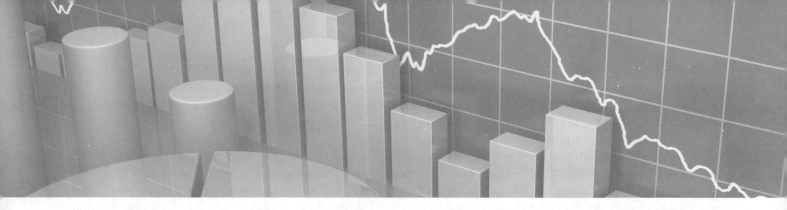

# CHAPTER 6

# Revenue Determination

## LEARNING OBJECTIVES

After studying this chapter, you should be able to do the following:

1. Define basic methods of payment for healthcare firms.
2. Understand the general factors that influence pricing.
3. Define the basic healthcare pricing formula.
4. Determine if prices are defensible.
5. Describe methods that are used to assess price defensibility prices in a real setting.
6. List some of the important considerations when negotiating a health plan contract.

## REAL-WORLD SCENARIO

Gary Bentham, CFO of Bartlett Community Hospital, is preparing for contract negotiation with his largest non-governmental payer, Antrim Healthcare. Antrim currently accounts for approximately 30% of all patient-care revenue at Bartlett and this percentage is growing. The current contract has been in force for 3 years and expires on June 30 of this year. Gary has given Antrim the required 180-day notification of his intent to terminate but is alarmed by the position taken by Antrim's chief negotiator, Alice Mullins. Alice has told Gary that Antrim is unwilling to increase its present payment schedule beyond 5%. Currently Antrim pays for inpatient care on a diagnosis-related group (DRG) basis using the relative weights employed by the centers for Medicare and Medicaid Services (CMS). The base payment for a case with weight of 1.0 is $4,800. Gary knows that Medicare currently pays the hospital $6,500 for a case with a weight of 1.0. While the outpatient payment from Antrim is more reasonable, Gary is concerned about the hospital's long-term financial position if the Antrim inpatient rate cannot be increased substantially.

Alice has told Gary that she believes the current inpatient rate is reasonable because Medicare patients are much more resource intensive than Antrim's younger patient population. To test this hypothesis, Gary compared the average charge by DRG for Medicare traditional patients and Antrim's patients. Gary was amazed at the similarity when the data analysis was completed. He discovered that on average an Antrim patient consumed 94.5% of the resources of a traditional Medicare patient. Gary further concluded that because the average cost of a traditional Medicare patient with a case weight of 1.0 was $6,200, he would need a payment of $5,859 (0.945 x $6,200) from Antrim to break even. If Alice is serious about their maximum rate increase of 5%, then the best rate that Gary could expect would be $5,040 (1.05 x $4,800), which is well below his estimated cost.

Even after Gary shared his cost analysis with Alice, Alice remains firm in her position. The best inpatient rate that Antrim will offer is $5,040. Alice has told Gary that any rate higher will compromise Antrim's market position and either destroy its margins or lead to a loss of market share.

Gary must now determine what position his hospital system should take with Antrim. He knows that his system controls about 40% of the capacity in their market, with the remaining 60% controlled by a competitive system. Both systems have some excess capacity, but that excess capacity has narrowed in the last few years as both hospitals have purchased smaller hospitals and consolidated them into their operations. There are also two major health plans that compete with Antrim. Both of these plans as well as Antrim have contracts with both systems. Gary knows that his present rates of payment from the other health plans are higher than Antrim's. He is also fairly certain that Antrim's rate of payment to his competitor is higher than their rates of payment to his hospital system.

Gary is attempting to answer the following questions before his next scheduled meeting with Alice. What is his marginal or incremental cost for the Antrim book of business? Could his competitor handle his present Antrim volume and at what cost? If Gary's system were not in Antrim's network, what percentage of his present Antrim volume would he retain? These issues and others are central to his negotiation posture with Alice and have profound implications for his hospital system.

---

▶ **Payment Methods and Their Relationship to Price Setting**

There are four generic methods of payment for healthcare firms: historical cost, bundled services, billed charges, and capitated rates. (See Chapter 3 for further discussion of payment methods.) **TABLE 6-1** presents a scheme for categorizing payment plans by two dimensions:

1. Payment basis
2. Unit of payment

The **payment basis** describes the manner by which a payer (Medicare, Medicaid, commercial health plans, and others) determines the amount to be paid for a specific healthcare claim. There are three payment bases: *cost, fee schedule,* and *price related.*

A **cost-payment basis** simply means that the underlying method for payment will be the provider's cost. The rules for determining cost will be specified in the contract between the payer and the healthcare provider. For example, payment may be defined as the provider's ratio of cost to charges (RCC) multiplied times the total charges for a specific healthcare claim. Payment for a claim with $1,000 of charges and a provider RCC of 50% would be paid $500 (50% times $1,000).

A **fee-schedule basis** means that the actual payment will be predetermined and will be unrelated to either the provider's cost or the provider's actual

**TABLE 6-1** Healthcare Payment Methods

| Unit of Payment | Payment Basis | | |
| | Cost | Fee Schedule | Price Related |
| --- | --- | --- | --- |
| Specific services | ■ High-cost drugs<br>■ Devices | ■ Resource-based relative value scale<br>■ Ambulatory payment classifications | ■ No contract<br>■ Self-pay<br>■ Outpatient |
| Bundled services | ■ Some government<br>■ clinics paid on an<br>■ annual budget | ■ DRGs<br>■ Per diem<br>■ Outpatient surgery groups | ■ Outliers |

prices. For example, Medicare payment to a hospital for a patient with a DRG assignment of 470 (major joint replacement or reattachment of lower extremity w/o MCC) will have a predetermined payment (e.g., $14,000). The actual charges, services provided, or the cost are not relevant once the DRG assignment has been made. The vast majority of physician payment from most payers is usually related to fee schedules. Usually fee schedules are negotiated in advance with the payer or are accepted as a condition of participation in programs such as Medicare and Medicaid.

A **price-related payment basis** means that the provider will be paid for services based on some relationship to its total charges or price for the services delivered to the patient. For example, a payer may negotiate payment with a healthcare provider at 75% of billed charges. In this situation, a claim with total charges of $10,000 would be paid $7,500 (75% times $10,000).

While there are three different payment basis methods, there are also two alternative methods for grouping the services provided to a patient that are referred to as the *unit of payment* (Table 6-1). These two different units of payment are called *specific services* or *bundled services*.

**Bundled services** aggregates services provided to a patient in an encounter of care into one payment unit. For example, many health plan contracts often pay for inpatient services on a per day or DRG basis. Payment is fixed in advance, based on an agreed fee schedule (e.g., $1,000 per day to cover all services provided) and is a bundled unit of payment because the provider's payment is the same regardless of the level of ancillary services per day.

In a **specific services** payment method the individual services provided to a patient in an encounter of care are not aggregated. An example of this might be a contract that makes payment for outpatient services based on a discount from billed charges (e.g., 75% of billed charges). This outpatient provision is related to the provider's prices and it is based on the prices of specific services that constitute the total claim for the patient, including radiology procedures, lab tests, and other procedures provided to the patient.

In many cases health plan contracts will have elements that may appear in more than one of the six cells displayed in Table 6-1. Many contracts that pay hospitals on a DRG basis will have a separate provision for outliers. Payment for outliers is often related to charges. For example, a contract may stipulate that for all claims in excess of $75,000 in billed charges, the payer will pay the claim not on a DRG basis, but at 80% of billed charges. Assume that a claim had a DRG payment of $15,000, but the patient incurred total charges of $90,000. The payer in this case would not pay $15,000, but 80% of $90,000, or $72,000. An interesting case is a health plan that has not negotiated a contract with a provider. In that case, the payment method would be billed charges and it would be related to the specific services provided. The apportionment of payment responsibility between the patient and their health plan would need to be worked out because the patient may have gone out of network, but the hospital in this case would expect payment based on billed charges.

## ▶ Methods for Controlling Revenue

Healthcare providers have three major ways that they can control their revenue function in today's economic climate:

1. Price setting
2. Payer contract negotiation
3. Billing/coding management

**Price setting** is the process of establishing specific prices for the services provided by the healthcare provider. The actual list of services to be priced can be quite large and could be as large as 80,000 in some hospitals. Pricing by healthcare firms is still a very important element of the revenue function even though the majority of revenue may not be related to prices. For example, a nursing home may have 80% of its revenue derived from Medicare and Medicaid that make payment on a fixed-fee-schedule basis that is unrelated to specific prices. The remaining 20% of the nursing home's business is affected by its set prices, and these prices may well mean the difference between a profit and a loss.

*Contract negotiation* is a critical activity for all healthcare firms that derive substantial portions of their revenue from commercial insurers. Any provider that negotiates a payment schedule that is lower than its costs is digging itself a deep hole, from which it may not be able to recover.

*Billing and coding* issues are very important in the current world of healthcare payment. Providers that fail to include delivered services on a claim are not paid for those services. For example, if an injectable drug is administered to a patient but the drug administration for that drug is not coded, lost payment will result. In a similar fashion, if secondary diagnosis codes are not included on a hospital claim, then the claim may be assigned to a lower weighted DRG, resulting in lost payment. See Chapter 2 for further discussion of coding and billing issues.

Our focus in this chapter is on the first two areas of revenue determination: pricing and payer contract negotiation. Improving performance in these areas will have a very positive impact on the firm's total revenue function.

---

### Learning Objective 2

Understand the general factors that influence pricing.

---

## ▶ Generic Principles of Pricing

**FIGURE 6-1** provides a schematic depicting the generic factors that influence pricing in any business. The three identified factors are *desired net income, competitive position*, and **market structure**. All of these factors will influence how a firm can change its prices and to what extent they are likely to control their pricing function.

### Desired Net Income

The first factor, desired net income, is the starting block for most short- and long-term pricing decisions. Net income is the difference between revenues and expenses. Every business must be able to generate enough revenue through its sales of products and services to sustain its operations and provide for the replacement of its physical assets as well as provide a return to its investors. Failure to realize adequate levels of pricing will result in eventual business failure. Deficiencies in levels of net income can be tolerated for short time frames, but long-term continuation of

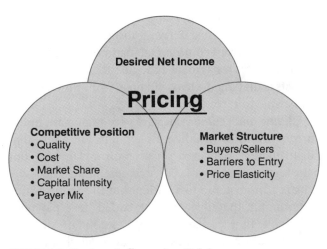

**FIGURE 6-1  Factors Influencing Pricing**

inadequate pricing will eventually result in business termination.

## Competitive Position

The competitive position of a business relative to its competitors has a significant influence on pricing policy. One of the most important factors in any business, but especially health care, is the perceived quality of the firm's products and services. Firms with higher perceived levels of *quality* can often price their products and services at a slightly higher level. Specific healthcare providers that are perceived as quality leaders in a marketplace often can realize higher prices in several ways. First, these firms may be able to negotiate more favorable payment terms with major health plans in the area. If the general community perceives one provider to be higher quality, employers may desire to have that provider in the plan's network of providers. It is also likely that the provider can establish prices that are above its local competitors because it knows that it has a premium quality advantage.

*Cost* is another critical factor that impacts a firm's relative competitive position. Lower-cost providers can afford to sell their products at lower prices and still generate adequate levels of profit, or they can sell their products at competitive prices but realize higher profits. In either case, it usually means market expansion for the lower-cost provider. If they establish lower prices, then they should be able to increase their market share. If they maintain competitive prices, the realization of greater profit may lead to expansion in the marketplace because of better access to capital, and they may even be in a position to acquire local competitors.

*Market share* is a critical determinant of price for any business. Most healthcare markets are regional in nature, and there are travel limits beyond which most consumers will not venture. Greater market share leads to greater leverage when negotiating health plan contracts. For example, if a hospital controlled 85% of the acute-care capacity in the region, virtually every health plan would be required to include that hospital in its network. This gives the hospital tremendous leverage when negotiating payment terms.

*Capital intensity* can also have an influence on pricing. Firms that are heavily capital intensive often have higher levels of fixed cost. It is also likely that their variable cost of production as a percentage of total cost may be lower, which may lead to marginal cost pricing in markets that have excess capacity. This behavior was seen in many urban hospital markets in the early days of health plan growth. Many hospitals would sign agreements with health plans at payment levels below their average total cost but above their variable or marginal cost. These hospitals were afraid that they might be excluded from a plan's network and lose critical volume so they agreed to payment levels that just barely covered their variable costs.

Of all the factors discussed to this point, none has a more pervasive influence on prices than *payer mix*, at least in the healthcare marketplace. Providers with heavy percentages of Medicaid and uninsured patients will usually experience large losses on these books of business no matter how efficiently they produce healthcare services. These providers must then be in a situation where they can increase levels of payment received from other patients to offset losses from Medicaid and uninsured patients. This payment inequity has been commonly referred to as *cost shifting*. This point is emphasized later in this chapter.

## Market Structure

The **market structure** in which a firm exists also influences pricing in a variety of ways. The number of *buyers and sellers* is a key dynamic that impacts pricing. Increasing the ratio of providers to health plans reduces the pricing flexibility of the provider. A worst-case scenario for a provider would be to be located in a market with many providers and only one buyer. Government is a major buyer in most healthcare markets through its Medicare and Medicaid programs. Providers have virtually no control over payment terms. Their only choice is to participate in the program and accept the payment rates or to exit and seek business with nongovernment patients. Given the sheer size of the programs, this is not a choice for many providers. It is the private market that represents the major area for pricing discretion. Ideally, providers would like to operate in a market where there were no or few other providers and many small health plans. Most healthcare markets are not like this, and there are usually a limited number of both providers and health plans. As health plans merge and consolidate, most providers feel a similar need to merge with other providers to keep the negotiation playing field level.

Most businesses would like to operate in an environment in which significant *barriers to entry* exist to protect them from new competitors. Large capital investment often serves as a barrier to entry. The actual level of investment required to either buy or build a hospital in an existing market can be more than $100 million. This level of capital will cause many potential competitors to think twice before entering a market where present capacity exists.

**Certificate-of-need (CON)** regulations can also prevent new healthcare providers from entering a market, as well as restrict growth for existing providers. CON programs are used by approximately 30 plus states to help maintain quality of care, control a portion of the healthcare costs of communities, and promote rational distribution of certain healthcare services. CON requires that individuals or healthcare facilities seeking to initiate or expand services submit applications to the state. Approval must be obtained before initiating projects that require capital expenditures above certain dollar thresholds, introduce new services, or expand beds or services.

The final factor affecting pricing under the market-structure umbrella is *price elasticity*. The concept of price elasticity describes the relationship between a change in price and demand for the service or product. Products or services whose ultimate demand is strongly influenced by price are said to be price elastic. Most products or services have some degree of price elasticity. Consumers will usually purchase fewer goods or services as their prices increase. For example, if the price of coffee rises, consumption would be expected to fall. Healthcare services, while not immune from the pressures of price elasticity, are usually less affected than other products. When someone needs to have his appendix removed, he is concerned less about price than he would be about the cost of a cup of coffee. The presence of health insurance has further insulated many consumers from the effects of price in healthcare markets. The cost of many procedures is either completely paid or is subject to relatively small deductibles and copayments. The rise of consumer-directed health plans has begun to affect price elasticity in healthcare markets. Many of these plans call for large initial deductibles of $1,000 or more. Patients in these types of plans are no longer insulated from the cost of health services, and price can become a more important factor in the decision to seek medical services.

---

### *Learning Objective 3*

Define the basic healthcare pricing formula.

---

## ▶ Price Setting for Healthcare Services

Healthcare firms must set rates at levels sufficient to maintain their financial viability. Prices must be set to cover the individual areas identified in **EXHIBIT 6-1**.

**EXHIBIT 6-1** Four Elements of Pricing

- Average costs
- Losses on third-party fee-schedule payments
  - Medicaid
  - Medicare
  - Other
- Discounts on billed-charge patients
  - Self-pay
  - Commerical
- Reasonable return on investment
  - Sustainable growth

Failure to develop pricing to cover all of these areas will result in eventual failure.

Before beginning the discussion of price setting it is important to define a few terms that often can cause some confusion in understanding pricing decisions and pricing behavior. Unless otherwise stated, the term *price* will represent the amount that exists in the healthcare firm's price list, commonly referred to as its **charge description master (CDM)**. Price then represents the amount that will be billed on a claim form that is sent to either the patient or their health plan. Prices and charges are often used interchangeably and represent the list price of services provided. These prices or charges are the same for everyone irrespective of payment status. Medicare, Medicaid, and even indigent patients have the same price or charge billed to their claim. Payment for services may be dramatically different from charges or prices and bear little or no relation to the total charges in a claim. For example, Medicare may receive a claim form from a physician for services provided to a Medicare beneficiary with $1,000 of charges but actual payment may be settled at $500 based on an existing fee schedule. In this section, the focus of discussion is on the determination of the price that will be used in the firm's CDM or price list.

It hardly seems necessary to state that any price must be set to cover the *average cost* of producing the product or service. If it costs $500 to perform a specific-imaging procedure, pricing that service at $400 would be a sure-fire formula for insolvency. We discussed earlier that on some occasions, firms may price a product at less than cost but more than average marginal cost. In our imaging-procedure example, the marginal cost of producing the image might be $250. In this case the firm might price the procedure at $250 or slightly more. This price would cover the marginal cost of production but would not cover the fixed costs

of operation, such as depreciation, interest expense on debt, and administrative costs. So-called marginal-cost pricing would, however, cover the incremental cost of production, and assuming excess capacity would contribute something to the coverage of fixed costs. In the long run, however, prices must be established to cover full costs of production.

Prices must be set to also recover any losses from third-party fee schedule payment. We referred to this practice as "**cost shifting**" earlier and is pervasive in the healthcare industry. For example, Medicaid may pay a nursing home $240 per day when the cost of one day of care is $300. Any price that is set must cover the cost of providing the service ($300) and it must also include the loss from Medicaid patients ($60 per day). It is not just governmental programs that may have payment rates below cost. A number of major health plans may have contracts that call for payment at levels below full cost. All of the collective losses incurred on these patients must be included in the price that is finally set. Losses incurred on these patients create an additional layer of cost which ultimately raises the price which is finally set.

Prices must also reflect **discounts from billed charges** that may be granted to health plans or uninsured patients. For example, a health plan may agree to pay a provider 85% of billed charges. A patient's claim with $100 of charges would therefore be paid 85% or $85. If $100 was needed to cover costs and losses from other third-party payers, the provider would need to set a price at $117.65 ($100/0.85), which when paid at 85% of billed charges, would equal $100. Uninsured patients are a growing problem for many healthcare providers, especially hospitals. Most hospitals in the United States collect only a small percentage of the billed charges for these patients, usually 5% or less. Although the Patient Protection and Affordable Care Act (ACA) has reduced the number of uninsured in the United States, about 10% of all Americans still do not have any form of health insurance coverage. The vast majority of the charges to the uninsured are written off as either charity care or bad debt. Uninsured patients are really patients who pay on a discount from billed charges, except their discount is usually very large.

The last requirement that needs to be included in price setting is some reasonable return on investment (ROI). Healthcare providers with either tax-exempt or taxable status need some return to insure their financial survival. A nursing home that only recovered the historical cost of its plant and equipment through depreciation expense would be unable to replace its plant and equipment if the replacement prices of those assets increased. In addition, all businesses need to cover so-called working capital costs, which are not recognized as expenses in a financial statement. Collections for many healthcare providers average 60 days or more, but payroll expenses and supply payments to vendors are paid on a more frequent basis. This difference, though not an accounting cost, must be financed, adding another element for required profit. Ultimately, any business firm needs to generate a ROI that will meet its requirement for sustainable growth. We will talk more about this topic in Chapter 11.

With this background on how prices should be set, let's examine a simple example to incorporate the four requirements for pricing just listed. We use the data in **TABLE 6-2** to illustrate the methodology of pricing. Note at the outset that we must set a price that will generate $105,000 of revenue, $100,000 of cost, and $5,000 of profit. We also know, given the current estimates of volume by payer and present payer rates, that we will receive $38,000 from Medicare (400 × $95), $7,500 from Medicaid (100 × $75), and $33,000 from Health Plan 1 (300 × $110). The total of these three fixed-fee schedule payers is $78,500. This means that we need to recover $26,500 ($105,000 less $78,500) from the two remaining payers that pay on a price or billed-charge basis. Health Plan 2 has 100 patients that will pay 80% of billed charges and the 100 uninsured patients will pay 10% of billed charges. Another way to look at the

**TABLE 6-3** Income Statement for Case Example

| Revenue | Computation | Amount |
|---|---|---|
| Medicare | 400 × $95 | $38,000 |
| Medicaid | 100 × $75 | 7,500 |
| Health Plan # 1 | 300 × $110 | 33,000 |
| Health Plan # 2 | 100 × 80% × $294.44 | 23,555 |
| Uninsured | 100 × 10% × $294.44 | 2,944 |
| Total | | $105,000 |
| Less costs | | 100,000 |
| Profit | | $5,000 |

billed-charge payers would be to state that we will have 80 patients from Health Plan 2 that will pay 100% of their charges and 20 patients who will pay nothing. We also have 10 uninsured patients who will pay 100% of the charges and 90 who will pay nothing. Viewed from this perspective, we will have 90 (80 + 10) patients who must cover the $26,500 of remaining financial requirement. Dividing the $26,500 by 90 yields a required price of $294.44. **TABLE 6-3** shows an income statement that proves the accuracy of our calculations.

The actual method for pricing can be reduced to a formula that is presented in **FIGURE 6-2**. The formula states that the average required price is derived from a series of computations. First, price must be set to include the average cost of production. **FIGURE 6-3** inserts the value of $100 into the average cost field using the example of Table 6-2. Second, the required level of net income must be defined, which was $5,000 in our example. Third, the total loss incurred on fixed-fee-schedule patients must be calculated. In Figure 6-3, this value is shown as $1,500. It is derived as follows:

Loss on Medicare = 400 patients × $5.00 per patient is $2,000

Loss on Medicare = 100 patients × $25.00 per patient is $2,500

Gain on Health Plan 1 = 300 patients × $10.00 is $3,000

The total loss on the three fixed-payer groups is thus $1,500 and is inserted in Figure 6-3. It is important

**TABLE 6-2** Price-Setting Example

| | |
|---|---|
| Total cost | $100,000 |
| Total volume | 1,000 |
| Average cost | $100 |
| Desired net income | $5,000 |
| **Payer volumes** | |
| Medicare (payment rate = $95) | 400 |
| Medicaid (payment rate = $75) | 100 |
| Health Plan 1 (payment rate = $110) | 300 |
| Health Plan 2 (pay 80% of charges) | 100 |
| Uninsured (pay 10% of charges) | 100 |
| Total all payers | 1,000 |

$$Price = \frac{Average\ Cost + \dfrac{Required\ net\ income + Loss\ on\ fee\ schedule\ payers}{Volume\ of\ charge\ payers}}{1 - Average\ discount\ experienced\ on\ charge\ payers}$$

**FIGURE 6-2  Pricing Formula**

$$Price = \frac{100 + \dfrac{\$5,000 + \$1,500}{200}}{1 - 0.55} = \$294.44$$

**FIGURE 6-3  Pricing Formula**

to note that the $3,000 gain from the health plan offsets the $4,500 loss incurred on the Medicare and Medicaid patients. In some situations this term can be negative, which means that there is no overall loss but a gain on fixed-fee-schedule patients. When this situation occurs, the actual required price that must be set actually can be decreased because the fixed-fee payers make a contribution toward the required profit level. The next step is to determine the number of total patients who pay on a charge basis. In our example, this value is 200: 100 Health Plan 2 patients and 100 uninsured patients. The patients of Health Plan 2 have a 20% discount while the uninsured patients have what amounts to a 90% discount. The final step is to derive the actual discount that is experienced on all combined charge-paying patients. This figure is defined by weighting the proportion of charge patients in a specific payer category to total charge patients by the appropriate discount rate of that charge payer. The value for our example is 0.55 and its computation is:

[% of Health Plan 2 × Health Plan 2 Discount %]
+ [% of Uninsured × Uninsured Discount %]

[(100/200) × 0.20] + [(100/200) × 0.90] = 0.55]

The formula yields a required price of $294.44, as we have previously determined. In this example, note that our markup from cost is 294%, which simply means that our charges ($294.44) are 2.94 times our average cost ($100). This seems like a very high markup and would cause many people to think that the healthcare firm is making an excessive amount of profit when in fact their margin is fairly small: $5,000 on a total cost of $100,000 (5%).

The formula of Figure 6-2 helps us to understand the effects of critical drivers on a healthcare firm's prices. In general prices will increase in the following situations:

- Costs increase
- Governmental programs pay less than cost
- Healthcare plans adopt fee schedules that do not pay at levels above cost

$$Price = \frac{100 + \dfrac{5,000}{1,000}}{1 - 0.09} = \$115.38$$

**FIGURE 6-4  Pricing Formula**

- The firm's required profit increases because of financial needs, such as debt-service obligations or capital replacement
- The proportion of charge-paying patients drops
- Levels of uninsured patients increase

It might be useful to see the effects of a system where every payer except the uninsured patients paid 100% of billed charges. If this were the situation, the required price in our example would fall to $115.38. This of course means that Medicare, Medicaid, and all healthcare plans would pay 100% of billed charges, and we would still experience a 90% write-off on the uninsured patients. **FIGURE 6-4** shows the computation of price in this revised payment scheme.

The results in our example are painfully obvious to every healthcare executive. Healthcare firms that lose money on Medicare, Medicaid, and healthcare contracts must raise rates sharply to a limited charge-related payer base. Large write-offs or discounts to the charge-related payer base can and often do escalate prices to levels that are well above costs. This is the nature of the economic environment facing healthcare firms today. Wishing it were not so will not change the facts, but it does create a need for many healthcare firms to justify their prices to the public because price appears so far from cost.

*Learning Objective 4*

Determine if prices are defensible.

## ▶ Justifying Healthcare Firm Prices

The rising visibility of healthcare firm prices in general and hospital prices in particular have focused attention on how best to both communicate and justify prices to the general public. There has been a dramatic increase in hospital prices over the last 20 years. **FIGURE 6-5** demonstrates that the relationship between hospital cost and hospital price has changed markedly during the period from 1996 to 2014. From our earlier discussion of pricing we learned that actual cost is only one factor that impacts price. Payer-mix variables such as percentage of billed-charge patients, level of

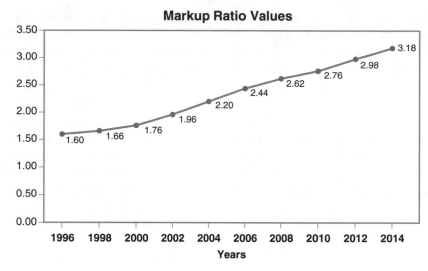

**FIGURE 6-5** **Median Hospital Mark-Ups—1996 to 2014**

Courtesy of Cleverley & Associates

uninsured patients, losses on Medicare and Medicaid, and payment patterns of health plans have a much more pervasive influence on prices than costs. This of course explains why the level of markups in the hospital industry has increased from 1.6 in 1996 to 3.18 in 2014.

The term *reasonable charges* is used by many people when they review healthcare firm pricing. Often, there is disagreement about the issue of reasonableness when the underlying data is the same. We believe that it is critical to bring a structured framework that may be used to assess the issue of reasonableness as it pertains to healthcare pricing. In our experience,

there are two generic ways that reasonableness of charges or prices has been used in the healthcare industry.

1. *Public utility regulatory.* Most public utility-type regulatory models permit the earning of a reasonable rate of ROI to ensure that capital can be replaced. Without adequate rates of return, capital will not be available to replace and renovate plant and equipment. Healthcare firms have a heavy investment in plant and equipment and must keep replacing that plant and equipment to keep pace with advances in medical technology.

   In addition, healthcare firms have sizable working capital needs that are not recognized as expenses but require cash outlays. For example, most healthcare firms pay employees on a biweekly basis but collect patient receivables on a 60-plus-day basis. Healthcare firms must set prices to generate a reasonable level of profit that will permit them to replace their capital-asset bases in a timely manner and to provide for working capital needs.

2. *Market-based comparisons.* Often, both payers and healthcare firms will assess the reasonableness of healthcare charges based on comparisons with similar and/ or other healthcare firms in the same geographic region. A number of states and local communities have reporting mechanisms for healthcare firms to report charges for either specific procedures or some

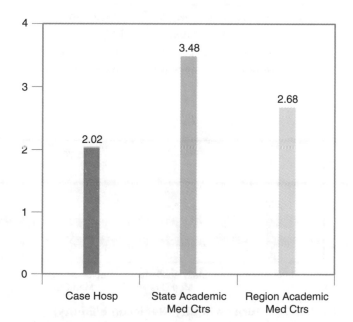

**FIGURE 6-6** **Return on Assets (Net Income/Assets) 5-Year Average—2012 to 2016**

aggregate measure of hospital output such as discharges. One of the difficulties with comparing hospital charges is that they may vary significantly across hospitals, not necessarily because of operating cost differences but because of payer differences. Hospitals with heavy percentages of Medicare, Medicaid, and indigent patients will need to have higher prices in order to realize minimal levels of profitability. Size, complexity, and teaching status will also impact charges.

We will now use a specific hospital example to develop a framework for assessing the reasonableness of charges in a specific setting, using these two methods.

---

### Learning Objective 5

Describe methods that are used to assess price defensibility prices in a real setting.

---

## Reasonableness of Charges for Case Hospital

### Public Utility ROI Method

Historically, many public utility rates were based on the fair-return-on-fair-value concept, manifested in an 1898 Supreme Court decision (*Smyth v. Ames et al.*). Implicitly, this permits a reasonable profit on the firm's underlying investment:

$$Retun\ on\ Investment = \frac{Net\ Revenue - Cost}{Investment}$$

To assess the reasonableness of Case Hospital's charges, using the above model, we will address three issues:

- Is ROI at Case Hospital reasonable?
- Are costs at Case Hospital reasonable?
- Is investment at Case Hospital reasonable?

The first question to be raised is whether returns at the Case Hospital are high in relation to hospital industry averages. Absolute levels of reported net income or profit margins, the ratio of net income to revenue, are not acceptable measures for assessing the adequacy of ROI because they do not relate net income to any measure of investment. We have chosen two alternative measures of investment for our analysis, total assets and equity. Total assets is simply the historical cost of all assets employed in the business

while equity is total assets less present liabilities. Our two measures of ROI are thus **return on total assets** (net income divided by total assets) and return on equity (net income divided by equity).

Case Hospital is a major academic medical center, and it will be compared with two peer groups of academic medical centers, one a state group and the other a regional group. **FIGURES 6-6** and **6-7** display values derived from Medicare cost reports for two comparative groups and Case Hospital for the period 2012 to 2016. The data suggest that Case Hospital has not realized excessive levels of profit based on values reported here. In some situations ROI levels may appear to be high relative to industry averages. In these situations it is important to determine whether other financial considerations may require greater levels of profitability. Specific areas would include low levels of cash and replacement reserves, high levels of debt, and older physical facilities. Conversely, a low level of ROI could in fact be acceptable if a firm has high levels of cash and replacement reserves, low levels of debt, and a young physical facility.

The second question to be answered is the reasonableness of costs at Case Hospital. In general, there are two methods of assessing hospital cost at the facility level. One method uses an adjusted-patient day or adjusted-discharge method. A second method relies on individual assessment of cost for inpatient and outpatient services. In our opinion, the second method provides superior accuracy. We will discuss this method further in Chapter 11. The methodology for defining a facility-wide measure of hospital cost involves weighting two measures:

1. *Medicare cost per discharge*: Case-mix- and wage-index adjusted (MCPD)
2. *Medicare cost per outpatient claim*: Relative-weight and wage-index adjusted (MCPC)

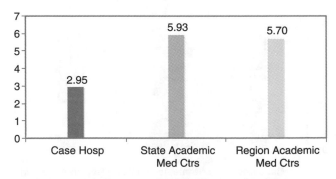

**FIGURE 6-7** **Return on Equity (Net Income/Equity) 5-Year Average—2012 to 2016**

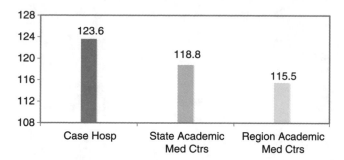

**FIGURE 6-8** **Hospital Cost Index—2016**

The hospital cost index (HCI) is then constructed as follows:

$$\text{HCI} = \% \text{ Inpatient revenue} \times \frac{\text{MCPD}}{\text{US avg}}$$

$$+ \% \text{ Outpatient revenue} \times \frac{\text{MCPC}}{\text{US avg}}$$

Values for these cost measures are presented in **FIGURES 6-8, 6-9**, and **6-10**. The data in Figure 6-8 show that Case Hospital has an overall cost structure that is very similar to that of the state academic medical centers and the median value for regional academic medical centers. Case Hospital appears to have slightly higher inpatient costs, as seen in Figure 6-9, but its outpatient costs are considerably lower than those of the comparison groups. We can conclude that Case Hospital is providing health services at levels of cost consistent with expected values. Therefore, based on this analysis, we can conclude that Case Hospital's costs are reasonable.

The third and final question relates to investment levels at Case Hospital. To assess investment reasonableness, we select a measure of investment productivity referred to as *fixed asset turnover*. This metric includes a measure of output (net revenue) in the numerator and a measure of input (net fixed assets)

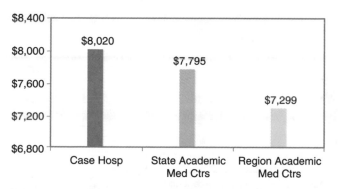

**FIGURE 6-9** **Medicare Cost per Discharge (CMI and WI Adj.)—2016**

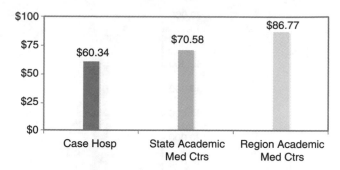

**FIGURE 6-10** **Cost per Medicare Visit (RW and WI Adj.)—2016**

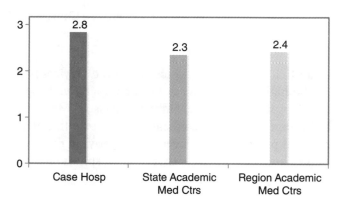

**FIGURE 6-11** **Fixed Asset Turnover (Net Revenue/Net Fixed Assets)—2016**

in the denominator. Review of investment levels show Case Hospital to have above-average efficiency with respect to investment in plant, property, and equipment (**FIGURE 6-11**).

All of these data indicate the following:

- Case Hospital is not realizing excessive profits
- Costs at Case Hospital are consistent with expected values and are reasonable
- Investment at Case Hospital is reasonable and not excessive

These three points show clearly that revenue and prices at Case Hospital are reasonable. This does not

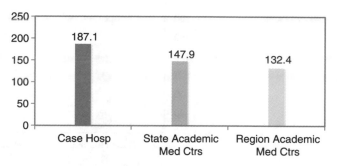

**FIGURE 6-12** **Hospital Charge Index—2016**

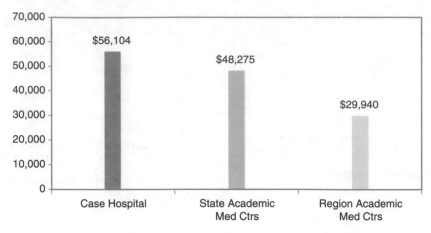

**FIGURE 6-13** **Medicare Charge per Discharge (CMI and WI Adj.)—2016**

mean that its individual prices for some services will not be higher than those at local comparative hospitals. Hospitals can have different levels of Medicaid and indigent-care or healthcare contracts with differences in payment. Whatever the underlying cause or causes, however, it is clear that Case Hospital's charges or prices are reasonable.

## Comparison-of-Charges Method

Often, both payers and hospitals will assess the reasonableness of their prices or charges based on comparisons with similar hospitals and/or other hospitals in the same geographic region. A number of states and local communities have mechanisms for hospitals to report charges for either specific procedures or some aggregate measure of facility output, such as discharges. Most recently, some states, including California, have made portions of hospital CDMs publicly available. One of the difficulties with comparing hospital charges is that they may vary significantly across hospitals, not necessarily because of operating cost

differences but because of payer differences. Hospitals with heavy percentages of Medicare, Medicaid, and indigent patients will have higher prices in order to realize minimal levels of profitability, as we previously discussed.

To provide some basis for comparison of charges at Case Hospital, we selected all academic medical centers in the state. We also included the regional average for academic medical centers, adjusting for cost-of-living differences. Academic medical centers often have both higher costs and charges because their patients are often more severely ill. Medicare has recognized this and provides greater levels of payment to compensate for their greater costs.

We examined the relative level of charges at Case Hospital from a global facility-level basis, using the same construction discussed earlier for costs. These comparisons are presented in **FIGURES 6-12, 6-13**, and **6-14**. The data reflected in these three graphs show charges at Case Hospital to be above those of the comparative groups. We believe that Case Hospital's charges are above the comparative groups because

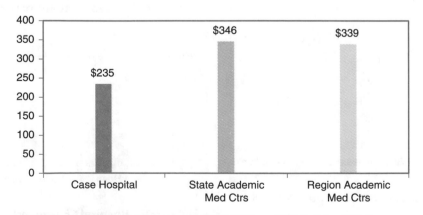

**FIGURE 6-14** **Average Charge per APC (RW and WI Adj.)—2016**

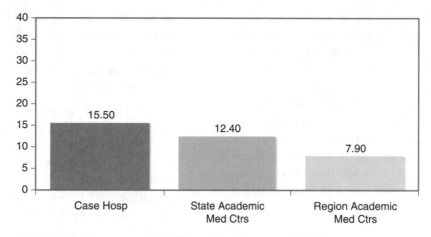

**FIGURE 6-15  Uncompensated Care Percentage—2016**

of its higher level of care provided to Medicaid and indigent patients. To see the effects of this patient mix on charges, **FIGURE 6-15** shows the **uncompensated care percentage**, which represents the cost of care delivered to indigent patients after subtracting any payments. The uncompensated care percentage for Case Hospital and the two comparative groups is presented in Figure 6-15. The uncompensated care percentage at Case Hospital is 25% above the state academic medical center average and 96% above the regional academic medical center average. In summary, we believe Case Hospital's charges are reasonable when compared to similar hospitals after payer-mix differences are considered.

*Learning Objective 6*

List some of the important considerations when negotiating a health plan contract.

## ▶ Health Plan Contract Negotiation

Having discussed pricing, we will now focus our attention on the last area of revenue management, the negotiation of health plan contracts. Negotiation of health plan contracts has become much more intense in recent years. An average hospital in the United States may be faced with the task of negotiating 30 health plan contracts or more. **EXHIBIT 6-2** shows a listing of payers for a medium-sized U.S. hospital.

**EXHIBIT 6-2**  Contracts for a Medium-Sized U.S. Hospital

### Contract/Payer Category

Aetna HMO
Aetna PPO
Beech Street
Blue Bell
Blue Cross/Blue Shield HMO/PPO
Blue Cross/Blue Shield Indemnity
Bravo Health
Champus/Tricare
Cigna HMO
Cigna LifeSource
Cigna PPO
Comm Health Choice Star
First Health
Galaxy
Great West–HMO/PPO
HAA Preferred Partners
Healthsmart
Humana–HMO
Humana–PPO
Integrated Health Plan
Medicaid
Medicare
Molina Healthcare–CHIP
Molina Healthcare–Star
Molina Healthcare–Star Plus
Multiplan
PHCS PPO
PPOnext
UHC HMO & PPO
Unicare HMO
USFHP
Workers' Compensation

Courtesy of Cleverley & Associates

In any health plan contract, there are two critical elements. First, there is the payment schedule, which describes the basis of payment and actual payment/fee schedules. Second, there is the actual contract language, which describes the administration of the contractual arrangement that determines how services are provided and paid. Most attention is focused on the actual payment schedules, but the actual administrative language is becoming more important. In the remainder of this section, we describe 10 important areas of health plan contract language.

## Remove Contract Ambiguity

It seems that a hallmark of many business relationships is to establish written agreements that no one except attorneys can understand. If contract language is unclear, it should be clarified.

## Eliminate Retroactive Denials

It has become increasingly common for health plans to deny claims for services that were either directly or indirectly approved by the plan. Contract clauses that permit retroactive denials should be removed from contract documents. An example of a retroactive denial clause follows:

> *Company, on its behalf and on behalf of other payers, reserves the right to perform utilization review (including retrospective review) and to adjust or deny payment for medically inappropriate services.*

## Establish a Reasonable Appeal Process

Medical necessity of services is a key element in payment approval. When services have been approved by the plan or the plan has been notified and did not protest the provision of services, claims should be paid. This is the basis of "retroactive denials," which we just discussed. In some cases, services may be provided because the member's physician believed they were necessary, but the plan protested. In these cases, a reasonable appeal process should be established that is not one sided. The following contract language came from an actual health plan contract and does not provide for any provider representation. These types of appeal arrangements should be modified to include both provider and plan representation.

### Level 1 Appeal

*Part 1: The matter will be reviewed by a physician selected by ABC. If the physician determines that the decision to deny payment is in error, payment of the Claim will be authorized. If the decision to deny payment is affirmed by physician, the Case will then automatically proceed to Part 2 of the Level 1 Appeal procedure.*

*Part 2: The matter will be reviewed by a physician, selected by ABC, who is currently practicing in a specialty relevant to the Case in question. If the physician determines that the decision to deny payment is in error, the payment of the Claim will be authorized. If the decision to deny payment is affirmed by the physician, no payment will be made.*

### Level 2 Appeal

*If HOSPITAL continues to dispute the payment decision, a Level 2 Appeal shall be available within the same timeframes as set forth above. The matter will be reviewed by a physician, selected by ABC, who is practicing in a specialty relevant to the Case in question and who was not involved in the Level 1 Appeal. If this reviewing physician determines that the decision to deny payment is in error, the payment of the Claim will be authorized. If the decision to deny payment is affirmed by the physician, no payment will be made. This level of appeal shall become final and binding upon both parties.*

## Define Clean Claims

In most health plan contracts, providers are required to submit claims on a standard form, usually a UB-04 for institutional providers or a HCFA 1500 for medical professionals. Some health plans often reject claims and return them to the provider for reasons that are not material to claim payment. For example, the claim may be missing the provider's address or it might have an incorrect patient zip code. While the claims may be paid eventually, it can cause cash flow hardships for providers. Many states have legislation requiring health plans to make payment for *clean claims* within specified time periods (e.g., 30 days). Claim denial for missing data is sometimes used as a stalling tactic.

Presented below is a language from a typical contract. Notice that it is the plan that determines if the claim is complete, and no specific standards are identified:

> *Any amount owing under this agreement shall be paid within thirty (30) days after receipt of a complete claim, unless additional information is requested within the thirty (30) day period.*

## Remove Most Favored Nation (MFN) Clauses

Some health plan contracts contain provisions that preclude a provider from contracting with any other health plan at rates lower than those defined in the current contract. These provisions are very hard to enforce and impair the provider's ability to conduct its business affairs in a reasonable manner. A simple response to the inclusion of a MFN clause in a contract is to make it reciprocal and require the health plan not to pay more for services to any other provider. While the health plan may argue this would be a violation of antitrust, it does point out the inequity of a one-sided MFN clause. The MFN clause can make it very difficult to negotiate new contracts. To illustrate this, assume a provider has just negotiated a new 3-year contract with a sizable price increase. If the new prices are above existing contract provisions in other older health plan contracts, the inclusion of a MFN could roll back payment terms to an existing old contract. MFN clauses are also very difficult to test. Payment terms are usually not identical across plans. One plan may pay on a per-diem and another on a case basis.

## Prohibit Silent PPO Arrangements

A common practice in the healthcare insurance marketplace is the leasing of networks. One health insurance plan may lease or rent its network to another plan for a sum of money. Members in that plan may then present themselves for medical services at the provider and claim the negotiated payment rate of the leased network. This will often extend payment discounts to a much larger group than originally intended. There should be specific contract language prohibiting this arrangement. Without specific language, it is inferred that the lease arrangement is valid. The contract language below extends the definition of the "Plan" to a potentially broad group, thereby allowing a large number of individuals access to favorable rates.

> *Plan. Any health benefit product or plan issued, administered, or serviced by the company or one of its affiliates, including but not limited to HMO, preferred provider organizations, indemnity, Medicaid, Medicare, and Workers' Compensation.*

## Include Terms for Outliers or Technology-Driven Cost Increases

Ideally, the contract will contain provisions increasing payments as time passes for increases in costs. Sometimes market forces or technology-driven changes in medical practice can cause major increases in costs. The use of stents in angioplasty is an example of a technology-driven change. Stents are used in most angioplasty cases today but were seldom used initially. One possible way to objectively link payment increases to costs is to relate actual payment to Medicare fee schedules. Payments for outliers should also be included to avoid the losses that result from treating catastrophic cases.

## Establish Ability to Recover Payment After Termination

Most health plan contracts will establish a term for the contract, usually 3 to 5 years. After that term, the contract will automatically renew for a year unless terminated. Termination in the initial term is often difficult unless there is a default or breach of the contract. After the initial term, either party usually can terminate the contract without cause, provided proper notification is given. A critical question to address is how will payment be made to the providers after the contract period? Providers must be careful to ensure that payment terms in the contract are not carried forward for a prolonged period of time after termination. The following contract language permits the plan to use existing payment terms for up to a full year in certain circumstances. This is not an ideal situation for the provider because it permits the plan an opportunity to seek other providers for their network without creating additional cost and it keeps members content because existing patient/provider relationships can be maintained.

> *Upon Termination. Upon termination of this Agreement for any reason, other than termination by Company in accordance with section 7.4 above, Hospital shall remain obligated at Company's sole discretion to provide Hospital Services to: (a) any Member who is an inpatient at Hospital as of the effective date of termination until such Member's discharge or Company's orderly transition of such Member's care to another provider; and (b) any Member, upon request of such Member or the applicable Payer, until the anniversary date of such Member's respective Plan or for one (1) calendar year, whichever is less. The terms of this Agreement shall apply to all services.*

## Preserve the Ability to be Paid for Services

Health plans are naturally interested in shielding their members from additional medical costs that are associated with services that were not medically necessary.

The critical question is how services that were deemed not medically necessary or not covered by the plan's benefits will be paid. We have already discussed the importance of removing the plan's ability to retroactively deny claims. In some situations, precertification by the plan for a member's treatment has been clearly denied. The provider in these situations should be free to provide services if requested by the patient and bill the patient directly. The following contract language appears to limit the provider's ability to do this without unnecessary bureaucracy. These kinds of clauses should be modified to still protect the patient but not destroy the legitimate right of the provider to be paid for services provided to the patient when consent is granted.

> HOSPITAL may seek payment from the Covered Individual for Health Services which are not provided in the Covered Individual's Health Benefit Plan when the non-coverage is due to reasons other than lack of Medical Necessity. HOSPITAL may seek payment from the Covered Individual for Health Services which are non-Covered Services because the services have been deemed not Medically Necessary, only if the Covered Individual has requested the Health Services to be provided notwithstanding Plan's determination, and only if HOSPITAL has provided Covered Individual notice in writing prior to the rendition of services of the approximate cost said Covered Individual will incur, and Covered Individual has agreed to the rendition of the service having had the benefit of said information. In such event, HOSPITAL may bill the Covered Individual at its customary rate for such services.

## Minimize Health Plan Rate Differentials

It is an interesting economic twist that providers seem to reward the worst-paying customers and punish their best-paying customers. The health plan that has negotiated the best rate or largest discount has a cost advantage over other health plans in the market. This should enable them to gain market share and drive out competitive plans. In turn, this gives the plan more negotiating leverage to receive even steeper discounts, which further enhances the plan's market position. The plans with smaller discounts—which means higher payments to providers—are forced out. Rather than continue this cycle, it may make sense for providers to establish a rate structure for all plans and grant discounts for administrative efficiencies only. This, of course, is much easier said than done, especially where a provider is facing financial ruin if 20% of its business

is lost. Payment equity across plans is, however, a goal and should be pursued where economically feasible.

## ▶ Health Plan Payment Schedules

From most providers' perspectives, the key element in a health plan contract is the payment or compensation schedule. **TABLE 6-4** presents a 2016 summary of over 4,000 health plan contract payment provisions for U.S. hospitals. The numbers presented are an average for all plans that make payment based on the unit identified.

**TABLE 6-4** Average Health Plan Payment Rates to Hospitals, 2016

| Services | Average |
|---|---|
| **INPATIENT SERVICES** | |
| All IP services paid at % | 77.7% |
| MS—DRG | $ 10,879 |
| Medical—per diem | $ 3,127 |
| Surgical—per diem | $ 3,377 |
| Psych | $ 1,225 |
| SNF | $ 1,049 |
| Normal vag del case rate (or 2-day stay) | $ 5,109 |
| C-section case rate (or 3-day stay) | $ 6,177 |
| Nursery level 1: Boarder—per diem | $ 947 |
| Stop loss: Threshold | $ 145,936 |
| Stop loss charges paid at % | 58.3% |
| Rate increase limit % | 4.6% |
| **OUTPATIENT SERVICES** | |
| All OP services paid at % | 76.5% |
| Emergency department paid at % | 72.3% |
| Emergency department: Case rate | $ 975 |
| Observation paid at % | 71.5% |

| Services | Average |
|---|---|
| Observation case rate: Per hour | $ 93 |
| Physical therapy paid at % | 72.6% |
| PT case rate: Per visit | $ 180 |
| MRI OP paid at % | 56.7% |
| MRI OP: Case rate | $ 1,321 |
| Outpatient surgery paid at % | 73.4% |
| OP Surg Group 1: Case rate | $ 1,707 |
| OP Surg Group 2: Case rate | $ 2,269 |
| OP Surg Group 3: Case rate | $ 3,000 |
| OP Surg Group 4: Case rate | $ 3,697 |
| OP Surg Group 5: Case rate | $ 4,505 |
| OP Surg Group 6: Case rate | $ 4,982 |
| OP Surg Group 7: Case rate | $ 6,184 |
| OP Surg Group 8: Case rate | $ 6,995 |
| OP Surg Group 9: Case rate | $ 9,107 |

Courtesy of Cleverley & Associates

For example, the average percentage of billed charges paid for hospital inpatient services was 77.7% in plans that paid for inpatient care on a percentage of charge basis. Hospitals that were not paid on a percentage of charge basis would most likely not have any separate payments on a per-diem or case basis. The data in Table 6-4 state that the average payment per case or DRG was $10,879 for a case weight of 1.0. For hospitals who paid on a per-diem basis for inpatient care there is often a mix of different per-diem rates. For example, the plan may pay a per-diem rate for all inpatients except a case rate for selected DRGs; most often these are high-cost surgical cases, such as coronary artery bypass. Outpatient care is often paid on either a fee-schedule or discount-from-charges basis. Again, a mix of the two may be present, and selected surgical and radiology procedures may be fee schedule, with all others being discounted charges.

Many hospital contracts have **outlier** or **stop-loss provisions**. This provision specifies that the hospital may pay on a basis other than per diem or case if charges exceed a specific limit. For example, Table 6-4 states that the average stop-loss threshold is $145,936 and any inpatient claim that has more than $145,936 would be paid on discount from billed-charge basis. In some cases, the entire claim would be paid as discount from billed charges (e.g., 66 percent). In other cases, only the charges that exceed the threshold would be paid on a billed-charge basis. For example, assume a claim with $200,000 of charges and a stop loss at $150,000 with payment at 70% of excess charges. Payment for this claim would consist of the original DRG fee and then an additional stop-loss payment of $35,000 [70% × ($200,000 − $150,000)].

Many health plan contracts that provide for payment of claims on a discount from billed charges include rate-increase-limit clauses. The overall objective of a rate-increase-limit provision is fairly straightforward. The rate-increase-limit provision is intended to prevent a hospital from raising its prices beyond reasonable levels. Significant increases in prices could cause a payer to lose large sums of money on existing negotiated contracts with employers and weaken the health plan's financial viability. In most cases the presence of a rate-increase limit can modify the historical discount from billed charges contained in the contract. The key contract provision is what is termed the *allowed rate of increase*. The allowed rate of increase is used in conjunction with the actual rate of increase to determine whether an adjustment in the discount

| TABLE 6-5 Physician Fee Schedule Example | | |
|---|---|---|
| **CPT Description** | **CPT Code** | **Fee Schedule** |
| Office/outpatient visit, new | 99205 | $403.58 |
| Implant neuroelectrodes | 64581 | 3,327.21 |
| Spinal fluid tap, diagnostic | 62270 | 704.34 |
| Resect/debride pancreas | 48105 | 12,523.25 |
| Shoulder arthroscopy/surgery | 29806 | 5,055.55 |
| Bone biopsy, trocar/needle | 20225 | 4,432.10 |

is necessary and, if so, to what extent. The usual payment adjustment can be stated as follows:

$$\text{New payment \%} = \frac{1 + \text{Allowed rate increase}}{1 + \text{Actual rate increase}}$$
$$\times \text{Present payment \%}$$

To illustrate this methodology, assume a present contract provides for payment at 70% of billed charges. The contract has a rate-increase limit of 5%, and the hospital has put a 10% rate increase into effect. The revised payment percentage would be 66.82% (1.05/1.10 × 70%). To see the actual effect of the adjustment, assume a present procedure is priced at $1,000 and its price is increased to $1,100 (a 10% increase). The hospital would have been paid $700 under the old arrangement (70% of $1,000). It will now be paid $735 ($1,100 × 66.82%). The actual payment increase is $35 or a 5% increase from the original $700 base payment, which is the maximum price increase allowed under the contract.

Medical groups are often paid on a fee-schedule basis, with limited capitation arrangements sometimes being used. The fee schedules are usually by current procedural terminology (CPT) and, in some cases, are directly related to Medicare's resource-based relative value scale (RBRVS) payment system. The health plan often contracts to pay some percentage, for example, 110% of Medicare RBRVS rates. A sample schedule of fees for a medical group is presented in **TABLE 6-5**.

## ▶ SUMMARY

The critical driver of any firm's financial solvency is usually its ability to generate reasonable levels of profit that can provide for the replacement and growth of capital in the firm. Because profit is simply the difference between revenue and cost, careful attention must be directed at both revenue management and cost control. This chapter has focused on revenue management. Revenue management is directly affected by three key areas: pricing, health plan contract negotiation, and billing and coding. Our focus in this chapter has been on pricing and health plan contract negotiation. Prices are currently receiving a lot of exposure in the healthcare industry, and the public is concerned about the relationship of prices to cost.

We have seen that healthcare firm prices are a function of four basic factors: costs, payment provisions of large third-party payers, levels of care provided to the uninsured, and required levels of profit. Because of inadequate payment from large governmental programs and rising levels of uninsured patients, many healthcare firms have prices that are multiples of cost, but profit levels are only marginal. Health plan contract negotiation can be a primary means to profit enhancement if reasonable rates of payment can be negotiated. It is also important, however, to examine specific contract language because reasonable payment rates mean very little if significant numbers of claims are denied.

## ASSIGNMENTS

1. You have been asked to comment on the reasonableness of a healthcare firm's prices using the ROI methodology described in this chapter. Your review has determined that the firm's costs are in line with industry averages and its overall investment is similar to other comparable healthcare firms, but its level of return on investment is 20% higher than industry averages. Are there any factors that the firm might be able to use to justify its higher-than-average rate of profitability?

2. You are trying to determine the average discount rate on charge payers to be used in the formula described in Figure 6-3. You have the following three payers with different discount rates: 200 uninsured patients who pay on average 5% of charges, 300 health plan patients who pay 85% of billed charges, and another block of 500 health plan patients who pay 75% of billed charges. What is the average discount rate that should be used in Figure 6-3?

3. Quality is usually described as a key factor in pricing. How can a healthcare firm with perceived higher levels of quality of care benefit from higher quality if 75% of its business is derived from Medicare and Medicaid patients who pay on a fixed-fee basis that does not adjust for quality differences?

4. Consumer-driven health plans often rely on large deductibles that are often funded via a health savings account framework. How might the presence of a large deductible affect price elasticity for health services?

5. In negotiating a health plan contract, why is it important to spell out precisely what constitutes a clean claim?

6. Your hospital has a contract with a large national health insurer that barely covers cost but does provide a small overall profit. Under the terms of this contract, the insurer may extend its contract terms to other plans when it leases its network to them. Why might it be desirable to remove this provision from your contract?

7. Using the example of Table 6-2, assume that the average cost has jumped from $100 to $105. All other factors in the example will remain the same. What will be the new required price?

8. Modifying the example in Assignment 7, assume that all fixed payers will raise their payment levels 5%: Medicare will pay $99.75, Medicaid will pay $78.75, and Managed-Care Plan 1 will pay $115.50. If costs have still increased 5% to $105, what rate would now be required?

9. Using the data of Table 6-2, assume that a new health plan has approached you with an opportunity to sign a contract with them that would pay on a fixed-fee schedule. The rate of payment would be $95 per unit and 200 new patient units would result. It is also assumed that the additional 200 new units would increase total cost from $100,000 to $112,000. This means that the marginal or variable cost per unit is $60. If the present price cannot be changed and will remain at $294.44 as determined in Table 6-3, what will be the effect on the firm's total profit? Should this contract be signed?

## SOLUTIONS

1. The best way to review the adequacy of current profit is to examine current and projected uses for the firm's profit. For example, a not-for-profit firm located in a growing market may need to earn above-average levels of profit to provide for larger capital expenditures to meet replacement and growth needs. A firm might also have a very high level of current debt financing, which calls for large payments of debt principal in the short term. Other possible areas might include a need to build current cash reserves because of present inadequacies. Major delays in claim payment might also cause a firm to increase profit levels to finance the larger balances of accounts receivable.

2. [(200/1,000 × 0.95) + [(300/1,000) × 0.15] + [(500/1,000) × 0.25] = 0.36. The average discount rate to be used for the three payers is 36% or, alternatively, the average rate of payment would be 64%.

3. Two possible benefits of higher quality still exist. First, higher quality may drive more patients to the firm. If the payment from Medicare and Medicaid patients exceeds the marginal cost of service delivery, the incremental profit will go up. Second, higher quality may permit the firm to negotiate more favorable payment rates from the remaining payers in either better managed-care contract terms or higher prices.

4. Large deductibles place the initial cost of many health services on the patient as opposed to traditional health insurance coverage, which provides payment for many health services. Because payment for health services is now coming directly from the patient and is not being paid by an insurance plan, many patients may delay or avoid seeking healthcare services or actively seek out the lowest-cost provider.

5. Without a definition of the requirements for a clean claim, payers can delay or completely avoid paying what is otherwise a legitimate claim.

6. This provision is often referred to as a silent PPO arrangement and extends the potential network far beyond the original expected patient population. Because the payment terms in this contract are not very favorable, the hospital could be in a situation where patients from other health plans might be receiving care under the national plan's favorable payment rates. Without this silent PPO arrangement patients from other health plans would be required to make higher payments to the hospital.

7. Note that the increase in average cost will have two effects on the resulting price. First, it will raise average cost to $105, and second, it will increase the loss on fee-schedule payers. The original loss on fee-schedule payers was $1,500, but with the $5.00 increase in average cost, the new loss on fee-schedule payers becomes $5,500 (the original loss of $1,500 + $5.00 × 800 units of Medicare, Medicaid, and Managed-Care Plan 1). The new required price is $350, 18.9% above the original price of $294.44.

$$Price = \frac{\$105 + \dfrac{(\$5,000 + \$5,500)}{200}}{1 - 0.55} = \$350.00$$

8. The increase in fixed-fee schedules will impact the loss on fee schedule payers as follows:

$$Medicare\ Loss = 400 \times (\$105.00 - \$99.75) = \$2,100$$

$$Medicaid\ Loss = 100 \times (\$105.00 - \$78.75) = \$2,625$$

$$Managed\text{-}Care\ Loss = 300 \times (\$105.00 - \$115.50) = -\$3,150$$

The total loss is now $1,575, which is added to the required net income of $5,000. The new required price is $306.39, 4.1% above the original $294.44.

$$Price = \frac{\$105 + \dfrac{(\$5,000 + \$1,575)}{200}}{1 - 0.55} = \$306.39$$

9. Because the contract calls for payment at a rate of $95, which is greater than the marginal cost ($60), we know that the contract will produce more profit, as **TABLE 6-6** shows. The firm will generate $7,000 in new profit ($12,000 less the original level of profit $5,000). Alternatively, the new profit is simply marginal revenue ($95 per unit) less marginal cost ($60 per unit) times the 200 new units. On the surface this seems like a favorable contract, but it might have negative long-term effects. Most specifically, perhaps the present health plan that pays $110 and provides 300 patient units may discover this payment arrangement and demand a similar rate.

**TABLE 6-6** Income Statement for Case Example

| Revenue | Computation | Amount |
| --- | --- | --- |
| Medicare | 400 × $95 | $38,000 |
| Medicaid | 100 × $75 | $7,500 |
| Health Plan 1 | 300 × $110 | $33,000 |
| New Health Plan | 200 × $95.00 | $19,000 |
| Health Plan 2 | 100 × 80% × $294.44 | $23,555 |
| Uninsured | 100 × 10% × $294.44 | $2,944 |
| Total | | $124,000 |
| Less Costs | | $112,000 |
| Profit | | $12,000 |

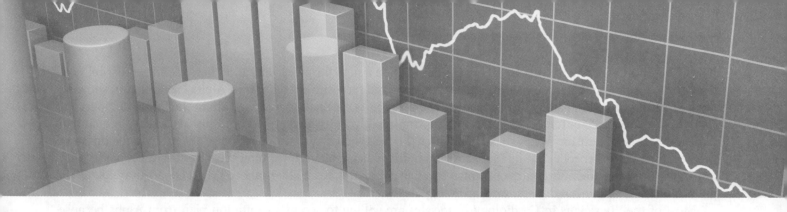

# CHAPTER 7
# Health Insurance and Managed Care

## REAL-WORLD SCENARIO

Archie Griffin, CEO of Cardiology Associates, has been approached by A. J. Hawk, a Vice President of Alpha Health Plans, to accept a capitation arrangement for all professional services associated with enrollees in Alpha's local market area. Currently, Cardiology Associates is being paid on an resource based relative value scale (RBRVS) fee schedule that gives them 110% of current Medicare rates. Mr. Hawk wants Archie to accept a capitation payment of $10.50 per month for every enrollee in Cardiology Associates' market area. Mr. Hawk has been explaining the many benefits of this payment methodology to Archie, but he is not certain whether all of Mr. Hawk's claims are true.

Archie has discussed this proposal with the principal partners in the practice and most of them are unclear whether this is a wise business move. Currently, Cardiology Associates captures about 40% of Alpha Health Plans' local enrollees and this figure would certainly increase to close to 100% of their enrollees. The firm believes that they have capacity to service this contract because last year they hired six new physicians who are not 100% productive at the present time.

The basic arrangement of the capitation plan is to have Cardiology Associates provide all professional services to the plan's enrollees for the fixed sum of $10.50 per member per month. Archie has explained to the physicians that this method of payment will essentially shift utilization risk to the physicians and offers them the possibility of greater returns if usage rates are controlled. Archie has asked for historical data from Alpha Health Plans, showing him historical utilization patterns by procedure code. Archie is especially concerned about the future demographics of Alpha Health Plans' enrollees. Alpha is growing rapidly in its marketplace and has established a qualified managed-care program for Medicare beneficiaries. Mr. Hawk's current proposal does not provide for different levels of payment for enrollees in its Medicare and non-Medicare plans. Cardiology services increase rapidly with age, and a shift in the demographics of Alpha's enrollee population to an older mix could accelerate usage patterns, quickly creating a financial disaster for Cardiology Associates.

Most of the physicians in Cardiology Associates are willing to accept a capitation plan from Alpha because they see a potential for capturing market share. They do want some age adjustment included in the capitation rate to protect them from **adverse risk selection**. Archie has scheduled a future meeting with Mr. Hawk to see if this is a possibility.

---

Managed-care, health maintenance organizations (HMOs), preferred provider organizations (PPOs), physician organizations (POs), physician hospital organizations (PHOs), capitation, medical service organizations (MSOs), consumer-directed health plans (CDHP), Accountable Care Organizations (ACOs), and integrated delivery systems (IDSs) are all terms and acronyms that are used freely in today's healthcare arena. These terms often represent different things to different people and often change in meaning over time. One common thread runs through all of these terms: the issue of change and market reform that is sweeping the healthcare industry. Our focus in this chapter will be primarily on the development of managed-care plans and the development of required premium payments for healthcare coverage.

> ### Learning Objective 1

Define a health maintenance organization (HMO).

## ▶ HMO and Managed-Care Development

Before describing the development of HMOs in the healthcare market, it is important to define what we mean by an HMO. HMOs are organizations that receive premium dollars from subscribers in exchange for a promise to provide all health care required by that subscriber for a defined period. They assume the risk of delivering both physician and hospital services to their enrolled populations for a fixed sum of money provided on a prepaid basis. HMOs are a type of health plan or health insurance company. In this regard, they are no different than any other type of health insurer.

**FIGURE 7-1** presents a view of the money flows from subscribers, to health plans, to providers of healthcare services.

Health plans receive premium dollars from buyers who may be employers, groups, or individuals on a prepaid basis in return for a promise to provide payment for covered healthcare services when needed. Payments for those services can be paid to the subscriber or to the healthcare provider. Indemnity plans make payments to the subscriber or indemnify the subscriber for covered healthcare services, but in most cases, payments are made directly to the provider.

Health plans must make a profit to remain in business, and it is easy to understand the principles of profitability in the health insurance marketplace. To earn positive profits, health plans must receive payments from subscribers greater than payments to healthcare providers. They must also cover their own internal administrative costs. Health plans also generate some additional revenue from the investment of prepaid health premiums. The amount of investment income earned by health insurers is relatively small compared to that of life insurance companies where the premium dollars are received far in advance of payment.

What functions do health plans perform to justify their position in the healthcare marketplace? There are four primary activities, and they are described next.

> ### Learning Objective 2

Describe the four main activities of health plans.

## Underwriting

Health plans accept risk much in the same way that any insurance company accepts risk. They agree to provide payment for services that at the time of contract are not certain. Greater-than-expected utilization can

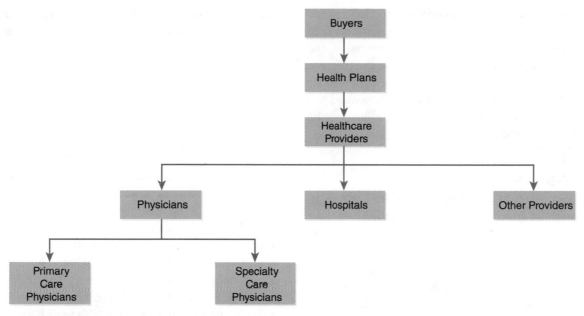

**FIGURE 7-1** **Healthcare Insurance Market**

easily destroy profits and cause payments to exceed receipts. Underwriting of risk is an important business function. Few of us would be willing to live in homes without homeowner's insurance because the occurrence of a fire could destroy us financially. Even though we may pay the insurance company much more in premiums over our lifetimes than we receive in payments, we are not willing to assume the risk of a fire. Health insurance is the same situation. Payment for open heart procedures, kidney transplants, and other sophisticated medical procedures are very expensive, and we all hope that we never need them; but, if we do, it is comforting to know that we have a source of payment for these procedures.

The United States is different from most other industrial countries regarding the percentage of private versus public financing. The United States relies on private financing of medical care to a much greater extent than do most other countries. This places a much greater emphasis on health insurance in our country and less on public financing programs such as Medicare and Medicaid.

## Utilization Review

Increasingly, health plans have sought to control escalating costs through a variety of utilization review techniques. Health plans employ doctors and nurses to review and approve the delivery of nonemergent medical care for necessity and appropriateness. Medical personnel at health plans also work with health providers to plan discharges from hospitals to less intense, subacute settings as soon as possible. **Case**

**management** of chronic conditions such as mental illness also is used by health plans to control costs. Much of the "managed" in managed care deals with health plan review and approval of treatment protocols.

## Claims Administration

Payments to healthcare providers for the provision of services to subscribers are a necessary administrative process. The health plan must verify that coverage for the services exists and that the services were in fact performed. In most cases, the health plan also must determine the amount of payment for the services, which is often different than the charges listed on a patient's bill or claim form. Verification of primary coverage also must be determined in cases when the individual has more than one insurer. The process of assigning payment responsibility when multiple insurers exist is called **coordination of benefits**.

HMOs are a subset of health plans and share all of the functions identified previously, but they are different in several areas, most notably regarding the pattern of relationships with their healthcare providers. First, most HMOs do not permit HMO subscribers to select providers who are out of network. For example, an HMO subscriber who wishes to use an orthopedic surgeon not in the HMO's network may not be covered for charges incurred by that surgeon. A hybrid form of an HMO package called **point of service (POS)** has a provision that permits subscribers to go out of network for services, but subscribers must pay a greater percentage of the cost. We review POS options later. Second, most HMOs rely on a **primary care gatekeeper** concept. The HMO uses the primary care physician as a central triage point for the referral and approval of services. Before a subscriber can see a specialist, the primary care physician must first approve the referral. The use of the primary care physician as a gatekeeper is a central concept underlying HMO success and has been adopted by other health plans that might not be characterized as HMOs.

## Marketing

Insurance companies in general and health insurers in particular must communicate the availability of their products to prospective buyers and convince buyers of the value of their product. Various media are used to accomplish this task, from individual salespersons to television and other media advertising. There are substantial costs associated with these efforts.

---

### Learning Objective 3

List the five types of health plans and their characteristics.

---

## Types of Health Plans

HMOs are often categorized by the pattern of provider relationships they maintain, especially physician–provider relationships. Health plans are usually categorized into five types. **TABLE 7-1** provides some data

on the five types of health plans and the distribution of healthcare coverage for employees in companies where healthcare benefits are provided. The most dramatic change between 1988 and 2015 is the reduction in conventional coverage—mostly indemnity-type plans. **TABLE 7-2** summarizes the key characteristics of alternative health plans.

## Health Maintenance Organizations

HMOs can take many forms but generally, there are four major HMO structures: staff model, group model, individual practice association (IPA) model, and network model. HMOs usually provide the broadest range of medical benefits, whereas indemnity or traditional plans are often the most restrictive. HMO members often have access to liberal outpatient and drug benefits that other health plans do not offer. The cost for increased benefits is most often limited access. HMO members cannot go to any doctor or hospital they wish but are limited to the panel listed in the benefits directory. HMO members are precluded from going out of network for services.

**Staff Model HMO**  In a **staff model HMO**, the physicians are either employees of the HMO or they provide most of their services to HMO members through a contractual relationship. The latter alternative is used in states where HMOs cannot employ physicians because of restrictions on employment of physicians by non-physician-owned companies. Not all physicians may be employees, nor may they be under direct

| **TABLE 7-1** Distribution and Premium Cost for Health Plans Among Covered Employees | | | | |
|---|---|---|---|---|
| | **Percentage** | | | |
| | **1988 (%)** | **1999 (%)** | **2015 (%)** | **Average Annual Premium for Single in 2015** |
| Conventional | 73 | 10 | 1 | NA |
| HMO | 16 | 28 | 17 | $6,212 |
| PPO | 11 | 39 | 50 | 6,575 |
| POS | 0 | 24 | 26 | 6,259 |
| HDHP/SO | 0 | 0 | 26 | 5,567 |
| Total | 100 | 100 | 100 | $6,251 |

"Employer Health Benefits 2015 Annual Survey" (#7936), The Henry J. Kaiser Family Foundation, September 2015.

Kaiser/HRET Survey of Employer-Sponsored Health Benefits, 2015.

contract, but the critical segment is the primary care physicians. The HMO must control the primary care physician network to be a true staff model HMO. A staff model HMO may own other related healthcare providers, such as hospitals, but ownership is not necessary.

**Group Model HMO** In a group model HMO, the HMO contracts with one or more medical groups to provide all necessary services to HMO members. Usually the groups are not exclusively bound to any one HMO and may provide services to several HMOs. The groups also may be primary care, specialty based, or multiple specialty based. The physicians in the groups, however, must come together and transfer all or most of their medical practice assets and liabilities to the group entity.

**IPA Model HMO** An **individual practice association (IPA) model HMO** is a much looser affiliation of independent physicians who have not come together and integrated their practices in any substantive way. The IPA contracts with the HMO for needed medical services, but the individual physicians maintain their own independent practices and use the IPA only to sign contracts with HMOs and other health plans. County medical societies often create an IPA for their physician members.

**Network Model HMO** Network model HMOs are really a hybrid of the previous three forms. A network model HMO may contract with both medical groups and IPAs, as well as employ individual physicians. The key to their success is the ability to access a pool of cost-effective physicians who can manage care.

## Conventional or Indemnity Plans

Indemnity plans, which are often referred to as traditional or conventional plans, provide their members with the greatest access to healthcare providers, both doctors and hospitals. Members are not restricted in terms of whom they can see for treatment of any medical disorders. In short, freedom of choice is the highest in indemnity plans. HMOs are usually the most restrictive in terms of choice and often limit access to hospitals and physicians that are part of the network. PPOs may be as restrictive as HMOs, but usually have larger panels of both doctors and hospitals. They attempt to select providers who have a good track record on both quality and cost effectiveness.

## Point of Service Plans

Point of service (POS) plans are really a hybrid form of an HMO. A POS provision will allow HMO members to seek medical services outside of the HMO panel of providers. In most situations, the cost of services to the HMO subscriber is higher when care is received out of network. Usually this higher cost is in the form of higher deductibles, higher copayments, or both. A *copayment* is a provision that specifies a percentage of the approved charge that must be paid by the member. For example, a 20% copayment would require a PPO member to pay 20% of the approved charge. The approved charge may be different from the charge made to the member for the service. A doctor may charge $2,000 for a procedure that the HMO/POS plan says is approved at $1,200. The member would be required to pay the doctor 20% of the approved charge of $1,200, or $240, plus the difference between the approved charge and the actual charge, or $800, for a total payment of $1,040.

## Preferred Provider Organizations Plans

Preferred provider organizations (PPOs) provide provisions for out-of-network services but require members to pay a portion of the cost for these benefits in the form of higher copayments and deductibles. In many respects their operation is very similar to HMO plans with a POS option.

## High-Deductible Health Plans with Savings Option Plans

There is current interest in the recent rise of high deductible health plans with a savings option (HDHP/SO), called consumer-directed health plans. These plans are relatively recent in origin and became viable alternatives with the 2003 Medicare Prescription Drug, Improvement, and Modernization Act. The act provided for the creation of **health savings accounts (HSAs)**. Individuals can fund HSAs using pretax dollars and use the money to pay for a variety of healthcare expenses, including deductibles and copayments. Most of HDHP/SOs have a HSA and usually have annual deductibles of more than $1,000 per individual or $2,000 per family.

The primary objective of these plans is to increase the involvement of patients in selecting cost-effective healthcare services. Most of the large health plans provide HDHP/SO option. As seen in Table 7-1, their growth has been dramatic and their market share will most likely grow as increased pressure for healthcare cost containment continues.

Many HDHP/SO plans are linked to a conventional health plan such as an HMO or PPO plan. The critical difference is not in the services that are covered but rather the source of payment. In a HDHP/SO plan the initial payment for services comes from the subscriber, either through the HSA or directly from the subscriber's personal accounts. When the deductible amount, often referred to as the bridge, is met, the traditional plan coverage begins for all additional covered health services in the benefit year.

## Health Exchange Plans

While not a separate type of health plan, it is important to reference the growth in health plans offered on state health exchanges. The Patient Protection and Affordable Care Act (ACA) was signed into law on March 23, 2010. The law required that health insurance exchanges commence operation in every state on October 1, 2013. In the first year of operation, open enrollment on the exchanges ran from October 1, 2013, to March 31, 2014, and insurance plans purchased by December 15, 2013, began coverage on January 1, 2014.

As of February 2016, about 12.7 million Americans have signed up for or been automatically renewed for 2016 marketplace coverage.

## Comparison of Health Plans

**TABLE 7-2** summarizes the key characteristics of the major health plan types and their relationships to subscribers, physicians, hospitals, and employers.

Indemnity or traditional plans usually pay providers, both hospitals and doctors, on the basis of charges. In some cases, there may be a fee schedule in effect that limits payment liability. PPOs usually negotiate some discount with the providers as a condition for participation in the network of providers. HMOs work in much the same way as PPOs and require a discount for participation in the network of providers. There is also a possibility of capitated payment to providers in an HMO arrangement. Capitation simply means the provider is not paid on the basis of services performed but rather on the basis of HMO members assigned to its organization. This means the provider may be paid on a **per-member-per-month (PMPM)** basis. Finally, HMOs use stringent utilization review (UR) procedures at both the hospital and physician levels to eliminate unnecessary services and to provide cost-effective treatment plans. PPOs use UR procedures, but at the present time most of their efforts are directed at hospitals. Indemnity plans are also beginning to use UR procedures to curtail unnecessary utilization.

Costs of healthcare coverage to the employer are usually lowest in a HDHP/SO plan because more of the cost has shifted to the subscriber. Most of these plans, however, are linked to an underlying conventional plan such as an HMO or PPO. HMOs usually have a lower cost than either PPOs or indemnity plans.

| **TABLE 7-2** Healthcare Insurance Alternatives | | | |
|---|---|---|---|
| | **Alternative Plans** | | |
| **Parties** | **HMOs** | **PPOs** | **Indemnity (Traditional)** |
| Subscribers | Restricted choice<br>Generous benefits | Choice from panel<br>Copayments<br>Out of network with reduced<br>  benefits and higher cost<br>Broader benefits | Free choice<br>Deductible and 80/20<br>  copayments<br>Major medical benefits<br>Limited outpatient coverage |
| Physicians | Limited access<br>Discounted reimbursement<br>  or capitation<br>Utilization review (UR)<br>  requirements | Access by contracting<br>Discounted charges or fee<br>  schedule<br>UR is mostly hospital based | All participate<br>Paid charges |
| Hospitals | Limited access<br>Discounted charges, per diems,<br>  case rates, or capitation<br>UR | Limited access<br>Discounted charges, per diem,<br>  or case rates<br>UR | All participate<br>Paid charges |
| Employers | Reduced cost | Reduced cost | Expensive, but most freedom<br>  for employees |

The reason for this observation is not hard to understand. HMOs try to reduce unnecessary utilization for both doctors and hospitals and they also try to curtail the amount paid for services to healthcare providers by restricting the network of providers. PPOs have tried to reduce costs primarily through reduced prices to providers by selective provider contracting, but utilization reductions have not been substantial relative to those achieved in an HMO setting. A major reason for the rapid growth of PPOs is related to the ease of organization and subscriber interest in choice of providers.

HMOs are not a new development and have been in existence for many years. Two of the earliest HMOs were Kaiser Permanente and Group Health of Puget Sound. Both of these HMOs could be described as staff model HMOs. Physicians and hospitals that participated in these HMOs derived most, if not all, of their business from the HMO. In the early 1970s, Dr. Paul Elwood of Interstudy, a consulting firm in Minneapolis, coined the term *health maintenance organization* to describe the kind of health plan represented by Kaiser and Group Health. The development of HMOs, although rapid, was not very impressive until the mid-1980s, when HMOs started to develop and grow. Most of the growth occurred in non–staff model HMOs. Newly formed HMOs simply could not put together the ownership structures necessary to employ physicians directly and relied on contractual relationships with groups and IPAs. Physicians also were reluctant to give up their independent status for employee positions.

> ### Learning Objective 4
>
> Describe the forces that influenced the development of integrated delivery systems.

# ▶ Integrated Delivery Systems

With the growth of HMOs and PPOs, buying power was concentrated in fewer purchasing groups, and hospitals and physicians sought some way to reduce the trend to greater and greater discounts granted for participation in managed-care contracts. To offset this concentration of purchasing power, hospitals and physicians began to develop integrated delivery system (IDS) structures to better position themselves and place themselves closer to the premium dollar. In some cases, these IDS organizations even approached employers directly to sell health insurance coverage. This eliminated the health plan, which they regarded as a middleman in the marketplace.

In the early 1990s, IDSs, which consisted of at least a hospital and physician component, began to develop. An IDS was thought of as a strategic alliance among doctors, hospitals, and other ancillary providers to deliver care to a defined population. There are few fully integrated delivery systems presently, and most consist of only hospital and doctor elements. IDS organizations initially sought to develop managed-care contracts on behalf of both the hospitals and the physicians and served primarily as a contracting vehicle.

A number of economic factors, however, created the stimulus for the formation of IDSs or other vertically integrated organizations, such as Accountable Care Organizations (ACOs). These factors are discussed next.

## Negotiation for Health Plan Contracts

One of the key driving forces behind current hospital–physician integration is related to financial concerns. Many of the early generation hospital-owned physician practices, which included a large proportion of primary care physicians, resulted in substantial losses for hospitals and healthcare systems. Losses were frequently in excess of $100,000 per employed physician. As a result, many of the practices were divested by hospitals soon after their creation.

Since 2005, there has been a renewed interest by both physicians and hospitals to create hospital-owned physician practices. The basic character of the acquisitions is changing, however. Physicians and physician practices are being acquired by hospitals and integrated delivery systems where a need for physicians exists, such as rural areas. Many physicians have actively sought hospital employment because of declining levels of reimbursement from major public and private payers. Current compensation models are now more directly related to physician productivity.

## Growing Importance of Payer Referrals

Physicians receive about 24% of each healthcare dollar in the United States, yet they control most of the expenditures. Hospitals and other institutional providers depend on physician referrals to keep utilization in their facilities at reasonable levels. Although physician referrals are still the primary source of business for most healthcare providers, there has been a subtle but growing increase in payer referrals. Physicians and hospitals suddenly have found that they are no longer acceptable providers for some health plans and that they have been dropped. Most of the reasons for their exclusion relate to the high cost of their practice patterns with only minimal, if any, attention presently paid to quality of care. Fear of being excluded has caused many hospitals and doctors to create larger corporate structures. It is believed the sheer size of these hospital–physician combinations will strengthen their negotiating position with health plans.

## Increasing Importance of Capitation

Under a capitated payment system, providers are paid a fixed amount for each person living in their covered service area. This is very different from the current practice of most payers (including most HMOs, who pay on the basis of services provided). The speed and extent to which the current system, which is largely dominated by retrospective payment for services, will be replaced with prospective capitation is debatable. It is not clear at the present time whether capitation payments to providers will increase. One thing is, however, very clear. Capitation payments will reverse present incentives that exist in fee-for-service payment methods. Supporters believe that this will encourage preventive care and reduce unnecessary utilization of services; others worry that it will create incentives for skimping on service or reducing quality.

A less comprehensive form of capitation that is gaining increasing attention is the use of "bundled payments" by Medicare and other commercial payers. Bundled payments for care improvement (BPCI) was officially launched in January of 2013. It was a voluntary program for hospitals and other designated healthcare providers that tested models for creating bundled payments for 48 specifically designated clinical episodes of care defined by the patient's Medicare Severity-Diagnosis Related Group (MS-DRG). On July 9, 2015, CMS proposed implementation of bundled payment for hip and knee replacements called comprehensive care for joint replacement (CCJR) that would require mandatory participation for most hospitals in 75 metropolitan areas in the United States. In the CCJR program Medicare provides a fixed sum of money to the hospital that performs the joint surgery to cover all payments for that episode of care. The hospital is responsible not only for its costs but also for the surgeon's costs and any related post-acute care for up to 90 days.

## Shift of Hospital Services to Outpatient

In 1988, about 88% of all hospital revenue was derived from traditional inpatient services. By 2014, that figure had fallen to 47%. This shift from inpatient to outpatient is related to tremendous cost pressures

to perform procedures on an outpatient basis when possible, technology that has made outpatient procedures more feasible, and a strong desire by patients to be treated on an outpatient basis. Cost pressures have forced hospitals to become more active in outpatient services that were traditionally the domain of the physician office, whereas new technology has enabled doctors to provide services in their offices that were historically performed in hospitals. The outpatient market can either be an area where hospitals and physicians can productively collaborate, or it can degenerate into a fierce competitive battleground between the two. For an integrated delivery system to succeed, it is imperative that collaboration, not competition, occurs. Only then can an appropriate continuum of care be assured for every patient.

## Integrated Data Systems

Technology has made it possible to share vast quantities of information among various potential users. Shared clinical data among physicians, hospitals, and other providers can enhance both the quality and effectiveness of medical care. Data that are shared also permit some economics in business functions such as billing. Although shared data is an objective sought by many parties, it is much easier to accomplish in organizations that are formally related, either through common ownership or business-related affiliations. Unfortunately, the healthcare industry is notoriously behind in using the power of modern computer systems to solve business and clinical problems. This is true partly because the hospital environment is complex and partly because the system is fragmented. For instance, a person who can get cash instantly from an ATM while traveling in the Philippines still cannot access his or her medical records if admitted to a hospital one county away from his or her home. A person can call a travel agent to schedule a complex trip itinerary involving multiple airlines yet cannot schedule a day's worth of diagnostic and treatment steps in a hospital without serious risk of delays or cancellations. The most important factor in the future success of the integrated delivery system likely will be its ability to use information as a competitive resource. Beginning in 2011, the electronic health records (EHR) incentive programs were developed to encourage eligible professionals and eligible hospitals to adopt, implement, upgrade (AIU), and demonstrate meaningful use of certified EHR technology. As of October 2015, more than 479,000 healthcare providers received payment for participating in Medicare and Medicaid EHR incentive programs.

## Vertical and Horizontal Integration Trends

There has been a concerted effort during the last few years to develop new entities that can dominate markets in selected areas. Major hospital chains have announced on a weekly basis some new merger that was designed to enhance their market position. HCA—The Healthcare Company (formerly Columbia/HCA)—through its mergers, quickly became the nation's largest hospital provider, with special strength in certain regions. This is an example of horizontal integration and can be a successful market strategy. Many other regional systems have chosen vertical integration as a means to market dominance. For example, Sentara Health System in Norfolk, Virginia, includes 12 hospitals, 9 outpatient campuses, 10 nursing homes, 380 employed physicians, and its own health plan with 452,000 members. The important lesson that most healthcare providers have realized is that it is dangerous to be small and unaffiliated in today's competitive markets. There is a major "shakeout" coming in the healthcare industry, and it will involve hospitals, physicians, and payers. Those who are incorporated into larger systems are the most likely to have greater access to consumer and capital markets and thus be better positioned for long-term survival.

## Productivity

Many economists believe that improvements in productivity are the primary means for realizing increases in the standard of living within a nation. The same is true in an economic enterprise. Over the long term, a hospital, medical group, or insurance company cannot increase its financial performance without continually enhancing productivity. One of the key potential benefits of creating integrated delivery systems is the opportunity to reengineer processes across what were formerly impregnable barriers to communication, thereby reducing redundancy and cost.

**FIGURE 7-2** presents a diagram of an IDS, or a collaborative group of providers, and shows its insertion among the health plan, the providers of medical services, and products that were shown in Figure 7-1. One of the developments discussed earlier that has led to the development of IDS organizations is the increasing importance of capitation or bundled payments as a form of payment to healthcare providers. Some health plans use some form of capitation for paying physicians and hospitals.

Health plans have a strong financial incentive to capitate providers whenever possible because this guarantees their profit and locks in a fixed return. For example, the illustration in Figure 7-2 depicts a situation where the health plan could guarantee itself a $46 return PMPM if it could negotiate a fixed PMPM payment of $254 to an IDS for all healthcare services. Although health plans would like to push capitation on healthcare providers, larger healthcare providers have asked themselves whether it is to their advantage to accept capitation from health plans or to directly market an insurance product to major employers, thus eliminating the middleman—the health plan—from the revenue stream. The providers assume that they can perform appropriate utilization review, administer claims, and market their product to employers. The only piece that they may be uncomfortable with is the assumption of risk or underwriting. If health plans push capitation downward to them, this is no longer an issue. They are already capitated and must assume the medical underwriting risk anyway. This

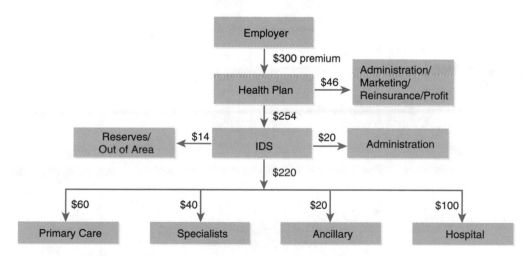

**FIGURE 7-2  IDS Funds Flow**

may partially explain why capitation is losing favor with many providers.

It is difficult to answer the question of who controls the IDS. In general, there are three alternatives. Hospitals can seek to control the IDS and protect their position in the healthcare marketplace as inpatient acute-care utilization falls. Physicians may think that they are in better position to control the IDS because the emphasis is increasingly on managing care, and this is a role that physicians are uniquely qualified to assume. Finally, organizers of health plans may believe that they are in the best position to control the IDS because of their closeness to the premium dollar and their historical interest in cost control. Health plans also presently have the cash reserves to finance much of the organizational development necessary to make this happen.

The primary vehicle for hospital control has been a Physician Hospital Organization (PHO). The PHO may serve as the IDS in Figure 7-2 and contract on behalf of physicians and hospitals. The development of PHOs is relatively new; most were not started until the 1990s or later. PHOs are, in theory, a partnership between hospitals and physicians. However, many have been tightly controlled by the hospital and do not always represent a true partnership. **FIGURE 7-3** presents two possible PHO organizational structures. PHOs formed between a hospital and a formal physician organization often are better suited to

tackle the issues of managed care because they have a structure in place to begin physician dialogue about cost-effective care. PHOs formed without a physician organization may simply represent shareholder interests of individual physicians or groups. This greatly diminishes physician control in the PHO. Significant physician involvement is needed to create an effective integrated delivery system. A loosely organized physician body may give effective control to the hospital but not really accomplish the physician–hospital integration that is essential for success.

PHOs may be formed on either a taxable or tax-exempt basis. There are pros and cons for either alternative, but if the objective is the eventual acquisition or employment of physicians, a taxable basis appears to have fewer problems. The creation of a tax-exempt, nonprofit PHO may raise the issue of inurement, which will be discussed later.

A PHO is not usually a fully integrated delivery system. The major difficulty with many PHOs is determining how to divide the payments from the health plan or HMO among the hospital and its contracting physicians. Each party most likely wants to protect its level of income, and without common ownership or control, this revenue allocation may doom many PHOs in the long term. Hospital-dominated PHOs often are considered by physicians as an attempt to protect the hospital's declining market share and to perpetuate hospital domination of the healthcare market.

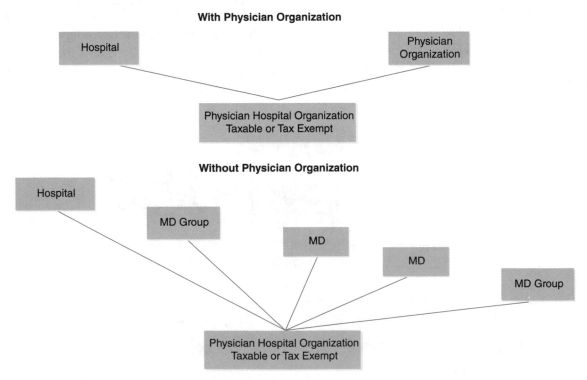

**FIGURE 7-3 Physician Hospital Organization Structure**

**Medical Service Organizations (MSOs)** are an alternative organizational structure to a PHO that also may serve as an IDS and contract for medical services with a health plan. MSOs are often formed to provide management services to medical groups and may or may not have any hospital ownership or control. If a MSO is formed without hospital interest, the MSO may have to contract with a hospital if the MSO wishes to contract for both hospital and physician services.

**Physician Organizations (POs)** are a relatively recent development. Most POs were developed in large part because of dissatisfaction with hospital-sponsored PHOs. They represent an attempt by physicians to take back control in the new managed-care world. The primary problem many physicians encountered when creating a PO was a lack of capital and organizational management skills. Investors have begun to pour capital dollars into the development of POs because they recognize the gigantic opportunities for cost savings in health care and the pivotal role that physicians play in the realization of those cost savings. National corporations, as well as the American Medical Association, have been aggressively organizing and funding POs to put them in a position where they can begin forming their own managed-care organizations (MCOs) and directly contract for healthcare services on a capitated basis.

Health insurers and HMOs are also actively entering the IDS arena and beginning to directly provide medical services, especially outpatient services. Acquisition of clinics and the employment of physicians have been undertaken by a number of insurers, and more are considering these types of ventures. Even large employers are beginning to ask the question, "Why should we buy health insurance when we believe that we can make our own delivery system and produce care cheaper than we buy it?" This is most often seen in the development of clinics for employees of a firm.

### Learning Objective 5

Describe some of the methods by which providers are paid by health plans.

▶ # Paying Providers in a Managed-Care Environment

One of the most difficult problems in a less than fully integrated delivery system is splitting the revenue between individual healthcare providers. Let's assume that the IDS represented in Figure 7-2 does not own the individual healthcare providers to which it is distributing premium dollars. How does it determine that primary care physicians get $60 PMPM and specialty care physicians get $40 PMPM? Or, on an even more basic level, how does the IDS decide if it will pay physicians on a capitated PMPM basis or use a fee schedule?

The decisions referenced previously are related to pricing and are ultimately related to costs. No business wishes to produce products that are priced at levels lower than costs. If a business continued to do this, it would ultimately be forced to close its doors. Healthcare providers and insurers are not an exception. The health plan or HMO in Figure 7-2 knows that in its marketplace it can sell healthcare insurance for $300 on a PMPM basis. Of that $300, $46 is needed to cover internal administrative costs and marketing costs. Additional costs are allocated for reinsurance and profit for the health plan's investors. Reinsurance represents the additional costs paid to other insurers for assumption of unusual risks. For example, the health plan may have to pay the IDS additional payments for treating high-risk patients, such as patients with AIDS.

The health plan then pays the IDS $254 PMPM to provide all healthcare benefits or some subset of benefits. The IDS needs $20 PMPM to cover its costs of administration and another $14 to create a reserve position to meet out-of-service-area costs. Reserves are needed because the IDS is obligating itself to pay for all healthcare costs that will be provided during the **benefit period**. The actual level of utilization is not certain. A reserve position will help them cover costs in situations when actual utilization exceeds estimates. Reserve requirements might also reflect a state requirement that the IDS entity be treated as an insurance company and, therefore, statutory reserve levels may be required. Out-of-area costs simply represent those payments that will be made to healthcare providers outside of the service area. A subscriber may be traveling in another state and require emergency medical attention that could not be provided by a network provider.

The IDS now has $220 to pay the providers of healthcare services that are part of its regional network. Each of those providers will develop a budget of what expected costs are likely to be incurred for the insured population. For example, assume that the primary care physicians have developed the following schedule to estimate their costs:

Unit of service: Office visits
Annual frequency per 1,000 members: 4,000
Unit cost: $75
Net PMPM cost: $25

The primary care physicians have estimated that approximately 4,000 visits per 1,000 members will be required per year. At this rate of utilization, approximately 4 office visits per year will be required per member with an estimated cost of $75 per office visit. Therefore, the average cost per member per year is 4 × $75, or $300 per year. Dividing by 12, the number of months in a year, yields a PMPM basis of $25. The primary care physicians would be willing to accept any amount greater than $25 PMPM to provide office visits for this insured population if they had confidence in their estimates, especially the estimated rate of utilization of four visits per year.

Estimating costs under a capitated contract basis is easy to understand from a conceptual basis. Cost can be expressed simply as follows:

$$\text{PMPM cost} = \frac{\text{Expected encounters per year} \times \text{Cost per encounter}}{12}$$

With this framework, the IDS (or the health plan if there is no intermediate IDS entity) has three primary forms of payment. These forms are discussed next.

## Salary or Budget

If the providers are owned by the IDS or health plan or are employees of the organization, there is no real revenue-sharing arrangement in effect. The IDS is merely trying to determine what costs it will incur when it treats the insured population for the budget period. A Kaiser-owned hospital receives a budget based on expected utilization during the coming year. Salaried physicians are not paid on a volume basis but are paid a salary with perhaps some incentives for above-average performance. The key relationship in this arrangement is determining the required physician and hospital staffing necessary to meet expected utilization.

## Fee for Service

Doctors and hospitals in this payment mode are paid on a volume-related basis. For doctors, there are two primary alternatives: charges or fee schedule. In a charge-based payment system, the doctor usually would be paid on the basis of total charges, most often some negotiated percentage of total charges such as 80 percent. In a fee-schedule arrangement, the doctor would be paid based upon some contractually specified fee structure. The Resource-Based Relative Value Scale (RBRVS) would be an example. (This scale is described further in Chapter 3.) Hospitals usually are paid on one of three bases: charges, per diems, or per case. As with physicians, a hospital being paid on a charge basis most likely would not receive 100% of charges, but rather some lower percentage. Per-diem payment is common among many health plans and simply guarantees the hospital so much per patient day, for example $900 for every medical-surgical patient day. Different rates may be in effect for maternity and intensive care days. Case payment may be similar to Medicare's diagnosis-related groups (DRGs) and could relate payment to specific DRGs. Case payment could be some aggregation of case categories such as medical cases, obstetrical cases, and surgical cases. Hospital outpatient services most often are based upon discounted charges, but ambulatory patient classification (APC) groups and other classification methods are becoming more popular and could be used to devise a fee schedule.

## Capitation

Presently, **capitation** arrangements are much more common for both physicians and hospitals, especially primary care physicians. Hospitals without direct control via common ownership with physicians may not be in a good position to control and manage costs because physicians control the amount of services provided.

In a flat-rate capitation arrangement, the provider would receive a flat amount, $30 PMPM, to provide all contracted services. A percentage arrangement pays the provider some fixed percentage, for example 25% of the PMPM premium payment. Floors or adjustments are sometimes included in capitated arrangements to protect the provider. For example, utilization is usually a function of age, gender, prior health status, and other variables. If an HMO contracted with a primary care group for $30 PMPM, that rate might be sufficient for insured individuals between 25 and 55 years old, but grossly inadequate for the population older than 65 years. The primary care group may therefore adjust its PMPM payment based upon age.

## Withholds and Risk Pools

The last element of provider payment that needs to be addressed is the presence of withholds and risk pools. Withholds are most common in fee-for-service arrangements and provide a mechanism for reducing the risk to the IDS or health plan. **TABLE 7-3** presents an example that we will use to illustrate the concept of withholds and risk pools. There are three categories of providers: primary care physicians who are paid $30 PMPM, specialty care physicians who are paid on a fee-schedule basis, and the hospital that is paid $850 per patient day. There are 10,000 people who are insured by the HMO, and budgets are projected for each category.

**TABLE 7-3** HMO Payment Example

| | Primary Care Physicians (PCP) | Specialty Care Physicians (SCP) | Hospital |
|---|---|---|---|
| Payment | $30 PMPM | Fee schedule | $850 per diem |
| Annual budget for 10,000 covered lives | $3,600,000 | $2,400,000 | $3,400,000 |
| Risk pool | 0 | $240,000 | $340,000 |
| Parties splitting risk pool | none | PCP, SCP, HMO | PCP, Hospital, HMO |
| Withhold | none | none | 10% |

The hospital budget is projected to be $3,400,000 and is derived as follows, assuming 400 patient days per 1,000 members with 10,000 members or 4,000 patient days of care:

$$= 4{,}000 \text{ Patient days} \times \$850$$
$$= \$3{,}400{,}000$$

The hospital also is subject to a 10% withhold, which means they will be paid $765 per diem (90% of $850). Now assume that actual days were 450 days per 1,000. Payments would be calculated as follows:

Initial hospital payment
(4,500 Days × $765) = $3,442,500

Risk pool (Budget – Paid)
($3,400,000 – $3,442,500) = –$42,500

Additional payments to hospital = 0

If actual days were 350 instead of 450, the following payments would result:

Initial hospital payment
(3,500 × $765) = $2,677,500

Risk pool (Budget – Paid)
($3,400,000 – $2,677,500) = $722,500

Additional payments to hospital
(one-third of risk pool) = $240,833

In the first example of excessive utilization, the risk pool is a negative value at the end of the year and the hospital would receive no additional moneys. An interesting question is whether the negative-risk pool balance would be divided among the primary care physician, the hospital, and the HMO. We will assume in this example that only the HMO is assuming the negative variance. In the second example, there is a surplus in the risk pool. The balance in the risk pool would be split equally among the three parties: the HMO, the hospital, and the primary care physicians. The critical factor in each situation is utilization. Some may wonder why the primary care physicians would be able to participate in the hospital-risk pool, but it is this group of decision makers that makes the referral and admission decisions that ultimately impact hospital utilization. Sharing in the risk pool gives them an incentive to keep utilization in check. The primary care physicians also share in the specialty care risk pool for the same reason. It is their referral decisions that will determine actual utilization; therefore, they determine the total payments, given a fixed-fee schedule for payment to specialty care physicians.

The use of withholds and risk pools can be confusing to even the most experienced financial analyst. It is important to work out several examples to make certain that all parties understand the contract language. The examples also may be part of the contract to help clarify actual interpretation.

*Learning Objective 6*

Describe how managed-care organizations establish their prices.

## ▶ Setting Prices in Capitated Contracts

Pricing in any market is a function of a variety of factors, but it ultimately rests on the relationship between costs and expected prices. In most markets, prices are already established within some narrow band. A health plan cannot decide to price a policy at $400 PMPM when its closest competitor is pricing a similar product at $300 PMPM. It would have few buyers, if any, and would be forced from that market. The health plan must therefore decide if it can provide coverage for approximately $300 PMPM to remain competitive in the marketplace.

**TABLE 7-4** presents some hypothetical data and shows average PMPM expenses. The table is useful to help identify the major categories of expense and their relative importance in the cost structures of HMOs.

Revenues for health plans consist of three categories: **premiums**, **copayments**, and **coordination of benefits**. The largest element is premiums received from health plan subscribers. In addition to those premiums, health plans also may receive additional revenues from copayments for selected services. Most copayments are not paid to the health plan but to the provider of services. The copayment amount is then used to reduce the contractual amount due the provider from the health plan for the services provided. For example, the health plan may have a $10 copayment for physician office visits, which is usually collected by the physician at the time of the visit. This copayment would then be offset against the amount due the provider from the health plan by $10. Copayments also provide an incentive for subscribers not to overuse health services. Coordination of benefits

relates to the recovery of payments from other insurers when two or more insurance policies are involved. For example, a health plan may have made payments to healthcare providers on behalf of a member for services rendered, but discovered later that the member also had coverage under a spouse's policy. The two insurance companies would work together to determine the amount that each insurance company is liable to pay and the health plan might receive some payment from the other insurance company for services that it has already paid.

The two largest categories of expense for health plans are inpatient expenses and physician payments. Inpatient expenses are mostly payments to hospitals for covered admissions, whereas physician payments reference amounts paid to both primary care and specialty care physicians. As discussed earlier, these payments could be fee for service or capitation. Other professional services relate to payments for diagnostic lab and radiology, home health, and other professional services. Outside referral payments are payments to physicians and others for services not contracted with existing providers. Emergency department payments are payments to hospitals for emergency department visits, and out-of-area payments relate to payments for services to members who become ill and need medical attention while traveling outside the plan's service area. Other expenses represent a "catch all" category designed to include expenses not previously included in the other categories. Lastly, administrative expenses refer to the marketing and administrative costs of plan management. Also included here are premium taxes charged against health insurance sales.

A health plan or an intermediate IDS that is attempting to either set a price or assess the profitability of an existing price will have to determine its expected costs of servicing the defined population. To do this, the following cost relationship would be used:

$$\text{PMPM} = \frac{\text{Expected encounters per year} \times \text{Cost per encounter}}{12}$$

Cost is a simple function of expected utilization and cost per type of encounter. We now discuss each of these factors in detail and use the pricing example of **TABLE 7-5**. Table 7-5 presents four categories of provider expenses: hospital inpatient, hospital outpatient, physician, and other. Each cost category in the table converts to a budgeted cost on a PMPM basis. To understand this more clearly, let's go through the first item, medical-surgical benefits. It is currently expected that 350 days per 1,000 lives (a utilization

**TABLE 7-4** PMPM Revenue and Expense Averages

| | |
|---|---|
| Revenue (including copayments and coordination of benefits) | $300.00 |
| Expenses | |
| Inpatient | $80.00 |
| Physician | 90.00 |
| Other professional | 18.00 |
| Outside referral | 15.00 |
| Emergency department and out-of-area | 8.00 |
| Other expenses | 42.00 |
| Administration | 26.00 |
| Total expenses | $279.00 |

rate of 0.350) will be used and that the health plan will pay the hospital(s) an average rate of $900 per day. To convert this to PMPM basis, the following calculation would be performed:

$$\$26.25 = \frac{0.350 \times \$900}{12}$$

There is also a copayment provision in this insurance package that requires a $100 copayment, but it is not expected that all 350 days will be subject to the copayment provision. Most likely, the copayment is in the form of a deductible payment that is paid upon admission. The expected copayment to be received for medical-surgical patients is 0.300 (the use rate) times

**TABLE 7-5** Development of PMPM Rate

| Category | Annual Frequency per 1,000 | Unit Cost | PMPM | Copay Frequency per 1,000 | Copay Amount | Copay PMPM | Net PMPM |
|---|---|---|---|---|---|---|---|
| **Hospital Inpatient** | | | | | | | |
| Medical-surgical | 350 | $900 | $26.25 | 300 | $100 | $2.50 | $23.75 |
| Maternity | 20 | 900 | $1.50 | 20 | 100 | $0.17 | $1.33 |
| Mental health | 30 | 300 | $0.75 | – | – | | $0.75 |
| *Subtotal* | | | **$28.50** | | | **$2.67** | **$25.83** |
| **Hospital Outpatient** | | | | | | | |
| Surgery | 70 | $1,200 | $7.00 | – | – | – | $7.00 |
| X-ray and lab | 400 | 250 | $8.33 | – | – | – | 8.33 |
| Emergency department | 120 | 250 | $2.50 | 80 | 50 | 0.33 | 2.17 |
| *Subtotal* | | | **$17.83** | | | **$0.33** | **$17.50** |
| **Physician** | | | | | | | |
| Inpatient visits | 200 | $100 | $1.67 | – | – | – | $1.67 |
| Inpatient surgery | 70 | 1,500 | $8.75 | – | – | – | $8.75 |
| Outpatient surgery | 400 | 200 | $6.67 | – | – | – | $6.67 |
| Maternity | 15 | 2,000 | $2.50 | 15 | 100 | $0.13 | $2.38 |
| Office visits | 4,000 | 75 | $25.00 | 3,000 | 10 | $2.50 | $22.50 |
| Emergency department | 120 | 100 | $1.00 | – | – | – | $1.00 |
| Mental health | 350 | 125 | $3.65 | 350 | 10 | $0.29 | $3.35 |
| *Subtotal* | | | **$49.23** | | | **$2.92** | **$46.31** |

*(continues)*

**TABLE 7-5** Development of PMPM Rate  *(continued)*

| Category | Annual Frequency per 1,000 | Unit Cost | PMPM | Copay Frequency per 1,000 | Copay Amount | Copay PMPM | Net PMPM |
|---|---|---|---|---|---|---|---|
| **Other** | | | | | | | |
| Home health | 50 | $200 | $0.83 | – | – | – | $0.83 |
| Diagnostic X-ray and lab | 700 | 125 | $7.29 | – | – | – | 7.29 |
| Durable medical Equipment | 30 | 300 | $0.75 | – | – | – | 0.75 |
| Ambulance | 35 | 400 | $1.17 | 35 | 50 | $0.15 | $1.02 |
| *Subtotal* | | | **$10.04** | | | **$0.15** | **$9.89** |
| **Total** | | | **$105.60** | | | **$6.06** | **$99.54** |
| Coordination of benefits (2%) | | | | | | | (1.99) |
| | | | | | | | **$97.55** |
| Net healthcare cost retention (15%) | | | | | | | $14.63 |
| PMPM requirement | | | | | | | **$112.18** |

$100, or $30, which is then converted to a PMPM basis of $2.50.

$$\$2.50 = \frac{0.300 \times \$100}{12}$$

The net PMPM cost of medical-surgical benefits is then $23.75 ($26.25 – $2.50). The copayment is subtracted from the expected payments to providers because this payment from the subscriber to the medical provider offsets provider payments. The health plan will pay $23.75 per member per month to providers, but the provider will receive $2.50 in direct payments from the subscriber. Similar methodology would be applied to the other cost categories.

The total cost of healthcare benefits expected to be paid using Table 7-5 is $99.54. This amount is net of copayments, but does not reflect any coordination of benefit (COB) recoveries. COB recoveries are expected to be 2% of the total and reduce the healthcare cost of this insurance package to $97.55. The HMO needs to mark up this amount by 15% to cover administrative costs and reserves and to build in a profit requirement. The required PMPM price is then $112.18.

The process of pricing is relatively easy, as the example shows. The most difficult part is forecasting, and the most difficult area is expected utilization. For example, how certain are we that 350 days of medical-surgical care will be delivered as the forecast states? If 400 days of medical-surgical care were required rather than the budgeted 350, the additional cost would be $3.75 PMPM:

$$[(50/1,000) \times \$900]/12 = \$3.75$$

This may seem like a small variance, but it should be remembered that margins in most HMOs are not large. Small variations in utilization can have disastrous effects on the financial performance of an HMO. **TABLE 7-6** provides some utilization averages from the Agency for Healthcare Research and Quality (AHRQ). The data clearly show the effects of

| **TABLE 7-6** Inpatient Utilization Data—2012 | | |
|---|---|---|
| | **Average length of Stay** | **Discharges per 1,000** |
| Total | 4.5 | 116.2 |
| <1 | 3.8 | 1079.9 |
| 1–17 years | 3.9 | 21.1 |
| 18–44 years | 3.6 | 78.4 |
| 45–64 years | 4.9 | 108.8 |
| 65–84 years | 5.2 | 260.9 |
| 85+ | 5.2 | 502.0 |
| | | |
| Male | 4.8 | 99.9 |
| Female | 4.3 | 132.0 |

age, gender, and income on hospital utilization. It is important to carefully assess and estimate utilization, incorporating all of the factors that are likely to drive usage rates.

For example, a policy with liberal benefits for mental health probably will have much greater mental health utilization than one with more stringent benefits. Perhaps the best source of information on expected utilization is prior utilization for the covered population. What were inpatient usage rates last year? How many office visits were made? What kinds of chronic conditions exist in the population? Have physician practice patterns changed or are they likely to change as a result of different financial incentives? The health plan should have data that answer these questions and others, and it should be willing to release those data in the contracting phase.

One of the first major effects of managed-care programs is often a reduction in inpatient usage. The biggest area of cost is in inpatient usage, and plans that provide financial incentives for reducing inpatient days almost always experience significant declines in inpatient days per 1,000. The use of withholds and risk pools described earlier provides strong financial incentives for physicians to decrease usage rates.

The cost per unit is not a terribly difficult item to forecast and usually is established in the contract. The health plan knows, for example, they will pay $900 per medical-surgical inpatient day, subject only to a withhold and/or risk pool. The only real issue confronted here is one of negotiation. The health plan wants to get the lowest possible price from the provider, and the provider wants to get the highest possible price from the health plan. If the provider is reasonably certain that dramatic reductions in utilization can occur, it might make sense to negotiate a capitation arrangement. For example, the hospital in Table 7-5 may decide that instead of receiving $900 per day for medical-surgical care, it would rather have $23.75 PMPM, subject to its collection of the copayment. If it can keep usage rates down, the hospital stands to make much more money. However, if usage rates increase above 350 days per 1,000, it will lose money. This is a fundamental principle behind risk–return tradeoffs. The entity assuming the risk gets the return or loss.

A provider or the provider's appointed IDS agent, however, needs to make an important decision during negotiation. Namely, the provider must decide whether to provide the services internally or buy contractually required services. For example, the hospital is scheduled to receive $300 per day for inpatient mental health services. Should it provide this service internally, assuming it has the delivery capability, or should it contract this service out to a specialized mental health provider? The hospital may decide that it is better off to contract out inpatient mental health benefits for $300 per day and divert its resources to areas where it has a significant competitive advantage, such as cardiology or orthopedics. In some cases, there is no choice, because the provider may not have the capability. For example, a primary care medical group that did not have any specialists would be required to negotiate contracts with specialty physicians to provide services if the primary care group contracted for all physician services.

Before we conclude this section on capitation pricing, there are several issues that are of paramount importance to providers or their IDS agents who are negotiating capitated rates with a health plan or directly with an employer.

## Delineation of the Set of Covered Services

A provider and health plan should carefully define the set of services covered under their agreement. For example, are transplants and AIDS patients included under the plan? A useful way to summarize this discussion is through a responsibility matrix. The responsibility matrix would list services in the rows and parties responsible in the columns. This matrix could be a part of the formal contract. Included in this category is the specific listing of "carve-outs" or services that are not included as part of the provider's responsibility, such as mental health.

## Determination of Break-Even Service Volumes

Providers that accept a capitation rate have a different break-even structure, as **FIGURE 7-4** shows. In a capitation environment, revenue is fixed, and costs vary with volume. For a fixed number of covered people, the provider wishes to minimize services or encounters. The provider accepting a capitation rate must carefully determine the maximum amount of service that could be provided before costs would exceed revenues.

## Cost and Use of Stop-Loss Coverage

Providers may have the option of buying stop-loss coverage from the health plan or another insurer to cover costs of patients with catastrophic illnesses. For example, a hospital may negotiate a $75,000 stop-loss on inpatient care. Whenever a patient incurred charges greater than $75,000, the stop-loss insurer would pay the hospital for all costs above the threshold. In a like manner, physicians may negotiate lower stop-loss limits of $7,500 per patient for physician charges.

## Adverse Selection Provisions

Some reference should be made to adverse selection of health plan members. If a significant number of chronically ill patients, such as patients with AIDS, are attracted to the health plan, both the health plan and the providers may lose. However, if the health plan has subcapitated all of its providers with no adverse selection provisions, it might be encouraged to market its policies to anyone at lower-than-required rates

because the health plan has a guaranteed cost because it has capitated its providers.

## Reporting Requirements

In capitated contracts, providers must closely monitor utilization rates. Small changes in usage rates can destroy profitability quickly. Data systems must be in place to collect and report this information frequently. Providers also must be aware of the potential for an unrecorded liability referred to as **incurred but not reported (IBNR)**. This covers situations when services have been delivered but no claim has been received to date. Providers under capitation may be obligated to pay for services not performed in their network and should be aware of this potential liability. For example, a hospital that contracted out mental health services may not, at any point in time, know the total outstanding liability. These amounts, although small in relationship to total cost, can produce severe distortions of estimated profitability on contracts unless information about these changes is reported promptly and reasonable estimates of expected costs are made.

## ▸ Medicare and Medicaid Risk Contracts

Perhaps the last frontier for major managed-care expansion is the Medicare and Medicaid markets. **TABLE 7-7** presents a table showing the recent growth in managed-care programs. Both Medicare and

| TABLE 7-7 Medicare and Medicaid Managed-Care Enrollment Percentage | | |
|---|---|---|
| | **Managed-Care Percentage** | |
| **Year** | **Medicare** | **Medicaid** |
| 1990 | 4% | 9% |
| 1995 | 8% | 29% |
| 2000 | 17% | 56% |
| 2005 | 14% | 63% |
| 2010 | 24% | 71% |
| 2015 | 31% | 77% |

Centers for Medicare and Medicaid Services.

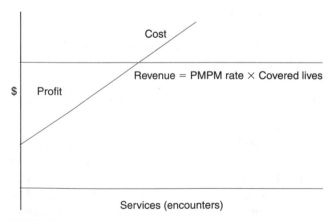

**FIGURE 7-4 Break-Even Analysis in a Capitated Environment**

Medicaid have experienced dramatic growth in managed care, but growth has been more rapid in the Medicaid program. The reason for the growth of managed care in Medicare and Medicaid is the potential for cost reduction, especially in inpatient areas. Medicare inpatient days per 1,000 are significantly higher in the traditional fee-for-service plans relative to managed Medicare programs, but there is some question whether part of the difference is related to adverse selection. Sicker patients may be more likely to enroll in the traditional fee-for-service plan rather than the Medicare-risk program.

Because Medicaid is a state-run healthcare program, there is no uniform program. Each state has defined its own program, and it will be different from programs in other states. Most states have received Section 1115 waivers that permit states to engage in Medicaid-demonstration projects. These waivers are largely used to expand Medicaid enrollment in HMOs. In many of these contracts, long-term care is eliminated or carved out because nursing-home expenditures are such a large percentage of the total Medicaid budget, and prediction of utilization can be speculative.

Medicare has been encouraging beneficiaries to drop fee-for-service arrangements and switch to its Medicare Advantage plan. The Medicare Advantage plan is at risk for all services provided by Medicare. Medicare reimburses health plans 95% of the estimated fee-for-service payment. The base rate is known as the adjusted average per capita cost (AAPCC) and is computed for each county in the United States. The AAPCC is the government's estimate of what fee-for-service costs would have been in the next fiscal year. Individual county rates are published in the Centers for Medicare and Medicaid Services (CMS) AAPCC rate book. Categories include demographic cost factors for Medicare Part A and Part B. These county rates are further adjusted for gender, age, Medicaid eligibility, work status, and institutionalized status. Rates can vary enormously by region of the country. For 2017, the range is from $1,305 PMPM in NW Arctic county Alaska to $574 PMPM in Ontario county New York. Potential contractors must review their projected costs using a format similar to the one presented in Table 7-5 and compare those with the allowed Medicare AAPCC.

---

*Learning Objective 7*

Discuss legal and regulatory issues that affect managed-care organizations.

---

# Legal and Regulatory Issues

There are a number of legal and regulatory issues that affect the formation and operation of provider-based MCOs, especially integrated delivery systems. Among them are the following.

## Antitrust

One concern with loose affiliations of physicians, such as an IPA, is the potential for price fixing. If the physicians do not share risk and have not commingled their assets and liabilities, the government may view an IPA arrangement that forms to negotiate prices with insurers as an attempt to fix prices. Similar arguments would apply to loose affiliations of hospitals or other providers who are not financially integrated but who merely created an association to negotiate prices.

## Inurement

If a nonprofit entity is involved in the creation of an IDS with physicians, it must be careful to ensure that it is not giving away more than it is receiving in value. This covers situations of physician-practice acquisition, rental of space, or the provision of other services to physicians or other groups. The nonprofit entity must not have its resources used to the benefit of any individual. A "commercially reasonable" test is often used to assess the potential of inurement. Did the nonprofit entity pay more for something that was commercially reasonable or provide services at a price that was less than commercially reasonable? In the areas of physician-practice acquisition, did the nonprofit entity pay more than fair market value for the practice?

## Licensure as an Insurer

It is not clear at this stage whether a provider or provider group, such as an IDS, is required to be licensed as an HMO if it accepts payment on a capitated basis for services that it does not provide. For example, if a primary care group contracted with an HMO for all physician services, not just primary care, would it be required to be licensed by the state as an HMO? Increasingly, many IDS organizations are being required to become licensed as HMOs if they contract out some of the medical services to organizations that are not part of its corporate system.

## Incentive Payments to Physicians to Reduce Services

Payments to physicians that provide incentives for fewer services may not be legal if they provide incentives to provide fewer services than are medically necessary. Nearly all HMO arrangements currently have financial rewards for reduced services and the pivotal point may be the term *medically necessary*.

## Intentional Torts

If physicians or other healthcare providers commit an act of malpractice because they wish to make more money, this may be construed as an intentional tort and their malpractice insurance may not be obligated to pay if wrongdoing was found to have occured. Physicians may be potentially liable under existing payment arrangements if their malpractice insurer could argue medical services were denied to make more money. For example, a doctor who failed to authorize a mammogram for a woman with a history of family breast cancer may be liable for an intentional tort if the physician were capitated and routinely scheduled mammograms for non-HMO patients with similar histories.

There are many other legal and regulatory issues that may affect business practices in managed-care relationships. Outside legal advice should be sought to investigate possible problems and solutions for those areas cited previously, as well as others.

## ▶ SUMMARY

This chapter has dealt with the topic of managed care and the evolving issues that affect financial management in managed-care situations. Managed care is not a new development in many respects. Health plans always have been in the business of accepting prepaid dollars in return for the promise to pay for any contractual medical benefits provided to the plan member. The new twist in managed care is really on the payment side. Health plans have historically paid providers, doctors, and hospitals on a fee-for-service basis. The health plan then assumed all the risk for utilization variances, whereas the provider assumed the risk of production, being able to provide services at costs less than negotiated prices. HMOs and other MCOs are trying to also shift utilization risk to providers by capitating payment.

Capitation payment systems require providers to know much more about the populations to which they are obligated to provide healthcare services and to do a much better job of forecasting. Pricing under a capitation payment system is easy to conceptualize but difficult to implement because most providers have little experience with utilization variation in a covered population. Historical use rates may be available, but managed care has created sizable shifts in utilization rates, and forecasting the magnitude of those changes is difficult.

IDSs have formed to try to place providers closer to the premium dollar flowing from the employer. At present, many of these IDS organizations are hospital-dominated, but physicians are increasingly asking why they should not take charge in the managed-care world because they have the most experience and the greatest ability to actually manage care and achieve cost savings. It is not clear whether the capital and organizational ability of the hospital or the patient-management ability of the physician will win or whether true partnerships will evolve.

## ASSIGNMENTS

1. High-deductible health plans with a savings option (HDHP/SO) have begun to gain market share in the last few years. What are the critical differences between these plans and more traditional health plans?
2. You have been hired as a consultant to a major health insurance company to help identify ways to reduce payments for healthcare benefits. Please identify some possible methods that may be useful in cutting costs.
3. You represent a medical group that is considering joining a Physician Hospital Organization (PHO) whose sole objective is to negotiate with health plans and employers for the provision of hospital and physician services on a capitated basis. If your state regards this PHO as a health insurance company and requires licensure, what possible effects might this have?
4. Your multispecialty group has been approached by an HMO that wishes you to contract with them for the provision of all physician services for a fixed capitated rate on a PMPM basis. How would you decide what to do in this situation?
5. You represent an integrated delivery system that is in negotiations with a health plan for a capitated rate to cover all hospital and physician services for a defined population. The following utilization data have been given to you, which detail last year's usage rates. You have included in this table your expected costs for selected services. Using

**TABLE 7-8**  Hospital and Physician Services Rates and Usage Rates

| Category | Annual Frequency per 1,000 | Unit Cost | PMPM | Copay Frequency per 1,000 | Copay Amount | Copay PMPM | Net PMPM |
|---|---|---|---|---|---|---|---|
| **Hospital Inpatient** | | | | | | | |
| Medical-surgical | 400 | $1,000 | | 0 | $0 | | |
| Maternity | 15 | 1,000 | | 0 | 0 | | |
| Mental health | 50 | 400 | | 0 | 0 | | |
| *Subtotal* | | | | | | | |
| **Hospital Outpatient** | | | | | | | |
| Surgery | 100 | $1,500 | | 0 | $0 | | |
| X-ray and lab | 500 | 300 | | 0 | 0 | | |
| Emergency department | 150 | 300 | | 150 | 50 | | |
| *Subtotal* | | | | | | | |
| **Physician** | | | | | | | |
| Inpatient surgery | 100 | $2,000 | | 0 | $0 | | |
| Outpatient surgery | 500 | 300 | | 0 | 0 | | |
| Office visits | 5,000 | 100 | | 5,000 | 10 | | |
| Inpatient visits | 250 | 150 | | 0 | 0 | | |
| Mental health | 400 | 150 | | 400 | 20 | | |
| *Subtotal* | | | | | | | |
| **Total** | | | | | | | |

the data presented in **TABLE 7-8**, calculate a required break-even rate for this contract, assuming that you need a 15% retention factor to cover administrative costs.

6. Memorial Hospital is trying to calculate its expected payments from a proposed fee structure with a local health plan. The health plan projects its hospital budget at 465 patient days per 1,000 members, with a payment rate of $1,000 per patient day. The covered population is 25,000 members, which produces a hospital budget of $11,625,000 [(465/1,000) × 25,000 × $1,000)]. The health plan proposes that a 10% withhold be put into effect, which translates to an actual per diem payment of $900. The risk pool would be shared equally by the doctors (one half) and the hospital (one half). Any negative balance in the risk pool would be assumed by the health plan. Calculate the amount of payment to Memorial Hospital under two assumptions: 550 patient days per 1,000 and 430 patient days per 1,000.

## SOLUTIONS

1. HDHP/SO plans differ from traditional health plans in several ways. First, HDHP/SO require the plan beneficiaries to pay for a specific level of healthcare services provided in a benefit year. This can amount to as much as $5,000 in some plans. Presumably, this creates better healthcare decision making by the beneficiaries because they seek more efficient medical services. Some have argued that some preventive services may be forgone because of high deductibles, which could result in costly care in the future. Covered services are often very similar in HDHP/SO plans because these plans are often related to traditional health plan coverage packages. Finally, many employers have viewed HDHP/SO plans as a means to shift cost to the employee for their healthcare benefits.

2. Healthcare benefit cost can be expressed as the product of utilization and price, which is the volume of services provided times the price paid for those services. Possible methods for reducing prices paid to providers would include selective contracting with the providers on a discounted basis, use of copayment provisions and deductibles to shift some of the cost to the insured health plan member, and development of a fee schedule for all providers that limit payments. Utilization options for reducing costs would include methods that either reduced the frequency of procedures or used less-expensive procedures. For example, better utilization review and prior authorization for medical procedures could be implemented. Case management of chronic conditions might also cut utilization by reducing the use of expensive inpatient procedures. Incentive structures for physicians, such as capitation payments or risk pools, might also be useful in decreasing utilization.

3. Aside from the legal filing requirements and increased government supervision of the PHO, it is also likely that certain reserve requirements must be maintained. These reserves may range from several hundred thousand dollars to several million dollars. This will create additional capital requirements for the PHO creation.

4. The critical issue to be resolved is the maximum amount of service that could be provided under the PMPM rate and still break even. In a fixed PMPM payment system, revenue is fixed, while costs vary with volume. The group needs to carefully consider the expected costs per unit. If total expected cost on a PMPM basis is less than the PMPM premium, it might make sense to accept the capitated rate.

5. **TABLE 7-9** calculates a required net PMPM rate of $138.50. When that rate is increased 15% to cover retention, the required PMPM rate would be $159.28.

6. **TABLE 7-10** provides the calculations for hospital payment under the two assumptions.

**TABLE 7-9** PMPM Rate Calculations

| Category | Annual Frequency per 1,000 | Unit Cost | PMPM | Copay Frequency per 1,000 | Copay Amount | Copay PMPM | Net PMPM |
|---|---|---|---|---|---|---|---|
| **Hospital Inpatient** | | | | | | | |
| Medical-surgical | 400 | $1,000 | 33.33 | 0 | $0 | – | 33.33 |
| Maternity | 15 | 1,000 | 1.25 | 0 | 0 | – | 1.25 |
| Mental health | 50 | 400 | 1.67 | 0 | 0 | – | 1.67 |
| *Subtotal* | | | 36.25 | | | – | 36.25 |
| **Hospital Outpatient** | | | | | | | |
| Surgery | 100 | $1,500 | 12.50 | 0 | $0 | – | 12.50 |
| X-ray and lab | 500 | 300 | 12.50 | 0 | 0 | – | 12.50 |
| Emergency department | 150 | 300 | 3.75 | 150 | 50 | 0.63 | 3.12 |
| *Subtotal* | | | 28.75 | | | 0.63 | 28.13 |

| Category | Annual Frequency per 1,000 | Unit Cost | PMPM | Copay Frequency per 1,000 | Copay Amount | Copay PMPM | Net PMPM |
|---|---|---|---|---|---|---|---|
| **Physician** | | | | | | | |
| Inpatient surgery | 100 | $2,000 | 16.67 | 0 | $0 | – | 16.67 |
| Outpatient surgery | 500 | 300 | 12.50 | 0 | 0 | – | 12.50 |
| Office visits | 5,000 | 100 | 41.67 | 5,000 | 10 | 4.17 | 37.50 |
| Inpatient visits | 250 | 150 | 3.13 | 0 | 0 | – | 3.13 |
| Mental health | 400 | 150 | 5.00 | 400 | 20 | 0.67 | 4.33 |
| *Subtotal* | | | 78.96 | | | 4.83 | 74.13 |
| **Total** | | | 143.96 | | | 5.46 | 138.50 |

**TABLE 7-10** Hospital Payment by Patient-Day Level

| Patient-Day Level | Hospital Payment (at $900 per Day) | Risk Pool (Budget Payment) | Hospital Share of Risk Pool (50%) | Total Hospital Payment |
|---|---|---|---|---|
| 550 PD per 1,000 | $12,375,000 | ($750,000) | negative/0 share | $12,375,000 |
| 430 PD per 1,000 | 9,675,000 | 1,950,000 | 975,000 | $10,650,000 |

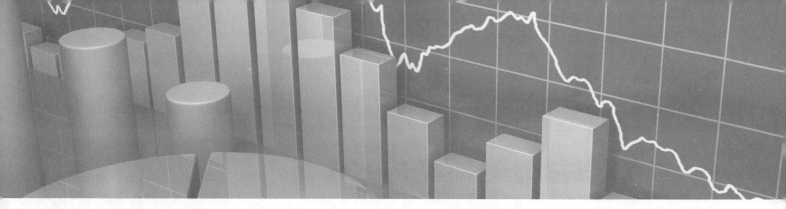

# CHAPTER 8

# General Principles of Accounting

## REAL-WORLD SCENARIO

Lindsay Harris was appointed recently to the Board of St. Thomas's Nursing Center, a religious nursing home in her community. Lindsay's first committee assignment was to the Finance Committee because of her prior business experience. Lindsay however has no understanding of accounting or financial issues because her career to date has been in the area of public relations. She is currently reviewing St. Thomas's quarterly financial statements in preparation for the Finance Committee's meeting. She is overwhelmed by the amount of detailed financial and operating data that is presented in the documents, but has noticed a dramatic decline in operating cash available. At the close of the most recent quarter St. Thomas's had consumed 50% of the beginning cash and currently had less than 10 days of average operating expenses available. Melody Ross, CFO at St. Thomas's, indicated in her narrative accompanying the quarterly statements that the recently completed quarter was outstanding from a financial perspective. Net income was up over 50% from the prior quarter and 75% above the same quarter last year. Melody explained that the primary reason for the improvement was the negotiation of a contract with a health plan to treat rehabilitation patients who would be transferred from local hospitals. This arrangement has led to a substantial increase in revenue, far above initial budgetary expectations. The provision of care is expected to be very profitable to St. Thomas's because the marginal cost of care provided to these patients is estimated to be less than 40% of the marginal revenue received. Patient accounting had difficulty, however, in implementing appropriate billing procedures and only recently were invoices sent to the health plan.

Melody made no mention of the erosion in cash position in her report to the Finance Committee, and Lindsay wonders how cash can decline so dramatically when profits are supposedly so strong. On further review of the financial statements she noted that St. Thomas's accounts receivable were up over 30% from beginning values. The increase in receivables almost matches the decline in cash. Lindsay is puzzled by this and wants to know if there is some relationship between cash balances and accounts receivable. She remembers from an accounting course taken more than 20 years ago that there was a difference between cash accounting and accrual accounting. Perhaps this could be the explanation for the erosion in cash position, but Lindsay is still concerned about St. Thomas's ability to pay near-term expenditures for payroll, supplies, and maturing debt.

---

Information does not happen by itself; an individual or a formally designed system must generate it. Financial information is no exception. The system and practice of accounting generates most financial information to provide quantitative data, primarily financial in nature, that are useful in making economic decisions about economic entities. In general, the term **accounting** refers to the process and principles for preparing and disseminating financial information. This chapter will present a general understanding of those principles and processes.

### Learning Objective 1

Describe the differences between financial and managerial accounting.

## ▶ Financial Versus Managerial Accounting

Accounting can be divided into two categories: financial accounting and managerial accounting. **Financial accounting** is the branch of accounting that provides general-purpose financial statements or reports to aid many decision-making groups, internal and external to the organization, in making a variety of decisions. The primary outputs of financial accounting are four financial statements that detail the organization's current financial position and how the organization reached that position over some period of time (usually 1 year). These statements will be described in detail in Chapter 9. The four statements are:

- Balance sheet
- Statement of operations (or income statement or statement of revenues and expenses)
- Statement of cash flows
- Statement of changes in net assets (or statement of changes in shareholders' equity)

The field of financial accounting is restricted in many ways regarding how certain events or business transactions may be accounted for. The term **generally accepted accounting principles (GAAP)** is often used to describe the body of rules and requirements that shape the preparation of the four primary financial statements. For example, an organization's financial statements that have been audited by an independent **certified public accountant (CPA)** would bear the following language in an unqualified opinion:

> We have audited the accompanying combined balance sheets of Harris Memorial Hospital and Harris Community Foundation and subsidiaries (the Foundation) as of December 31, 20X7 and 20X6, and the related combined statements of operations, changes in net assets, and cash flows for the years then ended.
>
> Management is responsible for the preparation and fair presentation of the consolidated financial statements in accordance with accounting principles generally accepted in the United States of America; this includes the design, implementation, and maintenance of internal control relevant to the preparation and fair presentation of consolidated financial statements that are free from material misstatement, whether due to fraud or error.
>
> Our responsibility is to express an opinion on these financial statements based on our audits. We conducted our audits in accordance with auditing standards generally accepted in the United States. Those standards require that we plan and perform the audit to obtain reasonable assurance about whether the financial statements are free of material misstatement.
>
> An audit involves performing procedures to obtain audit evidence about the amounts

and disclosures in the consolidated financial statements. The procedures selected depend on our judgment, including the assessment of the risks of material misstatement of the consolidated financial statements, whether due to fraud or error. In making those risk assessments, we consider internal control relevant to the Foundation's preparation and fair presentation of the consolidated financial statements in order to design audit procedures that are appropriate in the circumstances, but not for the purpose of expressing an opinion on the effectiveness of the Foundation's internal control. Accordingly, we express no such opinion. An audit also includes evaluating the appropriateness of accounting policies used and the reasonableness of significant accounting estimates made by management, as well as evaluating the overall presentation of the consolidated financial statements. We believe that the audit evidence we have obtained is sufficient and appropriate to provide a basis for our audit opinion.

In our opinion, the financial statements referred to above present fairly, in all material respects, the combined financial position of Harris Memorial Hospital and Harris Community Foundation and subsidiaries at December 31, 20X7 and 20X6, and the combined changes in their net assets and their cash flows for the years then ended in conformity with U.S. generally accepted accounting principles.

Financial accounting is not limited to preparation of the four statements. An increasing number of additional financial reports are being required, especially for external users for specific decision-making purposes. This is particularly important in the healthcare industry. For example, hospitals submit cost reports to a number of third-party payers, such as Blue Cross, Medicare, and Medicaid. They also submit financial reports to a large number of regulatory agencies, such as planning agencies, rate review agencies, service associations, and many others. In addition, CPAs often prepare financial projections that are used by investors in capital financing. These statements, although not usually audited by independent CPAs, are, for the most part, prepared in accordance with the same generally accepted accounting principles that govern the preparation of the four basic financial statements.

**Managerial accounting** is primarily concerned with the preparation of financial information for specific purposes, usually for internal users. Because this information is used within the organization, there is less need for a body of principles restricting its preparation. Presumably, the user and the preparer can meet to discuss questions of interpretation. Uniformity and comparability of information, which are desired goals for financial accountants, are clearly less important to management accountants. Where financial accounting has an emphasis on the recording and reporting of historical financial transactions, management accounting often has a focus on future periods. A budget is an example of a financial report that is often generated from a managerial accounting perspective.

---

### Learning Objective 2

Understand core principles of accounting that guide the preparation and dissemination of financial information.

---

## ▶ Principles of Accounting

In addressing the principles of accounting, we are concerned with both sets of accounting information—financial and managerial. Although managerial accounting has no formally adopted set of principles, it relies strongly on financial accounting principles. Understanding the principles and basics of financial accounting is therefore critical to understanding both financial and managerial accounting information.

In the text to follow, five specific principles of accounting are discussed:

1. Accounting entity
2. Money measurement
3. Duality
4. Cost valuation
5. Stable monetary unit

To better illustrate these principles, our discussion will include a case example of a newly formed, not-for-profit healthcare organization, which we refer to as "Alpha HCO."

### Principle One: Accounting Entity

Obviously, in any accounting there must be an entity for which the financial statements (balance sheet, statement of operations, etc.) are being prepared. Specifying the entity on which the accounting will focus defines the information that is pertinent. Drawing these boundaries is the underlying concept behind the accounting entity principle. Essentially, the accounting entity is the organization for which financial information will be recorded and reported.

Alpha HCO is the entity for which we will account and prepare financial statements. We are not interested in the individuals who may have incorporated Alpha HCO or other healthcare organizations in the community, but solely in Alpha HCO's financial transactions.

Defining the entity is not as clear-cut as one might expect. Significant problems arise, especially when the legal entity is different from the accounting entity. For example, if one physician owns a clinic through a sole proprietorship arrangement, the accounting entity may be the clinic operation, whereas the legal entity includes the physician and the physician's personal resources as well. A hospital may be part of a university or government agency, or it might be owned by a large corporation organized on a for-profit or not-for-profit basis. Indeed, as a result of corporate restructuring, many hospitals now have become subsidiaries of a holding company. Careful attention must be paid to the definition of the accounting entity in these situations. If the entity is not properly defined, evaluation of its financial information may be useless at best and misleading at worst.

The common practice of municipalities directly paying the fringe benefits of municipal employees employed in the hospital illustrates this situation. Such expenses may never show up in the hospital's accounts, resulting in an understatement of the expenses associated with running the hospital. In many cases, this may produce a bias in the rate-setting process. Clearly, a well-defined and communicated accounting entity is critical in recording and reporting financial information.

## Principle Two: Money Measurement

Accounting in general and financial accounting in particular are concerned with measuring economic resources and obligations and their changing levels for the accounting entity under consideration. The accountant's yardstick for measuring is not metered to size, color, weight, or other attributes; it is limited exclusively to money. However, there are significant problems in money measurement, which will be discussed in the following text.

Economic resources are defined as scarce means, limited in supply but essential to economic activity. They include supplies, buildings, equipment, money, claims to receive money, and ownership interests in other enterprises. The terms *economic resources* and assets may be interchanged for most practical purposes. Economic obligations are responsibilities

to transfer economic resources or provide services to other entities in the future, usually in return for economic resources received from other entities in the past through the purchase of assets, the receipt of services, or the acceptance of loans. For most practical purposes, the terms *economic obligations* and liabilities may be used interchangeably.

In most normal situations, assets exceed liabilities in money-measured value. Liabilities represent the claim of one entity on another's assets; any excess or remaining residual interest may be claimed by the owner. In fact, for entities with ownership interest, this residual interest is called owner's equity.

In most not-for-profit entities, including healthcare organizations, there is no residual ownership claim. Any assets remaining in a liquidated not-for-profit entity, after all liabilities have been dissolved, legally become the property of the state. Residual interest is referred to as fund balance or net assets for most not-for-profit healthcare organizations.

The use of the terms *assets, liabilities*, and *equity* (or net assets) can be easily understood in the common example of homeownership. To illustrate, let us assume that an individual purchases a $200,000 home. The individual uses $40,000 in personal cash and a bank mortgage of $160,000 to complete the purchase. At the end of the transaction, assuming no other financial information, the individual would have assets (historical value of items owned) of $200,000, liabilities (amount of items owed) of $160,000, and equity (the residual interest) of $40,000. As the individual pays off the mortgage balance, equity will increase. The relationship of assets, liabilities, and equity will be described in the "duality" principle discussion to follow.

In the Alpha HCO example, assume that the community donated $1,000,000 in cash to the healthcare organization at its formation, hypothetically assumed to be December 31, 20X2. At that time, a listing of its assets, liabilities, and net assets would have been prepared in a balance sheet and read as presented in EXHIBIT 8-1.

---

**EXHIBIT 8-1** Alpha HCO's Balance Sheet at Formation

Alpha HCO Balance Sheet
December 31, 20X2

| Assets | Liabilities and Net Assets |
|---|---|
| Cash $1,000,000 | Net assets $1,000,000 |

## Principle Three: Duality

One of the fundamental premises of accounting is a simple arithmetic requirement: the value of assets must always equal the combined value of liabilities and residual interest, which we have called net assets. This basic accounting equation, the **duality principle**, may be stated as follows:

$$Assets = Liabilities + Net\ assets$$

This requirement means that a balance sheet (where the values for assets, liabilities, and net assets are provided) will always balance: the value of the assets will always equal the value of claims, whether liabilities or net assets, on those assets.

Changes are always occurring in organizations that affect the value of assets, liabilities, and net assets. These changes are called *transactions* and represent the items that interest accountants. Examples of transactions are borrowing money, purchasing supplies, and constructing buildings. The important thing to remember is that cash transactions must be carefully analyzed under the duality principle to keep the basic accounting equation in balance.

To better understand how important this principle is, let us analyze several transactions in our Alpha HCO example:

- Transaction 1. On January 2, 20X3, Alpha HCO buys a piece of equipment for $100,000. The purchase is financed with a $100,000 note from the bank.
- Transaction 2. On January 3, 20X3, Alpha HCO buys a building for $2,000,000, using $500,000 cash and issuing $1,500,000 worth of 20-year bonds.
- Transaction 3. On January 4, 20X3, Alpha HCO purchases $200,000 worth of supplies from a supply firm on a credit basis.

If balance sheets were prepared after each of these three transactions, they would appear as presented in **EXHIBIT 8-2**. In each of these three transactions, the change in asset value is matched by an identical change in liability value. Thus, the basic accounting equation remains in balance.

It should be noted that, as the number of transactions increases, the number of individual asset and liability items also increases. In most organizations, there is a large number of these individual items, which are referred to as **accounts**. The listing of these accounts is often called a *chart of accounts*; it is a useful device for categorizing transactions related to a given healthcare organization. There is already significant uniformity among hospitals and other healthcare facilities in the chart of accounts used; however, there is also pressure, especially from external users of financial information, to move toward even more uniformity. You may not recognize each of the accounts listed in the transaction examples. However, the key thing to learn from these examples is that individual asset, liability, and net asset accounts will always create a balance through the duality principle.

## Principle Four: Cost Valuation

Many readers of financial statements make the mistake of assuming that reported balance sheet values represent the real worth of individual assets or liabilities. Asset and liability values reported in a balance sheet are based on their *historical* or *acquisition* cost. In most situations, asset values do not equal the amount of money that could be realized if the assets were sold. However, in many cases, the reported value of a liability in a balance sheet is a good approximation of the amount of money that would be required to extinguish the indebtedness.

Examining the alternatives to historical cost valuation helps clarify why the cost basis of valuation is used. The two primary alternatives to historical cost valuation of assets and liabilities are **market value** and **replacement cost** valuation.

Valuation of individual assets at their market value sounds simple enough and appeals to many users of financial statements. Creditors especially are often interested in what values assets would bring if liquidated. Current market values give decision makers an approximation of liquidation values.

The market value method's lack of objectivity, however, is a serious problem. In most normal situations, established markets dealing in secondhand merchandise do not exist. Decision makers must rely on individual appraisals. Given the current state of the art of appraisal, two appraisers are likely to produce different estimates of market value for identical assets. Accountants' insistence on objectivity in measurement thus eliminates market valuation of assets as a viable alternative.

Replacement cost valuation of assets measures assets by the money value required to replace them. This concept of valuation is extremely useful for many decision-making purposes. For example, management decisions to continue delivery of certain services should be affected by the replacement cost of resources, not their historical or acquisition cost—which is considered to be a **sunk cost**, irrelevant to future decisions. Planning agencies or other regulatory agencies also should consider estimates

**EXHIBIT 8-2** Alpha HCO's Balance Sheet, Transactions 1 Through 3

*Transaction 1*

Alpha HCO Balance Sheet
January 2, 20X3

| Assets | | Liabilities and Net Assets | |
|---|---|---|---|
| Cash | $1,000,000 | Notes payable | $100,000 |
| Equipment | 100,000 | Net assets | 1,000,000 |
| Total | $1,100,000 | Total | $1,100,000 |

Assets: Increase $100,000 (equipment increases by $100,000)
Liabilities: Increase $100,000 (notes payable increase by $100,000)

*Transaction 2*

Alpha HCO Balance Sheet
January 3, 20X3

| Assets | | Liabilities and Net Assets | |
|---|---|---|---|
| Cash | $500,000 | Notes payable | $100,000 |
| Equipment | 100,000 | Bonds payable | 1,500,000 |
| Building | 2,000,000 | Net assets | 1,000,000 |
| Total | $2,600,000 | Total | $2,600,000 |

Assets: Increase $1,500,000 (cash decreases by $500,000 and building increases by $2,000,000)
Liabilities: Increase $1,500,000 (bonds payable increase by $1,500,000)

*Transaction 3*

Alpha HCO Balance Sheet
January 4, 20X3

| Assets | | Liabilities and Net Assets | |
|---|---|---|---|
| Cash | $500,000 | Accounts payable | $200,000 |
| Supplies | 200,000 | Notes payable | 100,000 |
| Equipment | 100,000 | Bonds payable | 1,500,000 |
| Building | 2,000,000 | Net assets | 1,000,000 |
| Total | $2,800,000 | Total | $2,800,000 |

Assets: Increase $200,000 (supplies increase by $200,000)
Liabilities: Increase $200,000 (accounts payable increases by $200,000)

of replacement cost to avoid bias. Considering only historical cost may improperly make old facilities appear more efficient than new or proposed facilities and projects.

Replacement cost may be a useful concept of valuation; however, it too suffers from lack of objectivity in measurement. Replacement cost valuation depends on how an item is replaced. For example,

given the rate of technologic change in the general economy, especially in the healthcare industry, few assets today would be replaced with like assets. Instead, more refined or capable assets probably would replace them. What is the replacement cost in this situation? Is it the cost of the new, improved asset or the present cost of an identical asset that most likely would not be purchased? Compound this question by the large number of manufacturers selling roughly equivalent items and you have some idea of the inherent difficulty and subjectivity in replacement cost valuation.

Historical cost valuation, with all its faults, is thus the basis that the accounting profession has chosen to value assets and liabilities in most circumstances. Accountants use it rather than replacement cost largely because it is more objective. Over the years, there has been some fairly strong pressure from inside and outside the accounting profession to switch to replacement cost valuation, but it is still uncertain whether this pressure will be successful.

One final, important point should be noted: at the time of initial asset valuation, the values assigned by historical cost valuation and replacement cost valuation are identical. The historical cost value is most often criticized for assets that have long, useful lives, such as buildings and equipment. Over a period of many years, the historical cost and replacement cost values tend to diverge dramatically, in part because general **inflation** in our economy erodes the dollar's purchasing power. A dollar of today is simply not as valuable as a dollar of 10 years ago. This problem could be remedied, without sacrificing the objectivity of historical cost measurement, by selecting a unit of purchasing power as the unit of measure: transactions then would not be accounted in dollars but in dollars of purchasing power at a given point in time, usually the year for which the financial statements are being prepared. This issue is addressed in the next section, under Principle Five: Stable Monetary Unit.

## Required Return on Investment and Valuation Alternatives

Business firms, both voluntary not-for-profit and investor-owned, must produce returns on their investment greater than the cost of capital used to finance their investment. The **cost of capital** refers to the cost of debt or equity in financing the acquisition of an asset. Certainly, it would not be wise for a business to borrow money at 10% (cost of debt) and invest the proceeds in projects earning only 5%. Valuation of the investment at cost, market value, or replacement cost can have a significant effect on basic business decisions such as expansion or closure. To illustrate this point, consider James Nursing Home, a fictitious voluntary not-for-profit clinic, with the financial data presented in TABLE 8-1.

Return on investment (ROI) for James Nursing Home is 12.5% under a historical cost valuation

| TABLE 8-1 Financial Data for James Nursing Home—20X4 | |
|---|---|
| Cash flow | $10,000 |
| Cost of capital | 12% |
| Investment—Historical cost | $80,000 |
| Investment—Replacement cost | $150,000 |
| Investment—Market value | $60,000 |

($10,000 ÷ $80,000), 6.7% under replacement cost valuation ($10,000 ÷ $150,000), and 16.7% under a market value valuation ($10,000 ÷ 60,000). What should the management and board of James Nursing Home do?

First, the ROI calculated under cost valuation is meaningless for future decisions. An ROI based on historical cost tells you how well the investment has done, not how well it will do in the future. ROI calculated under replacement cost valuation will tell the decision maker the return using current replacement cost values. In our example, the James Nursing Home is not profitable given current replacement cost values and is not viable in the future. Unless expectations about future cash flows change, the nursing home should not receive significant new investment. ROI calculated under market values shows the James Nursing Home to be viable in the short run. It is

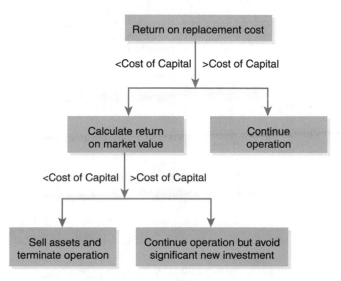

**FIGURE 8-1** **Return on Investment Relationships**

generating an ROI of 16.7%, which exceeds its cost of capital, 12%. **FIGURE 8-1** illustrates the decision framework.

## Principle Five: Stable Monetary Unit

The money measurement principle of accounting discussed earlier restricted accounting measures to money. In accounting in the United States, the unit of measure is the dollar. At the present time, no adjustment to changes in the general purchasing power of that unit is required in financial reports; a year-2007 dollar is assumed to be equal in value to a 2017 dollar. This permits arithmetic operations, such as addition and subtraction. If this assumption were not made, addition of the unadjusted historical cost values of assets acquired during different periods would be inappropriate, like adding apples and oranges. Current generally accepted accounting principles incorporate the stable monetary unit principle.

The stable monetary unit principle may not seem to pose any great problems. However, even modest rates of inflation at around 4% per year can quickly compound to produce major financial distortions. For example, $1.00 paid in the year 2025 would be equivalent to $0.67 paid in 2015 with a 4% annual inflation rate. To present an extreme example, imagine that the inflation rate in the economy is currently 100%, compounded monthly. Consider a neighborhood healthcare center that has all its expenses, except payroll, covered by grants from governmental agencies. Its employees have a contract that automatically adjusts their wages to changes in the general price level. (With a monthly inflation rate of 100%, it is no wonder.) Assume that revenues from patients are collected on the first day of the month after the one in which they were billed, but that the employees are paid at the beginning of each month. Rates to patients are set so that the excess of revenues over expenses will be zero. With the first month's wages set equal to $100,000, the income and cash flow positions presented in **TABLE 8-2** result for the first 6 months of the year.

Note the tremendous difference between income and cash flow. Although the income statement would indicate a break-even operation, the cash balance at the end of June would be a negative $3,150,000. Obviously, the healthcare center's operations cannot continue indefinitely in light of the extreme cash hardship position imposed.

Fortunately, the rate of inflation in our economy is not 100%. However, smaller rates of inflation compounded over long periods could create similar problems. For example, setting rates equal to historical cost depreciation of fixed assets leaves the entity with a significant cash deficit when it is time to replace the asset. Many healthcare boards and management organizations of not-for-profit firms do not adequately reflect increasing replacement costs in their pricing.

| **TABLE 8-2** Sample Income and Cash Flows, 100% Inflation | | | | | | |
|---|---|---|---|---|---|---|
| | **Income Flows** | | | **Cash Flows** | | |
| **Expense** | **Revenue** | **Net income** | **Inflow** | **Outflow** | **Difference** | **Income** |
| January | $100,000 | $100,000 | 0 | $50,000* | $100,000 | (50,000) |
| February | 200,000 | 200,000 | 0 | 100,000 | 200,000 | (100,000) |
| March | 400,000 | 400,000 | 0 | 200,000 | 400,000 | (200,000) |
| April | 800,000 | 800,000 | 0 | 400,000 | 800,000 | (400,000) |
| May | 1,600,000 | 1,600,000 | 0 | 800,000 | 1,600,000 | (800,000) |
| June | 3,200,000 | 3,200,000 | 0 | 1,600,000 | 3,200,000 | (1,600,000) |
| | $6,300,000 | $6,300,000 | 0 | $3,150,000 | $6,300,000 | ($3,150,000) |

Note: $50,000 is equal to the revenue billed in December.

Discuss the differences between the accrual- and cash-basis methods of accounting.

# ▶ Accrual Versus Cash Accounting

**Accrual accounting** is a fundamental premise of accounting. It means that transactions of a business enterprise are recognized during the period to which they relate, not necessarily during the periods in which cash is received or paid. The latter part of this definition refers to **cash-basis accounting**.

It is common to hear people talk about the differences between these two forms of accounting. Most of us think in cash-basis terms. We measure our personal financial success during the year by the amount of cash we realized. Seldom do we consider such things as wear and tear on our cars and other personal items or the differences between earned and uncollected income. Perhaps if we accrued expenses for items such as depreciation on heating systems, air conditioning systems, automobiles, and furniture, we might see a different picture of our financial well-being.

The accrual basis of accounting significantly affects the preparation of financial statements in general; however, its major impact is on the preparation of the statement of revenues and expenses. The following additional transactions for Alpha HCO illustrate the importance of the accrual principle:

- Transaction 4: Alpha HCO bills patients $100,000 on January 16, 20X3, for services provided to them.
- Transaction 5: Alpha HCO pays employees $60,000 for their wages and salaries on January 18, 20X3.
- Transaction 6: Alpha HCO receives $80,000 in cash from patients who were billed earlier in Transaction 4 on January 23, 20X3.
- Transaction 7: Alpha HCO pays the $200,000 of accounts payable on January 27, 20X3, for the purchase of supplies that took place on January 4, 20X3.

Balance sheets prepared after each of these transactions appear as presented in **EXHIBIT 8-3**. In Transactions 4 and 5, there is an effect on Alpha HCO's residual interest or its fund balance (also referred to as net assets or equity). In Transaction 4, an increase in net assets occurred because patients were billed for services previously rendered. Increases in net assets or owners' equity resulting from the sale of goods or delivery of services are called **revenues**. It should be noted that this increase occurred even though no cash was actually collected until January 23, 20X3, illustrating the accrual principle of accounting. Recognition of revenue occurs when the revenue is earned, not necessarily when it is collected.

In Transaction 5, a reduction in fund balance (net assets) occurs. Costs incurred by a business enterprise to provide goods or services that reduce net assets or owners' equity are called **expenses**. Under the accrual principle, expenses are recognized when assets are used up or liabilities are incurred in the production and delivery of goods or services, not necessarily when cash is paid.

---

**EXHIBIT 8-3**   Alpha HCO's Balance Sheet, Transactions 4 Through 7

*Transaction 4*

Alpha HCO Balance Sheet
January 16, 20X3

| Assets | | Liabilities and Net Assets | |
|---|---|---|---|
| Cash | $500,000 | Accounts payable | $200,000 |
| Accounts receivable | 100,000 | Notes payable | 100,000 |
| Supplies | 200,000 | Bonds payable | 1,500,000 |
| Equipment | 100,000 | Net assets | 1,100,000 |
| Building | 2,000,000 | | |
| Total | $2,900,000 | Total | $2,900,000 |

Assets: Increase $100,000 (accounts receivable increases by $100,000)
Net assets: Increase $100,000

*(continues)*

**EXHIBIT 8-3** Alpha HCO's Balance Sheet, Transactions 4 Through 7 *(continued)*

*Transaction 5*

Alpha HCO Balance Sheet
January 18, 20X3

| Assets | | Liabilities and Net Assets | |
|---|---|---|---|
| Cash | $440,000 | Accounts payable | $200,000 |
| Accounts receivable | 100,000 | Notes payable | 100,000 |
| Supplies | 200,000 | Bonds payable | 1,500,000 |
| Equipment | 100,000 | Net assets | 1,040,000 |
| Building | 2,000,000 | | |
| Total | $2,840,000 | Total | $2,840,000 |

Assets: Decrease by $60,000 (cash decreases by $60,000)
Net assets: Decrease by $60,000

*Transaction 6*

Alpha HCO Balance Sheet
January 23, 20X3

| Assets | | Liabilities and Net Assets | |
|---|---|---|---|
| Cash | $520,000 | Accounts payable | $200,000 |
| Accounts receivable | 20,000 | Notes payable | 100,000 |
| Supplies | 200,000 | Bonds payable | 1,500,000 |
| Equipment | 100,000 | Net assets | 1,040,000 |
| Building | 2,000,000 | | |
| Total | $2,840,000 | Total | $2,840,000 |

Assets: No change (cash increases by $80,000; accounts receivable decrease by $80,000)

*Transaction 7*

Alpha HCO Balance Sheet
January 27, 20X3

| Assets | | Liabilities and Net Assets | |
|---|---|---|---|
| Cash | $320,000 | Accounts payable | $0 |
| Accounts receivable | 20,000 | Notes payable | 100,000 |
| Supplies | 200,000 | Bonds payable | 1,500,000 |
| Equipment | 100,000 | Net assets | 1,040,000 |
| Building | 2,000,000 | | |
| Total | $2,640,000 | Total | $2,640,000 |

Assets: Decrease by $200,000 (cash decreases by $200,000)
Liabilities: Decrease by $200,000 (accounts payable decrease by $200,000)

The difference between revenue and expense is often referred to as *net income*. In the hospital and healthcare industry, this term may be used interchangeably with the term **excess of revenues over expenses** or *revenues and gains in excess of expenses*.

The income statement, or statement of operations, summarizes the revenues and expenses of a business enterprise over a defined period. If an income statement is prepared for the total life of an entity, that is, from inception to dissolution, the value for net income would be the same under both an accrual and a cash basis method of accounting.

In most situations, frequent measurements of revenue and expense are demanded, creating some important measurement problems. Ideally, under the accrual accounting principle, expenses should be matched to the revenue that they helped create. For example, wage, salary, and supply costs usually can be easily associated with revenues of a given period. However, in certain circumstances, the association between revenue and expense is impossible to discover, necessitating the accountant's use of a systematic, rational method of allocating costs to a benefiting period. In the best example of this procedure, costs such as those associated with building and equipment are spread over the estimated useful life of the assets through the recording of depreciation.

To complete the Alpha HCO example, assume that the financial statements must be prepared at the end of January. Before they are prepared, certain adjustments must be made to the accounts to adhere fully to the accrual principle of accounting. The following adjustments might be recorded.

- Adjustment 1: There are currently $100,000 of patient charges that have been incurred but not yet billed.
- Adjustment 2: There are currently $50,000 worth of unpaid wages and salaries for which employees have performed services.
- Adjustment 3: A physical inventory count indicates that $50,000 worth of initial supplies have been used.
- Adjustment 4: The equipment of Alpha HCO has an estimated useful life of 10 years, and the cost is being allocated over this period. On a monthly basis, this amounts to an allocation of $833 per month.
- Adjustment 5: The building has an estimated useful life of 40 years, and the cost of the building is being allocated equally over its estimated life. On a monthly basis, this amounts to $4,167.
- Adjustment 6: Although no payment has been made on either notes payable or bonds payable, there is an interest expense associated with using money for this 1-month period. This interest expense will be paid later. Assume that the note payable carries an interest rate of 8% and the bond payable carries an interest rate of 6%. The actual amount of interest expense incurred for the month of January would be $8,167 ($667 on the note and $7,500 on the bond payable).

The effects of these adjustments on the balance sheet of Alpha HCO and on the ending balance sheet that would be prepared after all the adjustments were made, are presented in **EXHIBIT 8-4** (with explanations in **TABLE 8-3**). It is also possible to prepare the statement of revenues and expenses presented in **EXHIBIT 8-5**.

Note that the difference between revenue and expense during the month of January was $26,833, the exact amount by which the net assets of Alpha HCO changed during the month. Alpha HCO began the month with $1,000,000 in its net asset account and ended with $1,026,833. This illustrates an important point to remember when reading financial statements: the individual financial statements are fundamentally related to one another.

---

**EXHIBIT 8-4**  Alpha HCO Balance Sheet: January 31, 20X3

| Assets | | Liabilities and Net Assets | |
|---|---|---|---|
| Cash | $320,000 | Wages and salaries payable | $50,000 |
| Accounts receivable | 120,000 | Interest payable | 8,167 |
| Supplies | 150,000 | Notes payable | 100,000 |
| Equipment | 99,167 | Bonds payable | 1,500,000 |
| Building | 1,995,833 | Net assets | 1,026,833 |
| Total | $2,685,000 | Total | $2,685,000 |

**TABLE 8-3** End of Period Adjusting Entries and End of Month Balance Sheet

| Adjustment | Change | Account(s) Increased | Account(s) Decreased |
|---|---|---|---|
| 1 | $100,000 | Net assets and accounts receivable | None |
| 2 | $50,000 | Wages and salaries payable | Net assets |
| 3 | $50,000 | None | Net assets and supplies |
| 4 | $833 | None | Net assets and equipment |
| 5 | $4,167 | None | Net assets and building |
| 6 | $8,167 | Interest payable | Net assets |

**EXHIBIT 8-5** Alpha HCO Statement of Revenue and Expenses: For Month Ended January 31, 20X3

| | |
|---|---|
| Revenues | $200,000 |
| Less expenses | |
| Wages and salaries | $110,000 |
| Supplies | 50,000 |
| Depreciation | 5,000 |
| Interest | 8,167 |
| Total | $173,167 |
| Excess of revenue over expenses | $26,833 |

*Learning Objective 4*

List the three categories of net assets.

## ▶ Fund Accounting

Fund accounting is a system in which an entity's assets and liabilities are segregated in the accounting records. Each fund may be considered an independent entity with its own self-balancing set of accounts. The basic accounting equation discussed under "duality" must be satisfied for each fund: assets must equal liabilities plus net assets for the particular fund in question.

The Financial Accounting Statement Board (FASB) pronouncement 117 changed the nature of fund accounting for voluntary not-for-profit healthcare organizations. It stipulated that only three classifications of fund balance or net assets be used:

1. Unrestricted net assets
2. Temporarily restricted net assets
3. Permanently restricted net assets

The last two categories of net assets, temporarily and permanently restricted net assets, are related to the existence of a *donor-imposed restriction*. The difference between the two is based on the nature of the donor's restriction. **Temporarily restricted net assets** are funds that can be used for a specific purpose only, funds that may be released for a specific purpose only, or funds that may be released for general purposes after a passage of time. **Permanently restricted net assets** are often of an endowment nature. Only the income of the fund can be used, and the principal cannot be used to fund any purpose. Generally, donor-restricted net assets can consist of the following three common types:

- Specific-purpose funds
- Plant replacement and expansion funds
- Endowment funds

**Specific-purpose funds** are donated by individuals or organizations and restricted for purposes other than plant replacement and expansion or endowment. Monies received from government agencies to perform specific research or other work are examples of specific-purpose funds.

**Plant replacement and expansion funds** are restricted for use in plant replacement and expansion. Assets purchased with these monies are not recorded in the fund. When the monies are used for plant purposes, the amounts are transferred to the unrestricted net assets. For example, if $200,000 in cash from the plant replacement fund were used to acquire a piece of equipment, equipment and unrestricted net assets would be increased.

**Endowment funds** are contributed to be held intact for generating income. The income may or may not be restricted for specific purposes. Some endowments are classified as "term" endowments. That is, after the expiration of some period, the restriction on use of the principal is lifted. The balance is then transferred to the general fund.

---

### Learning Objective 5

Discuss the accounting conventions that affect the application of accounting principles.

---

## ▶ Conventions of Accounting

The accounting principles discussed up to this point are important in the preparation of financial statements. However, several widely accepted conventions modify the application of these principles in certain circumstances. Three of the more important conventions are discussed next:

1. Conservatism
2. Materiality
3. Consistency

*Conservatism* affects the valuation of some assets. Specifically, accountants use a "lower of cost or market" rule for valuing inventories and marketable securities. The lower of cost or market rule means that the value of a stock of inventory or **marketable securities** would be the actual cost or market value, whichever is less. For these resources, there is a deviation from cost valuation to market valuation whenever market value is lower.

*Materiality* permits certain transactions to be treated out of accordance with generally accepted accounting principles. This might be permitted because the transaction does not materially affect the presentation of financial position. For example, theoretically,

paper clips may have an estimated useful life greater than 1 year. However, the cost of capitalizing this item and systematically and rationally allocating it over its useful life is not justifiable; the difference in financial position that would be created by not using generally accepted accounting principles would be immaterial.

*Consistency* limits the accounting alternatives that can be used. In any given transaction, there is usually a variety of available, generally acceptable, accounting treatments. For example, generally accepted accounting principles permit the use of double-declining balance, sum-of-the-years' digits, or straight-line methods for allocating the costs of depreciable assets over their estimated useful life; but the consistency convention limits an entity's ability to change from one acceptable method to another.

## ▶ SUMMARY

In this chapter, we discussed the importance of generally accepted accounting principles in deriving financial information. Although these principles are formally required only in the preparation of audited financial statements, they influence the derivation of most financial information. An understanding of some of the basic principles is critical to an understanding of financial information in general.

The following five specific principles of accounting were discussed in some detail:

1. Accounting entity
2. Money measurement
3. Duality
4. Cost valuation
5. Stable monetary unit

In addition to these, the importance accrual and fund accounting as it relates to the hospital and healthcare industry was discussed. The chapter concluded with a discussion of three conventions that may modify the application of generally accepted accounting principles in specific situations.

---

### ASSIGNMENTS

1. ABC Medical Center has undergone a recent corporate reorganization. The structure presented in **FIGURE 8-2** resulted. What difficulties might be experienced in preparing financial statements for the ABC Hospital?
2. Does the value of total assets represent the economic value of the entity?
3. What is the difference between stockholders' equity and net assets or unrestricted net assets?
4. A home healthcare firm has purchased five automobiles. Each automobile costs $24,000 and has an estimated useful life of 3 years. Each year, the replacement cost of the automobiles is expected to increase 10%. At the end of the third year, replacement cost is $31,944. The firm anticipates that each automobile will be used to make 1,500 patient visits per year. If the firm prices each visit to recover just the historical cost of the automobiles, it will include a capital cost of $5.33 per visit ($24,000 divided by 4,500 total visits). Assuming the revenue generated

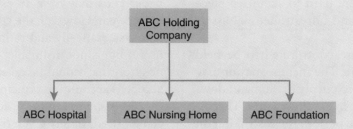

FIGURE 8-2  **ABC Medical Center's Reorganization**

from this capital charge is invested at 10%, will the firm have enough funds available to meet its replacement cost? How would this situation change if price-level depreciation were used to establish the capital charge?

5. A health maintenance organization (HMO) has just been formed. During its first year of operations, the organization reported an accounting loss of $500,000. Cash flow during the same period was a positive $500,000. How might this situation exist, and which measure better describes financial performance?

6. What is the difference between restricted and unrestricted net assets?

7. Why is consistency in financial reporting critical to fairness in financial representation?

8. Describe the primary differences between financial and managerial accounting.

## SOLUTIONS AND ANSWERS

1. It may be difficult to associate specific assets and liabilities for the ABC Hospital. For example, debt may have been issued by the holding company to finance projects for both the hospital and the nursing home. In addition, commonly used assets may be involved, such as a dietary department providing meals for both hospital and nursing home patients. Some expenses also may be difficult to trace to either the hospital or the nursing home. For example, how should expenses that are common to the hospital, the nursing home, and the foundation (such as administrative expenses of the holding company) be allocated? Thus, many problems of "jointness" may make preparation of the financial statements for the hospital difficult, but such statements are still likely to be a necessity for adequate planning and control.

2. Only coincidentally would the value of total assets equal the economic value of the entity. Total assets, as reported in the balance sheet, represent the undepreciated historical cost of assets acquired by the entity. Economic value of an entity is related to the discounted value of future earnings or the market value of the entity if sold.

3. Both stockholders' equity and net assets or unrestricted net assets represent the difference between total assets and total liabilities. Stockholders' equity is used in investor-owned corporations to designate the residual owners' claims. Net assets are used in not-for-profit corporations in which there is no residual ownership interest.

4. **TABLE 8-4** presents data relevant to the pricing decision of the home healthcare firm regarding the five automobiles. Funds available are shown with historical cost depreciation per automobile. **TABLE 8-5** presents

**TABLE 8-4**  Historical Cost Depreciation for Home Healthcare Firm's Automobiles

|  | Depreciation | Years Invested (10%) | Value, End of Third Year |
|---|---|---|---|
| Year 1 | $8,000 | 2 | $9,680 |
| Year 2 | 8,000 | 1 | 8,800 |
| Year 3 | 8,000 | 0 | 8,000 |
|  | $24,000 |  | $26,480 |

Shortage = $31,944 − $26,480 = $5,464 per automobile

**TABLE 8-5** Price-Level Depreciation for Home Healthcare Firm's Automobiles

|  | Depreciation | Years Invested (10%) | Value, End of Third Year |
|---|---|---|---|
| Year 1 | $8,800 | 2 | $10,648 |
| Year 2 | 9,680 | 1 | 10,648 |
| Year 3 | 10,648 | 0 | 10,648 |
|  | $29,128 |  | $31,944 |

Price-level depreciation in year $t = (\$24,000\ [1.10]^t) \div 3$ Shortage $= \$31,944 - \$31,944 = 0$

funds available with price-level depreciation per automobile. Thus, the prices should be set equal to expected replacement cost. Clearly, pricing services to recover capital costs is critical to long-term financial survival.

5. The HMO could have received large payments in advance for providing health services to major employers. This would mean that a liability to provide future services exists. Both accounting loss and cash flow are important in assessing financial performance. The accounting loss is symbolic of a critical operational problem regarding revenue and expense relationships. The positive cash flow may be temporary unless revenue exceeds expenses in future periods.

6. A restricted fund has a third-party donor restriction placed on the use of the funds. An unrestricted fund has no such restriction.

7. Changes in financial reporting can impair the comparability of financial results between years for a given firm.

8. Financial accounting has its primary focus on external financial reporting through the preparation and dissemination of the four primary financial statements. Managerial accounting is more internally focused, providing information within the organization to measure, monitor, and facilitate performance improvement.

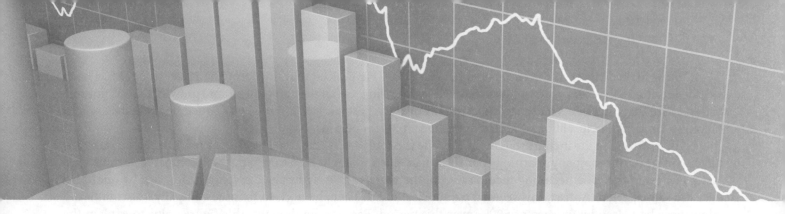

# CHAPTER 9

# Financial Statements

## LEARNING OBJECTIVES

After studying this chapter, you should be able to do the following:

1. Explain why it is important to know the scope of business being reviewed when using financial statements.
2. Understand the format and content of the balance sheet.
3. Understand the format and content of the statement of operations.
4. Understand the format and content of the statement of changes in net assets.
5. Understand the format and content of the statement of cash flows.

## REAL-WORLD SCENARIO

Ed Adams, a 2004 graduate of a well-respected health administration graduate program, recently accepted a job offer to work as a financial analyst in the controller's office at Northern Healthcare Corporation (NHC), an investor-owned provider of outpatient and rehabilitative healthcare services. Ed, who will start his job next month, has obtained the company's financial statements for the past several years so that he can better understand the company's recent financial position and performance.

Ed already knew that NHC owns nearly 200 rehabilitation facilities and ambulatory surgery centers across the United States. In recent years NHC had expanded rapidly through multiple acquisitions, new facilities, and growth at existing facilities. Yet, even with this rapid growth, Ed knew that the financial performance had been unsatisfactory in recent years and that management was feeling intense pressure by shareholders to improve its performance.

Upon his first inspection of NHC's financial statements, Ed noticed that the financial statements were in accordance with the provisions of Statement of Financial Accounting Standards (SFAS) No. 131, "Disclosures about Segments of an Enterprise and Related Information," which were issued by the Financial Accounting Standards Board (FASB) in 1997. Ed had learned in school that SFAS 131 requires an enterprise to report operating segments based on the way its operations are managed. This approach defines operating segments along the lines used by management to assess performance and to make operating and resource allocation decisions. Among other requirements, Ed knew that segments must be segregated by product and service, by geographic area, by legal entity, and by type of customer. In the case of NHC, based on its management and reporting structure, segment information was presented for inpatient and other clinical services and outpatient services.

Ed now looked closer at the company's balance sheet. He noticed that the company's cash balance has been steadily declining in recent years, while inventories were rising. Given the company's rapid growth, Ed was not surprised to see that total assets had risen substantially over the past few years. But he was concerned that the amount of long-term debt had just about doubled over a recent 2-year period.

Ed then turned to the income statement. Despite the company's increased leverage, as reflected by the substantial rise in debt, the company's earnings per share had fallen by about 80% in recent years compared with its high just a few years ago. The declining income was all the more surprising because revenues had risen by one-third over the same period. At first, this seemed paradoxical to Ed. Then, he noticed that the company's discounts and allowances had risen by upward of 500% over this period. Perhaps, he thought, this figure helps to explain the recent poor performance.

Ed realized that trying to more fully understand the company's financial performance would require a lot of time and effort. He would have to study the company's four major financial statements in greater detail. Additionally, he would need to read the accompanying footnotes to the financial statements and would need to supplement with additional knowledge of economic, regulatory, and other factors to get a more accurate sense of why NHC's financial performance had deteriorated so much in recent years.

---

Previously, we presented the principles of accounting that are necessary in organizing and preparing financial statements for an organization. These statements tell a story of where the organization is financially, and, how it arrived there. To many people, financial statements seem confusing. However, a general understanding of the format and content of these statements can yield financial literacy. At the conclusion of this chapter, you should be able to read and understand the four primary financial statements.

First, let's briefly discuss what the four statements are and what information is available in each. The **balance sheet** presents a record of an organization's assets, liabilities, and net assets (equity) at a specific point of time. In essence, it is a financial snapshot of the organization at a certain date. The **statement of operations** (also known as the income statement or statement of revenues and expenses) details the organization's revenues and expenses during the **accounting period**—typically, 1 year. If the balance sheet is a snapshot, the statement of operations can be thought of as a video clip showing the running total of funds generated and expended during the period. The **statement of changes in net assets** (or statement of changes in shareholders' equity) lists how net assets (or equity) changed during the period, and the **statement of cash flows** describes how cash was generated and used. Finally, the **notes to the financial statements** provide detail on the organization's structure, accounting practices, and financial standing. The notes are not considered to be a part of the four primary statements; however, they are critical in any financial assessment of an organization. When the statements above are prepared and reviewed by an external, independent accounting firm they are collectively referred to as **audited financial statements**.

In order to learn the format and content of audited financial statements, we will use a case example for a not-for-profit healthcare entity: Harris Memorial Hospital and Harris Community Foundation (jointly abbreviated HCF). The complete audited financial statements can be found in **Appendix 9-A**. Although the document's size appears overwhelming, our step-by-step discussion will hopefully make the information manageable and useful.

| *Learning Objective 1* |
|---|

Explain why it is important to know the scope of business being reviewed when using financial statements.

## ▶ Organizational Structure

The first information available in any audited financial statement is the organization for which the statements represent. As seen in our case example, the name of the organization is Harris Memorial Hospital and Harris Community Foundation. You may wonder what the relationship is between these two entities. The answer to this question can almost always be found in the beginning of the notes to the financial statements. The description of the entity from the notes follows:

**Organization and Basis of Combination**
Harris Memorial Hospital (the Hospital) and Harris Community Foundation (the Foundation) are a hospital and charitable foundation located in Jersey, Ohio. The Hospital and Foundation are exempt from federal income

taxes under Section 501(c)(3) of the Internal Revenue Code (IRC). The Hospital and Foundation are collectively referred to herein as the Foundation.

The Foundation owns and operates the Renee Center, which has 27 skilled nursing beds; Harris Assurance, Ltd. (Assurance), a for-profit, wholly owned insurance subsidiary; and Harris Properties (Condit Inn), a for-profit, wholly owned subsidiary. During 20X6, the Foundation formed the Harris Community Hospital Corporation (dba Harris Hospital) located in Oldstone, Ohio and the Harris Long Term Acute Care Hospital Corporation (dba Harris Continuing Care Hospital) located in Jersey, Ohio. The 60-bed Harris Continuing Care Hospital opened in May 20X7. Harris Hospital, with 92 beds, opened in late July 20X7. At December 31, 20X7, the Foundation has remaining commitments totaling approximately $7,360,000 under construction contracts for these and other capital projects.

The Foundation is affiliated with the Harris Health Plan (the Health Plan). The Health Plan's financial statements are not included in these combined financial statements. The Foundation provides healthcare services in the central Ohio region. All appropriate intercompany accounts have been eliminated in combination.

What we learn from this reading is that Harris Memorial Hospital and Harris Community Foundation are not-for-profit organizations that are effectively presented as one entity (referred throughout the remainder of the statements as the Foundation). This combined entity not only represents the hospital and charitable foundation, but also a host of other business interests: a skilled-nursing facility, an insurance firm, a real estate company that runs a hotel, and two other smaller hospitals. Some of these interests are for-profit even though the parent is not-for-profit (as understood by the tax-free status). The Foundation also has an affiliation with a health plan; however, the financial details of this relationship are not provided.

The Harris Foundation (HCF) presents a great example for our discussion of modern healthcare organizations (HCOs). Clearly, HCOs can be complex entities that represent a variety of business interests. As such, prior to reviewing the four core financial statements, it is imperative to understand who and what those statements are representing.

Understand the format and content of the balance sheet.

# ▶ Balance Sheet

As discussed previously, the balance sheet presents a record of an organization's assets, liabilities, and net assets (equity) at a specific point of time. You will recall these terms from the previous chapter. Assets are things that an organization owns (e.g., buildings, equipment, and cash). Liabilities and net assets describe how the assets are financed. When an organization uses debt (loans, mortgages, etc.) to purchase an asset, this is referred to as a liability. The owner is liable to someone else for the funds used to purchase the asset. Net assets or fund balance, also known as equity, refer to the remaining interest the owner(s) has after the liabilities have been paid. Recalling the duality principle, a balance sheet will always balance: assets = liabilities + net assets (equity). The balance sheet will always show this relationship for one point in time, typically the end of the accounting period.

In our case example, the accounting period for HCF is 1 year ending on December 31. Most audited financial statements present 2 years of information for comparison purposes. Examining the balance sheet for HCF we confirm that assets of $1,305,046 equal the sum of liabilities ($620,427) and net assets ($684,619). Note that the values have been listed "in thousands"; this is a common practice in audited financial statements.

Although it is nice to see that the balance sheet balances (as, of course, it should), it is more interesting to learn about the types of assets, liabilities, and net assets the entity possesses. The following paragraphs will explore these areas that are applicable in most audited financial statements.

## Current Assets

Assets that are expected to be exchanged for cash or consumed during the operating cycle of the entity (or 1 year, whichever is longer) are classified as **current assets** on the balance sheet. The operating cycle is the length of time between acquisition of materials and services and collection of revenue generated by them. Because the operating cycle for most HCOs is significantly less than 1 year (perhaps 3 months or less), current assets are predominantly those that may be expected to be converted into cash or used to reduce expenditures of cash within 1 year.

## Cash and Cash Equivalents

**Cash** consists of coin, currency, and available deposited funds at banks. Negotiable instruments such as money orders, certified checks, cashier's checks, personal checks, or bank drafts are also viewed as cash. **Cash equivalents** include savings accounts, certificates of deposit, and other temporary marketable securities. Categorization as a cash equivalent requires that two criteria be met. First, management must intend to convert the investment into cash within 1 year or during the operating cycle, whichever is longer. Second, the investment must be readily marketable and capable of being transformed into cash easily. HCF had $82,815,000 in cash and cash equivalents in 20X7, which was an increase over the prior year. In a subsequent chapter we will discuss if HCF's cash position is appropriate.

## Accounts Receivable

**Accounts receivable** represent legally enforceable claims on customers for prior services or goods. HCF has net patient accounts receivable of $70,025,000 at the end of 20X7. This value represents the amount of money that HCF expects to collect in the next year (20X8) from services provided to patients and other customers in 20X7 that as yet have not been paid. HCF also has nonpatient accounts receivable in the amount of $28,990,000 at the end of 20X7.

A characteristic of hospitals and other HCOs that makes their accounts receivable different from those of most other organizations is that the charges actually billed to patients are often settled for substantially lower amounts. The differences are known as allowances. The following four major categories of allowances are used to restate accounts receivable to expected, realizable value:

1. Charity allowances
2. Courtesy allowances
3. Doubtful account allowances
4. Contractual allowances

A **charity allowance** is the difference between established service rates and amounts actually charged to indigent patients. Most healthcare facilities have a policy of scaling the normal charge by some factor based on income in relationship to a standard, usually the Federal Poverty Level values. The difference between the initial price and the discounted price is the amount of the charity allowance. A **courtesy allowance** is the difference between established rates for services and rates billed to special patients, such as employees, physicians, and clergy. Again, the difference between initial price and discounted price for these special patients represent the courtesy allowance.

A **doubtful account allowance** is the difference between rates billed and amounts expected to be recovered. For example, a medically indigent patient might actually receive services that have an established rate of $100, but be billed only $50. If it is anticipated that the patient will not pay even the $50, then that $50 will show up as a doubtful account allowance. HCF had a doubtful account allowance of $25,302,000 for its accounts receivable in 20X7. This means that the organization had uncollected net patient charges of $95,327,000 ($70,025,000 + $25,302,000) but only expected to collect $70,025,000 (the amount listed in accounts receivable for 20X7).

In most situations, **contractual allowances** represent the largest deduction from accounts receivable. A contractual allowance is the difference between rates billed to a third-party payer, such as Medicare, and the amount that actually will be paid by that third-party payer. For example, a Medicare patient may receive hospital services priced at $4,000 but actually pay the hospital only $3,000 for those services, based on a prearranged agreement between the payer and the hospital. If this account is unpaid at the fiscal year end, the financial statements would include the net amount of cash expected to be received ($3,000), not the gross prices charged ($4,000). Accounts receivable represent the amount of cash expected to be received, not the gross prices charged. Because most major payers, such as Medicare, Medicaid, and Blue Cross, have a contractual relationship that permits payment on a basis other than charges, contractual allowances can be, and usually are, very large.

The allowances are estimates and will, in all probability, differ from the actual value of accounts receivable that eventually will be written off. Because estimation of allowances is so critical to the reported value of accounts receivable, the methodology should be scrutinized. Just how was the estimate developed? Has the estimating method been used in the past with any degree of reliability? An external audit performed by an independent certified public accountant can usually provide the required degree of reliability and assurance.

## Inventories and Supplies

**Inventories** in a healthcare facility represent items that are to be used in the delivery of healthcare services. They may range from normal business office supplies to highly specialized chemicals used in a laboratory.

## Prepaid Expenses

**Prepaid expenses** represent expenditures already made for future service. Although these do not appear in the HCF balance sheet, they may represent prepayment of insurance premiums for the year, rents on leased equipment, or other similar items. For example, an insurance premium for a professional liability insurance policy may be $600,000 per year, due 1 year in advance. If this amount were paid on January 1, then on June 30, $300,000 (one-half of the total) would be shown as a prepaid expense.

## Plant, Property, and Equipment (PPE)

Property and equipment are sometimes called **fixed assets** or shown more descriptively as **plant, property, and equipment**. Items in this category represent investment in tangible, permanent assets; they are sometimes referred to as the capital assets of the organization. These items are shown at the historical cost or acquisition cost, reduced by allowances for depreciation. Details regarding the elements of fixed assets are often shown in the footnotes. Footnote number 3 in Appendix 9-A provides this detail for HCF.

## Land and Improvements

**Land and improvements** represent the historical cost of land owned by the healthcare facility and the historical cost of any improvements erected on it. Such improvements might include water and sewer systems, roadways, fences, sidewalks, shrubbery, and parking lots. Although land may not be depreciated, land improvements may be depreciated. Land held for investment purposes is not shown in this category but appears as an investment in the other assets section.

## Buildings and Equipment

Buildings and equipment represent all buildings and equipment owned by the entity and used during the normal course of its operations. These items are also stated at historical cost. Buildings and equipment not used in the normal course of operations should be reported separately. For example, real estate investments would not be shown in the fixed asset or plant property and equipment section but in the other assets section. Equipment in many situations is classified into three categories: (1) fixed equipment—affixed to the building in which it is located, including items such as elevators, boilers, and generators; (2) major movable equipment—usually stationary but capable of being moved, including reasonably expensive items such as automobiles, laboratory equipment, and X-ray

apparatuses; and (3) minor equipment—usually low in cost with short estimated useful lives, including such items as wastebaskets, glassware, and sheets.

## Construction in Progress

**Construction in progress** represents the amount of money that has been expended on projects that are still not complete when the financial statement is published.

## Allowance for Depreciation

**Allowance for depreciation** represents the **accumulated depreciation** taken on the asset to the date of the financial statement. The concept of depreciation is important and useful regarding a wide variety of decisions. **TABLE 9-1** illustrates the depreciation concept: A $500 desk is purchased and depreciated over a 5-year life.

In the case of HCF, there is $493,814,000 of accumulated depreciation as of December 31, 20X7 (this value is found in Appendix 9-A under footnote 3, Property and Equipment). The historical cost base for this amount is $1,057,163,000, the historical cost value of buildings and equipment. This means that 46.7% of the historical cost of present facilities has been depreciated in prior years. As the ratio of allowance for depreciation to building and equipment increases, it usually signifies that a physical plant will need to be replaced in the near future.

## Assets That Have Limited Use

Most organizations will have some amounts listed under **assets that have limited use**. Often these assets are cash and investments that can only be spent for specific purposes. At the end of 20X7,

**TABLE 9-1** Balance Sheet Values

| | Year | | | | |
|---|---|---|---|---|---|
| | 1 | 2 | 3 | 4 | 5 |
| Historical equipment cost | $500 | $500 | $500 | $500 | $500 |
| Allowance for depreciation | 100 | 200 | 300 | 400 | 500 |
| Net | $400 | $300 | $200 | $100 | $0 |

HCF had $512,986,000 in limited funds. The nature of the asset limitation usually derives from one of two possibilities. First, the board of directors for the organization may restrict certain funds to be used only in designated ways. HCF had $382,835,000 in board-designated funds at the end of 20X7 (see Appendix 9-A, footnote 8). At times, no additional detail is provided for what areas the board is restricting funds. However, the HCF audit has further breakout of these funds in the notes section under Assets Limited as to Use (Appendix 9-A, footnote 8). The section details funded depreciation (to replace aging physical assets), professional liabilities, institutional research, subsidiary investments, and other board-designated purposes as the primary fund areas. In sum, board-designated funds must receive approval from the board prior to being expended.

Second, aside from a board restriction, a third party also may restrict funds. Two major types of third-party restrictions are seen in the HCF audit: donor-restricted and trustee restrictions for bond agreements. Donor-restricted funds are typically tied to a specific building campaign or community service function. Bond-restricted funds are primarily held to assure investors that sufficient money is available to repay the bond commitment.

## Other Assets

Finally, other assets are those that are neither current nor involve property and equipment. Typically, they are either investments or intangible assets. Several categories exist. For example, deferred financing costs are listed in the other asset area. Deferred financing costs are costs incurred initially by a borrower to issue bonds. Such costs include legal fees, accounting fees, and underwriter's costs. The costs are amortized over the life of the bonds, much like depreciation.

Two other intangible asset items that may be included in some healthcare facility balance sheets are goodwill and organization costs. Goodwill represents the difference between the price paid to acquire another entity and the fair market value of the acquired entity's assets, less any related obligations or liabilities. Goodwill is included mainly in balance sheets of proprietary facilities, although increasingly, it is also being seen in balance sheets of voluntary not-for-profit organizations as they acquire other healthcare entities, especially physician practices. Organization costs are expended for legal and accounting fees and other items incurred at the formation of the entity. The cost of these items is usually amortized over some allowable life.

## Current Liabilities

Current liabilities are obligations that are expected to require payment in cash during the coming year or operating cycle, whichever is longer. Like current assets, they are generally expected to be paid in 1 year.

## Accounts Payable

Accounts payable may be thought of as the counterpart of accounts receivable. They represent the entity's promise to pay money for goods or services it has received.

## Accrued Liabilities

Accrued liabilities are obligations that result from prior operations. They are thus a legal obligation to make future payment. The expense of accruing interest is an example. (This is discussed further in Chapter 8.) Other examples of accrued expenses are payroll, vacation pay, tax deductions, rent, and insurance. In some cases, especially payroll, accrued liabilities are desegregated to show material categories.

## Due to Third-Party Payers

Similar to accounts receivable on the asset side of the balance sheet, amounts listed under due to third-party payers represent money that is due an intermediary payer (Medicare, Blue Cross, etc.) from the organization that is, as yet, unpaid. HCF has a relatively small current liability for this area. The values for both due to and from third-party payers usually reflect differences between interim payments for medical services in the preceding year and estimated final payments. For example, a large payer such as Blue Cross may agree to make biweekly payments of $1,000,000 for services to its beneficiaries. At year-end, a final accounting will be made to determine the actual amounts that should have been paid based on actual utilization and cost. In the case of HCF, a large balance ($7,380,000) is due to the payers, which may be offset against future payments from the payer.

## Current Portion of Long-Term Debt

Current portion (or maturities) of long-term debt represents the amount of principal that will be repaid on the indebtedness within the coming year. It does not equal the total amount of the payments that will be made during that year. Total payments include both interest and principal; current portion of long-term debt includes just the principal portion. For example, if at the June 30 fiscal year close, a total of $360,000 ($30,000 per month) will be paid on long-term indebtedness during the coming year and of this amount, only $120,000 is principal payment, then $120,000 would be shown as a current portion of the long-term debt.

## Noncurrent Liabilities

**Noncurrent liabilities** include obligations that will not require payment in cash for at least 1 year or more. Harris Community Foundation shows five types of noncurrent liabilities: contingent professional liabilities; due to broker; postretirement obligation, other than pensions; long-term debt; and other liabilities. Often, these areas can be described further in the notes to the financial statements. The largest area by far for HCF is long-term debt.

## Long-Term Debt

**Long-term debt** represents the amount of long-term indebtedness that is not due in the next year. HCF reported $439,597,000 in 20X7. When the current portion of long-term debt ($4,692,000) is added to the long-term portion, the total amount of long-term debt is determined. The notes to the financial statements usually provide additional information on maturities, interest rates, and types of outstanding debt (Appendix 9-A, footnote 4).

## Net Assets

**Net assets** (or equity), as discussed earlier, represent the difference between assets and the claim to those assets by third parties or liabilities. It is helpful to remember that assets and liabilities are more "material" in nature. Cash, buildings, and loans (examples of assets and a liability) are physical things that are easier to understand for most people. The concept of equity is perhaps, less clear because it is the result of a mathematical equation and is not truly material or physical in nature. Essentially, equity represents the net worth of an entity after all liabilities have been paid. Let us use an illustration to make this point more clear. Assume two individuals own homes each with a $200,000 value. The first individual has $150,000 remaining on his loan, while the second individual only has $30,000 left on her loan. Assuming no other assets or liabilities, the second individual would obviously have the greater net worth (or equity position) at $170,000 versus the first individual with only $50,000 in equity. Increasing equity is a primary financial goal for individuals and organizations. This will be discussed in more detail in Chapter 11.

We know from our discussion on limited use assets that there are restrictions placed on certain asset areas. As a result, net assets are typically categorized into one of three types: (1) unrestricted, (2) temporarily restricted, and (3) permanently restricted. (See further discussion in Chapter 8.) This is represented in the net asset categorization for HCF, as well. Unrestricted net assets are by far the largest of the three types for HCF ($600,179,000 of the total $684,619,000).

Increases in net assets usually arise from one of two sources: (1) contributions or (2) earnings. In the nonprofit healthcare industry, there is usually no separation in the fund balance account (net assets or equity) to recognize these two sources. Thus, there is no indication of how much of HCF's unrestricted net assets of $600,179,000 were earned and how much were contributed. Financial statements prepared for proprietary entities do show this breakdown. Earnings of prior years, reduced by dividend payments to stockholders, are shown in an account labeled "retained earnings." In any given year, however, it is possible to determine the sources of change in unrestricted net assets by examining the statement of changes in net assets, as will be discussed.

*Learning Objective 3*

Understand the format and content of the statement of operations.

## ▶ Statement of Operations (Revenues and Expenses)

Previously defined, the statement of operations (also known as the income statement or statement of revenues and expenses) details the organization's revenues and expenses during the accounting period—typically, 1 year. The statement of operations has become increasingly important in both the proprietary and nonproprietary sectors. It represents operations in a given period better than a balance sheet does. A balance sheet summarizes the wealth position of an entity at a given point by delineating its assets, liabilities, and net assets. An income statement provides information concerning how that wealth position was changed through operations.

An entity's ability to earn an excess of revenue over expenses (also commonly referred to as net income or profit) is an important variable in many external and internal decisions. A series of income statements indicates this ability well. Creditors use income statements to determine the entity's ability to pay future and present debts; management and rate-regulating agencies use them to assess whether current and proposed rate structures are adequate.

The entity principle is an important factor in analyzing and interpreting the statement of revenue and expense. Income, the excess of revenue over expenses, comes from a large number of individual operations within a healthcare entity and is aggregated in the statement of revenues and expenses. For example, HCF has aggregated the revenues and expenses from its subsidiaries to create a consolidated statement of revenues and expenses. Individuals interested in details about any of the individual entities that constitute HCF would need to see income statements for those organizations. Information about revenues and expenses by product line also often are needed when making managerial decisions. Here, however, our focus is on the general-purpose statement of revenues and expenses, which is an aggregate of individual product lines.

## Revenue

Generally speaking, revenue in a healthcare facility comes from three sources:

1. Patient services revenue
2. Other revenue
3. Nonoperating gains (losses)

## Patient Services Revenue

Patient services revenue represents the amount of revenue that results from the provision of healthcare services to patients. It is often shown on a net basis in the statement of revenues and expenses with additional detail in the footnotes. Net patient revenue is the residual of gross patient revenue less allowances. Gross revenue is the "list price" for services provided to the patient. However, most third-party payers or uninsured individuals do not pay list price for services. Instead, the hospital discounts the services to a lesser price for major payers (Medicare, Blue Cross, etc.) and to individuals who meet certain income standards described in the hospital's charity care policy. The hospital may also choose to grant discounts to other individuals or parties, as well, based on established criteria. The discount, or allowance, is subtracted from the gross price to arrive at the amount the hospital expects to collect from the payer or individual. HCF reported net patient services revenue of $829,005,000 in fiscal year 20X7. This value is the amount that HCF expects to collect from the patient services it has provided.

Bad-debt (doubtful account) provisions recognize the amount of charges that will not be collected from patients from whom payment was expected. It should be emphasized that bad debts are different from charity care. Bad debts are incurred on patients for whom services were provided and payment *was* expected, but no payment was forthcoming. For example, if a patient had commercial insurance coverage that paid 80% of the patient's bill of $10,000 and required the patient to pay the residual balance, the hospital would bill the patient for $2,000. If the patient refused to pay the $2,000 and no payment was expected, the $2,000 charge would be written off as a bad debt. Bad debts are reported as a deduction from net patient services revenue. As shown in the statement of operations, HCF had $55,851,000 of bad debt in 20X7. This value represents the amount of net payment due to the hospital that has been determined to be uncollectable. Accounting for this amount of bad debt leaves HCF with $773,154 in net patient service revenue.

The value that is reported for net patient service revenue is part fact and part estimate. At the close of the fiscal year, someone must estimate what amounts actually will be paid by third-party payers under existing contracts. This is not an easy task in most situations, and there is likely to be some error. This is important to recognize when revenue figures are examined for periods shorter than 1 year (for example, monthly) and when those statements are not audited by an independent auditor. This does not mean that the data are not valid, only that some caution should be exercised in using them.

## Other Revenue

Other revenue is generated from normal day-to-day operations not directly related to patient care. Harris Community Foundation reports $27,055,000 of other revenue for 20X7. There is no indication regarding the source of this revenue in the financial statements, but the usual sources include revenue from the following:

- Educational programs
- Research and grants
- Rentals of space or equipment
- Sales of medical and pharmacy items to nonpatients
- Cafeteria sales
- Gift shop sales
- Parking lot sales
- Investment income on borrowed funds held by a trustee
- Investment income on malpractice trust funds

It is not entirely clear in all cases whether an item should be categorized as other revenue or as nonoperating gain or loss. The general rule is that items are categorized as nonoperating gains or losses when they are peripheral or incidental to the activities of the healthcare provider. For example, donations could be classified as a gain to some organizations and as other revenue to other organizations.

## Nonoperating Gains (Losses)

**Nonoperating gains and losses** result from peripheral or incidental transactions. The definitions of peripheral and incidental transactions are not exactly clear, and the terms could be treated inconsistently. For example, HCF reports $30,453,000 of investment income in 20X7. Most likely, these earnings resulted from funds restricted by the board for internally designated purposes. Is the investment of funded depreciation or capital replacement reserves incidental to HCF? HCF must believe that it is, but another organization with exactly the same situation might choose to categorize it differently.

In general, the following items are often categorized as nonoperating gains or losses:

- Contributions or donations that are unrestricted income from endowments
- Income from the investment of unrestricted funds
- Gains or losses on sale of property
- Net rentals of facilities not used in the operation of the facility

## Operating Expenses

In these days of increasing concern regarding healthcare costs, decision makers are paying more attention to healthcare facilities' operating expenses. Generally speaking, there are two ways that expenses may be categorized: (1) by cost or responsibility center or (2) by object or type of expenditure.

In most general-purpose financial statements, costs are reported by cost object. HCF breaks down expenses into the following categories:

- Salaries and wages
- Employee benefits
- Supplies and purchased services
- Advertising
- Staff enrichment
- Occupancy cost
- Depreciation and amortization
- Interest

Many of the expense areas are easily understood. **Salaries and wages** represent the amount paid to staff (either salaried or hourly workers). **Employee benefits** represent amounts for employee benefits and tax payments. Among items included are social security, unemployment tax, workers' compensation, retirement costs, health insurance, and other fringe-benefit programs.

Other items, such as staff enrichment, may not be as easily understood. There is no further detail in the notes to the financial statements that elaborate on the content of this expense area.

**Depreciation** and **interest** are two special accounts that have great importance in financial analysis. They are both discussed in Chapter 10. In general, depreciation is a noncash expense that represents the financial value that an asset loses over some period of time (usually defined by the asset's useful life). Interest is the expense paid as part of debt financing.

Accumulated depreciation on the balance sheet and depreciation expense on the income statement are related, but are not the same. Depreciation expense is the amount depreciated for the accounting period (usually 1 year) while accumulated depreciation on the balance sheet represents the sum of these expenses for prior periods.

Finally, it should be noted that **expense** and **expenditure** (or payment of cash) may not be equivalent in any given period. For example, a healthcare facility may incur an expenditure of $1,000,000 to buy a piece of equipment but may charge only $200,000 as depreciation expense in a given year. In general, expenditure reflects the payment of cash, whereas expense recognizes prior expenditure that has produced revenue. The following three major categories of expenditures usually are not treated as expenses:

1. Retirement or repayment of debt
2. Investment in new fixed assets
3. Increases in working capital or current assets

One major category of expense—depreciation of fixed assets—does not involve a cash expenditure. In addition, other normal accruals, such as vacation and sick leave benefits, may be recognized as expense but involve no immediate cash outlay.

---

### Learning Objective 4

Understand the format and content of the statement of changes in net assets.

---

## ▸ Statement of Changes in Net Assets

The statement of changes in net assets (or statement of changes in shareholders' equity in for-profit settings) merely accounts for the changes in net assets (or equity) during the year. HCF's financial statement shows that the majority of the change in unrestricted net assets is attributed to excess of revenues over expenses, or net income. HCF does, however, show sizable values for contributions, gifts, and bequests. Donations are typically included in the statement of changes in net assets as opposed to the statement of operations because of established accounting reporting standards. This is primarily the result of the restrictions placed on most donations and the delayed ability to use the donated funds.

Another major area for changes in net assets is changes in net unrealized gains and losses on other than trading securities. These changes represent valuation adjustments for nontrading securities, usually equity investments, with objective market values, such as publicly traded values. When the securities are finally sold, the difference between the sales price and acquisition cost will be recognized as a realizable gain.

Some HCOs will consolidate the statements of operations and changes in net assets into one financial statement. The driving factor for this is that there is often little activity beyond net income that changes net assets for a nonprofit healthcare provider. This serves as a powerful reminder that the primary method that a nonprofit healthcare provider employs to grow net assets is through net income performance. Whereas for-profit providers can generate additional equity through shareholder investments, a nonprofit provider must impact this important financial element through its operating and nonoperating gains. This point will be emphasized in Chapter 11, where we will discuss the primary long-term financial objective for organizations.

---

*Learning Objective 5*

Understand the format and content of the statement of cash flows.

---

## ▶ Statement of Cash Flows

The statement of cash flows is designed to give additional information on the flow of funds within an entity. As we have noted, the concept of expense does not necessarily give decision makers information on

funds flow. The statement of cash flows is designed to give information on the flow of funds within an entity, and to summarize the sources that make funds available and the uses for those funds during a given period.

In general, there are three activities that generate or use cash flows for an organization: (1) operating activities, (2) investing activities, and (3) financing activities. HCF derived $59,885,000 of cash flow from operating activities during 20X7. It then spent $142,793,000 on investments, primarily property, and equipment. It also generated $106,027,000 for **financing activities** during 20X7. The difference is the net increase in cash and cash equivalents during the year, or $23,119,000. A statement of cash flows can be thought of simply as a statement that explains the sources for changes in the cash accounts during the year.

The amount of cash flow generated from operating activities can be thought of as the amount of excess of revenues over expenses subject to several adjustments, the first of which is for expenses that did not involve an actual outlay of cash. The biggest items here are depreciation and provision for bad debts. **Provision for bad debts** is added back because the expense did not involve an outlay of cash, merely a write-off of a receivable.

## ▶ SUMMARY

In this chapter, we have discussed the contents of the following four general-purpose financial statements:

1. Balance sheet
2. Statement of revenues and expenses
3. Statement of cash flows
4. Statement of changes in unrestricted net assets

Primary attention was directed at the first two, balance sheet and statement of revenues and expenses, which provide a basis for most financial information.

This chapter focused on understanding the basic information available in these four financial statements. Later chapters describe how this information can be interpreted and used in actual decision making.

---

**ASSIGNMENTS**

1. Consider a hospital that is introducing a new service anticipated to have 1,000 patient visits per year at an average cost of $2,200 and average billed charges of $4,500. Determine the amount of gross revenue, contractual deductions, net patient revenue, and net operating income that would result given the payer mix and terms shown in **TABLE 9-2**.

**TABLE 9-2**

| Payer Class | Number of Patients | Payment per Case |
|---|---|---|
| Medicare | 400 | $2,050 per case |
| Medicaid | 150 | $1,650 per case |
| Payers with a hospital contract | 280 | $3,000 per case |
| Payers without a hospital contract | 100 | 90% of gross (billed) charges |
| Self-pay patients | 50 | 5% of gross (billed) charges |
| Charity care patients | 20 | $0 per case |
|  | 1,000 |  |

2. How could you determine the amount of debt principal that will be retired during the next year through an examination of the financial statements for HCF?
3. What are the titles of the four financial statements that are usually included in an audited financial report?
4. Shady Rest nursing home has just acquired a home health firm for $850,000 in cash. The balance sheet of the home health firm looked as follows just before the acquisition:

| | |
|---|---|
| Current assets | $200,000 |
| Net fixed assets | 100,000 |
| Total | $300,000 |
| Current liabilities | $100,000 |
| Shareholder's equity | 200,000 |
| Total | $300,000 |

   Assume that the fair market value of the net fixed assets is $300,000 and fair market value of current assets is $200,000. Describe how this acquisition might be reflected on the balance sheet of Shady Rest.

5. Describe several items that are treated as expenses in the income statement but do not require any expenditure of cash in the present period.
6. A major medical supplier has donated $45,000 worth of medical supply items to your firm. These items are then used in the treatment of patients. Explain how this transaction would be recorded in your firm's financial statements.
7. Your HMO is experiencing a critical shortage of funds. Using the statement of cash flows as a framework for discussion, explain how you might attempt to reduce the need for additional funds.
8. Your hospital has experienced negative levels of net income for the last 5 years. The total amount of accumulated deficits is $5 million, but you have noticed that unrestricted net assets have increased $2 million during the same period. How might this situation be explained?
9. You have been reading the footnotes to your hospital's financial statements and were surprised to see that the actuarial present value of accumulated pension plan benefits is $4,500,000. A footnote cites a fund of $8,500,000 that has been established to pay these benefits. However, you can find no mention of either the liability or the fund in the balance sheet. What might explain this situation?

## SOLUTIONS AND ANSWERS

1. The calculations to determine the hospital's net operating income are shown in **TABLE 9-3**.

### TABLE 9-3

| Payer Class | Number of Patients | Payment per Case | Gross Revenue | Contractual Deductions | Net Patient Revenue | Total Costs | Net Operating Income |
|---|---|---|---|---|---|---|---|
| Medicare | 400 | 2,050 | 1,800,000 | (980,000) | 820,000 | 880,000 | (60,000) |
| Medicaid | 150 | 1,650 | 675,000 | (427,500) | 247,500 | 330,000 | (82,500) |
| Payers with a hospital contract | 280 | 3,000 | 1,260,000 | (420,000) | 840,000 | 616,000 | 224,000 |
| Payers without a hospital contract | 100 | 4,050 | 450,000 | (45,000) | 405,000 | 220,000 | 185,000 |
| Self-pay patients | 50 | 250 | 225,000 | (212,500) | 12,500 | 110,000 | (97,500) |
| Charity care patients | 20 | — | 90,000 | (90,000) | — | 44,000 | (44,000) |
| | 1,000 | | 4,500,000 | (2,175,000) | 2,325,000 | 2,200,000 | 125,000 |

2. The value reported for current maturities of long-term debt in the balance sheet should represent the value of debt principal that will be retired during the next fiscal year. For HCF that value is $4,692,000.
3. The four financial statements are the balance sheet, the statement of revenues and expenses or statements of operations, the statement of cash flows, and the statement of changes in unrestricted net assets.
4. First, fair market value of the assets acquired by Shady Rest would be determined. In this example, we will assume that the current asset value would not change, but that the fixed assets would be restated to $300,000 at fair market value. Shady Rest is thus acquiring total assets worth $500,000 and assuming liabilities of $100,000 for a net book value of $400,000. Because Shady Rest is paying $850,000 for these assets, there would be a goodwill account of $450,000 created for the residual. The following account changes would occur:

   - Cash—decrease of $850,000
   - Current assets—increase of $200,000
   - Net fixed assets—increase of $300,000
   - Goodwill—increase of $450,000
   - Current liabilities—increase of $100,000

   The goodwill value would be charged to expense in future periods.

5. Pension expense would not require an actual expenditure of cash at the present time, although a payment may be made to a trustee for investment. Other accruals, such as vacation benefits, sick leave benefits, and FICA (Federal Insurance Contributions Act) accruals, may not require immediate cash expenditures.
6. The fair market value of the items donated would be treated as other revenue. In this case, if $45,000 is the fair market value, that amount would be shown as other revenue.

7. Major categories of fund usage in the statement of cash flows are the following:

   - Repayment of debt
   - Purchase of fixed assets
   - Increase in working-capital items, such as accounts receivable

   Conservation of funds could occur in any one of these three areas. For example, the HMO could postpone or delay new fixed asset acquisitions. It also could try to restructure its debt, especially in situations when a large proportion of the debt is short term. Finally, it could attempt to reduce the amount of funds necessary for working capital increases. This could be accomplished through a reduction in the HMO's receivable cycle or through an increase in its payable cycle.

8. In this example, the hospital has increased its total equity by $7 million through sources other than income. The most likely sources of these funds are transfers from restricted net assets, such as from plant replacement, or from direct equity transfers from related parties, such as a holding company. It is important to note that the funds were not derived from unrestricted contributions. Unrestricted contributions would have been shown as revenue and thus included in the computation of excess of revenues over expenses. It is also possible that unrealized gains on other than trading securities could have taken place.

9. Pension funds in a defined benefit plan are often held by a trustee and are not shown on the firm's financial statements. This is most likely the situation here. It is important to periodically examine the relationship between the pension fund and the actuarial present value of the pension fund liability. Changes in actuarial assumptions— for example, in mortality, investment yield, or inflation rates—can have a dramatic influence over the size of the liability. The relevant information can be found in the footnotes to the financial statements.

# Appendix 9-A

## Case Example Audited Financial Statement

### ▶ Combined Financial Statements

Harris Memorial Hospital and Harris Community Foundation

*Years Ended December 31, 20X7 and 20X6*

#### Contents

### Report of Independent Auditors— Pennypacker & Vandelay, LLC

The Board of Trustees
Harris Memorial Hospital and
Harris Community Foundation

We have audited the accompanying combined balance sheets of Harris Memorial Hospital and Harris Community Foundation and subsidiaries (the Foundation) as of December 31, 20X7 and 20X6, and the related combined statements of operations, changes in net assets, and cash flows for the years then ended.

Management is responsible for the preparation and fair presentation of the consolidated financial statements in accordance with accounting principles generally accepted in the United States of America; this includes the design, implementation, and maintenance of internal control relevant to the preparation and fair presentation of consolidated financial statements that are free from material misstatement, whether due to fraud or error.

Our responsibility is to express an opinion on these financial statements based on our audits. We conducted our audits in accordance with auditing standards generally accepted in the United States. Those standards require that we plan and perform the audit to obtain reasonable assurance about whether the financial statements are free of material misstatement.

An audit involves performing procedures to obtain audit evidence about the amounts and disclosures in the consolidated financial statements. The procedures selected depend on our judgment, including the assessment of the risks of material misstatement of the consolidated financial statements, whether due to fraud or error. In making this risk assessment, we consider internal control relevant to the Foundation's preparation and fair presentation of the consolidated financial statements in order to design audit procedures that are appropriate in the circumstances, but not for the purpose of expressing an opinion on the effectiveness of the Foundation's internal control. Accordingly, we express no such opinion. An audit also includes evaluating the appropriateness of accounting policies used and the reasonableness of significant accounting estimates made by management, as well as evaluating the overall presentation of the consolidated financial statements. We believe that the audit evidence we have obtained is sufficient and appropriate to provide a basis for our audit opinion.

In our opinion, the financial statements referred to above present fairly, in all material respects, the combined financial position of Harris Memorial Hospital and Harris Community Foundation and subsidiaries at December 31, 20X7 and 20X6, and the combined changes in their net assets and their cash flows for the years then ended in conformity with U.S. generally accepted accounting principles.

| **TABLE 9A-1** Harris Memorial Hospital and Harris Community Foundation Combined Balance Sheets (in Thousands) | | |
|---|---|---|
| | **December 31, 20X7** | **December 31, 20X6** |
| Assets | | |
| Current assets | | |
| Cash and cash equivalents | **$82,815** | $59,696 |
| Assets limited as to use, current portion | **5,327** | 5,088 |
| Accounts receivable | | |
| Patients, less allowance for doubtful accounts ($25,302 in 20X7 and $23,014 in 20X6) | **70,025** | 59,939 |
| Other | **28,990** | 24,995 |
| Supplies | **7,078** | 6,663 |
| Total current assets | **194,235** | 156,381 |
| Assets limited as to use | | |
| For donor-restricted purposes | **84,440** | 67,826 |
| Board designated for specific purposes | **382,835** | 378,413 |
| Held by trustees under bond agreements | **51,038** | 25,937 |
| | **518,313** | 472,176 |
| Less current portion | **5,327** | 5,088 |
| | **512,986** | 467,088 |
| Property and equipment, net | **563,349** | 458,829 |
| Other assets | **34,476** | 34,302 |
| Total assets | **$1,305,046** | $1,116,600 |
| Liabilities and net assets | | |
| Current liabilities | | |

| | | |
|---|---|---|
| Accounts payable | **$32,572** | $24,631 |
| Accrued expenses and other liabilities | **58,878** | 53,725 |
| Due to third-party payers | **7,380** | 12,633 |
| Current maturities of long-term debt | **4,692** | 5,908 |
| Total current liabilities | **103,522** | 96,897 |
| Long-term debt, less current maturities | **439,597** | 332,354 |
| Contingent professional liabilities | **33,260** | 48,487 |
| Due to broker | **15,128** | 19,608 |
| Other liabilities | **20,713** | 5,298 |
| Postretirement benefit obligation, other than pensions | **8,207** | 7,694 |
| Total liabilities | **620,427** | 510,338 |
| Net assets | | |
| Unrestricted | **600,179** | 538,436 |
| Temporarily restricted | **55,213** | 40,393 |
| Permanently restricted | **29,227** | 27,433 |
| Total net assets | **684,619** | 606,262 |
| Total liabilities and net assets | **$1,305,046** | $1,116,600 |

**TABLE 9A-2** Harris Memorial Hospital and Harris Community Foundation Combined Statements of Operations (in Thousands)

| | **December 31, 20X7** | **December 31, 20X6** |
|---|---|---|
| Operating revenues and other support | | |
| Net patient service revenue | **$829,005** | $774,662 |
| Provision for doubtful accounts | **(55,851)** | (57,975) |
| Net patient service revenue less provision for doubtful accounts | **773,154** | 716,687 |
| Other operating revenue | **27,055** | 29,334 |
| Total operating revenue | **800,209** | 746,021 |

*(continues)*

**TABLE 9A-2** Harris Memorial Hospital and Harris Community Foundation Combined Statements of *(continued)* Operations (in Thousands)

| Operating expenses | | |
|---|---|---|
| Salaries and wages | **$371,449** | $329,668 |
| Employee benefits | **81,532** | 77,231 |
| Supplies and purchased services | **228,244** | 225,497 |
| Advertising | **3,072** | 2,376 |
| Staff enrichment | **10,767** | 8,591 |
| Occupancy cost | **14,346** | 13,442 |
| Depreciation | **44,392** | 41,627 |
| Interest | **10,974** | 6,145 |
| Operating expenses | **764,776** | 704,577 |
| Excess of revenue over expenses | **35,433** | 41,444 |
| Nonoperating gains (losses) | | |
| Contributions, gifts, and bequests | **3,189** | 1,318 |
| Net assets released from restrictions for research expenditures | **14,070** | 14,474 |
| Research, education, and other nonoperating expenses | **(22,980)** | (24,773) |
| Change in interest rate swap value and put agreements | **1,578** | 9,397 |
| Investment income | **30,453** | 18,402 |
| | **26,310** | 18,818 |
| Excess of revenues and gains over expenses and losses | **$61,743** | $60,262 |

**TABLE 9A-3** Harris Memorial Hospital and Harris Community Foundation Combined Statements of Changes in Net Assets (in Thousands)

| | **December 31, 20X7** | **December 31, 20X6** |
|---|---|---|
| Unrestricted net assets | | |
| Excess of revenues and gains over expenses and losses | **$61,743** | $60,262 |
| Net assets released from restrictions for capital expenditures | **—** | 119 |

| | | |
|---|---|---|
| Cumulative effect of change in accounting principle | — | (3,943) |
| Increase in unrestricted net assets | **61,743** | 56,438 |
| Temporarily restricted net assets | | |
| Contributions, gifts, and bequests | **20,435** | 15,512 |
| Investment income | **8,455** | 3,972 |
| Net assets released from restrictions for research expenditures | **(14,070)** | (14,474) |
| Net assets released from restrictions for capital expenditures | — | (119) |
| Increase in temporarily restricted net assets | **14,820** | 4,891 |
| Permanently restricted net assets | | |
| Contributions, gifts, and bequests | **1,794** | 3,218 |
| Increase in permanently restricted net assets | **1,794** | 3,218 |
| Net assets at beginning of year | **606,262** | 541,715 |
| Net assets at end of year | **$684,619** | $606,262 |

**TABLE 9A-4** Harris Memorial Hospital and Harris Community Foundation Combined Statements of Cash Flows (in Thousands)

| | December 31, 20X7 | December 31, 20X6 |
|---|---|---|
| Operating activities | | |
| Increase in net assets | **$78,357** | $64,547 |
| Adjustments to reconcile increase in net assets to net cash provided by operating activities | | |
| Change in net unrealized gains and losses on investment securities | **(26,358)** | 11,432 |
| Cumulative effect of change in accounting principle | — | (3,943) |
| Depreciation | **44,392** | 41,627 |
| Gain on sale or disposal of assets, net | **(6,119)** | — |
| Provision for bad debts | **55,851** | 57,975 |
| Change in interest rate swap value and put agreements | **(1,578)** | (9,397) |

*(continues)*

**TABLE 9A-4** Harris Memorial Hospital and Harris Community Foundation Combined Statements of Cash *(continued)* Flows (in Thousands)

| | December 31, 20X7 | December 31, 20X6 |
|---|---|---|
| Changes in operating assets and liabilities | | |
| Assets limited as to use | **(19,779)** | (14,274) |
| Accounts receivable | **(65,937)** | (51,251) |
| Other assets | **(7,071)** | (43) |
| Supplies | **(415)** | 840 |
| Accounts payable | **7,941** | 10,613 |
| Accrued expenses and other liabilities | **20,568** | 8,430 |
| Due to third-party payers | **(5,253)** | (4,877) |
| Contingent professional liabilities | **(15,227)** | 3,743 |
| Postretirement benefit obligation, other than pensions | **513** | 456 |
| Net cash provided by operating activities | **59,885** | 115,878 |
| Investing activities | | |
| Property and equipment acquired | **(142,793)** | (159,943) |
| Cash used in investing activities | **(142,793)** | (159,943) |
| Financing activities | | |
| Repayment of long-term debt | **(177,294)** | (5,545) |
| Proceeds from borrowing | **283,321** | 57,614 |
| Net cash provided by financing activities | **106,027** | 52,069 |
| Net increase in cash and cash equivalents | **23,119** | 8,004 |
| Cash and cash equivalents at beginning of year | **59,696** | 51,692 |
| Cash and cash equivalents at end of year | **$82,815** | $59,696 |

# Harris Memorial Hospital and Harris Community Foundation

Notes to Combined Financial Statements
December 31, 20X7

1. **Organization and Significant Accounting Policies**

**Organization and Basis of Combination**

Harris Memorial Hospital (the Hospital) and Harris Community Foundation (the Foundation) are a hospital and charitable foundation located in Jersey, Ohio. The Hospital and Foundation are exempt from federal income taxes under Section 501(c)(3) of the Internal Revenue Code (IRC). The Hospital and Foundation are collectively referred to herein as the Foundation.

The Foundation owns and operates the Renee Center, which has 27 skilled nursing beds; Harris Assurance, Ltd. (Assurance), a for-profit, wholly owned insurance subsidiary; and Harris Properties (Condit Inn), a for-profit, wholly owned subsidiary. During 20X6, the Foundation formed the Harris Community Hospital Corporation (dba Harris Hospital) located in Oldstone, Ohio and the Harris Long Term Acute Care Hospital Corporation (dba Harris Continuing Care Hospital) located in Jersey, Ohio. The 60-bed Harris Continuing Care Hospital opened in May 20X7. Harris Hospital, with 92 beds, opened in late July 20X7. At December 31, 20X7, the Foundation has remaining commitments totaling approximately $7,360,000 under construction contracts for these and other capital projects.

The Foundation is affiliated with the Harris Health Plan (the Health Plan). The Health Plan's financial statements are not included in these combined financial statements. The Foundation provides healthcare services in the central Ohio region. All appropriate intercompany accounts have been eliminated in combination.

**Cash Equivalents**

The Foundation considers all undesignated highly liquid investments with maturities of 3 months or less when purchased to be cash equivalents.

**Supplies**

Supplies are stated at cost (first-in, first-out method), which is not in excess of market value.

**Patient Accounts Receivable**

Patient accounts receivable are stated at estimated net realizable value. Significant concentrations of patient accounts receivable were 20% and 19% at December 31, 20X7 and 20X6, respectively, from government-related programs. Patient accounts receivable from the Health Plan were 25% and 29% at December 31, 20X7 and 20X6, respectively.

The Foundation maintains allowances for uncollectable accounts for estimated losses resulting from a payer's inability to make payments on accounts. The Foundation uses a balance sheet approach to value the allowance account based on historical write-offs, payer type, and the aging of the accounts. Accounts are written off when collection efforts have been exhausted. Management continually monitors and adjusts, as necessary, allowances associated with its receivables. The majority of uncollectable accounts are from uninsured and the patient portion of accounts receivable.

**Assets Limited as to Use**

Assets limited as to use at December 31, 20X7, include 76% and 9% held under master trust agreements with Liberty Eagle Trust and Highbanks, respectively, and 15% held in government-insured time deposits and other financial instruments. Assets limited as to use at December 31, 20X6, include 78% and 5% held under master trust agreements with Liberty Eagle Trust and Highbanks, respectively, and 17% held in government-insured time deposits and other financial instruments. The investments held under the master trust agreements are diversified among equity, debt, and money market instruments and are reported at estimated fair value. The fair value of these investments is generally based on quoted market prices on national exchanges.

**Property and Equipment**

Property and equipment are recorded at cost at the date of acquisition or estimated fair value at the date of donation. Depreciation is computed on the straight-line method using the estimated economic lives of the depreciable assets, generally ranging from 3 to 40 years. Expenditures that materially increase values, change capacities, or extend useful lives are capitalized. Routine maintenance and repair items are charged to operating expenses.

The Foundation evaluates whether events and circumstances have occurred that indicate the remaining estimated useful life of long-lived assets may warrant revision or that the remaining balance of an asset may not be recoverable. The assessment of possible impairment is based on whether the carrying amount of the asset exceeds the expected total undiscounted value of cash flows expected to result from the use of the assets and their eventual disposition. No amounts were recognized in 20X6.

In 20X7, the Foundation recorded a charge of $4,000,000, net of reimbursement, for unrecoverable costs incurred in connection with repair and maintenance costs of the Condit Inn.

### Derivative Financial Instruments

The Foundation accounts for its derivatives under Statement of Financial Accounting Standards No. 133, *Accounting for Derivative Instruments and Hedging Activities,* or SFAS No. 133. SFAS No. 133 requires that all derivative financial instruments that qualify for hedge accounting be recognized in the financial statements and measured at fair value regardless of the purpose or intent for holding them. Changes in the fair value of derivative financial instruments are recognized periodically either in operations or in changes in unrestricted net assets. The Foundation's policy is to not hold or issue derivatives for trading purposes and to avoid derivatives with leverage features.

### Restricted Support

The Foundation records unconditional promises of cash or other assets at estimated fair value on the date the promises are received. The Foundation reports gifts of cash and other assets as restricted support if they are received with donor stipulations that limit the use of the donated assets. When a donor restriction expires, that is, when a stipulated time restriction ends or a purpose of restriction is accomplished, temporarily restricted net assets are reclassified to unrestricted net assets and reported in the combined statements of operations or combined statements of changes in net assets (based on nature of restriction) as net assets released from restrictions.

The Foundation reports gifts of land, buildings, and equipment as unrestricted support unless explicit donor stipulations specify how the donated assets must be used. Gifts of long-lived assets with explicit restrictions that specify how the assets are to be used and gifts of cash or other assets that must be used to acquire long-lived assets are reported as restricted support. The Foundation reports expirations of donor restrictions when the donated or acquired long-lived assets are placed in service.

Permanently restricted net assets have been restricted by donors to be maintained by the Foundation in perpetuity. The income from permanently restricted net assets is recorded as unrestricted unless explicitly restricted by donors. Donor-restricted income on permanently restricted net assets is generally available to support research and education and is reported as temporarily restricted.

The Foundation's temporarily restricted net assets are restricted primarily for research, education, capital projects, and medical care programs and its permanently restricted net assets are primarily restricted for endowment purposes.

### Net Patient Service Revenue

Net patient service revenue is reported at estimated net realizable amounts from patients, third-party payers, and others for services rendered and includes estimated retroactive revenue adjustments due to future audits, reviews, and investigations. Retroactive adjustments are considered in the recognition of revenue on an estimated basis in the period the related services are rendered, and such amounts are adjusted in future periods as adjustments become known or as years are no longer subject to such audits, reviews, and investigations.

### Charity Care

The Foundation provides care without charge or at amounts less than its established rates to patients who meet certain criteria under its charity policy. Because the Foundation does not pursue collection of amounts determined to qualify as charity care, they are not reported as revenue. Hospital charges foregone for charity care, based on established rates, were approximately $35,200,000 in 20X7, prior to application of disproportionate share funds of approximately $4,800,000 received from the State of Ohio, and $35,300,000 in 20X6, prior to application of disproportionate share funds of approximately $5,800,000 received from the State of Ohio. Clinic charges forgone for charity care, based on established rates, were $12,525,000 and $10,216,000 in 20X7 and 20X6, respectively.

### Health Insurance Program Reimbursement

Revenue from the Medicare and Medicaid programs accounted for approximately 45% and 8%, respectively, of the Foundation's net patient service revenue for the year ended December

31, 20X7, and 51% and 11%, respectively, for the year ended December 31, 20X6. Laws and regulations governing the Medicare and Medicaid programs are extremely complex and are subject to interpretation. Federal regulations require the submission of annual cost reports covering medical costs and expenses associated with services provided to program beneficiaries. Medicare and Medicaid cost report settlements are estimated in the period services are provided to beneficiaries. As a result, there is at least a reasonable possibility that recorded estimates will change by a material amount in the near term. The 20X7 and 20X6 net patient service revenue increased (decreased) approximately $10,340,000 and $(1,332,000), respectively, due to changes in allowances previously estimated as a result of the final settlements for years that are no longer subject to audits, reviews, and investigations. The Foundation believes that it is in compliance with all applicable laws and regulations and is not aware of any pending or threatened investigations involving allegations of potential wrongdoing.

Medicare cost reports filed by the Hospital for all years before 20X4 have been audited and settled as of December 31, 20X7. Medicare cost reports filed by the Clinic for all years before 20X0 have been audited and settled as of December 31, 20X7. Amounts due to the Medicare and Medicaid programs totaled approximately $7,380,000 and $12,633,000 at December 31, 20X7 and 20X6, respectively, and are included in due to third-party payers in the accompanying combined balance sheets.

### Nonoperating Gains and Losses

Nonoperating gains and losses include unrestricted contributions, gifts and bequests, interest earnings on investments, net assets released from restrictions for research and education expenditures (net of contributions for such expenditures), change in interest rate swap value and put agreements, and other gains and losses unrelated to the Foundation's primary operations.

### Excess of Revenues and Gains over Expenses and Losses

Included in excess of revenues and gains over expenses and losses in the accompanying combined statements of operations are all changes in unrestricted net assets other than net assets released from restrictions for capital expenditures, unrealized gains and losses on investments other than trading investment securities, and investment returns restricted by donors.

### Use of Estimates

The preparation of financial statements in conformity with accounting principles generally accepted in the United States requires management to make estimates and assumptions that affect the amounts reported in the combined financial statements and accompanying notes. Actual results could differ from those estimates.

### Other

Certain reclassifications of donor trust liabilities, previously included in assets limited as to use, were made to the 20X6 combined financial statements to conform to the 20X7 presentation.

Additionally, in previous years, the Foundation's investment portfolio (see Note 7) was classified as other than trading. As such, unrealized gains and losses that were considered temporary were excluded from excess of revenues and gains over expenses and losses. During fiscal year 20X7, the Foundation determined that substantially all of its investment portfolio was more accurately classified as trading with unrealized gains and losses included in excess of revenues and gains over expenses and losses. Therefore, a reclassification was made in the accompanying 20X6 combined financial statements to reflect this change in classification. A net unrealized loss of approximately $9,183,000 was reclassified from change in net unrealized gains and losses on investment securities to investment income.

### 2. Contingent Professional Liabilities

The Foundation self-insures substantially all of its professional liability risk through its wholly owned insurance subsidiary. A commercial insurance policy is maintained to insure claims exceeding $7,000,000 individually or $35,000,000 in the aggregate in 20X7 on a claims-made basis. Contingent professional liabilities are recorded for incurred but not reported claims and reported claims based on estimates by independent actuaries. Management established a fund for the purpose of setting aside assets based on estimates made by independent actuaries, and these funds are reported in the combined balance sheets as assets limited as to use.

### 3. Property and Equipment

**TABLE 9A-5** Property and Equipment and Related Accumulated Depreciation (in Thousands)

|  | December 31, 20X7 | December 31, 20X6 |
|---|---|---|
| Land and improvements | $26,945 | $26,610 |
| Buildings and improvements expenditures | 447,897 | 265,965 |
| Fixed and movable equipment | 469,441 | 427,882 |
| Construction-in-progress | 112,880 | 189,807 |
|  | 1,057,163 | 910,264 |
| Less accumulated depreciation | 493,814 | 451,435 |
|  | $563,349 | $458,829 |

### 4. Long-Term Debt

In July 20X7, the Foundation issued the Series 20X7 LTACH Revenue Bonds totaling $15,700,000. The Series 20X7 LTACH Revenue Bonds are due July 20X2 with principal and interest payments due monthly. Interest accrues at 65% of LIBOR plus 100 basis points. Effective with the issuance of the bonds, the Foundation entered into a fixed rate swap agreement for the amount of the bonds by which the Foundation pays a fixed rate of interest of 4.55%. The change in fair value for the period ended December 31, 20X7 was not significant to the increase in net assets.

In November 20X6, the Foundation issued Series 20X6 Revenue Bonds with a par amount of $233,350,000. Proceeds were used to advance refund $31,280,000 of the Series 20X0A Revenue Bonds, current refund $58,410,000 of the Series 20X1 Revenue Bonds, and finance and/or refinance expansion projects. The Series 20X6 Bonds were issued as Auction Rate Securities and generally bear interest for successive 7-day auction periods at interest rates determined through Dutch auctions on the business day preceding the auction period. Any series or subseries of the Series 20X6 Revenue Bonds may be converted at the option of the Foundation, subject to certain restrictions, to bonds that bear interest in different rate periods, including daily, weekly, flexible, term, or fixed rate periods. The Series 20X6 Revenue Bonds contain certain restrictive covenants, including minimum levels of debt service coverage. Management believes the Foundation is in compliance with all covenants.

**TABLE 9A-6** Long-Term Debt (in Thousands)

|  | December 31, 20X7 | December 31, 20X6 |
|---|---|---|
| Revenue bonds, LTACH Series 20X7; interest at 65% of LIBOR plus100 basis points (4.647% at December 31, 20X7); principal and interest payable monthly through July 20X2 | $15,679 | $— |
| Revenue bonds, Series 20X6A-1; interest accrues for successive 7-day auction periods at interest rates determined through Dutch auctions (3.800% at December 31, 20X7) | 42,375 | — |
| Revenue bonds, Series 20X6A-2; interest accrues for successive 7-day auction periods at interest rates determined through Dutch auctions (3.800% at December 31, 20X7) | 42,400 | — |

| | | |
|---|---:|---:|
| Revenue bonds, Series 20X6B; interest accrues for successive 7-day auction periods at interest rates determined through Dutch auctions (3.850% at December 31, 20X7) | **56,550** | — |
| Revenue bonds, Series 20X6C; interest accrues for successive 7-day auction periods at interest rates determined through Dutch auctions (3.850% at December 31, 20X7) | **55,275** | — |
| Revenue bonds, Series 20X6D; interest accrues for successive 7-day auction periods at interest rates determined through Dutch auctions (3.900% at December 31, 20X7) | **36,750** | — |
| Revenue bonds, Series 20X1; interest accrues at a daily rate determined by the remarketing agent (3.960% at December 31, 20X7); interest and principal payable annually through 20X1 (principal payments began in 20X6) | **90,360** | 151,800 |
| Revenue bonds, Series 20X0A; interest at 5.375%; interest and principal payable annually through 20X9 | **2,700** | 35,230 |
| Revenue bonds, Series 20X0B; interest accrues at a daily rate determined by the remarketing agent (3.960% at December 31, 20X7); interest and principal payable annually through 20X9 | **83,200** | 84,500 |
| Line of credit | **19,000** | 46,686 |
| Interim construction loan | **—** | 7,000 |
| Other | **—** | 13,046 |
| | **444,289** | 338,262 |
| Less current maturities | **4,692** | 5,908 |
| | **$439,597** | $332,354 |

In January 20X6, the Foundation entered into a revolving line of credit with Bank of Central Ohio to fund interim construction costs and provide for liquidity and other short-term needs. In accordance with terms of the loan agreement, the total available for borrowing was decreased from $70,000,000 to $30,000,000 30 days following the issuance of the Series 20X6 Revenue Bonds. The total amount drawn as of December 31, 20X7 was $19,000,000. Interest is payable quarterly at a rate equal to the lesser of the maximum lawful rate or LIBOR plus 15 basis points (5.71% at December 31, 20X7). Amounts drawn are due in full June 25, 20X9.

The Foundation issued Series 20X1 Revenue Bonds with a par amount of $158,000,000 that were partially refunded in November 20X6. The net proceeds were used to fund expansion projects.

The Foundation issued Series 20X0A Revenue Bonds with a par amount of $42,025,000 that were partially refunded in November 20X6 and Series 20X0B Revenue Bonds with a par amount of $91,200,000. The majority of the proceeds from the Series 20X0A and Series 20X0B Revenue Bonds were used to refund the current Series 19X8 Revenue Bonds with an outstanding balance of $19,147,000 and a note payable with an outstanding par amount of $88,000,000.

The Series 20X0A and Series 20X0B Revenue Bonds and the Series 20X1 Revenue Bonds contain certain restrictive covenants, including minimum levels of debt service coverage. Management believes the Foundation is in compliance with all covenants.

The Series 20X0B Revenue Bonds and the Series 20X1 Revenue Bonds are variable rate bonds in a daily mode and can be tendered by holders upon demand. A remarketing agent selected by the Foundation determines the interest rates and remarkets both series of bonds. The Series 20X0B Revenue Bonds and the Series 20X1 Revenue Bonds are supported by Standby Bond Purchase Agreements (the Agreements) with liquidity providers pursuant to which the providers will purchase any bonds the remarketing agent is unable to market. The termination date of the two Agreements related to the Series 20X0B Revenue Bonds was December 6, 20X7. On October 18, 20X7, these Agreements were extended to December 4, 20X8. There are also two Agreements associated with the Series 20X1 Revenue Bonds. The termination date of the first Agreement related to the Series 20X1 Revenue Bonds was December 6, 20X7, and on October 18, 20X7, was extended to December 4, 20X8. The termination date of the second Agreement related to the Series 20X1 Revenue Bonds is December 15, 20X5, as extended in November 20X4. All Agreements include covenants that are customary in credit agreements of this nature. Repayment of bonds purchased under the Agreements is subject to a 5-year payout beginning July 20X6, if other liquidity facilities, as defined in the bond agreements, are not executed. The maturities of long-term debt, net of unamortized premium, as of December 31, 20X7, are shown below (in thousands):

| | |
|---|---|
| 20X8 | $4,692 |
| 20X9 | 23,902 |
| 20X0 | 5,136 |
| 20X1 | 5,353 |
| 20X2 | 19,896 |
| Thereafter | 385,310 |
| | **$444,289** |

Total interest costs incurred during fiscal 20X7 and 20X6 were $16,779,140 and $9,339,000 respectively, including $5,805,140 and $3,194,000 of capitalized interest costs in 20X7 and 20X6,

respectively. Interest paid during fiscal 20X7 and 20X6 was $16,937,249 and $9,084,500, respectively, net of amounts capitalized.

5. **Concentrations of Credit Risk**

Harris Memorial grants credit without collateral to its patients, most of whom are local residents and are insured under third-party payer agreements. The mix of receivables from patients and third-party payers was as follows:

**TABLE 9A-7**  Mix of Receivables

| | December 31, 20X7 | December 31, 20X6 |
|---|---|---|
| Medicare | **21%** | 19% |
| Medicaid | **2** | 2 |
| Major payer 1 | **15** | 15 |
| Major payer 2 | **11** | 11 |
| Major payer 3 | **11** | 13 |
| Other third-party payers | **28** | 28 |
| Private pay | **12** | 12 |
| Total | **100%** | 100% |

6. **Interest Rate Swap Agreements**

Effective December 20X1, the Foundation entered into an interest rate swap agreement with an initial notional amount of $150,000,000. The interest rate swap agreement converts a notional amount of $150,000,000 of floating rate borrowings to fixed rate borrowings. The Foundation pays a fixed rate of interest (5.17%) and receives, from the counterparty, a variable rate of interest based on the SIFMA Municipal Swap Index (SIFMA Index) on the outstanding principal balance of the Series 20X1 Revenue Bonds until 2031. The Foundation has elected not to apply hedge accounting; therefore, the change in fair value is included in nonoperating (gains) losses. The fair value of the interest rate swap at December 31, 20X7 and 20X6, is a liability of approximately $9,498,000 and $16,530,000, respectively, and is included in due to broker in the accompanying combined balance sheets. The change in the fair value of the interest rate swap is included in non-operating gains (losses) and totaled approximately $(7,032,000) and $(6,885,000) for the years ended December 31, 20X7 and 20X6, respectively. The change in fair value for the year ended December 31, 20X7 includes the amendment fee paid to the counterparty of $7,037,000, realized as a part of the Series 20X1 Revenue Bond refunding.

Simultaneous with entering into the interest rate swap agreement, the Foundation also entered into a put agreement with the counterparty. The counterparty may exercise this put agreement if the daily weighted average of the SIFMA Index is greater than 7.00% for the 180-day period ending on the day the counterparty exercises the put option. Under this agreement, the Foundation pays a variable rate of interest, based on the SIFMA Index, on the outstanding principal balance of the proposed bonds until 2031. For this put agreement, the counterparty pays the Foundation an annual premium of 77.30 basis points on an initial notional amount of $150,000,000 over the term of the put agreement, for a net effective combined annual payment by the Foundation to the counterparty for the swap agreement and the put agreement of approximately 4.39%. The premium payment, however, will cease upon exercise of the put agreement. This put agreement, if exercised, will offset the cash flows of the interest rate swap agreement noted above. The fair value of the put agreement at December 31, 20X7 and 20X6, is an asset of $4,200,000 and $7,016,000, respectively, and has been included in other assets. The change in the fair value of $(2,816,000) and $(552,000) for the years ended December 31, 20X7 and 20X6, respectively, has been included in nonoperating gains (losses) since the put agreement is not a hedge and must be adjusted to fair value through the performance indicator. A portion of the change in fair value for the year ended December 31, 20X7 includes the amount related to the partial refunding of the Series 20X1 Revenue Bonds. The amendment fee received from the counterparty was $2,005,000.

On October 30, 20X2, the Foundation entered into an interest rate swap agreement with an initial notional amount of $96,400,000 ($88,400,000 Series 20X0A and Series 20X0B and $8,000,000 Series 20X1). The interest rate swap agreement converts a notional amount of $96,400,000 of floating rate borrowings to fixed rate borrowings. The Foundation pays a fixed rate of interest (4.34)%

and receives, from the counterparty, a variable rate of interest based on the SIFMA Index on the outstanding principal balance of the Revenue Bonds until 2031. The Foundation has elected not to apply hedge accounting; therefore, the change in fair value is included in nonoperating (gains) losses. The fair value of the interest rate swap at December 31, 20X7 and 20X6, is a liability of approximately $3,020,000 and $3,078,000, respectively, and is included in due to broker in the accompanying combined balance sheets. The change in the fair value of the interest rate swap is included in nonoperating gains (losses) and totaled approximately $(58,000) and $(3,639,000) for the years ended December 31, 20X7 and 20X6, respectively. The change in fair value includes the amendment fee of $176,000 paid to the counterparty to terminate the portion of the interest rate swap agreement associated with the Series 20X1 Revenue Bonds. Simultaneous with entering into the interest rate swap agreement, the Foundation also entered into a put agreement with the counterparty. The counterparty may exercise this put agreement if the daily weighted-average of the SIFMA Index is greater than 6.00% for the 180-day period ending on the day the counterparty exercises the put option. Under this agreement, the Foundation pays a variable rate of interest, based on the SIFMA Index, on the outstanding principal balance of the related bonds until 2031. For this put agreement, the counterparty pays the Foundation an annual premium of 110.10 basis points on an initial notional amount $96,400,000 over the term of the put agreement, for a net effective combined annual payment by the Foundation to the counterparty for the swap agreement and the put agreement of approximately 3.24%. The premium payment, however, will cease upon exercise of the put agreement. This put agreement, if exercised, will offset the cash flows of the interest rate swap agreement noted above. The fair value of the put agreement at December 31, 20X7 and 20X6, is an asset of approximately $4,970,000 and $5,056,000, respectively, and has been included in other assets. This change in fair value of $(86,000) and $(575,000) for the years ended December 31, 20X7 and 20X6, respectively, has been included in nonoperating gains (losses) since the put agreement is not a hedge and must be adjusted to fair value through the performance indicator. The change in fair value includes the amendment fee of $198,000 received from the counterparty to terminate the portion of the put agreement associated with the Series 20X1 Revenue Bonds.

In anticipation of the issuance of the Series 20X6 Bonds, the Foundation entered into five interest rate swap transactions in October 20X6 with an initial notional amount totaling $233,350,000.

The swap transactions serve to substantially fix the expected net interest expense associated with the Series 20X6 Bonds by converting floating rate borrowings with a notional amount of $233,350,000 to fixed rate borrowings. For the swaps related to the Series 20X6A and 20X6B Bonds, the Foundation pays a fixed rate of 3.502% per annum, and the counterparty pays a variable rate of interest at a rate equal to 57.4% of the 1-month LIBOR rate plus a spread of 0.33%. For the swaps related to the Series 20X6C Bonds and 20X6D Bonds, the Foundation pays a fixed rate of 3.496% per annum, and the counterparty pays a variable rate of interest at a rate equal to 57.4% of the 1-month LIBOR rate plus a spread of 0.33%.

The Foundation has elected not to apply hedge accounting; therefore, the change in fair value is included in nonoperating (gains) losses. The fair value of the interest rate swaps at December 31, 20X7 is a liability of approximately $2,610,000, which equates to the change in fair value from inception of the swaps through the year ended December 31, 20X7.

The Foundation can terminate any of these agreements at any time at current market value. The Foundation would make or receive a payment depending on market value on the date of termination.

The Foundation is exposed to credit losses in the event of nonperformance by the counterparty to the agreements. The counterparty is a creditworthy financial institution, and the Foundation anticipates that the counterparty will be able to fully satisfy its obligation under the agreements.

### 7. Pension Plans

The Foundation implemented a 401(a) defined contribution plan and a 403(b) voluntary savings plan covering substantially all employees. The Foundation contributes from 6% to 13% of participating employees' compensation. Prior to January 1, 20X6, the Foundation's contributions were based on participating employees' age. The plan was amended January 1, 20X6 and these contributions are now based on years of service. The Foundation's contribution expense was approximately $28,495,000 and $26,121,000 in 20X7 and 20X6, respectively.

The Foundation sponsors a defined benefit postretirement plan that provides medical and dental benefits to retirees who meet specific eligibility requirements upon termination of active service. The plan is unfunded and requires covered retirees to contribute a portion of the cost of benefits. The Foundation uses an incremental cost approach in estimating the annual accrued cost related to postretirement benefits other than pensions, which is based on estimates by independent actuaries. Such an approach is considered appropriate since substantially all of the healthcare benefits are provided by the Foundation to retirees, using the Health Plan to manage the care provided. Plan expenses incurred by the Foundation were $880,000 and $822,000 for the years ended December 31, 20X7 and 20X6, respectively.

### 8. Assets Limited as to Use

Certain cash and investments, where their use is limited due to board designations or other purposes as set forth below, are reported as assets limited as to use. The carrying values (in thousands) are at estimated fair values, which are summarized in **TABLE 9A-8**.

| **TABLE 9A-8** Assets Limited as to Use | | |
|---|---|---|
| | **December 31, 20X7** | **December 31, 20X6** |
| Assets limited as to use and long-term investments | | |
| For donor-restricted purposes, such as research, lectureships, and capital projects | **$84,440** | $67,826 |
| Board designated for specific purposes | | |
| Funded depreciation | **133,028** | 118,618 |

| | | |
|---|---|---|
| Contingent professional liabilities | **33,357** | 46,566 |
| Institutional research | **18,072** | 16,241 |
| Investments held by subsidiary | **19,925** | 16,019 |
| Other board designated | **178,453** | 180,969 |
| | **382,835** | 378,413 |
| Held by trustees under bond agreements | **51,038** | 25,937 |
| | **518,313** | 472,176 |
| Less current portion of assets limited as to use | **5,327** | 5,088 |
| | **$512,986** | $467,088 |

Investment income or loss is included in the excess of revenues and gains over expenses and losses, and includes realized and unrealized gains and losses, interest, and dividends.

**TABLE 9A-9** The Foundation's Assets Limited as to Use at December 31 (in Thousands)

| | December 31, 20X7 | December 31, 20X6 |
|---|---|---|
| Carried at fair value | | |
| Money market accounts | **$83,900** | $58,833 |
| Certificates of deposit | **1,651** | 2,151 |
| U.S. Treasury securities | **74,896** | 75,195 |
| Corporate debt securities | **53,412** | 82,657 |
| Equity securities | **304,454** | 253,340 |
| | **518,313** | 472,176 |
| Less current portion of assets limited as to use | **5,327** | 5,088 |
| | **$512,986** | $467,088 |

## 9. Commitments and Contingencies

The Foundation leases equipment and a medical office building under operating leases. These payments are due monthly through December 2012. Rent expense totaled approximately $7,426,000 and $8,715,000 in 20X7 and 20X6, respectively.

Future minimum lease commitments under operating leases that have initial or remaining lease terms in excess of 1 year are as follows as of December 31, 20X7 (in thousands):

| | |
|---|---|
| 20X8 | $3,410 |
| 20X9 | 3,544 |
| 20X0 | 3,252 |
| 20X1 | 2,886 |
| 20X2 | 2,287 |
| | **$15,379** |

### Sale of Medical Office Building

On December 29, 20X7, the Foundation sold a medical office building to Ross Acquisition of Alexandria (RA) for approximately $22,200,000. The building had a book value of approximately $10,900,000. The transaction included a ground lease with a term of 50 years and HR prepaid the rent totaling approximately $900,000. The Foundation entered into lease-back agreements for space within the building. The Foundation recognized an immediate gain of approximately $6,100,000 and a deferred gain of approximately $4,300,000 to be recognized over a period equal to the operating lease term.

### Other

The Foundation is a defendant in various legal proceedings arising in the ordinary course of business. Although the results of litigation cannot be predicted with certainty, management believes the outcome of pending litigation will not have a material adverse effect on the Foundation's combined financial statements.

On February 21, 20X3, the Foundation entered into a 10-year Master Customer Agreement with COTC, for the provision of services, supplies, and equipment. The agreement provides a platform for the development of the Zuber Center as a fully integrated, all-digital facility. COTC will support the Foundation in five core areas: healthcare information technology applications and infrastructure, medical equipment, telecommunications power, and "smart" building technologies. The agreement provides for a commitment of approximately $200,000,000 from the Foundation to purchase certain goods and services at favorable prices. The Foundation has certain minimum yearly purchase commitments ranging from $10,000,000 to $25,000,000 over the 10-year term of the agreement. For the years ended December 31, 20X7 and 20X6, the Foundation purchased approximately $22,353,000 and $26,372,000, respectively, in goods and services from Siemens and affiliated companies, which exceeded the purchase commitments in those years. Goods and services purchased under the contract total approximately $137,400,000.

The Foundation invests in short-term instruments as part of its money management program. These instruments include short-term government securities and investment grade commercial paper. Generally, an investment firm on behalf of the Foundation manages these investments, and the Foundation has invested in a number of short-term investment grade commercial papers over the years. On October 29, 20X1, the Foundation sold approximately $10,000,000 in MGMTMatrix commercial paper prior to maturity. MGMTMatrix filed a voluntary petition for

relief under Chapter 11 on February 17, 20X1. On October 6, 20X3, the Foundation learned that the bankruptcy counsel for MGMTMatrix filed, in U.S. Bankruptcy Court in the District of New York, an attempt to nullify the redemption of certain MGMTMatrix commercial paper including that divested by the Foundation. The case was settled in December 20X7 for approximately $3,900,000 and is included in accrued expenses and other liabilities in the accompanying combined balance sheets. The Foundation paid the settlement amount in October 20X7.

### 10. Fair Values of Financial Instruments

Generally accepted accounting principles established a framework for measuring fair value that provides a fair value hierarchy that prioritizes the inputs to valuation techniques used to measure fair value. The hierarchy gives the highest priority to unadjusted quoted prices in active markets for identical assets or liabilities (Level 1 measurements) and the lowest priority to unobservable inputs (Level 3 measurements).

The three levels of the fair value hierarchy under Accounting Standards Codification (ASC) 820-10-50, Fair Value Measurement—Overall, are described here:

- Level 1: Valuation is based on quoted prices for identical instruments traded in active markets. Level 1 securities include primarily overnight repurchase agreements, money market funds, and mutual funds.
- Level 2: Valuation is based on quoted prices for similar instruments in active markets, quoted prices for identical or similar instruments in markets that are not active, and model-based valuation techniques for which all significant assumptions are observable in the market. At Level 2 securities include an unregistered mutual fund.
- Level 3: Valuation is generated from model-based techniques that use significant assumptions not observable in the market. These unobservable assumptions reflect the Hospital's estimates of assumptions that market participants would use in pricing the asset or liability. Valuation techniques include use of discounted cash flow models and similar techniques. Level 3 securities include an equity fund limited partnership.

Fair value is based on the price that would be received to sell an asset or paid to transfer a liability in an orderly transaction between market participants at the measurement date. The Hospital maximizes the use of observable inputs and minimizes the use of unobservable inputs when developing fair value measurements.

Fair value measurements for assets and liabilities where there is limited or no observable market data and, therefore, are based primarily on estimates calculated by the Hospital, are based on the economic and competitive environment, the characteristics of the asset or liability and other factors. Therefore, the results cannot be determined with precision and may not be realized upon an actual settlement of the asset or liability. There may be inherent weaknesses in any calculation technique, and changes in the underlying assumptions used, including discount rates and estimates of future cash flows that could significantly affect the results of the current or future values.

The following methods and assumptions were used by the Foundation in estimating the fair value of its financial instruments:

*Cash and cash equivalents*: The carrying amount reported in the combined balance sheet for cash and cash equivalents approximates its fair value.

*Investments*: Fair values, which are the amounts reported in the combined balance sheet, are based on quoted market prices.

*Interest rate swap agreements*: Fair values, which are the amounts reported in the combined balance sheet as due to broker and other assets, are based on market rates.

*Long-term debt*: The carrying amount of the Foundation's borrowings under its revolving line of credit and auction rate security bond issues approximates fair value. The fair value of the Foundation's other long-term debt is estimated using discounted cash flow analyses, based on the Foundation's current incremental borrowing rates for similar types of borrowing arrangements.

11. **Functional Expenses**

The Foundation provides healthcare services to residents within its geographical service area.

**TABLE 9A-10** The Carrying Amounts and Fair Values of the Foundation's Financial Instruments in the Combined Balance Sheets at December 31 (in Thousands)

| | Carrying Amount | Fair Value |
|---|---|---|
| 20X7 | | |
| Cash and cash equivalents | $82,815 | $82,815 |
| Assets limited as to use | 518,313 | 518,313 |
| Due to broker | 15,128 | 15,128 |
| Long-term debt | 444,289 | 444,349 |
| 20X6 | | |
| Cash and cash equivalents | $59,696 | $59,696 |
| Assets limited as to use | 472,176 | 472,176 |
| Due to broker | 19,608 | 19,608 |
| Long-term debt | 338,262 | 340,809 |

**TABLE 9A-11** Expenses Related to Providing These Services for the Years Ended December 31, 20X7 and 20X6 (in Thousands)

|  | December 31, 20X7 | December 31, 20X6 |
|---|---|---|
| Healthcare services | $619,596 | 562,186 |
| General and administrative | 143,293 | 140,546 |
| Fundraising | 1,887 | 1,845 |
| Total operating expenses | $764,776 | 704,577 |

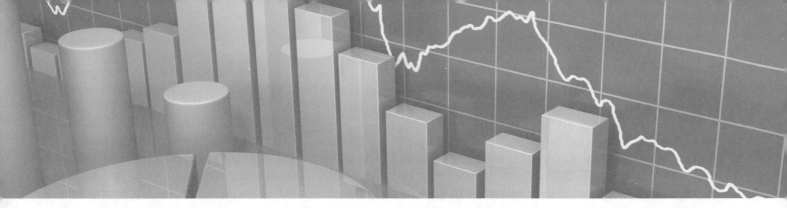

# CHAPTER 10

# Accounting for Inflation

## REAL-WORLD SCENARIO

Lydia Renee is the CEO of a large metropolitan hospital. She has recently come under attack from the local press regarding profit levels at the hospital. Last year Renee's hospital earned more than $10 million, which was described in the local press as "obscene" because the hospital is tax-exempt. Renee tried to explain that all of the earnings for the hospital were earmarked for future investment and replacement of physical facilities, but the local reporter was adamant about profiteering at the hospital.

Renee's CFO, William Olin, has told her that the need for profit is directly related to the existence of inflation in the cost of plant and equipment that the hospital needs to purchase. For example, a new digital mammography unit was recently acquired for $750,000 to replace an older unit acquired 5 years ago for $350,000. The hospital recognized historical cost depreciation on this older mammography unit of $70,000 per year ($350,000/5) but the real replacement cost of the equipment was much higher.

Olin showed Renee that firms with heavy investments in plant and equipment, such as hospitals, must make positive profits because the historical accounting costs of depreciation grossly understate true replacement costs. Olin then recast the hospital's financial statements using the principles of "constant purchasing power accounting" to demonstrate that the hospital actually incurred a modest loss of $1 million in the most recent year. Renee understands the nature of the purchasing power adjustments that Olin made but is seeking a way to communicate this in a clear manner to the local press.

To adjust for the effects of changing price levels, the Financial Accounting Standards Board (FASB) has issued a number of pronouncements over the last 40 years. In September 1979, the FASB issued Statement 33, which required large public enterprises to provide supplemental information on the effects of changing price levels in their annual financial reports. In particular, Statement 33 required firms to disclose primarily current cost and constant dollar earnings; certain other income statement items; and current cost of inventory, property, plant, and equipment, in notes to the financial statements. This was a major step for the FASB and represented for the first time that firms were required to report price-level effects in their financial reports.

In 1986, when the inflation rate had subsided to less than 5%, the FASB substantially modified its initial position set forth in Statement 33 with the publication of Statement 89. This pronouncement left much of Statement 33 intact, except that it designated the reporting as voluntary. Consequently, most publicly traded companies stopped disclosing inflation-adjusted earnings. In Statement 89 business enterprises were encouraged, but not required, to report supplementary information on the effects of changing prices in the following areas for the most recent 5 years:

- Net sales and operating revenues, using constant purchasing power
- Income from continuing operations on a current cost basis
- Purchasing power gains or losses from holding monetary items
- Increases in specific prices of net plant, property, and equipment, net of inflation
- Foreign currency translation adjustments on a current cost basis
- Net assets (assets less liabilities) on a current cost basis
- Income per common share from continuing operations on a current cost basis
- Cash dividends per common share
- Market price per common share at year end

The rationale for these changes in financial reporting stems from the inaccuracy and inability of present historical cost reporting to measure financial position accurately in an inflation-riddled economy. Although the U.S. inflation rate has been low in recent years, inflationary pressures can increase at any time and will never be removed entirely. Many countries around the world still experience high inflation. Mexico and Brazil have required some accounting inflationary adjustments for over 20 years. Thus, inflation accounting will continue to be relevant.

Most people understand the effects that general inflation has on their purchasing power and they realize that a dollar in 2006 is not equivalent to a dollar in 2016. Most of us will intuitively make price-level adjustments to account for differences. A person who had a salary of $50,000 in 2006 and a salary of $50,000 in 2016 knows that their overall financial position has eroded because of increases in the Consumer Price Index (CPI). The accounting profession's task is to make its financial statement adjustments easy to understand by the vast majority of people who use and rely on these statements as scorecards of business success.

The major purpose of this chapter is to discuss and describe the major alternatives for reflecting the effects of inflation in financial statements. Specific methods are described and the adjustments that need to be made to convert historical cost statements are illustrated. This discussion should provide a basis for understanding and using financial statements that have been adjusted for inflation.

### *Learning Objective 1*

Discuss the major types of asset valuation.

## ▶ Reporting Alternatives

Methods of financial reporting can be categorized using two dimensions: (1) the method of asset valuation and (2) the unit of measurement. In chapter 8 we discussed five major principles of accounting. That list of five included the following two principles: cost valuation and a stable monetary unit. When historical cost values do not change and inflation or deflation does not exist, accountants can feel very comfortable using unadjusted historical cost as the method for valuing assets acquired by the firm. If asset values do change or the monetary unit is not stable, then alternative asset valuation rules may be needed. Two alternative methods of asset valuation are (1) **acquisition (or historical) cost** and (2) **current (or replacement) value**.

Asset valuation at acquisition cost means that the value of the asset is not changed over time to reflect changing market values. Amortization of the value may take place, but the basis is the acquisition cost. Depreciation is recorded, using the acquisition (historical) cost of the asset. Use of an acquisition cost valuation method postpones the recognition of gains or losses from holding assets until the point of sale or retirement.

Current valuation of assets revalues the assets in each reporting period. The assets are stated at their current value rather than their acquisition cost.

Likewise, depreciation expense is based on the current value, not the historical cost. Current valuation recognizes gains or losses from holding assets before sale or retirement. If it were easy to obtain objective measures of current asset values, all assets would be restated to current value, but in many cases objective measures of current value may not be obtainable.

### Learning Objective 2

Describe the alternative units of measurement in financial reporting.

There are also two major alternative units of measurement in financial reporting: (1) **nominal (unadjusted) dollars** and (2) **constant dollars** measured in units of general purchasing power. Use of a nominal dollar unit of measurement simply means that the attribute being measured is the number of dollars. From an accounting perspective, a dollar of one year is no different from a dollar of another year. No recognition is given to changes in the purchasing power of the dollar because purchasing power is not measured. The major outcome associated with the use of this measurement unit is that gains or losses, regardless of when they are recognized, are not adjusted for changes in purchasing power. For example, if a piece of land that was acquired for $1 million in 1996 were sold for $3 million in 2016, it would have generated a $2 million gain, regardless of changes in the purchasing power of the dollar during the 20-year period.

A constant dollar measuring unit reports the effects of all financial transactions in terms of constant purchasing power. The unit that is usually used is the purchasing power of the dollar at the end of the reporting period or the average during the fiscal year. The measurement is made by multiplying the unadjusted, or nominal, dollars by a price index to convert to a measure of constant purchasing power. During periods of inflation, when using a constant dollar measuring unit, gains from holding assets are reduced, whereas losses are increased. Thus, in the previous land sale example, the initial acquisition cost would be restated to 2016 purchasing power units to reduce the gain, as shown in **EXHIBIT 10-1**. Because the Consumer Price Index or CPI increased from 158.6 in 1996 to 239.2 in 2016, we restate the 1996 cost by the conversion factor (239.2/158.6 or 1.508).

Constant dollar measurement has a further significant effect on financial reporting: the gains or losses created by holding **monetary liabilities** or **monetary assets** during periods of purchasing power changes are recognized in the financial reporting.

**EXHIBIT 10-1** Restatement of Land Cost

| Unadjusted historical cost | |
|---|---|
| Sale of land in 2016 (CPI = 239.2) | $3,000,000 |
| Purchase of land in 1996 (CPI = 158.6) | $1,000,000 |
| Unadjusted gain on sale | $2,000,000 |
| **Purchasing power cost** | |
| Sale of land in 2016 (CPI = 239.2) | $3,000,000 |
| Conversion factor (CPI 2016/CPI 1996) | 1.508 |
| Restated cost of land | $1,508,000 |
| Adjusted gain on sale | $1,492,000 |

Monetary assets and liabilities are defined as those items that reflect cash or claims to cash that are fixed in terms of the number of dollars, regardless of changes in prices. Almost all liabilities are monetary items, whereas monetary assets consist primarily of cash, marketable securities, and receivables.

Purchasing power gains or losses are recognized on monetary items because there is an assumption that the gains or losses are already realized, because repayments or receipts are fixed. For example, an entity that owed $25 million during a year when the purchasing power of the dollar decreased by 10% would report a $2.5 million (0.10 × $25 million) purchasing power gain. All gains or losses would be recognized, regardless of the asset valuation basis used.

### Learning Objective 3

Define the major financial reporting alternatives.

The interfacing of the valuation basis and the unit of measurement basis produces four alternative financial reporting methods (**TABLE 10-1**). Each of the four methods is a possible basis for financial reporting. The **unadjusted historical cost (HC)** method represents the present method used by accountants; the other three methods are alternatives that would provide some degree of inflationary adjustment not present in the HC method. The **HC–general price level adjusted (HC–GPL)** method is often referred to as *constant dollar accounting*, whereas the **current value–general price level adjusted (CV–GPL)** method is referred to as *current cost accounting*.

**TABLE 10-1** Alternative Financial Reporting Bases

| | Asset Valuation Method | |
|---|---|---|
| **Unit of Measurement** | **Acquisition Cost** | **Current Value** |
| Nominal dollars | Unadjusted historical cost (HC) | Current value (CV) |
| Constant dollars | Historical cost–general price level adjusted (HC–GPL) | Current value–general price level adjusted (CV–GPL) |
| | Constant dollar accounting | Current cost accounting |

TABLE 10-2 summarizes the effects the four reporting methods would have on the three critical income statement items assuming price inflation: (1) depreciation expense, (2) purchasing power gains or losses, and (3) unrealized gains in replacement values.

*Learning Objective 4*

Describe the uses of financial report information.

▶ **Uses of Financial Report Information**

The measurement of financial position is an important function, and its results are useful to a great variety of decision makers, both internal and external to the organization. Changes in financial reporting methods unquestionably will alter the resulting measures of financial position reported in financial statements. These changes are likely to produce changes in the decisions that are based on the financial reports (FIGURE 10-1).

Lenders represent an important category of financial statement users who may change their decisions on the basis of a new financial reporting method. The lender's major concern is the relative financial position of both the individual firm and the industry. A decrease in the relative financial position of the industry could seriously affect both the availability and the cost of credit. If, for a variety of reasons, new measurements of financial position make the healthcare industry appear weaker than other industries, financing terms could change. Particularly for the healthcare industry, which is increasingly dependent on debt financing, the importance of changes in financial

**TABLE 10-2** Major Effect of Alternative Reporting Methods on Net Income Measurement

| | Impact Variables | | |
|---|---|---|---|
| **Reporting Methods** | **Depreciation Expense** | **Purchasing Power Gains/ Losses** | **Unrealized Gains in Replacement Value** |
| HC | No change | No change/not recognized | No change/not recognized |
| HC-GPL | Increase/GPL depreciation recognized | Gain or loss/depends on the net monetary asset position | No change/not recognized |
| CV | Increase/will recognize replacement cost | No change/not recognized | Gain/will recognize increase in replacement cost |
| CV-GPL | Increase/will recognize current replacement cost | Gain or loss/depends on the net monetary asset position | Gain/will recognize increase in replacement cost but will reduce amount by changes in the GPL |

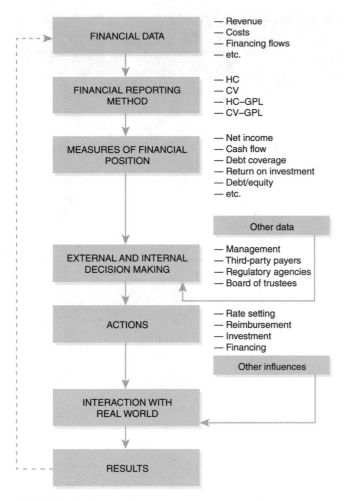

FINANCIAL DATA
— Revenue
— Costs
— Financing flows
— etc.

FINANCIAL REPORTING METHOD
— HC
— CV
— HC–GPL
— CV–GPL

MEASURES OF FINANCIAL POSITION
— Net income
— Cash flow
— Debt coverage
— Return on investment
— Debt/equity
— etc.

Other data

EXTERNAL AND INTERNAL DECISION MAKING
— Management
— Third-party payers
— Regulatory agencies
— Board of trustees

ACTIONS
— Rate setting
— Reimbursement
— Investment
— Financing

Other influences

INTERACTION WITH REAL WORLD

RESULTS

**FIGURE 10-1 Financial Data in Decision Making**

reporting methods cannot be overstated. Research on the results of changing to an HC–GPL or constant dollar accounting method has shown that the relative financial positions of individual firms and industries are also likely to change.

Changes in financial reporting methods also could have an effect on decisions reached by regulatory and rate-setting organizations. As a result of such changes, comparisons of costs across institutions may be more meaningful than they were previously. For example, depreciation in firms that operate in relatively new physical plants cannot be compared with the unadjusted historical depreciation costs of older facilities. Without financial reporting adjustments, new facilities may appear to have higher costs and thus be less efficient, whereas, in fact, the opposite may be true.

The actions of interested community leaders who have access to, and make decisions based on, financial statements also might be affected by reporting method changes. For example, suppose that individual, corporate, and public agency giving is in part affected by reported income. Many, in fact, regard reported income as a basic index of need, and the relationship between

income and giving seems logical. Thus, because each of the alternative financial reporting methods we have discussed will produce a different measure of income, total giving in each case could be affected.

Internal management decisions also might change with a new financial reporting method. Perhaps the most obvious example of such a change would be rate setting. Organizations that have control over pricing decisions and are not reacting to market-determined prices should set prices at levels at least high enough to recover their costs. The use of any of the three alternative methods of reporting will increase reported cost levels and therefore increase rates.

## ▶ Case Example: Williams Convalescent Center

In the remainder of this chapter, we show how adjustments are made in the income statement and balance sheet of Williams Convalescent Center, a 120-bed skilled and intermediate care facility, to take into account the effects of inflation. The center's two financial statements are shown in **TABLES 10-3** and **10-4**. You will note that values are reported for each of the following three reporting methods: (1) HC, (2) HC–GPL, and (3) CV–GPL. In this discussion, we do not describe or apply the CV method. The accounting profession presently is not seriously considering this method, and it is not likely to be considered in the future. The CV method suffers from a serious flaw: it does not recognize the effects of changing price levels on equity. In short, the CV method treats increases in the replacement cost of assets as a gain and does not restate them for changes in purchasing power.

**TABLE 10-5** presents values for the CPI. The CPI is the price index that is presently used by the accounting profession to adjust financial statements for the effects of inflation.

### Price Index Conversion

Both of the two methods we have selected to adjust the financial statements of the Williams Convalescent Center (CV–GPL and HC–GPL) use purchasing power as the unit of measurement. This means that unadjusted dollars are not the measurement unit for reporting accounting transactions. This means that all reported values in the financial statements are expressed in dollars of a specified purchasing power. Usually, the purchasing power used is the period end value. In our case example, Williams Convalescent Center uses purchasing power as of December 31,

**TABLE 10-3** Statement of Income for Williams Convalescent Center (in Thousands)

| | HC 20Y4 | Constant Dollar (HC–GPL) 20Y4 | Current Cost (CV–GPL) 20Y4 |
|---|---|---|---|
| Operating revenue | $3,556 | $3,625 | $3,625 |
| Operating expenses | 3,253 | 3,316 | 3,316 |
| Depreciation | 74 | 164 | 185 |
| Interest | 102 | 104 | 104 |
| Net income | $127 | $41 | $20 |
| Purchasing power gain from holding net monetary liabilities during the year | — | $43 | $43 |
| Increase in specific prices of property, plant, and equipment during the year | — | — | $136 |
| Less effect of increase in general price level | — | — | $144 |
| Increase in specific prices over (under) increase in the general price level | — | — | ($8) |
| Change in equity due to income transactions | $127 | $84 | $55 |

**TABLE 10-4** Balance Sheet for Williams Convalescent Center (in Thousands)

| | HC | | Constant Dollar (HC–GPL) 20Y4 | Current Cost (CV–GPL) 20Y4 |
|---|---|---|---|---|
| | 20Y3 | 20Y4 | | |
| Current assets | | | | |
| Cash | $98 | $21 | $21 | $21 |
| Accounts receivable | 217 | 249 | 249 | 249 |
| Supplies | 22 | 27 | 27 | 27 |
| Prepaid expenses | 36 | 36 | 36 | 36 |
| Total current assets | $373 | $333 | $333 | $333 |
| Property and equipment | | | | |
| Land | 200 | 200 | 530 | 525 |
| Building and equipment | 2,102 | 2,228 | 4,948 | 5,570 |

| | | | | |
|---|---|---|---|---|
| Total land and building and equipment | 2,302 | 2,428 | 5,478 | 6,095 |
| Less accumulated depreciation | 783 | 844 | 1,874 | 2,186 |
| Investments | 161 | 596 | 596 | 596 |
| Total assets | $2,053 | $2,513 | $4,533 | $4,838 |
| Current liabilities | 412 | 493 | 493 | 493 |
| Long-term debt | 1,203 | 1,478 | 1,478 | 1,478 |
| Partner's equity | 438 | 542 | 2,562 | 2,867 |
| Total liabilities and equity | $2,053 | $2,513 | $4,533 | $4,838 |

**TABLE 10-5** Consumer Price Index, Year-End Values

| Year | CPI |
|---|---|
| 20X0 | 119.1 |
| 20X1 | 123.1 |
| 20X2 | 127.3 |
| 20X3 | 138.5 |
| 20X4 | 155.4 |
| 20X5 | 166.3 |
| 20X6 | 174.3 |
| 20X7 | 186.1 |
| 20X8 | 202.9 |
| 20X9 | 229.9 |
| 20Y0 | 258.4 |
| 20Y1 | 283.4 |
| 20Y2 | 292.4 |
| 20Y3 | 303.5 |
| 20Y4 | 315.5 |

20Y4, as its unit of measurement. This means that we will restate all accounts to a purchasing power of 315.5, the CPI value at 20Y4.

Restatement of nominal or unadjusted dollars to constant dollars is a relatively simple process, at least conceptually. All that is required are the following three pieces of information:

1. The unadjusted value of the account in historical or nominal dollars
2. A price index that reflects the purchasing power in which the unadjusted value is currently expressed
3. A price index that reflects the purchasing power at the date the account is to be restated

For example, Williams Convalescent Center's long-term debt at December 31, 20Y3, is $1,203 (see Table 10-4). To express that amount in constant dollars as of December 31, 20Y4, the following adjustment would be made:

Unadjusted amount $\times$ 20Y4 CPI/20Y3 CPI

or

$$\$1,203 \times \frac{315.5}{303.5} = \$1,251$$

The value of the beginning long-term debt for the center would be $1,251, expressed in purchasing power as of December 31, 20Y4. The previously described adjusted method is the same for all other accounts. The price index to which the conversion is made is usually the price index at the ending balance sheet date (December 31, 20Y4, in our example). The price index from which the conversion is made represents the purchasing power in which the account is currently expressed. This value will vary depending on the classification of the account as either monetary or nonmonetary.

---

### Learning Objective 5

Describe the difference between monetary and nonmonetary accounts.

---

## Monetary Versus Nonmonetary Accounts

When restating financial statements from a system based on an HC method to one based on a constant dollar method, it is critical to distinguish between monetary accounts and nonmonetary accounts. Monetary accounts are automatically stated in current dollars and therefore require no price-level adjustments. Monetary items, discussed earlier in this chapter, consist of cash, claims to cash, or promises to pay cash that are fixed in terms of dollars, regardless of price-level changes. Nonmonetary accounts require price-level adjustments to be stated in current dollars.

Because of the fixed nature of monetary items, holding them during a period of changing price levels creates a **gain or loss**. For example, if a firm holds cash during a period of inflation, the firm will experience a monetary loss because the purchasing power of the cash has eroded over the holding period. Conversely, if a firm has a monetary liability during a period of inflation, it will experience a gain because it will repay the liability with dollars of a lower purchasing power. In constant dollar accounting, purchasing power is the unit of measurement, not unadjusted dollars. This can be seen in **TABLE 10-6**, which includes data from the Williams Convalescent Center (in thousands).

The data in Table 10-6 assume that a repayment of long-term debt and new issue occurred at the midpoint of the year, June 30, 20Y4. The price index at that point would have been approximately 309.5. This resulted from taking the average of the beginning and ending values (303.5 + 315.5) ÷ 2. In constant dollars, the Williams Convalescent Center would have reported $1,531 of long-term debt as of December 31, 20Y4. However, the actual value of the long-term debt at that date was $1,478. The difference of $53 represents a purchasing power gain to the center during the year. Because the price level increased during 20Y4, the value of the long-term debt actually owed by the center declined when measured in constant purchasing power.

Nonmonetary asset accounts must be restated to purchasing power as of the current date. The price index at the time of acquisition represents the price index from which the conversion is made. To illustrate the adjustment, assume that the building and equipment account of the Williams Convalescent Center has the age distribution presented in **TABLE 10-7**.

The data in Table 10-7 show that assets with a historical cost of $2,228 represent $4,948 of cost when stated in dollars as of December 31, 20Y4. The latter value is much more meaningful than the former as a measure of actual asset cost in 20Y4. It provides the center with a measure of cost that is expressed in dollars as of the current date and thus better represents its actual investment. Depreciation expense also should be restated in 20Y4 dollars to accurately portray the center's actual cost of using its building and equipment in the generation of current revenues.

---

### TABLE 10-6 Computation Purchasing Power Gains and Losses

| | Unadjusted Historical Dollars | Conversion Factor | Constant Dollars |
|---|---|---|---|
| Beginning long-term debt (12/31/Y3) | $1,203 | 315.5/303.5 | $1,251 |
| – Repayment (6/30/Y4) | 152 | 315.5/309.5 | 155 |
| + New debt (6/30/Y4) | 427 | 315.5/309.5 | 435 |
| Ending long-term debt (12/31/Y4) | $1,478 | | $1,531 |
| – Actual ending long-term debt (12/31/Y4) | | | $1,478 |
| Purchasing power gain | | | $53 |

**TABLE 10-7** Restatement of Nonmonetary Assets

| Year | Acquired Cost | Conversion Factor | Constant Dollar Cost (12/31/Y4) |
|---|---|---|---|
| 20X0 | $1,500 | 315.5/119.1 | $3,974 |
| 20X8 | 401 | 315.5/202.9 | 624 |
| 20Y1 | 201 | 315.5/283.4 | 224 |
| 20Y4 | 126 | 315.5/315.5 | 126 |
| | $2,228 | | $4,948 |

## Adjusting the Income Statement

### Operating Revenues

If one assumes that revenues are realized equally throughout the year, the restatement is significantly simplified. If the assumption is valid—and in most cases it is—it means that the revenues can be considered realized at the midpoint of the year, in our case, June 30, 20Y4. As already noted, the price index at June 30, 20Y4 can be assumed to be the average of the beginning and ending price index, or 309.5. The restated **operating revenue** would be calculated as follows:

Operating revenues × 20Y4 CPI ÷ 20Y4 mid-year CPI

or

$$\$3,556 \times 315.5 \div 309.5 = \$3,625$$

### Operating Expenses

Based on the same assumption that we used with operating revenues, the adjustment for **operating expenses** would be as follows:

$$\$3,253 \times 315.5 \div 309.5 = \$3,316$$

Operating expenses do not include depreciation or interest. Separate adjustments for these two items may be required.

### Depreciation

The depreciation expense adjustment is different from the earlier adjustments in two ways. First, depreciation expense represents an amortization of assets purchased over a long period, usually many years. This means that the midpoint conversion method used for operating revenues and operating expenses clearly is

not appropriate. Second, the adjustment methods for the HC–GPL or constant dollar and CV–GPL or current cost methods diverge. Depreciation expense may vary considerably because the current cost of the assets may differ dramatically from the constant dollar cost. Remember, a price index represents price changes for a large number of goods and services; specific price changes of individual assets may vary significantly from that index. For example, the general price level may have increased 20% in the last 5 years, but the cost of a specific piece of equipment may have increased 50% during the same period.

### Constant Dollar Adjustment

We estimate the depreciation expense value for Williams Convalescent Center under the constant dollar method by using the relationship of constant dollar buildings and equipment cost in Table 10-7 to historical cost. This gives us a multiplier of restated cost to historical cost that we can then apply to historical cost depreciation. The multiplier from Table 10-7 is calculated as:

$$\frac{\text{Constant dollar cost}}{\text{Historical cost}} = \$4,948/\$2,228 = 2.221$$

We then multiply this factor times the historical depreciation expense of $74 to yield a constant dollar depreciation expense of $164.

### Current Cost Adjustment

The identification of the current cost of existing physical assets is a subjective and complex process. To many individuals, the current cost method provides little additional value compared with the constant dollar method. Whether it will be eventually eliminated and replaced by the constant dollar method is not clear at this time.

The first issue to address is the definition of current cost. By and large, current cost can be equated to the replacement cost of the assets. In short, we must determine what the cost of replacing assets in today's dollars would be. This could be estimated through a variety of techniques using, for example, insurance appraisals or specific price indexes. In the case of Williams Convalescent Center, we assume that a recent insurance appraisal indicated a replacement cost of $5,570 for buildings and equipment. With this estimate, depreciation expense could be adjusted as follows:

$$\frac{\text{Appraisal cost}}{\text{Historical cost}} \times \text{Depreciation expense}$$
$$= \text{Restated depreciation expense}$$

or

$$\frac{\$5,570}{\$2,228} \times \$74 = \$185$$

## Interest Expense

We again assume that interest expense is paid equally throughout the year. This assumption produces the following interest expense adjustment:

$$\$102 \times 315.5 \div 309.5 = \$104$$

## Purchasing Power Gains or Losses

A purchasing power gain results if one is a net debtor during a period of increasing prices, whereas a purchasing power loss results if one is a net creditor during such a period. In most healthcare firms, purchasing power gains result because liabilities exceed monetary assets. A firm is thus paying its debts with dollars that are of less value than the ones it received.

To calculate purchasing power gains or losses, net monetary asset positions must first be calculated. The net monetary position for Williams Convalescent Center is presented in **TABLE 10-8**.

The actual calculation of the purchasing power gain for Williams Convalescent Center is presented in **TABLE 10-9**.

Because the center was in a net monetary liability position during the year, it experienced a purchasing

**TABLE 10-8** Net Monetary Asset Schedule

| | Beginning (12/31/Y3) | Ending (12/31/Y4) |
|---|---|---|
| Monetary assets | | |
| Cash | $98 | $21 |
| Accounts receivable | 217 | 249 |
| Prepaid expenses | 36 | 36 |
| Investments | 161 | 596 |
| Total monetary | $512 | $902 |
| Monetary liabilities | | |
| Current liabilities | $412 | $493 |
| Long-term | 1,203 | 1,478 |
| Total monetary liabilities | $1,615 | $1,971 |
| Net monetary assets | ($1,103) | ($1,069) |

**TABLE 10-9** Purchasing Power Gain (Loss) Schedule

| | Actual Dollars | Conversion Factor | Constant Dollars |
|---|---|---|---|
| Beginning net monetary liabilities | $1,103 | 315.5/303.5 | $1,147 |
| – Decrease | 34 | 315.5/309.5 | 35 |
| Ending net monetary liabilities | $1,069 | | $1,112 |
| – Actual | 1,069 | | |
| Purchasing power gain | | | $43 |

power gain of $43. This value is not an element of net income; it is, rather, shown below the net income line in Table 10-3. It thus affects the change in equity.

## Increase in Specific Prices over General Prices

The adjustment to consider—an increase in specific prices over general prices—is made only in the current cost method. The constant dollar method does not recognize any increases (or reductions) in prices that are different from the general price level. In short, no gains or losses from holding assets are permitted in the constant dollar method.

The calculations involved in this adjustment can be complex. In our Williams Convalescent Center example, we will make some assumptions to simplify the arithmetic without impairing the reader's conceptual understanding of the adjustment. We will assume the following data:

> Insurance appraisal of buildings and equipment, 12/31/Y3: $5,015
> Insurance appraisal of buildings and equipment, 12/31/Y4: $5,570
> Appraised value of land, 12/31/Y3: $500
> Appraised value of land, 12/31/Y4: $525
> New equipment bought on 12/31/Y4: $126

**TABLE 10-10** shows the increase in specific prices over general prices. These data show that, during 20Y4, the value of physical assets held by Williams Convalescent Center did not increase more than the general price level. In fact, there was an $8,000 decline in the specific prices of assets held by the firm when compared to the increase in general price level during the year. This may be a positive sign for the center if it is not contemplating a sale. The replacement cost for its assets is increasing less than the general price level. Therefore, revenues could increase less than the general price level and replacement could still be ensured.

## Adjusting the Balance Sheet

### Monetary Items

None of the monetary items—cash, accounts receivable, prepaid expenses, investments, current liabilities, or long-term debt—requires adjustment. The values of these items already reflect current dollars.

### Land

In our discussion of the increase in specific prices over the general price level in the Williams Convalescent Center's income statement, we assumed an appraisal value for land of $525. That value will be used here with the current cost method. With the constant dollar method, we will assume that the land was acquired in 20X0 for $200. To restate that amount to purchasing power as of December 31, 20Y4, the following calculation would be made:

$$\$200 \times 315.5 \div 119.1 = \$530$$

| **TABLE 10-10** Increase in Specific over General Prices Schedule | | | |
|---|---|---|---|
| | **Building and Equipment** | **Land** | **Total** |
| Ending appraised value less acquisitions of $126 | $5,444 | $525 | $5,969 |
| – Accumulated depreciation on appraised value | 2,186 | 0 | 2,186 |
| Ending net appraised value | $3,258 | $525 | $3,783 |
| Beginning appraised value | $5,015 | $500 | $5,515 |
| – Accumulated depreciation on appraised value | 1,868 | — | 1,868 |
| Beginning net appraised value | $3,147 | $500 | $3,647 |
| Beginning net appraised value restated for general price level (315.5/303.5) | | | $3,791 |
| Increase in specific prices over general price level ($3,783 less $3,791) | | | ($8) |

## Buildings and Equipment

Values for the center's buildings and equipment and the related accumulated depreciation already have been cited for the current cost method. We will assume those same values here. This produces a value for buildings and equipment of $5,570 (000s omitted) based on an appraisal. The value for accumulated depreciation was derived as follows:

Adjusted accumulated depreciation

= Unadjusted accumulated depreciation

$$\times \frac{\text{Appraised value} - \text{Current year acquisitions}}{\text{Historical cost} - \text{Current year acquisitions}} =$$

or

$$\$2,186 = \$844 \times \frac{(\$5,570 - \$126)}{(\$2,228 - \$126)}$$

## Equity

Equity calculations are not discussed in any detail here. It is enough for our purposes to recognize that equity is a derived figure. Equity must equal total assets less liabilities. In our Williams Convalescent Center example, this generates values of $2,562 for the constant dollar method and $2,867 for the current cost method.

## ▶ SUMMARY

Financial reporting suffers from its current reliance on the HC valuation concept. Inflation has made many of the reported values in current financial reports meaningless to decision makers. The example used in this chapter illustrates this point. The total asset investment of Williams Convalescent Center is approximately 100% larger when adjusted for inflation under the current cost or constant dollar method. Net income, however, decreased. The result is a dramatic deterioration in return on investment—the single most important test of business success.

**TABLE 10-11** summarizes return on assets and return on equity for Williams Convalescent Center.

These reductions are so drastic that they would prompt an investor to seriously question the continuation of the present investment, let alone replacement. More profitable avenues of investment very likely may be available.

To the extent that the Williams Convalescent Center example is representative of many healthcare firms (and it probably is), decisions regarding healthcare business continuation must be evaluated seriously. It is imperative that healthcare companies, like all other businesses, adjust their financial reports to reflect inflation. Whether the method used is current cost or constant dollar is not the issue. The important point is that ignoring the effects of inflation is unwise at best.

**TABLE 10-11** Effect of Alternative Reporting Methods on Financial Measures

| | Historical Cost | Constant Dollar | Current Cost |
|---|---|---|---|
| Return on assets (ROA) | | | |
| Net income/total assets | 5.1% | 0.9% | 0.40% |
| Revised ROA | | | |
| Change in equity due to income transaction/total assets | 5.1 | 1.9 | 1.1 |
| Return on equity (ROE) | | | |
| Net income equity | 23.4 | 1.6 | 0.7 |
| Revised ROE | | | |
| Change in equity due to income transactions/equity | 23.4 | 3.4 | 1.9 |

## ASSIGNMENTS

Use the data and information presented in **EXHIBIT 10-2** to answer the following questions:

1. What index was used to restate to constant dollars?
2. What method was used to determine current cost values?
3. Is the American Medical Firm (AMF) a net debtor or a net creditor?
4. In 2001, AMF showed a minus $24 million value for the increase in specific prices over general prices. What does this mean?
5. Why are AMF's net operating revenues in 2004 identical for the HC, constant dollar, and current cost methods of reporting?
6. Why is depreciation expense greater in the current cost method than in the constant dollar method?

## SOLUTIONS AND ANSWERS

1. AMF used the CPI, which is required by FASB 33 to restate historical costs to constant dollars.
2. AMF used specific price indexes to restate historical costs to current costs. This method contrasts with the use of appraisals discussed in the chapter example.
3. AMF is a net debtor. It has experienced a purchasing power gain in each year from 2000 to 2004. Because prices were increasing during that period, AMF must have had a net monetary liability position in each year.
4. In 2001, the specific prices of AMF's fixed assets must have increased less than the general price level as determined by using the CPI.
5. AMF does not restate revenues or expenses to the fiscal year end, December 31. Instead, they restate to the midpoint of the fiscal year, June 30. Because it is usually assumed that revenues are received equally throughout the year, the midpoint (June 30) would represent the index from which the conversion is made. Because AMF is converting to the midpoint index, the adjustment is 1.0.
6. Depreciation expense under the current cost method exceeds depreciation expense under the constant dollar method because the current cost value of depreciable assets exceeds the constant dollar value of depreciable assets.

**EXHIBIT 10-2** Supplementary Financial Information for American Medical Firm (AMF)

**Effects of Changing Prices**

The company's financial statements have been prepared in accordance with generally accepted accounting principles and reflect historical cost. The goal of the supplemental information that follows is to reflect the decline in the purchasing power of the dollar resulting from inflation. This information should be viewed only as an indication, however, and not as a specific measure of the inflationary impact.

The constant dollars were calculated by adjusting historical cost amounts by the CPI. Current costs, however, reflect the changes in specific prices of land, buildings, and equipment from the date acquired to the present; they differ from constant dollar amounts to the extent that prices in general have increased more or less rapidly than specific prices. The current cost of buildings and equipment was determined by applying published indices to the historical cost.

Net income has been adjusted only for the change in depreciation expense. Other operating expenses, which are the result of current transactions, are, in effect, recorded in amounts approximating purchasing power on the primary financial statements. Depreciation index was determined by applying primary financial statement depreciation rates to restated building and equipment amounts. Because only historical costs are deductible for income tax purposes, the income tax expense in the primary financial statements was not adjusted.

During a period of inflation, the holding of monetary assets (cash, receivables, etc.) results in a purchasing power loss, whereas owing monetary liabilities (current liabilities, long-term debt, deferred credits, etc.) results in a gain. Net monetary gains or losses are not included in the adjusted net income amounts reported.

| Consolidated Statement of Income Adjusted for Changing Prices ($ IN MILLIONS) | | | |
|---|---|---|---|
| | For the Year Ended December 31, 2004 | | |
| | As reported in Primary Statements (Historical Cost) | Adjusted for General Inflation (Constant $) | Adjusted for Changes in Specific Prices (Current Costs) |
| Net operating revenue | $2,065 | $2,065 | $2,065 |
| Operating and administrative expenses | $1,698 | $1,698 | $1,698 |
| Depreciation and amortization | 84 | 98 | 111 |
| Interest | 91 | 91 | 91 |
| Total cost and expenses | $1,873 | $1,887 | $1,900 |
| Income from operations | $192 | $178 | $165 |
| Investment earnings | $24 | $24 | $24 |
| Income before taxes on income | $216 | $202 | $189 |
| Taxes on income | $95 | $95 | $95 |
| Net income | $121 | $107 | $94 |
| Effective income tax rate | 44% | 47% | 50% |
| Changing price gains not included in adjusted income: Increase in specific prices (current cost) of property, plant, and equipment held during the year* | | | $139 |
| Less effect of increase in general price level | | | 68 |
| Excess of increase in specific prices over increase in the general price level | | | $71 |

| Financial Data Adjusted for Effects on Changing Prices ($ IN MILLIONS) | | | | | |
|---|---|---|---|---|---|
| | 2004 | 2003 | 2002 | 2001 | 2000 |
| Net operating revenues | | | | | |
| Adjusted for general inflation | $2,065 | $1,852 | $1,271 | $1,070 | $832 |

| Net income | | | | | |
|---|---|---|---|---|---|
| Adjusted for general inflation | 107 | 85 | 73 | 54 | 36 |
| Adjusted for changes in specific prices | 94 | 73 | 64 | 46 | 27 |
| Earnings per share | | | | | |
| Adjusted for general inflation | 1.54 | 1.29 | 1.18 | .95 | .82 |
| Adjusted for changes in specific prices | 1.35 | 1.12 | 1.04 | .82 | .61 |
| Purchasing power gain from holding net monetary liabilities during the year | 28 | 15 | 16 | 22 | 32 |
| Increase in specific prices of property, plant, and equipment over (under) increase in the general price level | 71 | 85 | 16 | (24) | .77 |
| Net assets at year end (total assets less total liabilities) | | | | | |
| Adjusted for general inflation | 1,095 | 972 | 756 | 657 | 413 |
| Adjusted for changes in specific prices | 1,332 | 1,162 | 894 | 809 | 470 |
| Cash dividends declared per common share | $0.43 | $0.39 | $0.34 | $0.28 | $0.21 |
| Adjusted for general inflation | | | | | |
| Market price per common share at year end: adjusted for general inflation | $20.24 | $29.41 | $12.39 | $24.30 | $11.66 |
| Average CPI—all urban consumers | 303.9 | 293.4 | 280.3 | 257.5 | 230.0 |

*As of December 31, 2004, current cost of property, plant, and equipment, net of accumulated depreciation, was $1,915 (his- torical cost $1,349). "Property, plant, and equipment" in both the previous and following data includes land held for expansion.

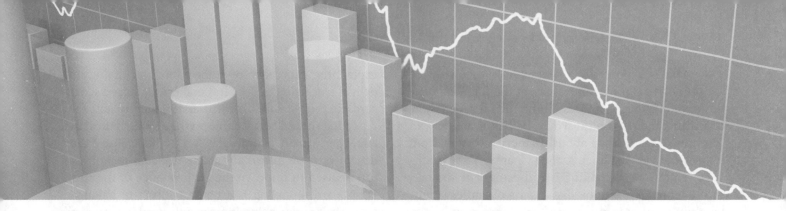

# CHAPTER 11

# Analyzing Financial Position

## REAL-WORLD SCENARIO

Michael Dean has been recently appointed to the board of Kenyon Medical Center, a 300-bed not-for-profit community hospital. Mike is an attorney who specializes in labor law and is the firm's primary litigation expert in this area. He is reviewing the financial information that was sent to him this morning in preparation for his first board meeting this evening. His total financial package includes 28 pages of financial information consisting of current monthly income statements, a balance sheet, and other monthly actual-to-budget comparisons of performance with some selected financial ratios.

Tonight's meeting is a critical one because the board's major item for discussion is related to a proposed bond issue to finance a major hospital renovation. Mike recognizes that he has a fiduciary responsibility to protect the assets of the hospital and to ensure its continued financial viability, but he does not know how to determine if the hospital can afford to take on this additional debt. There is so much information and no apparent pattern regarding what really is important. He is also concerned about assessing how the proposed financing would impact the hospital's financial performance and thus its ability to repay both interest and principal on the debt. He recently read a report on "dashboard reporting" and wonders if some structure like this would help him and other board members to get a better appreciation for the financial performance of the hospital.

The major purpose of this chapter is to introduce some analytical tools for evaluating the financial condition of healthcare entities. Think for a moment how confusing and difficult it would be, without a key, to reach any conclusions about financial position from many financial statements. (See Chapter 9 for examples.) Unless your training is in business or finance, the statements may look like a mass of endless numbers with little meaning. In short, there may be too much information in most financial statements to be digested easily by a general-purpose user.

During the last 30 years, there has been an explosion in the adoption and integration of information technology to financial reporting. Financial data are collected, analyzed, and distributed to decision makers in a more accurate and timely manner and in greater quantity than ever before. However, many people believe that the technology has not had a positive impact on performance. While we have made important strides in the technology of information collection and distribution, we have failed to realize significant improvements in the decision-making value of that information.

What accounts for the failure to take advantage of information technology advances? We think the answer is very clear and is one that most executives would readily acknowledge. We have been using the technology to deliver data, and more of it, to decision makers more rapidly, but we have ignored the issue of information relevance. As a result, we have in many cases simply used technology to deliver irrelevant or inappropriate data more quickly. Bad data delivered more quickly is not likely to improve performance in either the short run or the long run.

---

### Learning Objective 1

Describe the balanced scorecard and dashboard reporting.

---

In order to improve the collection and communication of financial and operating information **balanced scorecards** and **dashboards** were created. Essentially, these tools are neatly formatted reports that provide information on the organization's performance in a limited number of areas. The reports help focus attention to key performance indicators (also referred to as key metrics or measures) that are typically defined by senior leadership.

The concept of balanced scorecards developed by Robert Kaplan and David Norton represents an attempt to enhance the value of information and

exploit the capability of information technology to deliver true value to decision makers. Balanced scorecards, in their stripped-down version, simply state that reporting should be available on the key attributes that affect performance. More data are of little value if they do not provide information to a decision maker that can be used to improve the performance of the firm. Dashboard reporting is a natural subset of balanced scorecards and is being increasingly used in almost all sectors of the economy to keep managers focused on critical areas that will affect overall firm performance.

---

### Learning Objective 2

Describe the four key elements of dashboard reporting.

---

## ▶ Developing an Effective Financial Reporting System

Assuming that many healthcare providers are interested in developing a dashboard reporting system for key executives and board members, what needs to be done? In general, four critical questions must be answered:

1. What is most important to the firm's success?
2. What are the critical drivers that influence performance attainment?
3. What are the most relevant measures that reflect critical driver relationships?
4. What relevant benchmarking data are available to assess performance?

In the remainder of this chapter, we will answer these four questions with respect to financial performance. We will then examine a specific hospital example to illustrate the definition and utilization of financial indicators to assess financial performance and to identify critical opportunities for management intervention.

### Question One: What Is Most Important for Success?

Understanding financial performance in any business requires some global or summary measure of financial success. For many healthcare organization executives, this measure is often the operating margin (**operating income** divided by revenues). While **operating margin** is important, we believe that relying on this number as a measure of success can be misleading in many situations. For example, low operating margins may not always be bad and high operating margins may not always be good.

### Learning Objective 3

Explain what is most important in long-term financial success.

---

What should be the primary criterion for financial success in healthcare organizations? We believe that a financially successful organization is capable of generating the resources needed to meet its mission. This creates two immediate questions. First, what are resources? Second, what level of resources is needed to fulfill the mission? Economic resources that are owned or controlled by a business firm are referred to as *assets* and would include such items as supplies, equipment, buildings, and other factors of production that must be present to produce health services. Human resources are not usually shown as assets because the firm does not own an individual, but human resources also are required in the production of products or services. Resources or assets owned by a healthcare organization are shown in its balance sheet, which provides a listing of its assets and the pattern of financing used to acquire those assets. The level of resources required by a healthcare organization depends largely on the range and quantity of health services envisioned in the **mission statement**. In situations when there is no scientific standard for resource requirements, benchmarking against other healthcare organizations may be used to partially address the issue of resource need. A hospital or healthcare firm can find itself in a situation in which it may have too little investment in assets to meet the production needs for services, or it may have excessive investment in assets of a certain category.

Resources can be financed with either debt or equity funds, as any balance sheet clearly shows. A financially successful organization must therefore be capable of generating the amount of funds through debt and/or equity that is needed to finance the required level of resources. **FIGURE 11-1** depicts a simple balance sheet that illustrates these concepts. In this example, our healthcare organization needs to increase its investment in assets, or resources, by $100 million (to a total of $200 million) over the next 7 years to fulfill its mission. This level of future investment should be a byproduct of the firm's strategic plan. A strategic plan should provide some

information about projected service levels, which in turn should drive expected investment. Strategic financial planning is the topic of Chapter 13. The rate of annual compounded asset growth for the example in Figure 11-1 is approximately 10% per year. This rate equals the average rate of asset growth in many voluntary not-for-profit hospitals during the last 5 years. Although this growth rate may seem high, remember that this rate incorporates replacement of assets at higher prices, new technology, entry into new product lines requiring new investment, and increases in working capital such as accounts receivable. The healthcare organization depicted in Figure 11-1 has chosen a **financing mix** of 50% equity and 50% debt. This means that 7 years later, the target financing mix will be $100 million of debt and $100 million of equity to finance the $200 million investment in assets.

If an organization must grow to meet its mission then, given our discussion, it must be sensitive to how quickly it grows (the asset growth rate) and how it grows (the mix of debt and equity financing). The principle of **sustainable growth** states that no business entity can generate a growth rate in assets (10% in our example) that is greater than its growth rate in equity (also 10% in our example) for a prolonged period. It may be possible to generate new asset growth of 15% for several years when equity growth is only 5% by changing the percentages of equity and debt financing. There is no mystery in the principle of sustainable growth, and it is not some esoteric finance concept that bears no relationship to reality. Any business will have its asset growth rates limited by its ability to generate new equity growth. To not believe in

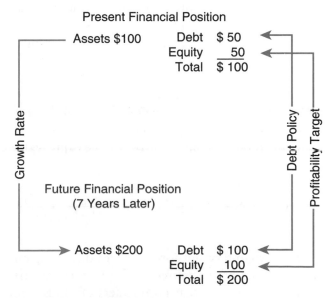

**FIGURE 11-1 Sustainable Growth**

the validity of this concept would imply that a firm could always increase its percentage of debt financing to any level. There are no exceptions to this theorem. It is not something that represents a nice target; it is a fundamental principle of business from which no one is exempt. Some governmental healthcare organizations may argue that they always generate growth rates in equity less than their asset growth because they get capital funds directly from their governmental sponsors. Those transfers represent a transfer of equity and are a part of equity growth. To be clear, the most important aspect of long-term financial success is sustainable growth.

---

*Learning Objective 4*

Explain what a firm's primary financial objective should be.

---

If sustainable growth (equity growth that meets or exceeds asset growth) is an organization's long-term financial goal, then there is no other financial objective that is more important than **equity growth**. Healthcare organizations that expect low rates of equity growth in the future most likely will not be able to provide the level of resources sufficient to meet their mission. If your healthcare organization anticipates growth rates in equity of only 5% over the next decade, it is almost certain that your asset growth potential will be no greater than 5%. Although the objective is not to add assets or investments for the sake of growth, healthcare organizations that remain viable must add new investments. Healthcare organizations with low rates of growth in equity most likely will experience most of their asset growth in working-capital areas, such as accounts receivable and supplies. These firms will invest very little in renovation and replacement of existing equipment and plant and very little in new capital required for entry into new markets. If they are surrounded by firms that are not experiencing low equity growth rates, their market share will decrease as their relative delivery capability deteriorates.

Growth rate in equity (GRIE) can be expressed as follows:

$$\frac{\text{Change in equity}}{\text{Equity}} = \frac{\text{Net income}}{\text{Equity}} \times \frac{\text{Change in equity}}{\text{Net income}}$$

Most voluntary not-for-profit healthcare organizations do not have a source of equity other than net income. This means that no transfers of funds from government or large restricted endowments exist to increase the firm's change in equity from the level of reported net income. In these situations, the term change in equity/net income equals 1; therefore, GRIE can be defined as net income divided by equity, or **return on equity (ROE)**. ROE is therefore the primary financial criterion that should be used to evaluate and target financial performance for voluntary not-for-profit healthcare organizations when transfers of new equity are not likely. ROE is also the primary financial criterion that should be used to evaluate and target financial performance for taxable for-profit firms.

In sum, to answer our first question of "what is most important" in dashboard creation, we believe that organizations must focus on sustainable growth in order to be viable long term. Sustainable growth, and equity growth in particular, can be measured by ROE. Therefore, the most important long-term financial metric that can be included on a financial dashboard is ROE. In the remaining portions of this chapter, we will explore how the relationships that drive ROE impact the rest of the financial dashboard.

---

*Learning Objective 5*

Describe the critical drivers of financial performance.

---

## Question Two: What Are the Critical Drivers of Performance?

At present, we only have one measure on our financial dashboard: return on equity (ROE). If improving ROE is our goal it is important to understand the underlying performance relationships that will impact that growth. ROE is simply defined as:

$$\text{ROE} = \frac{\text{Net income}}{\text{Equity (or Net assets)}}$$

However, ROE can be factored into a number of components that help executives analyze and improve their ROE values. The following equation also defines ROE:

$$\text{ROE} = \frac{\text{Operating income} + \text{Nonoperating income}}{\text{Revenue}} \times \frac{\text{Revenue}}{\text{Assets}} \times \frac{\text{Assets}}{\text{Equity}}$$

This alternative formula tells us that there are a variety of ways that an organization can improve its ROE. First, it can improve its operating margins (operating income divided by revenue). Second, it can increase its nonoperating gain ratio (nonoperating income divided by revenue). Third, it can increase its **total asset turnover** (revenue divided by assets). Fourth, it can reduce its equity-financing ratio (equity divided by assets). Operating margin improvement is an important strategy for improving ROE, but it is not the only way that ROE can be increased and sustainable growth achieved. **FIGURE 11-2** depicts the critical relationships affecting financial performance in most healthcare firms.

If we assume that ROE, or business unit value, is the primary measure of financial-performance success, the schematic in Figure 11-2 provides a road map of the critical drivers of performance. The schematic shows that the three primary determinants of value are profit, investment, and cost of capital. These three primary determinants of value can be related to a set

of macro drivers, and then ultimately to a number of micro value drivers that will enable measurement and modeling for effective dashboard reporting.

It is important for every healthcare firm interested in developing a set of measures to monitor and evaluate performance to start with a model similar to the one defined in Figure 11-2. Without this type of framework, many executives simply try to define a set of measures from those that currently exist or could be created. Defining measures without understanding key relationships can be dangerous. For example, reporting man-hours per discharge without adjusting for case-mix intensity can lead to erroneous conclusions and potentially bad decisions. Know your business before you determine how best to capture the essence of its performance.

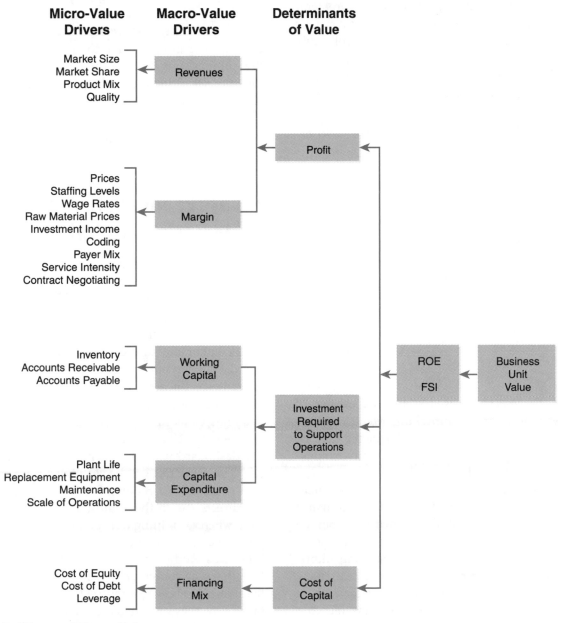

**FIGURE 11-2 Micro and Macro Drivers**

Discuss the importance of and types of performance measures.

## Question Three: What Are the Most Relevant Metrics?

Understanding the relationships that drive performance permits one to define **performance measures** that should focus management attention on areas that need correction. There is always a dilemma encountered in the definition of the measures that will be used for reporting. First, the absolute number of measures used must be limited. The measures used should have a high probability of problem/opportunity detection. For example, in our sample hospital's dashboard report, we assess the probability of a supply or drug cost problem by examining costs for four high-profile DRGs. Second, the measures should be naturally related to the key driver map developed earlier (Figure 11-2). In the case of our dashboard report we identify 13 critical performance driver categories:

1. Market factors
2. Pricing
3. Coding
4. Contract negotiation
5. Overall cost
6. Labor costs
7. Departmental costs
8. Supply and drug costs
9. Service intensity
10. Nonoperating income
11. Investment efficiency
12. Plant obsolescence
13. Capital position

Third, the measures used should be capable of external validation or benchmarking. Measuring current performance against past performance may be helpful in some cases, but ideally comparative industry benchmarks should be available.

Our hospital dashboard report contains 49 measures that are related to the 13 critical performance driver categories. Each of these measures can be related to external comparative data as well as to comparisons with individual market area competitors. Benchmarking data from competitors is extremely valuable. We discuss the measures used for each of the 13 performance drivers when we begin our case discussion.

## Question Four: What Benchmarking Data Should Be Used?

Comparative **benchmarking data** are crucial ingredients to the success of any dashboard-reporting system. Ideally, a business would like some comparative reference points. How am I doing with respect to similar firms in my industry? How am I doing relative to my primary competitors?

Identifying measures that are able to capture the nuances of revenue or cost drivers is nice, but it may be of little value if no external comparative benchmarks can be found. For example, most hospitals would like to measure and compare nursing cost on an acuity-adjusted basis, but uniform benchmarks are not currently available. In this situation, direct nursing cost per patient-day may be the best that one can do.

The measures that are used in this chapter for our case hospital allow external comparisons and competitor comparisons because the databases employed in measure definition are publicly available from the following sources:

- Medicare Cost Reports
- Standard analytical outpatient file (SAOF)
- MedPAR File

## ▶ Case Example: Harris Memorial Hospital

For the remainder of this chapter, we illustrate the use of financial analysis techniques through a case example: Harris Memorial Hospital and Harris Community Foundation (HCF). You will recall HCF from Chapter 9. We will be using the audit for HCF in Appendix 9-A to calculate many of the financial ratios in our dashboard. HCF has one primary competitor in its market: Eastside Healthcare. The primary hospital for HCF is Harris Memorial Hospital, a 430-bed facility. The primary hospital for Eastside Healthcare is Eastside Medical Center, a 170-bed facility. Many of the metrics on our dashboard will relate only to the primary hospitals. These metrics will be calculated from the public data sources (cost reports, SAOF, MedPAR) and will not directly tie to the audit. (See Appendix 9-A.) In sum, when examining our sample dashboard you can practice calculating the metrics when the data source is listed as "Audit," but cannot practice calculations for the other data sources. In the end, it is most important to understand how to interpret the metrics, not simply know how they are calculated. The dashboard can be found in **TABLE 11-1**.

**TABLE 11-1** Dashboard for Harris Memorial Hospital

| Data Element | Data Source | Formula | Harris Memorial Hospital | Eastside Medical Center | U.S. Median |
|---|---|---|---|---|---|
| **Overview** | | | | | |
| Return on equity | Audit | Excess of revenue over expenses/Net assets | 9.0 | 13.8 | 8.5 |
| Financial strength index® | Audit | [Total margin – 4%/4%] + [Days cash on hand – 120/120] + [50% – Debt financing%/50%] + [9 – Average age of plant/9] | 1.7 | 2.4 | −0.3 |
| Total margin | Audit | Excess of revenues over expenses/Operating revenue + Nonoperating gains | 7.5 | 8.3 | 5.0 |
| **Market factors** | | | | | |
| Inpatient revenue % | Public | Gross IP revenue/Gross patient revenue | 30.5 | 61.9 | 46.2 |
| Surgical cases % | Public | Medicare surgical discharges/Medicare total discharges | 35.6 | 38.3 | 23.7 |
| Market share % | Public | Net patient revenue/Sum of net patient revenue in county | 65.5 | 34.5 | 57.4 |
| Medicaid days %** | Public | Medicaid patient-days/Total patient-days | 23.2 | 12.4 | 19.4 |
| Medicare days %** | Public | Medicare patient-days/Total patient-days | 42.3 | 59.7 | 54.1 |
| Revenue growth (last year) % | Audit | (Operating revenue current year – Operating revenue prior year)/Operating revenue prior year | 7.3 | 10.5 | 5.4 |
| **Pricing** | | | | | |
| Average charge per Medicare discharge (CMI = 1.0)* | Public | All Medicare inpatient charges/(Number of discharges × CMI) | 25,052 | 27,506 | 22,506 |
| Average charge per visit (RW = 1.0)* | Public | Average Medicare visit charge/Average relative weight | 307 | 410 | 353 |
| Routine room rate* | Public | Average charge for routine care | 640 | 1,667 | 1,372 |
| Chest x-ray (71020)* | Public | Average charge for chest x-ray | 291 | 385 | 301 |
| **Coding factors** | | | | | |
| Change in Medicare CMI % | Public | Percentage change in Medicare case-mix index (2 years) | −1.9 | 3.4 | 2.1 |

*(continues)*

**TABLE 11-1** Dashboard for Harris Memorial Hospital    *(continued)*

| Data Element | Data Source | Formula | Harris Memorial Hospital | Eastside Medical Center | U.S. Median |
|---|---|---|---|---|---|
| Medicare CMI | Public | Measure of the costliness of cases treated by a hospital relative to the national average of all Medicare hospital cases, using DRG weights as a measure of relative costliness of cases | 1.7644 | 1.7439 | 1.5243 |
| CC/MCC capture rate | Public | The number of Medicare cases in MS-DRGs with a CC or MCC designation divided by the total Medicare cases | 67.0 | 68.0 | 60.0 |
| Average relative weight per outpatient visit (SMI) | Public | Based on weights for all CPT/HCPCS codes | 4.6 | 7.7 | 9.2 |
| Injectable drug without administration % | Public | Claim chosen if pharmaceutical item requiring injection or infusion present without the administration procedure | 24.1 | 8.1 | 10.0 |
| Contract negotiation | | | | | |
| Nongovernment payers % | Public | Percent of revenue from sources other than Medicare or Medicaid | 34.4 | 27.9 | 23.9 |
| Markup (charges/cost) | Public | (Gross patient revenue + Other operating revenue)/Total operating expenses | 2.8 | 3.8 | 3.3 |
| Deduction % | Public | Contractual allowances/Gross patient revenue | 72.6 | 67.5 | 69.9 |
| Net patient revenue per equivalent discharge™* | Public | Net patient revenue/Equivalent discharges™ | 6,683 | 8,701 | 7,798 |
| Cost position | | | | | |
| Hospital cost index* | Public | [(Average cost per Medicare discharge/U.S. median) × IP revenue%] + [(Average cost per visit/U.S. median) × Average OP revenue %] | 99.5 | 107.2 | 101.2 |
| Average cost per Medicare discharge (CMI = 1.0)* | Public | Medicare inpatient costs/(Medicare discharges average CMI) | 7,345 | 7,084 | 6,858 |
| Average cost per visit (RW = 1.0)* | Public | Average Medicare visit costs/Average relative weight | 76 | 92 | 79 |

| Labor costs | | | | | |
|---|---|---|---|---|---|
| Net patient revenue per FTE* | Public | Net patient revenue/FTEs | 179,127 | 141,281 | 172,373 |
| Man-hours per equivalent discharge™ | Public | Paid hours/Equivalent discharges™ | 68.3 | 105.5 | 102.0 |
| Salary per FTE* | Public | Salaries/FTEs | 75,171 | 69,181 | 60,809 |
| Departmental cost | | | | | |
| Direct cost per routine day* | Public | Direct routine costs/Routine patient-days | 411 | 509 | 451 |
| Direct cost per ICU/CCU day* | Public | Direct ICU and CCU Costs/ICU and CCU patient-days | 788 | 862 | 881 |
| Overhead cost % | Public | Overhead expenses/Total expenses | 37 | 34 | 34 |
| Capital costs per equivalent discharge™* | Public | Capital-related costs/Equivalent discharges™ | 768 | 469 | 572 |
| Supply and drug costs | | | | | |
| MS-DRG 247 supply cost | Public | Perc cardiovasc proc w drug-eluting stent w/o MCC | 2,895 | 4,764 | 3,839 |
| MS-DRG 470 supply cost | Public | Major joint replacement or reattachment of lower extremity w/o MCC | 4,668 | 6,346 | 5,667 |
| MS-DRG 194 pharmacy cost | Public | Simple pneumonia & pleurisy w CC | 1,166 | 585 | 787 |
| MS-DRG 603 pharmacy cost | Public | Cellulitis w/o MCC | 1,337 | 852 | 820 |
| Service intensity | | | | | |
| Medicare LOS (CMI = 1.0) | Public | Medicare inpatient-days/(Medicare discharges × CMI) | 2.7 | 2.5 | 3.0 |
| Ancillary cost per Medicare discharge (CMI = 1.0)* | Public | Medicare ancillary costs/(Medicare discharges × CMI) | 5,360 | 3,906 | 3,635 |
| Nonoperating income | | | | | |
| Days cash on hand† | Audit | (Cash and cash equivalents + Long-term investments)/[(Total expenses – Depreciation)/365] | 236 | 220 | 33 |

*(continues)*

| TABLE 11-1 | Dashboard for Harris Memorial Hospital *(continued)* | | | | |
|---|---|---|---|---|---|
| **Data Element** | **Data Source** | **Formula** | **Harris Memorial Hospital** | **Eastside Medical Center** | **U.S. Median** |
| Investment income/ investment % | Audit | Investment income/Total investments | 5.9 | 0.0 | 0.7 |
| Portfolio in equities % | Audit | Equity investments/Total investments | 58.7 | N/A | 50.0 |
| Investment efficiency | | | | | |
| Days in accounts receivable | Audit | Net accounts receivable/(Net patient revenue/365) | 30.8 | 72.0 | 53.0 |
| Inventory/Net patient revenue % | Audit | Inventory/Net patient revenue | 0.9 | 2.9 | 2.0 |
| Revenue/Net fixed assets | Audit | Operating revenue/Net fixed assets | 1.4 | 2.9 | 2.5 |
| Plant obsolescence | | | | | |
| Average age of plant | Audit | Accumulated depreciation/Depreciation expense | 11.1 | 8.2 | 11.1 |
| Two-year change in net fixed assets | Audit | [Net fixed assets − Net fixed assets (2 yr prior)]/ Net fixed assets (2 yr prior) | 37.2 | 44.6 | −2.4 |
| Capital position | | | | | |
| Long-term debt/ Equity % | Audit | Long-term debt/Net assets | 72.1 | 37.8 | 15.0 |
| Average cost of equity % | Public | Risk-free rate on U.S. government obligations + Estimated beta of firm × Market risk premium | 9.1 | 7.8 | 5.7 |
| Debt financing % | Audit | (Total assets − Net asets)/Total assets | 47.5 | 31.6 | 42.1 |
| Cash flow to total debt % | Audit | (Net income + Depreciation)/Total liability | 17.1 | 29.6 | 10.5 |
| Debt service coverage | Audit | (Net income + Depreciation + Interest)/ (Principal payment + Interest) | 6.9 | N/A | N/A |

CMI, case-mix index; MCC, major compication and comorbidity.

*Wage index adjusted metric to remove differences in cost of living.

**Medicaid and Medicare days % include government-sponsored health maintenance organization (HMO) days.

†DCOH for Eastside and U.S. median based on Medicare cost report (Worksheet G) and may be understated.

## Dashboard: Overall Performance

Three measures of overall performance are identified in Table 11-1:

- Return on equity (ROE)
- Financial strength index® (FSI)
- Total margin (TM)

For all three of these measures, larger values are desirable. A quick review of the data in Table 11-1 reveals a strong position for Harris when compared to U.S. medians. However, Eastside has better performance in all three measures. Before we discuss these measures, we will define them and compute values for 20X7.

$$ROE = \frac{\text{Excess of revenue over expenses}}{\text{Net assets}} = \frac{61{,}743}{684{,}619} = 9.0\%$$

$$TM = \frac{\text{Excess of revenues over expenses}}{\text{Operating revenue} + \text{Nonoperating gains}} = \frac{61{,}743}{800{,}209 + 26{,}310} = 7.5\%$$

$$FSI = \left[\frac{\text{Total margin} - 4.0}{4.0}\right] = \frac{7.5 - 4.0}{4.0} = 0.88$$
$$+$$
$$\left[\frac{\text{Days cash on hand} - 120}{120}\right] = \frac{236 - 120}{120} = 0.97$$
$$+$$
$$\left[\frac{50 - \text{Debt financing }\%}{50}\right] = \frac{50.0 - 47.5}{50.0} = 0.05$$
$$+$$
$$\left[\frac{9.0 - \text{Average age of plant}}{9.0}\right] = \frac{9.0 - 11.1}{9.0} = -0.23$$

$$= 0.88 + 0.97 + 0.05 + (0.23) = -1.67$$

Harris' value for ROE is 9.0%, which indicates that the firm has a positive bottom line. A review of the data shows that Harris has reported sizable balances of both operating and nonoperating income in 20X7 and 20X6. Also note the sizable increases in equity that resulted from unrealized gains on investments ($2,171,000 in 20X7 and $8,354,000 in 20X6). (See data in Appendix 9-A.) While these gains will not impact net income until the securities are sold, they did raise the level of total equity at Harris.

**Total margin** measures the return on revenue from both operating and nonoperating sources. Harris is realizing positive returns in both areas, but nonoperating returns in 20X7 were lower than those in 20X6.

The final overall measure is the **financial strength index®** (FSI). FSI attempts to measure the four areas of financial position that collectively determine a firm's financial strength:

- Profits—measured by total margin (normalized average target: 4%)
- Liquidity—measured by days cash on hand (normalized average target: 120 days)
- Debt expense—measured by debt financing percentage (normalized average target: 50%)
- Age of physical facilities—measured by average age of plant (normalized average target: 9 years)

Simply stated, firms that have high profits, lots of cash, little debt, and new plants have great financial strength. Firms with losses, little cash, lots of debt, and old physical facilities will not be in business long. Each of the four measures is "normalized" around a predefined average for the measure. This permits us to add the four measures to create a composite indicator

of total financial strength. Harris has a very strong overall financial strength index (FSI) due primarily to its favorable total-margin position and its strong cash position. Harris's strong cash position is also a factor that impacts total margin. In 20X7 nearly 50% of Harris's total net income was derived from investment income. Debt levels at Harris are also below normative values, which further enhances its overall financial strength.

A critical objective for Harris in coming years will be to maintain its current financial position and figure out how to better compete with Eastside, which has better ROI, margin, and overall financial strength. We now focus our attention on reviewing the 13 critical drivers of performance listed earlier to identify possible areas of opportunity for Harris.

## Market Factors

There are many factors that influence the financial performance of a healthcare provider, as the schematic in Figure 11-2 shows. Market factors play an important role in the final financial performance of any business. There are six measures of market factors identified in Table 11-1:

1. Inpatient revenue percentage
2. Surgical cases percentage
3. Market share percentage
4. Medicaid days percentage
5. Medicare days percentage
6. Revenue growth

*Inpatient revenue* at Harris is only 30.5% compared with 61.9% at its Eastside and 46.2% nationwide. In most situations, a higher percentage of inpatient revenue is desirable because profit margins are usually higher on inpatient product lines. For example, many U.S. hospitals make positive margins on Medicare inpatients but most hospitals lose money on Medicare outpatients.

Harris does a lot of surgery compared to U.S. averages but less than Eastside does. Usually, *surgical inpatient cases* are more profitable than are medical cases.

**Market share** is perhaps the most critical measure of performance in the market-factor category. High market share often leads to higher realized prices and lower cost per unit. If a healthcare provider had no competitors and operated as a monopoly, it could conceivably dictate price to all payer groups except Medicare and Medicaid. The market share position of Harris is higher than that of Eastside. Harris enjoys greater market share, which should give it a better contract-negotiation position. Because only two providers dominate this market, both hospitals should be able to demand and receive favorable contract terms because neither hospital has the capacity to service the entire market. We explore this further in the contract negotiation section.

In addition to the ability to negotiate more favorable reimbursement terms, higher market share also can provide significant improvements in profits because of lower cost per unit. Greater volume will spread fixed costs among more patients.

*Medicare and Medicaid percentages* provide an indication of payer-segment importance. Usually, Medicaid is perceived as a less desirable payer while Medicare in many hospitals is a desirable payer, especially for acute inpatient care. Harris appears to have an unfavorable relationship here. It has much higher Medicaid volume compared with its competitor and U.S. averages, while it has lower percentages of Medicare. Harris's geographical location has placed it closer to the Medicaid population than its primary competitor. Losses on Medicaid patients are substantial and, when combined with Medicare losses, create a need for higher payments from the limited private-payer base.

*Revenue growth* at Harris is above U.S. averages but below Eastside. This is most likely a result of Harris's greater growth in Medicaid volume. While revenue growth is desirable, revenue growth in profitable product lines is critical. Harris has experienced growth in some less profitable lines such as Medicaid, and this can hurt overall profitability.

Conclusions reached from our review of market factors are:

- Harris must concentrate growth strategies in product lines that are profitable, especially inpatient surgical areas.
- If market-share enhancement is not feasible, cost cutting must be pursued or unprofitable product lines must be eliminated.
- Reduced reliance on Medicaid business is desirable.

## Pricing Factors

Pricing can still have a sizable influence on a healthcare firm's profitability, even considering that many payers have fixed-fee reimbursement schedules. Of concern to many is the **price elasticity** of healthcare services. In simple terms, will volume drop if I raise prices? This is a difficult question to answer, but in many cases, price elasticity is believed to be negligible for many healthcare services. If a healthcare firm's prices are lower than those of its competitors, the issue of price elasticity becomes of less importance. The first objective is, therefore, to determine whether your prices are above or below those of your competitors. The four pricing measures are all developed from public data sets and are presented in Table 11-1. The data show that Harris has prices below its competitor's and the national average in all four metrics.

**Average charge per Medicare discharge** (CMI = 1.0) defines the average price for a Medicare discharge with a case-mix weight of 1.0. **TABLE 11-2**

| **TABLE 11-2** Illustration of Case-Mix Weighting | | | | |
|---|---|---|---|---|
| DRG | Case Weight | Number of Cases | Aggregate Case Weight | Total Charges |
| 1 | 0.80 | 10 | 8.00 | $64,000 |
| 2 | 1.20 | 10 | 12.00 | 96,000 |
| 3 | 1.60 | 10 | 16.00 | 128,000 |
| | | 30 | 36.00 | $288,000 |

$$\text{Average charge per case} = \frac{\$288,000}{30} = \$9,600$$

$$\text{Average charge per case} \left(\text{CMI} = 1.0\right) = \frac{\$288,000}{36} = \$8,000$$

$$\text{Average case weight} = \frac{36}{30} = 1.2$$

provides a simple example to illustrate how this measure is developed. Adjusting charges or cost to a case weight of 1.0 permits meaningful comparisons across firms. Table 11-1 also indicates that this measure for the U.S. median is stated in the hospital's wage index of 0.9246. This removes potential cost-of-living issues that might impair comparability. Charges for a specific discharge or an outpatient encounter are the product of two factors:

- Intensity of service
- Charges for specific procedures

An inpatient discharge has a large number of services provided, such as routine nursing, laboratory procedures, surgical procedures, drugs, and many others. Total charges may be high not because of high procedure prices but because of high utilization of services, for example, a long length of stay. A high total charge can also result from high procedure-level prices even in situations of low service intensity. Harris's inpatient charge per case is below that of Eastside and the U.S. average on a case- and wage-index adjusted basis. It is unusual that Harris has been able to maintain lower charges given its high Medicaid volume. High percentages of Medicaid are often associated with large indigent populations, which often increase prices to the private payer base. It is likely that Harris has been able to keep charges lower because of its higher market share.

**Average charge per Medicare visit** adjusted for relative weight is a concept similar to the average charge per Medicare discharge case-mix adjusted measure just described. It uses the weights assigned by Medicare to pay for outpatient procedures to case-mix adjust individual claims. We will discuss this measure further when we review cost measures. Data for the outpatient charge measure are similar to the inpatient measure just discussed. Harris has a charge structure below the U.S. average and its local competitor.

The last two measures, *routine room rate* and *chest x-ray* represent two specific high-volume procedures. Harris has lower prices for both.

Since prices at Harris are low compared to its competitor, a rate increase might be initiated with little or no damage to its competitive position. A rate increase of 5% would most likely keep Harris's prices in its same relative position because many hospitals change rates annually by about this percentage, but how much profit would result? The answer depends on the percentage of patients who pay for services on a charge or discounted-charge basis. **TABLE 11-3** provides some results for alternative charge-payer percentages. The possible improvement in profit from a price increase is large and could maintain Harris's profitability. Most hospitals have charge-payer percentages that are between 10 and 20%, so the range is realistic. In fact, many managed-care contracts provide for fixed case or per diem inpatient payments but more percentage-of-charge payments for outpatient care. Even in situations where payments are all set at fixed rates, most contracts contain charge-based components through outlier (where claims are paid on a charge basis once a certain dollar amount is reached)

**TABLE 11-3** Profit Resulting from Pricing Increase

| | Percentage-of-Charge Payers | |
| --- | --- | --- |
| | **10%** | **20%** |
| Present gross charges | $2,109,427,000 | $2,109,427,000 |
| *times* charge payer % | 10% | 20% |
| Charge-driven revenue | $210,942,700 | $421,885,400 |
| *times* rate increase % | 5% | 5% |
| Potential new charges | $10,547,135 | $21,094,270 |
| *times* average recovery % | 30% | 30% |
| **Profit Change** | **$3,164,141** | **$6,328,281** |

or lesser-of (where charges are paid unless the claim reaches the specific fixed payment rate) clauses that lead to net revenue impact from pricing changes. The price-setting function is described in greater depth in Chapter 6.

The conclusion reached from our pricing review is:

■ Harris should initiate a rate increase, approximately 5%, to put its rates closer to its competitor's. An increase of this size could generate close to $6 million in profit.

## Coding Factors

Coding can have a significant effect on the actual payment received in almost every healthcare sector, from physician services to hospitals, and for almost every type of payer, from self-pay to Medicare. Coding can also be a two-edged sword. Code too aggressively or fraudulently, and you may be prosecuted. Undercode patient services, and you will lose sizable legitimate payments.

In our hospital dashboard in Table 11-1, we identified five primary coding measures that assess Medicare inpatient and outpatient coding. Data for these measures are provided from publicly available sources.

**Medicare case-mix index** (CMI) provides an indication of the average complexity of Medicare inpatients seen. Table 11-2 provides a simple example to illustrate the computation of a case-mix index. In that example, the average case-mix index for the 30 patients was 1.2. Harris has a Medicare CMI of 1.7644, which approximates its competitor's value (1.7439) but is above the U.S. median (1.5243).

Of special interest is the 2-year decline in Harris's Medicare case mix. This decline compares to a 2.1% increase nationally and 3.4% increase at Eastside.

A more specific way to assess coding reasonableness is to review so-called **Medicare severity diagnosis-related groups (MS-DRG)** families—the payment classification system used by Medicare for inpatient hospital services. These are groups (usually two or three per group) of MS-DRGs in which possible missed information in the medical records could affect MS-DRG assignment. One of the most critical relationships to evaluate is the frequency at which patients are assigned into the higher weighted MS-DRGs. A patient is assigned to the higher weighted MS-DRG when the patient presents with a comorbidity or complication (CC or MCC). The **CC/MCC capture rate** shows that Harris assigns patients into the higher MS-DRGs 67% of the time— very close to Eastside and above the U.S. average. This

finding would suggest that Harris is likely not upcoding or downcoding, although there may be opportunities by individual MS-DRG families.

The last two measures in the coding area evaluate outpatient performance. The first is the **average relative weight per outpatient visit (service mix index)**. Similar to CMI for inpatient services, the SMI measures the resource intensity of outpatient services by measuring the number of paid HCPCS codes on each claim. Consider a patient that has an emergency room visit that carries an APC weight of 2.3 and a chest x-ray with a weight of 0.8. The total relative weight for this patient would be 3.1. To calculate the SMI, an organization would sum all the relative weights and divide by the sum of the patient visits. This metric shows that Harris has an average of 4.6 paid APC procedure weights per visit, which is below Eastside and the U.S. average. This implies that Harris has fewer Medicare-paid services per claim. A portion of this could be due to different services (perhaps Harris does more clinic visits that carry lower weights). However, it also could be that Harris is not capturing all of the services it is providing to patients when it is billing for them on patient claims. To evaluate the latter, we look at one example of outpatient charge capture: the percentage of Medicare outpatient claims with an injectable drug present but with no drug-administration code (injection procedure) present. This metric represents one of many where hospital administrators can tell charges were missed because one service demands another be performed. At Harris, this specific situation was present 24.1% of the time. In essence, nearly 25% of the time Harris missed the reimbursement it was due for administering a drug to a patient simply because the hospital failed to report it on the patient claim. This amount is significantly higher than Eastside and the U.S. average. Conclusions reached from our coding review are:

■ Harris should evaluate the sources of case-mix index decline.
■ Harris should pursue an outpatient claims assessment to determine where potential missed reimbursement opportunities are present.

## Contract Negotiation Factors

A popular saying in many management circles is, "You don't get what you deserve, but rather what you negotiate." The same appears to be true in the large number of managed-care contracts that healthcare providers negotiate with health plans. The contract terms are especially important to most healthcare providers because favorable terms here often spell the difference between financial success or failure. For most health-care providers, there is no opportunity to negotiate terms for Medicare and Medicaid payment. The terms are fixed and are made on a take-it-or-leave-it basis. The magnitude of patient volume in these two payer categories makes it a must for most providers. The real opportunity comes in negotiation of nongovernment payer terms.

We have provided four measures for contract negotiation assessment. Collectively, these measures help assess any possible weakness in current contract terms. The first measure is **nongovernment payers' percentage** and represents the percentage of revenues not derived from Medicare or Medicaid patients. A high number indicates greater relative importance of effective contract negotiation. Harris has a relatively high percentage of nongovernment payers (34.4%) relative to Eastside (27.9%) and the U.S. average (23.9%).

Harris has a lower **mark-up ratio** relative to both its competitor and the U.S. average. Because prices at Harris are below those of its competitor, the lower mark-up ratio is understandable. Most troubling for Harris, though, is that even with these lower charges the **deduction percentage** measure is higher. Deduction percentage shows the amount of contractual allowances deducted from gross charges. A lower percentage is clearly more desirable because additional net revenue would result with the lower value. Negotiating net payment closer to charges would reduce this value. Clearly, Eastside has an advantage because it has higher charges and lower deductions.

To summarize many of these elements we see, on a per patient basis, that Harris has a lower average payment through the **net patient revenue per equivalent discharge™** metric. This metric divides net patient revenue by equivalent discharges, which is a value meant to replace adjusted discharges for total patient volume. Problems with adjusted discharge metrics, which are common in hospital benchmarking, are described in the next section. The equivalent discharge™ (equivalent patient unit) methodology is further described in *Healthcare Financial Management* March 2011 issue titled, "A better way to measure volume and benchmark costs." The value for Harris suggests that payment per patient encounter is lower than the national average and significantly below Eastside. Four factors will influence this metric: payer mix, payer terms, pricing, and patient service utilization. We have seen issues in three of these factors: high Medicaid patient mix, low prices, and charge capture

issues would all drive down average payment. What can also be suggested is that contract terms could also be an issue, given that Harris has more market share and more nongovernment patients but significantly lower average payment levels.

Conclusions reached from our review of contract negotiation factors are:

- Harris does have lower average payment per patient encounter due, in part, to higher Medicaid and lower pricing and charge capture.
- Renegotiation of commercial contract terms to higher rates could be possible given its lower prices and higher market share.

Introduce the hospital cost-index measure.

## Cost Position: A Different Approach

We have already seen that Harris has lower relative revenue levels than Eastside. Still, the hospital has had good financial performance. What is the explanation? Costs must be a bright spot for the organization. To better assess relative cost positions, we can introduce a construct for reviewing total hospital cost. This construct is further described in a July 2002 article published in *Healthcare Financial Management*, "The hospital cost index: A new way to assess hospital efficiency." **FIGURE 11-3** provides a schematic of the methodology. Most hospitals currently use an adjusted-discharge or adjusted-patient-day output measure

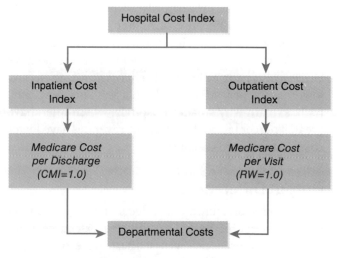

**FIGURE 11-3  Analysis of Overall Cost**

to compare costs on a per unit basis. We believe the adjusted output measures are flawed for reasons we discuss next.

## Problems with Adjusted-Discharge Measures of Cost

Most U.S. hospitals can divide their patient operations into inpatient and outpatient areas. Gross patient revenue is often subdivided along these lines. In the last 25 years, outpatient activity has gone from under 20% in most hospitals to close to 50% in 2008. This dramatic increase in outpatient revenue has caused more individuals to question the validity of incorporating outpatient activity into a consolidated measure of cost, using adjusted discharges or adjusted patient-days.

The critical measurement concept in an adjusted discharge or day measure is the weighting for outpatient revenue. The usual methodology for defining adjusted discharges or days is expressed as a formula:

$$\text{Adjusted discharges(days)} = \text{Inpatient discharges(days)}$$
$$\times \left[ 1 + \frac{\text{Gross outpatient revenue}}{\text{Gross inpatient revenue}} \right]$$

## Procedure Pricing

The computation of adjusted discharges is heavily influenced by specific procedure prices in the hospital's charge description master (CDM). Some hospitals may price procedures with high outpatient utilization at higher levels to take advantage of the greater presence of "percentage of billed charges" payment arrangements. Other hospitals may keep high outpatient procedures at lower levels because of a large self-pay presence, implying greater price elasticity. Some data suggest that the majority of hospitals overstate outpatient costs because of higher procedure prices. If this is so, hospitals with heavier percentages of outpatient activity or higher outpatient prices would have larger values for adjusted discharges and, therefore, lower costs per adjusted discharge. This may partially explain why smaller hospitals, which often have greater percentages of outpatient revenue, have lower costs per adjusted discharge.

## Output Differences

Another major factor that affects the comparability of cost measures using an adjusted-discharge basis is output differences. Even if there were only inpatient discharges and no outpatient activity, discharges would not be an ideal measure to make comparisons

of cost across hospitals because of case-mix differences. Many cost-per-adjusted-discharge measures are further adjusted by dividing by the case-mix index of the hospital for the time period. There are two alternative case-mix indexes that are often used:

- All-payer case-mix index
- Medicare case-mix index

Obviously, the all-payer case-mix index will do a better job of reflecting output differences than will a Medicare-only case-mix index. There is one major issue, however, with the utilization of all-payer case-mix-index adjustments. You may be able to adjust your cost for case-mix effects, but will the external comparative cost measures be adjusted in similar fashion? Competitor data extracted from public-use files such as Medicare Cost Reports will not have all-payer case-mix-index values. For controlled subscriber-based benchmarking services, the all-payer case-mix-index adjustments may be accurate, but the comparisons will be limited to other subscribing hospitals and will exclude specific competitor comparisons.

For the above reasons, Medicare case-mix-index adjustments are often utilized in a number of comparative reports. In many cases, the Medicare case-mix index can remove cost variance and better isolate possible problems. The Medicare case-mix-index adjustment will be an issue, however, when the non-Medicare patient population differs dramatically from the Medicare patient population. For example, a hospital that specialized in orthopedics and obstetrics would present problems. Using the Medicare case-mix index would grossly overstate case-mix complexity because all of the obstetric cases, which would be lower case weighted, would be non-Medicare.

## Geographical Cost-of-Living Differences

The final area affecting the comparability of cost-per-adjusted-discharge (CPAD) measures is geographic cost-of-living differences. Hospitals in Oakland, California, have higher operating costs than do hospitals in rural North Dakota. The usual method of adjustment is to divide the unadjusted cost measure by the local area cost-of-living index. This division would restate costs into a cost-of-living index equal to 1.0. The wage index used by Medicare is the most often-used index and may be applied to total cost or some percentage of total cost. The rationale for a percentage is that some portion of hospital costs, for example, supplies, may not be affected by cost-of-living differences. Medicare assumes that the wage index affects 71% of total cost. The remaining 29% is presumed to be unaffected by wage variation.

Cost-of-living differences are important, and the adjustments can be easily handled. Of the three problems affecting cost comparability (procedure pricing, output differences, and geographical cost-of-living differences), cost-of-living differences can be resolved. The problems with procedure pricing and output differences are still present in a CPAD measure, even after case-mix indexes have been applied.

## Hospital Cost Index® (HCI)

We believe that a better measure of facility-wide hospital costliness can be constructed by weighting two measures:

1. Medicare cost per discharge, case-mix and wage-index adjusted (MCPD)
2. Medicare cost per outpatient visit, relative value unit and wage-index adjusted (MCPV)

The HCI is then constructed as follows:

$$HCI = \% \text{ Inpatient revenue} \times \frac{MCPD}{U.S. \text{ median}}$$
$$+ \% \text{ Outpatient revenue} \times \frac{MCPV}{U.S. \text{ median}}$$

**Medicare Cost per Discharge (MCPD)** MCPD is a good reflection of inpatient cost. Data for computing this measure can be derived from the public-use files: MedPAR and Medicare Cost Reports. Each Medicare inpatient claim is costed using the relevant departmental ratio of cost-to-charge (DRCC) values derived from the Medicare Cost Report applied to charges from the inpatient claim. The DRCC values are mapped to specific revenue codes in the claims file. Finally, a wage index assigned to the hospital by Medicare is used to restate costs to an index of 1.0. This process results in

a unique publicly available number for most hospitals in the United States.

The MCPD is not a perfect measure of relative inpatient costs, but we believe it is better than any other publicly available measure of cost or inpatient cost at the facility level for several reasons.

- The output unit is more comparable than any other.
- There is no application of outpatient-equivalent discharges to distort output similarity.
- The case-mix index used to adjust is specific to those patients and is not extended to non-Medicare patients.
- The cost measures are adjusted using department-specific cost-to-charge ratios, not facility-wide cost-to-charge ratios.
- The costs are adjusted for cost-of-living differences.

The major problem with MCPD is its comprehensiveness. In short, the measure may or may not be reflective of costs in other non-Medicare areas. We believe that this is not a major issue for the following reasons. First, Medicare represents the largest payer for most hospitals: approximately 54% of all inpatient-days. Second, with fixed payment per DRG, there is an incentive to keep costs low. If costs are high in the Medicare area, they will most likely be high in other non-Medicare areas.

**Medicare Cost per Outpatient Visit (MCPV)** We use MCPV to assess costliness on the outpatient side of hospital operations. We can construct this measure from public-use files (Medicare Outpatient Claims and Medicare Cost Reports), which makes its availability a reality for most U.S. hospitals. To derive the measure, we divide the cost per claim defined through the DRCC extensions by the relative value units of the claim. We estimate RVUs based on the taxonomy presented in **TABLE 11-4**.

**TABLE 11-4** Determination of Relative Value Units

| Line-Item Type | Relative Value Unit Assignment |
|---|---|
| APC | APC weight |
| Fee schedule | Fee schedule/national price per APC = 1.0 |
| Pass-through drug and biologicals | Average wholesale price/national price per APC = 1.0 |
| Pass-through device | Estimate payment/national price per APC = 1.0 |

APC, ambulatory payment classification.

We believe the introduction of the Medicare outpatient prospective payment system (OPPS) has provided an opportunity to adjust outpatient costs for relative value unit differences in a manner similar to case-mix-index adjustment on the inpatient side. We do not know of any other measure of facility-wide outpatient cost that incorporates relative value unit adjustment to this degree. Medical groups have used resource-based relative value scales (RBRVS) measure, but these were not applicable to hospital outpatient operations.

The MCPV is not a perfect measure of outpatient costliness. Like the MCPD, the MCPV does not necessarily reflect cost for non-Medicare patients. Medicare patients are, however, a significant percentage of total outpatient business. Medicare also pays on a fixed-fee basis now, so a strong incentive should exist to keep costs low. If costs are high for Medicare outpatients, it seems reasonable to conclude that they would be high for other categories.

**Merging the MCPD and the MCPV** The final step in the development of the HCI is to combine the MCPD and MCPV. To combine these two measures, we must weight them by the percentage of business activity. The MCPD is, therefore, multiplied by the percentage of inpatient revenue, and the MCPV is multiplied by the percentage of outpatient revenue. The total of inpatient revenue and outpatient revenue percentages should equal 1.0. Data for these values can be taken from Medicare Cost Reports.

The final step is to "normalize" the MCPD and MCPV around some central value. We use the current U.S. median values for both measures.

## Overall Cost Factors

Using the three measures just described (HCI, MDPD, and MCPV), we can see from Table 11-1 that Harris is a lower-cost hospital with respect to both its primary competitor and the U.S. average. Harris's HCI is currently at 99.5, which is slightly below the U.S. average (101.2) and its primary competitor (107.2). However, the data does show us that Harris has a greater opportunity for cost reduction in the inpatient arena where its cost per discharge on a case-mix basis is above both its competitor and U.S. averages.

## Labor Cost Factors

Healthcare providers in general and hospitals in particular are labor-intensive operations. More than 50% of their costs are connected to staffing. To analyze labor costs, we have selected two measures of productivity and one measure of compensation.

Collectively, the labor-cost measures communicate a mixed message. *Salary costs* at Harris are higher compared to U.S. averages and also high relative to its competitor. While some of the difference is due to higher physician employment at Harris, the sizable gap should be explored further.

**Labor productivity** at Harris is better on both measures when compared to its competitor. The two productivity measures (**net patient revenue per FTE** and **man-hours per equivalent discharge**™) show that Harris generates more revenue dollars with fewer full-time-equivalent employees and/or employee hours.

Conclusions reached from our review of labor cost factors are:

- Compensation costs appear out of line with U.S. averages and those of its competitor. Harris should explore department-specific compensation standards to ensure appropriate payment levels.
- Labor productivity appears to be better than competitor values.

## Departmental Cost Factors

We have included four measures of departmental cost:

1. Nursing cost measures
   a. Direct cost per routine day
   b. Direct cost per ICU/CCU day
2. Overhead measures/adjusted patient-day
   a. Capital-related cost per equivalent discharge™
   b. Overhead cost percentage

*Direct routine nursing costs* are below Eastside's values in the routine and ICU/CCU areas. These cost measures include only the direct cost of the department and do not include overhead allocations. The cost data are extracted from filed Medicare Cost Reports.

The two overhead measures of cost suggest some inefficiency. Harris appears to have higher **overhead costs** (costs in nonrevenue-producing departments) than Eastside. In addition, Harris has higher **capital costs** (investment in equipment and facilities) when compared to Eastside and the U.S. median. These areas should be targeted for further review.

Conclusions reached from the review of departmental cost factors are:

- Harris has lower direct nursing costs per day. This is a result of increased productivity as there appears to be higher salaries.
- Overhead costs at Harris are high, especially in the capital-related area.

## Supply and Drug Costs

Supply and drug costs can be significant factors for a large number of medical and surgical procedures. The magnitude of total supply and drug costs is complicated because of the underlying factors that influence cost. Total supply and drug costs are a product of quantity used and price paid. Lower costs can be realized by either reducing the intensity of usage or reducing the price paid. The issue is often complicated by physician preferences. Healthcare executives can attempt to influence physician behavior in supply or drug selection, but ultimately, the physician will determine which drug or supply item will be used and in what quantity.

We have provided four measures of inpatient supply and drug costs. Two of these measures define supply costs for MS-DRGs whose supply costs are usually sizable:

- MS-DRG 247—Percutaneous cardiovascular procedure with drug-eluting stent w/o MCC
- MS-DRG 470—Major joint replacement or reattachment of lower extremity w/o MCC

Both measures indicate that Harris has costs much lower than U.S. averages and also much lower than competitor values. While the variance exists, the explanation is not clear without further review. Possible explanations could be:

- Better negotiated purchase contracts, which result in lower prices
- Use of less expensive supply items by physicians
- Quantity of medical supplies used throughout the patient encounter

Two MS-DRG drug-cost measures are also reviewed:

- MS-DRG 194—Simple pneumonia and pleurisy w CC
- MS-DRG 603—Cellulitis w/o MCC

Harris appears to have higher drug costs than the U.S. average and its competitor. The underlying issues exist in higher rates for the drugs either due to contracted price or physician selection and/or higher quantity of drugs used.

Conclusions reached from our review of drug and supply costs are:

- Drug costs appear to be high compared to its competitor and national data.
- Review of drug costs with the pharmacy department and selected physicians should be undertaken with the desired outcome of drug price reductions and usage standardization.

## Service Intensity

Service intensity is a critical driver of healthcare cost. Cost per encounter of service can be defined as:

$$\frac{\text{Services}}{\text{Encounters}} \times \frac{\text{Inputs}}{\text{Services}} \times \text{Prices of resources}$$

Each of these three factors will drive total healthcare costs. The first term (services/encounters) is referred to as **service intensity**. The two major drivers of service intensity for inpatient care are **length of stay** and **ancillary service usage**. We have, therefore, included two measures to help assess service intensity:

- Medicare length of stay, case-mix-index adjusted
- Medicare ancillary cost per discharge, case-mix-index adjusted

Both of these measures are taken from Medicare data and are case-mix adjusted to 1.0. The use of these measures assures that there will be comparability across hospitals because the measures are "apple-to-apple" comparisons

Harris has a low length of stay on a case-mix-adjusted basis when compared to the U.S. median. Its value, however, is above its primary competitor's. Its low length of stay is a reason its cost per discharge is comparable to the national average.

Ancillary costs are above U.S. averages and warrant review. Prior discussion has already disclosed high prices paid for drug items. This is most likely the cause for the variance. It should also be noted that a higher length of stay, relative to Eastside, may also affect the ancillary cost comparison.

The conclusion reached from our service intensity review is:

- Harris has significant opportunity for ancillary savings. Higher drug costs, as seen previously, may explain a sizable portion of the difference.

## Nonoperating Income

Many not-for-profit healthcare providers, especially hospitals, derive a large percentage of their total net income from nonoperating sources. The usual source of nonoperating income for most hospitals is investment income. Data show this to be especially true for Harris. (See Appendix 9-A.)

We have defined three measures to assess performance in the nonoperating income area:

1. Days cash on hand
2. Investment yield
3. Portfolio in equities

Harris has a very sizable investment in securities, as seen from its **days cash on hand** (DCOH) value of 236 days. Only investments that are not restricted by donors or third parties are included. This explains why trustee-held funds ($51,038) and donor-restricted funds ($84,440) are excluded. DCOH measures the number of days an organization could continue to operate given its current level of cash and operating expenses.

Harris also has a very sizable percentage of its investment in equities: 58.7%. This high percentage of equity investment can increase yields, but risk is also increased. Investment income includes both interest and dividend income, as well as realized gains or losses on securities sold during the period.

Conclusions for Harris with respect to its investment portfolio are:

- Review current investment strategy and perhaps place equity investment in funds that replicate broad market segments such as the Standard and Poor's 500 or the Wilshire 5000.
- Determine if Harris is willing to assume the relatively high risk of equity investments or whether a reduced reliance on equity funds is more consistent with projected needs for these funds.

## Investment Efficiency Factors

As discussed earlier in this chapter, it is not the amount of profit realized that is of prime concern but rather the amount of profit in relation to investment. For most healthcare providers, the three critical areas of control are plant, property, and equipment; accounts receivable; and inventory. To assess performance in these three areas, we have defined three measures that assess the productivity of investment:

1. Days in accounts receivable
2. Inventory to net patient revenue
3. Revenue to net fixed assets (fixed asset turnover)

Harris has good investment productivity with respect to both accounts receivable. High values for *receivables* can be the result of many factors but, in general, result from three primary causes:

- Payment delays by payers, especially commercial health plans
- Large balances of old accounts whose collection is suspect
- Billing delays that prevent prompt invoicing of provided care

However, the very low number of days in accounts receivable could also present a problem for Harris.

At times, collections managers may close delinquent accounts and write off the claim balance to bad debt. At times, managers are incentivized to keep days in accounts receivable low, and this action could prohibit collection from accounts that would pay if given more time.

Harris appears to have excess *investment in net fixed assets*. It currently generates 1.42 of operating revenue per dollar of investment in net fixed assets compared to a U.S. average of 2.45 and a competitor value of 2.93. Determining the desired level of investment in fixed assets is not an easy decision and is heavily influenced by a large number of stakeholders in the firm, including doctors, board members, employees, and the community. **Long-term investment** levels in property and equipment are often a part of the firm's strategic plan and reflect perceived community needs as well as financial and marketing objectives. Many not-for-profit healthcare executives often forget that capital has a real cost and excessive fixed-asset investment can impair the firm's long-term financial viability.

What is the potential cost of Harris's excessive investment in fixed assets? There are several ways that this could be measured. First, we could isolate the direct costs of the excessive investment in terms of depreciation and interest expense. Second, we could impute some opportunity cost of the excess investment, using the expected yield on alternative investments. Third, we could multiply the firm's estimated cost of capital times the excess investment.

To determine the amount of excess investment in fixed assets, we need a target revenue to fixed assets standard. For this purpose, let's use the U.S. median of 2.45. The desired level of investment in fixed assets would be:

$$\frac{\text{Operating revenue}}{\text{Target revenue to fixed assets}} = \frac{\$800,209}{2.45} = \$326,616$$

Harris has $236,733,000 in excess investment ($563,349,000 − $326,616,000). This surplus investment represents 42% of Harris's present investment in net fixed assets. Assuming that 42% of the firm's depreciation and interest is not necessary produces one estimate of annual cost:

$$0.42 \times (\$44,392,000 + \$10,974,000) = \$23,253,720$$

Alternatively, we could assume a possible yield on risk-free investment of 6.0% as our opportunity cost. This would produce an annual savings of $14,203,985 ($0.06 \times \$236,733,000$).

No matter what method of cost savings is used, Harris has a heavy cost associated with its excess investment in fixed assets. Much of this surplus is a direct result of intense physician pressure to finance new investment in clinic facilities to support the integrated network of services provided by Harris.

Conclusions reached from our investment efficiency review are:

■ Receivables are low at Harris, primarily due good management. However, claims should be reviewed to ensure that accounts are not being closed too quickly.
■ Fixed asset investment at Harris is $237 million above typical U.S. averages. This surplus investment could cost Harris somewhere between $14 million and $23 million annually. Tighter capital expenditure review policics need to be implemented to prevent this problem from getting worse.

## Plant Obsolescence Factors

While excessive investment in fixed assets can impair the realization of reasonable return on investment, investment in old facilities and outdated technology can be fatal. If a healthcare firm, especially a hospital, has old and outdated facilities, it will likely affect the quality of care rendered to its patients. It may also lead medical staff to practice at facilities where they believe the welfare of their patients may be better served. We have defined two measures to assess the issue of plant obsolescence:

1. Average age of plant
2. Two-year capital expenditure growth rate

Harris has been spending more on fixed assets than U.S. averages in the last 2 years, a likely response to its significantly older plant age and to keep pace with Eastside's significant investments.

The conclusion regarding plant obsolescence is:

■ Harris has made some large investments to keep up with current technology and has been replacing its current physical facilities and investing in new areas.

## Capital Position

The last area of performance factors to be reviewed is capital position. Successful firms have profitable operations with reasonable levels of investment. They also keep their cost of financing at a reasonable level. Capital funds in any firm are provided from either debt or equity, and each has a cost. Debt has an explicit cost

that can be easily determined by either examining current financing documents or obtaining present bond market yields. Debt also affects the cost of equity capital. Higher levels of debt or financial leverage increase the risk of business failure and lead to higher required returns for invested equity capital, irrespective of its source. A religious, government, community, or investor-owned firm must obtain higher returns on its equity as it raises the level of risk through increased borrowing. We have identified five measures of capital position:

1. Debt financing percentage
2. Long-term debt-to-equity percentage
3. Average cost of equity percentage
4. Cash flow to debt percentage
5. Debt service coverage

Harris has a reasonable overall level of liabilities with 47.5% of its assets financed through current and long-term debt. This value is consistent with the U.S. average but is well above Eastside. Of more concern, however, is the higher long-term debt to equity percentage. Harris has borrowed extensively to finance its capital investment program but has also used its extensive capital reserves. This increased debt has raised the cost-of-equity capital. Harris's cost-of-equity capital is explained in **FIGURE 11-4**. The cost of a firm's equity increases as debt financing rises, but the firm's weighted cost of capital may not increase. Weighted cost of capital is defined as:

$$\{[\text{Long-term debt} / (\text{Long-term debt} + \text{Equity})]$$
$$\times \text{Interest rate on debt}\} +$$
$$\{[\text{Equity}/(\text{Long-term debt} + \text{Equity})] \times \text{Cost of equity}\}$$

$$\{[493,597 / (439,597 + 684,619)] \times 5.1\%\} + \{[684,619 /$$
$$(439,597 + 684,619)] \times 10.2\%\} = 8.2\%$$

Harris has increased its debt position. Most of its debt is variable rate, with average rates running less than 1%. We have chosen to use a 5.1% rate on debt, which better reflects what Harris would pay on non-variable-rate debt, and also aligns with the organization's true borrowing rate when the effect of swap agreements is factored.

Conclusions regarding the capital position of Harris are:

■ Harris has growing levels of debt.
■ Its ability to meet debt-service obligations is excellent.

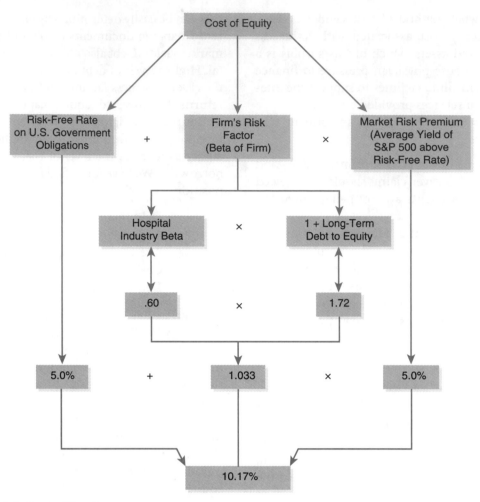

**FIGURE 11-4 Harris's Cost of Equity**

## ▶ SUMMARY: HARRIS CASE

Our financial review of Harris suggests possible improvements in profitability. Most of the opportunity for profit enhancement at Harris will likely be related to both revenue and cost issues. Areas identified for improvement include the following:

- Harris has lower inpatient and outpatient charges, and higher market share. Harris should use this position to negotiate better contracts with major payers and implement a modest price increase to generate additional revenue.
- Decreasing case-mix index should be monitored and addressed, as well as charge capture opportunities in the outpatient area.

- Hospital costs are reasonable but appear to be higher for inpatient services. Higher inpatient ancillary costs, especially in pharmaceuticals, could be driving this finding.
- Harris appears to be strong financially, but has borrowed extensively to invest in its aging facility. Total plant investment appears to be high and utilized inefficiently.

The dashboard approach used in this case can be very helpful in focusing management attention on either potential problems or areas of opportunity. Ultimately however, management must make changes. The best dashboard design, combined with accurate and timely reporting and without actual management intervention, will accomplish nothing.

## ASSIGNMENTS

1. Operating margins in your hospital have been consistently below national norms for the past 3 years. Discuss the factors that might have created this situation and the ways in which you might determine specific causes.
2. Your firm reported net income of $5,000,000, but the change in equity was only $3,000,000. What could account for this difference?

3.  Determine the amount of incremental profit that would be realized with a 10% across-the-board rate increase at Thunderbird Hospital. Thunderbird's present payment composition is 80% fixed fee and 20% charges or discounted charges. Present operating income is defined below:

| | |
|---|---:|
| Gross patient revenue | $100,000,000 |
| *less* Contractual allowances | 40,000,000 |
| Net patient revenue | $60,000,000 |
| *less* Expenses | 59,000,000 |
| Operating income | $1,000,000 |

4.  You have been reviewing documentation in your medical records department for the last week and have discovered a potential issue with respect to documentation for MS-DRG 193 (Simple Pneumonia & Pleurisy w MCC) and MS-DRG 194 (Simple Pneumonia & Pleurisy w CC). You have discovered 20 cases that were coded as MS-DRG 194, when in fact these patients did have diagnosis to support the major comorbidity and complication assignment. If the hospital's base payment rate for a case weight of 1.000 is $5,000, determine the incremental payment the hospital would have received. Assume the case weight for is 1.000 for MS-DRG 194 and 1.4378 for MS-DRG 193.

5.  Your firm's investment portfolio was valued at $100,000,000 at the beginning of the year. Approximately 60% of the portfolio was invested in fixed-income securities, primarily U.S. government bonds. The remaining 40% was invested in mutual funds selected by your firm's portfolio manager. During the year U.S. government bonds yielded 6.0%, and the change in the Standard and Poor's 500 index was 10.0%. Reported investment income during the year was $6,000,000 including realized gains. The firm also reported an unrealized loss of $1,000,000. Total yield on the portfolio was thus $5,000,000. What value would you have expected given the facts above?

6.  Your present length of stay on Medicare patients is 6.3 days for 2,000 Medicare admissions. This value is unadjusted for case-mix effects. You have discovered that a normal length of stay should have been 5.0 days. If this level had been realized, you would have had 2,600 fewer days of care for Medicare patients. You are trying to determine the amount of actual savings that would be realized if the shorter length of stay could be achieved. You have been told that a shorter length of stay would affect only direct costs of nursing. Your present direct cost of nursing per day is $300. Some of this cost is considered fixed and would not be changed. If 60% of the nursing cost were considered variable, how much saving would be realized through the length of stay reduction?

7.  Charles S. Lewis has just been named the CEO of Community Hospital, a 230-bed hospital located in an agricultural community of approximately 150,000. There is one other similar-size hospital in the community. C.S. Lewis has been told by his CFO, J.R. Tolkien, that the hospital is in excellent financial condition, but Lewis is not convinced. He has requested and received summary financial statements presented in **TABLE 11-5**. You have been asked to help Mr. Lewis identify the trends in financial position for the hospital in the last 5 years. Please compute the values for the financial ratios described in Chapter 10 and provide Lewis with your assessment of Community Hospital's financial position.

**TABLE 11-5** Summary Financial Information Community Hospital* 20X3–20X7 (data in thousands)

| | 20X3 | 20X4 | 20X5 | 20X6 | 20X7 |
|---|---:|---:|---:|---:|---:|
| **Balance sheet accounts** | | | | | |
| Cash and cash equivalents | $34,402 | $30,444 | $45,848 | $46,010 | $73,711 |
| Patient accounts receivable | 39,506 | 38,878 | 35,444 | 38,853 | 35,647 |
| Inventory | 2,133 | 2,318 | 2,398 | 3,197 | 3,279 |

*(continues)*

**TABLE 11-5** Summary Financial Information Community Hospital* 20X3–20X7 (data in thousands) *(continued)*

|  | 20X3 | 20X4 | 20X5 | 20X6 | 20X7 |
|---|---|---|---|---|---|
| Gross fixed assets | 187,278 | 221,548 | 240,988 | 256,652 | 276,458 |
| Accumulated depreciation | 73,227 | 79,523 | 89,324 | 101,007 | 113,851 |
| Net fixed assets | 114,051 | 142,025 | 151,664 | 155,645 | 162,607 |
| Unrestricted capital funds | 10,720 | 13,625 | 20,160 | 25,615 | 17,716 |
| Total assets | $238,365 | $265,784 | $276,965 | $287,193 | $311,140 |
|  |  |  |  |  |  |
| Current maturities of LTD | 111 | 1,794 | 1,431 | 2,211 | 1,143 |
| Current liabilities | $37,426 | $38,492 | $33,240 | $31,699 | $35,862 |
| Long-term debt | 2,032 | 12,821 | 11,720 | 9,578 | 9,570 |
| Net assets | $188,743 | $204,262 | $222,606 | $237,022 | $251,241 |
|  |  |  |  |  |  |
| **Income Statement Accounts** |  |  |  |  |  |
| Net patient revenue | $208,861 | $225,950 | $244,976 | $257,784 | $282,461 |
| Other revenue | 1,569 | 1,756 | 1,929 | 2,170 | 1,757 |
| Total operating revenue | $210,430 | $227,706 | $246,905 | $259,954 | $284,218 |
|  |  |  |  |  |  |
| Total operating expenses | $203,043 | $219,768 | $233,867 | $254,382 | $278,629 |
| Operating income | 7,387 | 7,938 | 13,038 | 5,572 | 5,589 |
| *plus* Nonoperating revenue | 6,806 | 7,579 | 8,971 | 8,430 | 8,696 |
| Excess of revenue over expenses | $14,193 | $15,517 | $22,009 | $14,002 | $14,285 |
|  |  |  |  |  |  |
| Depreciation | $10,588 | $11,161 | $11,659 | $12,184 | $12,524 |
| Interest | 115 | 611 | 471 | 419 | 392 |

* Note that not all asset and liability items are shown. The totals do not, therefore, foot to the individual account values.

## SOLUTIONS AND ANSWERS

1. Low operating margins are the result of either low prices or high costs. Low prices may be difficult to change in either competitive markets or situations involving high percentages of fixed-price payers, such as Medicare. High costs may result from excessive length of stay, poor productivity, or high salaries.

2. A transfer of funds from the entity may have taken place. This is often the case in investor-owned companies, because of the payment of dividends. It also may occur in a voluntary entity because of corporate restructuring. Unrealized losses on the firm's investment portfolio may have occurred.

3. The amount of incremental profit is equal to:

$$\text{Percentage of charge patients} \times \text{Price increase} \times \text{Present gross patient revenue}$$

   The increase in charges is $10,000,000, or 10% times $100,000,000. Of that amount 20%, or $2,000,000, will be to charge or discounted-charge payers.

4. The difference in payment would be 20 patients × $5,000 × (1.4378 − 1.000), or $43,780.

5. The expected yield should have been $7,600,000:

$$\text{Expected fixed-income yield} = \$60,000,000 \times 6.0\% = \$3,600,000$$
$$\text{Expected equity yield} = \$40,000,000 \times 10\% = \$4,000,000$$

6. The estimated savings would be:

$$\text{Days saved} \times \text{Direct cost of nursing} \times \text{Variable cost percentage}$$
$$(2,600 \times \$300 \times 60\%) = \$468,000$$

7. Only selected financial ratios for Community Hospital can be calculated for the period 20X3 through 20X7. These values are shown in **TABLE 11-6**, which presents a number of financial ratios. Major observations that would result include the following:

   - Present financial position at Community Hospital is strong. Current financial strength is a result of two primary factors: minimal levels of long-term debt and above-average total margins.
   - The trend in margins is downward, however. The primary cause is an erosion in operating-income levels. Expenses have been growing more rapidly than revenues since 20X5.

**TABLE 11-6** Selected Financial Ratios

|  | 20X3 | 20X4 | 20X5 | 20X6 | 20X7 |
|---|---|---|---|---|---|
| **Overall** | | | | | |
| ROE % | 7.5 | 7.6 | 9.9 | 5.9 | 5.7 |
| Total margin % | 6.5 | 6.6 | 8.6 | 5.2 | 4.9 |
| Financial strength index | 2.2 | 1.9 | 3.1 | 2.2 | 2.3 |
| **Nonoperating Income** | | | | | |
| Days cash on hand | 86 | 77 | 108 | 108 | 125 |

*(continues)*

**TABLE 11-6** Selected Financial Ratios    *(continued)*

|  | 20X3 | 20X4 | 20X5 | 20X6 | 20X7 |
|---|---|---|---|---|---|
| **Investment Efficiency** | | | | | |
| Days in accounts receivable | 69 | 63 | 53 | 55 | 46 |
| Revenue to net fixed assets | 1.9 | 1.7 | 1.7 | 1.7 | 1.8 |
| **Plant Obsolescence** | | | | | |
| Average age of plant | 6.9 | 7.1 | 7.7 | 8.3 | 9.1 |
| **Capital Position** | | | | | |
| Debt financing % | 20.8 | 23.1 | 19.6 | 17.5 | 19.3 |
| Cash flow to debt % | 49.9 | 43.4 | 61.9 | 52.2 | 44.8 |

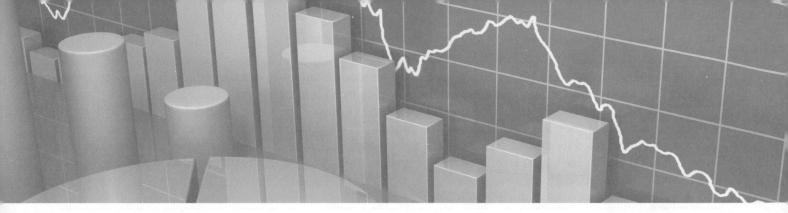

# CHAPTER 12

# Financial Analysis of Alternative Healthcare Firms

## LEARNING OBJECTIVES

After studying this chapter, you should be able to do the following:

1. List some of the major nonhospital and nonphysician sectors of the healthcare industry.
2. Discuss the sources of revenue for the nursing home industry.
3. Discuss the major sources of revenue and expenses of medical groups.
4. List and describe the major organizational types of physician groups.
5. Describe alternative HMO organizational arrangements.

## REAL-WORLD SCENARIO

Laura Rose has recently been appointed to the Board of ElderCare, a large, for-profit operator of skilled nursing facilities (SNFs) around the country. Rose's first committee assignment is to the Treasury Committee because of her prior business experience. Although Laura had extensive experience as a hospital administrator, she had relatively little familiarity with the SNF industry. Upon reviewing ElderCare's recent financial statements, she was concerned about the dramatically declining financial position. She noticed that revenues were declining on per facility and per patient bases. Meanwhile, the company's debt had been downgraded and its borrowing costs had risen substantially.

She is aware that Medicare and Medicaid establish fixed fees that they reimburse SNF providers. Payment increases by Medicare and Medicaid have not kept pace with increases in costs in recent years. She wonders whether this might be a factor in the company's financing issues. In general, profitability in the long-term care industry has declined significantly in recent years, and several industry leaders had filed for bankruptcy protection. While some believe that the SNF Prospective Payment System (PPS) was largely to blame, other factors, such as ill-advised acquisitions, excessive long-term debt, and poor balance sheets, probably contributed as well. In essence, she is unsure whether ElderCare's financing difficulties are unique to management issues at ElderCare or whether they reflect more general market conditions and economic and reimbursement trends.

To understand the issue better, Rose needs to be able to estimate the direct financial impact of SNF reimbursement. She asked the ElderCare treasury and controller's office staff to prepare an analysis of the financial performance of selected long-term care facilities over the period 2012 to 2016. In particular, she wants to know how SNF bond ratings have been affected by PPS and what other factors might have contributed to the industry's deteriorating financial performance.

Previously, we discussed the measures and concepts of financial analysis in some detail, but most of the examples and industry standards were from the hospital sector. (See Chapter 11.) The hospital industry is by far the largest sector in the healthcare industry, but it is not the only sector; its rate of growth in recent years has been slower than in other areas. This chapter will provide some additional information about alternative healthcare firms.

| Learning Objective 1 |
| --- |
| List some of the major nonhospital and nonphysician sectors of the healthcare industry. |

First, we will discuss the financial characteristics of the following three specific alternative sectors:

1. Nursing homes
2. Medical groups
3. Health plans

It is impossible to describe all of the specific operating characteristics for these three sectors in one chapter, but we will try to highlight the important differences that affect financial measures. It is important to remember that the financial measures and concepts discussed previously are still applicable. (See Chapter 11.) For example, the concept and measurement of liquidity is the same for a hospital as it would be for a health plan. However, operating differences between health plans and hospitals will produce different values and standards. Health plans have much lower days in receivables than do hospitals, and are required to carry much higher cash balances to meet transaction needs, namely claims payment.

It is not just the higher relative growth rates of nonhospital sectors that cause us to separately examine the topic of financial analysis for alternative healthcare firms. Many of the alternative healthcare firms have been consolidating through both horizontal and vertical mergers and have now become major corporations in our nation's economy. For example, UnitedHealth Group, Aetna, and Anthem are among the largest corporations in the country, employing large numbers of people and absorbing significant amounts of capital to finance their continued growth. Much financial analysis and discussion are now devoted to these firms because of their almost continuous need for financing. Major brokerage houses now have analysts who devote their time to narrow sectors of the healthcare industry, such as home health firms or medical groups.

**TABLE 12-1** presents 2015 financial ratio medians for two of the three sectors, along with comparative values for the investor-owned hospital-industry sector. We have calculated ratio averages by computing the ratio average for three large publicly traded firms in each industrial group. **TABLE 12-2** shows the composition for each of the three groups.

## ▶ Long-Term Care Facilities and Nursing Homes

It is not always clear what types of firms individuals are referring to when they talk about the long-term care industry. For our purposes, we will be referring primarily to nursing homes, both skilled and intermediate-care facilities. The nursing home industry has experienced significant growth during the last decade, and expectations about the aging of America have led many analysts to project even more rapid growth in the future. Growth in the nursing home industry is inextricably linked to government payment and regulatory policy.

As of 2015, there were over 15,000 nursing homes in the United States, and of those, 68% were investor owned. Investor-owned presence in the nursing home industry is much larger than it is in the hospital industry, where only 17% of hospital capacity is investor owned. Many of the investor-owned nursing homes are part of large national chains, such as Kindred Healthcare. However, there still are many investors that may own as few as 1 or 2 nursing homes to as many as 20. Most of the large investor-owned chains became involved in the industry when the government started

| Financial Ratio | Nursing Homes | Health Insurers | Hospitals |
|---|---|---|---|
| **TABLE 12-1** Financial Ratio Medians, 2015 | | | |
| Liquidity | | | |
| Days in receivables | 52 | 31 | 58 |
| Days-cash-on-hand | 44 | 124 | 21 |
| Capital structure | | | |
| Debt financing percentage | 53 | 41 | 88 |
| Long-term debt to capital | 35 | 49 | 86 |
| Cash flow to debt percentage | 16.3 | 13.1 | 12.2 |
| Activity | | | |
| Total asset turnover | 1.25 | 1.12 | 0.96 |
| Fixed asset turnover | 4.47 | 95.70 | 2.31 |
| Current asset turnover | 4.17 | NA | 4.41 |
| Profitability | | | |
| Total margin percentage | 2.87 | 3.64 | 4.57 |
| Return on equity percentage | 5.03 | 14.45 | 9.98 |

to finance a sizable percentage of nursing home care through the Medicaid program. Heavy government financing provided a stable source of payment that was not present before Medicaid.

### Learning Objective 2

Discuss the sources of revenue for the nursing home industry.

Financing of nursing home care is a critical driver of nursing home supply as it is for most other healthcare sectors. **TABLE 12-3** summarizes sources of financing trends for nursing homes as of 2014.

The data in Table 12-3 reflect the dramatic increase in the percentage of nursing home financing that is derived from public sources and a corresponding reduction in private financing. The percentage of Medicare financing increased sharply in the first half of the 1990s as hospitals discharged more patients into

nursing home settings to cut their costs per case and to maximize their profit per Medicare case. Much of this shift probably was related to the financial incentives created by the Medicare program when the government shifted to a per case payment system in 1983 for hospitals.

Although the federal government pays more than 50% of Medicaid nursing home costs, actual nursing home payments for Medicaid patients are set by the states. There is wide variation among the states between retrospective and prospective systems. In many states, there may be a mix of both systems. For example, capital costs may be paid on a retrospective basis, whereas all other costs may be paid on a prospective basis. Many states also use a case-mix-adjustment methodology to provide higher payments for nursing homes treating more severely ill patients.

Medicaid payments from states are usually the second largest state expenditure and, as a result, are subject to dramatic changes based on economic conditions in the state. When economic times are bad and

## TABLE 12-2 Industry Composition, 2015

| Industry/Firm | Stock Symbol | 2015 Revenue (Millions) |
|---|---|---|
| Health insurance | | |
| UnitedHealth Group | (UNH) | $157,107 |
| Anthem | (ANTM) | $79,240 |
| Aetna | (AET) | $53,789 |
| Nursing homes | | |
| Kindred Healthcare | (KND) | $7,055 |
| Ensign Corp. | (ENSG) | $1,342 |
| National Healthcare | (NHC) | $907 |
| Hospitals | | |
| Universal Health Services | (UHS) | $9,043 |
| Community Health Systems | (CYH) | $19,437 |
| HCA Holdings | (HCA) | $39,678 |

Reprinted from the Centers for Medicare and Medicaid Services

## TABLE 12-3 Financing Percentages for Nursing Home Expenditures

| | 1990 | 2000 | 2010 | 2014 |
|---|---|---|---|---|
| Private financing | 54 | 46 | 40 | 40 |
| Insurance | 6 | 9 | 8 | 8 |
| Out-of-pocket | 40 | 32 | 27 | 27 |
| All other | 8 | 5 | 5 | 5 |
| Public financing | 46 | 54 | 60 | 60 |
| Medicare | 4 | 13 | 23 | 23 |
| Medicaid | 37 | 37 | 33 | 32 |
| All other | 5 | 4 | 4 | 5 |

Reprinted from the Centers for Medicare & Medicaid Services, National Health Expenditure Data. Retrieved July 6, 2010, from http://www.cms.gov.

states have a difficult time meeting their budgets, one of the areas usually affected is nursing home payments.

On a national basis the number of nursing home beds per 1,000 persons older than 85 was 282.9 in 2012, but great variations by state exist. The *Nursing Home Data Compendium 2013 Edition* published by the Department of Health and Human Services shows 10 states with values between 119 and 222 and 10 states with values between 375 and 491. Some states have used the supply of nursing home beds as a means to control state expenditures for nursing home care. Licensure laws and certificate of need (CON) have been the primary means for controlling the number of nursing home beds in most states. Rates of payment for Medicaid patients also serve as an indirect method of controlling nursing home capacity. As rates are held down, less capital becomes available for expansion and renovation. Major national nursing home chains have been known to sell all of their nursing homes in certain states where they believed that reasonable profits would be difficult to obtain because of restrictive state payment policies.

It is expected that demand for nursing home care will increase dramatically in the next 20 years as the baby boomers reach the age of 75 plus, which is the age at which nursing home demand peaks. Nursing homes are also diversifying and expanding their product lines. For example, many nursing homes are becoming **continuing care retirement communities (CCRCs)**. In a CCRC, there is a continuum of care that runs the gamut from independent living, to assisted living, to skilled care.

Continuing care retirement communities also have discovered that their resident populations are desirable targets for HMOs that are seeking to expand their Medicare risk contracts. The CCRC is in a strong position to market itself to a managed-care group because of the economies of scale provided from its continuum of care and its personal relationship to a Medicare population. At the same time, hospitals are looking for ways to expand their revenue base and have begun to develop skilled-care units and other subacute units that can expand their business along the continuum of care and compete with existing nursing homes. Increasing emphasis on "bundled payments" by both Medicare and Medicaid have also provided a strong incentive for hospitals and nursing homes to either merge or to establish affiliation arrangements. In many respects, some of the historical distinctions among healthcare industry segments are becoming blurred as vertical integration accelerates.

The financial statements in **TABLES 12-4** and **12-5** reflect the operations of Friendly Village, a church-owned CCRC. A review of these financial statements

| **TABLE 12-4** Friendly Village and Subsidiary Consolidated Balance Sheets | | |
|---|---|---|
| | **June** | |
| | **2016** | **2015** |
| **Assets** | | |
| General funds | | |
| Current assets | | |
|    Cash and cash equivalents | $228,693 | $173,134 |
|    Investments (at cost-approximate market value of $293,000 in 2016 and $530,000 in 2015) | 199,811 | 409,393 |
|    Cash and investments that have limited use | 634,918 | 310,629 |
|    Receivable-Friendly Church entrance-fee fund | 2,151,994 | 2,169,635 |
|    Resident and patient accounts receivable, less allowance for doubtful accounts (2016: $195,000; 2015: $115,000) | 803,634 | 445,291 |
|    Mortgage escrow deposits | 30,891 | 81,961 |
|    Inventories, prepaid expenses, and other assets | 118,565 | 144,093 |
| **Total current assets** | **$4,168,506** | **$3,734,136** |
| Assets that have limited use | | |
|    Cash and investments (at cost, which approximates market value) | | |
|       Under bond indenture agreement—held by trustee | $5,103,399 | $662,217 |
|       Repair and replacement—held by trustee | 283,179 | 355,392 |
|       Resident deposits | 292,762 | 284,749 |
| | $5,679,340 | $1,302,358 |
|       *Less* cash and investments required for current liabilities | (634,918) | (310,629) |
| | $5,044,422 | $991,728 |
|       Receivable-Friendly Church fee-fee fund, *less* portion classified as current assets | 5,862,673 | 5,142,678 |
| | $10,907,095 | $6,134,406 |
|       Property and equipment, *less* allowances for depreciation | $13,312,799 | $10,747,006 |

*(continues)*

**TABLE 12-4**  Friendly Village and Subsidiary Consolidated Balance Sheets    *(continued)*

| | June | |
|---|---|---|
| | **2016** | **2015** |
| Unamortized debt financing costs | 551,700 | 226,100 |
| Total general funds | $28,940,101 | $20,841,648 |
| Donor-restricted funds | | |
| Cash and investments (at cost-approximate market value of $1,121,000 in 2016 and $1,210,000 in 2015) | $1,206,604 | $1,075,115 |
| Receivable-Friendly Foundation | 198,414 | 189,608 |
| **Due from general funds** | **196,594** | **188,578** |
| Due from nurse scholarship recipients | 14,357 | 6,064 |
| Due from employee hardship recipients | 3,266 | |
| **Total donor-restricted funds** | **$1,619,235** | **$1,459,364** |
| **Liabilities and fund balances** | | |
| General funds | | |
| Current liabilities | | |
| Accounts payable | $888,489 | $694,390 |
| Interest payable | 340,460 | 220,318 |
| Salaries, wages, and related liabilities | 759,495 | 696,458 |
| Funds held for others | 30,562 | 30,077 |
| Due to donor-restricted funds | 196,594 | 188,597 |
| Estimated third-party settlement | 45,842 | 441 |
| Current portion of deferred entrance fees | 824,000 | 987,251 |
| Current portion of note payable to Friendly | | |
| Church fee-fee fund | 28,291 | 40,889 |
| Current portion of long-term liabilities | 426,163 | 374,663 |
| **Total current liabilities** | **$3,539,897** | **$3,233,083** |

| | | |
|---|---:|---:|
| Deferred entrance fees, *less* current portion | 2,975,343 | 4,284,149 |
| Deposits—residents | 288,040 | 274,578 |
| Note payable to the fee-fee fund, *less* current portion | 635,776 | 666,549 |
| Long-term liabilities, *less* current portion | 15,972,531 | 8,265,908 |
| Refundable entrance fees | 28,110 | 29,907 |
| Obligation to provide future services and use of facilities | 190,550 | 190,550 |
| General fund balance | 5,309,854 | 3,942,682 |
| **Total general funds** | **$28,940,101** | **$26,365,697** |
| Donor-restricted funds | | |
| Fund balances | | |
| Sustaining fund | $751,708 | $692,320 |
| Foundation fund | 198,413 | 189,608 |
| Medical memorial fund | 344,657 | 336,169 |
| Specific purpose fund | 196,595 | 188,597 |
| Nurse scholarship fund | 47,451 | 45,624 |
| Employee hardship fund | 12,227 | 7,066 |
| Pooled income fund | 68,184 | |
| **Total donor-restricted funds** | **$1,619,235** | **$1,459,383** |

will give the reader some idea of the nature of business operations in this type of healthcare organization. A CCRC usually provides three levels of care: nursing home care, assisted living, and independent living. Often, residents progress through these three levels of care. An elderly person may enter the CCRC in an independent-living status and occupy one of the independent-living apartments. These apartments often are similar to apartments in other settings except that the residents are all retired and there are usually a variety of social activities to keep the residents active and united. As the health of a resident erodes, that resident may move to an assisted-living environment. In an assisted-living environment, some healthcare services are provided to enable the resident

to maintain daily activities. For example, medication administration, medical monitoring, or some help with daily living functions such as bathing, toileting, and cooking may be required. Many residents are prolonging admission into an assisted-living center, and assisted-living residents are becoming similar to the nursing home residents of 10 years ago. The last level of care is nursing home services, either intermediate or skilled. Many CCRCs also may have specialized units to treat patients with Alzheimer's disease or who have experienced a stroke.

The income statement of Table 12-5 reports revenues from a variety of sources. The largest share is from the nursing home and is referred to as routine healthcare center services ($6,214,764 in 2016).

**TABLE 12-5** Friendly Village and Subsidiary Consolidated Statements of Revenues and Expenses of General Funds

| | Year Ended June 30 | |
| --- | --- | --- |
| | **2016** | **2015** |
| Revenues | | |
| Routine healthcare center services—net | $6,214,764 | $5,863,469 |
| Care and service fees—net | 4,039,897 | 3,795,875 |
| Amortization of entrance fees | 1,080,635 | 987,252 |
| Other medical services | 690,593 | 676,216 |
| Applicant fees | 6,386 | 6,077 |
| Investment income on restricted funds | 287,261 | 97,265 |
| Other | 284,761 | 209,449 |
| **Total revenues** | **$12,604,296** | **$11,635,603** |
| Expenses | | |
| Salaries and wages | $5,903,470 | 5,581,287 |
| Employee benefits | 1,052,944 | 964,048 |
| Purchased services | 1,023,900 | 976,639 |
| Other medical services | 780,176 | 763,314 |
| Supplies | 1,076,176 | 953,586 |
| Repairs and maintenance | 137,898 | 109,047 |
| Utilities | 600,423 | 534,664 |
| Equipment rental | 7,757 | 4,881 |
| Interest and amortization | 1,312,727 | 793,622 |
| Provision for doubtful accounts | 65,718 | 25,415 |
| Taxes | 388,164 | 370,308 |
| Insurance—property, liability, and general | 78,830 | 93,782 |
| Other | 84,098 | 87,618 |
| **Total expenses** | **$12,512,281** | **$11,258,211** |

| | | |
|---|---|---|
| Gain from operations before depreciation and other operating revenues | $92,015 | $377,392 |
| Other operating revenues and expenses | | |
| Unrestricted contributions | 19,807 | 67,504 |
| Investment income on entrance-fee fund, net | 2,174,411 | 774,901 |
| Gain from operations before depreciation | $2,286,233 | $1,219,797 |
| Provision for depreciation | (922,501) | (825,221) |
| Gain from operations | $1,363,732 | $394,577 |
| Nonoperating loss | | |
| Loss on disposal of property and equipment | (51,082) | (10,096) |
| *Excess of revenues over expenses and nonoperating loss* | ***$1,312,651*** | ***$384,480*** |

The second largest source of revenue is fees generated from care and services provided to residents of the assisted-living center or the independent-living apartments ($4,039,897 in 2016). Some other revenue is generated from entrance fees and consists of $1,080,635 from an amortization of entrance fees and $287,261 from investment income earned on the entrance-fee fund. Some residents pay entrance fees upon entrance into the independent-living or assisted-living center. These deposits guarantee that a nursing home bed will be available if needed and that the rate for that nursing home bed will be less than the nursing home's current rates. For example, the CCRC may guarantee that the resident would have to pay only 50% of the posted rate for a nursing home bed if needed.

The amount of the entrance fee may be based on age at entrance. The fund is then amortized or recognized as income as the patient ages or dies. There is also income earned on the deposits that is recognized as income each year. The entrance-fee fund is listed several times in the balance sheet depicted in Table 12-4. On the asset side, there is a receivable from the church, which holds the entrance fees, in both the current asset and assets that have limited-use sections. On the liability side, there are accounts in both the current and noncurrent sections that represent deferred entrance fees. We will discuss shortly what these accounts represent because they are one of the most confusing accounting aspects of CCRCs.

The expense structure of a CCRC or nursing home is similar to other healthcare providers and is labor intensive. At Friendly Village, salaries and wages plus benefits constitute slightly more than 50% of total expenses. Also, notice that depreciation is not shown in the expense section but is separately shown as other expense. This is not uncommon for not-for-profit CCRCs, which often regard capital as a gift and do not regard replacement of the existing assets as an operating expense.

Perhaps the most unusual feature of a CCRC's financial statement relates to the entrance-fee fund and the **deferred revenue** that results from the receipt of those moneys upon admission to the retirement community. To understand the concepts of entrance fees and their amortization and deferred-revenue recognition, we will use a simple example and then relate those concepts to the data for Friendly Village. Let us assume that a resident enters the CCRC at the beginning of the year and contributes $35,000 to the entrance-fee fund. This amount will be amortized over the expected life of the resident, which we will assume to be 7 years. During the year, the resident spends 20 days in the skilled nursing facility and is required to pay only 60% of the $150 per day charge, or $90 per day. This means that a payment of $60 per day for 20 days, or $1,200, will be paid to the skilled nursing facility for 40% of the residents' charges by the entrance-fee fund. Finally, assume that the $35,000 entrance-fee fund earned investment income during the year in the amount of $2,000. The following entries would be made:

Entry No. 1.   Record receipt of the $35,000 entrance fee

Increase entrance-fee fund by $35,000

Increase deferred revenue by $35,000

Entry No. 2.   Record transfer of money to skilled nursing facility

Increase unrestricted cash by $1,200

Decrease entrance-fee fund by $1,200

Entry No. 3.   Record annual amortization of entrance-fee fund

Increase revenue account amortization of entrance fees by $5,000

Decrease deferred revenue by $5,000

Entry No. 4.   Record the investment income earned during the year

Increase entrance-fee fund by $2,000

Increase investment income on entrance-fee fund by $2,000

These are the accounting entries that would be made to reflect activities related to the entrance-fee fund and the deferred revenue account relating to the entrance-fee fund. The entrance-fee fund is an asset account that represents the funds available to meet contractual commitments to provide future healthcare services to residents. The deferred revenue account is a liability account that represents the estimated present value of future contractual obligations to provide healthcare services to residents.

---

*Learning Objective 3*

Discuss the major sources of revenue and expenses of medical groups.

---

▶ **Medical Groups**

Expenditures for physician and clinical services amounted to approximately $604 billion in 2014 and are second only to hospital expenditures. Physician expenditures have been increasing more rapidly than expenditures of most other sectors of the healthcare industry, which has increased the relative importance of physicians. However, it is not just the absolute level of expenditures made to physicians that make doctors an important element in our healthcare industry. It is

widely believed that doctors directly or indirectly control up to 85% of all healthcare expenditures. Doctors admit and discharge patients to hospitals; they prescribe drugs, order expensive diagnostic imaging services, and schedule rehabilitative services. The stroke of a doctor's pen directs a massive amount of healthcare resources to or away from an individual patient. Managed-care plans realized the demand-influencing behavior of physicians early and have attempted to incorporate incentives for cost control in physician payment plans.

Although few would debate the importance of physicians in controlling healthcare costs, physicians have yet to realize their importance in the medical marketplace because of their lack of organization. Of the 900,000 physicians in the United States, many still operate in one- to five-person practices. Physicians are slowly realizing this weakness and are now becoming part of larger organizations that are being developed by hospitals, health plans, large practice management companies, and large physician-controlled medical groups.

**TABLE 12-6** presents some data on sources of financing for the physician sector of the healthcare industry. Perhaps the most significant trend is the dramatic reduction in the percentage of physician expenditures financed by out-of-pocket payments from patients. In the period from 1990 to 2014, the percentage dropped from 19 to 9. It is not exactly clear what has caused this decrease, but the decline of indemnity

**TABLE 12-6** Financing Percentages for Physician Expenditures

|  | 1990 | 2000 | 2010 | 2014 |
|---|---|---|---|---|
| Private financing | 68% | 66% | 61% | 59% |
| Insurance | 42% | 47% | 45% | 42% |
| Out-of-pocket | 19% | 11% | 9% | 9% |
| All other | 7% | 8% | 7% | 7% |
| Public financing | 32% | 34% | 39% | 41% |
| Medicare | 19% | 20% | 22% | 23% |
| Medicaid | 4% | 7% | 8% | 11% |
| All other | 8% | 7% | 8% | 8% |

Reprinted from the Centers for Medicare and Medicaid Services coverage and the corresponding increase in HMO and PPO plans may be possible causes. Many HMO plans require a low copayment or no copayment for routine office visits, whereas most traditional indemnity programs have a coinsurance and deductible provision. For example, indemnity programs may require a subscriber to make all routine physician payments until some deductible is met, for example $500. This might change in the years ahead if consumer-driven health plans with large deductibles become more pervasive.

Physicians do receive a much larger percentage of their **total revenue** from the private sector than do most other major healthcare sectors. In 2014, physicians received 59% of their total revenues from the private sector, whereas hospitals received only 47%. Medicare covers nearly 100% of hospital service charges for the elderly, but is subject to a 20% coinsurance payment for most physician services. Most Medicare beneficiaries will finance this payment with supplemental insurance, which creates a shift from public to private financing.

Physician expenditures are increasing because there is increasing usage of physician services. **TABLE 12-7** documents the increasing number of healthcare visits as people get older. As the population ages, demand for physician services is expected to increase sharply. The substitution of ambulatory care for inpatient care also further accelerates demand for physicians.

As we discussed earlier, physicians are beginning to align themselves with larger groups and are moving quickly from one- or two-person practices to these larger groups. Some of this movement is a reflection of personal tastes. Physicians who practice in larger groups can make arrangements for weekend or evening coverage. Large group practices often provide their doctors with better consultative services and also reduce administrative burden, permitting greater patient-contact time. Lifestyle considerations may be an important cause of physicians joining larger groups, but the primary cause is related to economics. Physicians have seen hospitals and health plans merge and become more and more dominant in the local healthcare marketplace. Prior to increasing physician organization to counterbalance these large bargaining entities, physicians perceived themselves as being at a disadvantage.

### Learning Objective 4

List and describe the major organizational types of physician groups.

Physicians can choose whether to align with other physicians or to remain independent. If they choose to align with other physicians, there are four primary organizational alternatives for them to consider:

- Alignment with other medical groups
- Alignment with hospitals
- Alignment with health plans
- Alignment with physician practice management firms

Alignment with other physicians is, in some respects, most appealing to physicians because their control is maximized in this type of organizational setting. Often the critical limitation is capital. To achieve large-scale integration and development of new information systems and administrative structures, massive amounts of both financial and human capital are required. For integration with other physicians to be successful, a physician activist is needed who not only arranges the financing of capital needs but who also provides the administrative leadership.

Hospitals have the financial capital to create large groups, but in some cases their administrative experiences with physician practice management are limited. This limitation, coupled with differing incentives, can lead to organizational conflict. In a managed-care environment, the objective is to empty hospital beds, not fill them, and this often leads to conflict between hospitals and doctors. Additionally, hospitals have

**TABLE 12-7** Office Visits per Year, 2012: Distribution by Age Group

| Age Group | Number of Visits (in Thousands) | Percentage Distribution | Number of Visits (per 100 Persons) |
|---|---|---|---|
| Under 15 | 147,387 | 15.9% | 241.2 |
| 15 to 24 | 71,451 | 7.7% | 166.3 |
| 25 to 44 | 186,852 | 20.1% | 231.5 |
| 45 to 64 | 275,307 | 29.6% | 335.5 |
| 65 to 74 | 126,436 | 13.6% | 532.2 |
| Over 75 | 121,197 | 13.1% | 669.9 |
| **Total** | **928,630** | **100.0%** | **300.8** |

Reproduced from National Center for Health Statistics

been dominated by specialists, whereas primary care physicians are the key in managed-care markets. Primary care physicians often believe that hospitals do not understand them or their needs.

Health plans have the capital to put together large medical groups, but a conflict may arise between the incentives of health plans and its employee doctors. The health plan has a strong incentive to reduce fees or salaries of its doctors, while also controlling utilization. Physicians do not react favorably to lower income; they also object to mandates or controls over their practice patterns.

Physician practice management firms formed in the early and mid-1990s to meet the needs of both the physicians and the marketplace. Some of these firms were quite large and were publicly traded. Most of these firms closed or went bankrupt in the early 2000s. Most of their problems were linked to exorbitant premiums paid for physician practice acquisitions and later disenchantment by the acquired physicians serving in an employee relationship. Success in the capital markets required growth coupled with earnings. The earnings growth was not sufficient to merit the high valuation multiples accorded these firms.

The financial statements in **TABLES 12-8** and **12-9** provide financial information for Waverly Health Clinic (WHC), a hospital-owned network of 8 primary care clinics with 24 full-time physicians and 122 nonphysician employees. The clinic recorded 101,542 patient encounters during the past year with an average resource-based relative value scale relative value unit (RBRVS RVU) of 1.5 per patient encounter. WHC is a separately incorporated for-profit subsidiary of the hospital, and all of its physicians are salaried with profit and productivity incentives.

The financial statements of WHC provide some interesting information about physician practices, especially those owned by hospitals. We can see that the practices lost $1,825,716 in the current year. It is not unusual for hospital-owned physician practices to lose money. Revenues from the practice are often less than expenses. Many hospital executives argue that although the direct revenues and expenses of the practice may show a loss, there are substantial benefits realized from operating the practice. These benefits result from the admitting and referral patterns of the acquired physician practices, which raise volume at the hospital. Greater integration with the physicians themselves also may result in better cost control, which is important for managed-care contracts. Although all of these facts may be true, in many cases, it is simply poor management that creates

**TABLE 12-8**  Balance Sheet, Waverly Health Clinic, December 31, 2016

| Assets | |
|---|---|
| Current assets | |
| Cash | $375,570 |
| Net accounts receivable | $1,453,343 |
| Prepaid expenses | $147,785 |
| Other current assets | $753,497 |
| Total current assets | $2,730,195 |
| Net property, plant, and equipment | $1,911,545 |
| Intangible assets | $194,609 |
| Total Assets | $4,836,350 |
| Liabilities and equity | |
| Current liabilities | |
| Accounts payable | $173,175 |
| Withheld taxes | $87,235 |
| Employee benefits withheld | $3,379 |
| Accrued salaries and wages | $345,578 |
| Other current liabilities | $101,436 |
| Total current liabilities | $710,804 |
| Equity | |
| Contributed capital | $8,481,937 |
| Retained earnings | ($4,356,391) |
| Total equity | $4,125,546 |
| **Total liabilities and equity** | **$4,836,350** |

the financial loss. Before hospital acquisition most of these acquired practices were profitable, yet once they become hospital-owned and operated, they suddenly become unprofitable. A review of the financial

**TABLE 12-9** Income Statement, Waverly Health Clinic, Year Ending December 31, 2016

| Revenue | |
|---|---|
| Gross physician charges | $13,691,347 |
| Other revenue | $2,952,073 |
| Adjustments and write-offs | ($3,170,855) |
| *Net revenue* | *$13,472,565* |
| Operating expenses | |
| Personnel expense | $6,179,382 |
| Supplies expense | $540,956 |
| Occupancy expense | $2,530,195 |
| Purchased services | $275,422 |
| General and administrative expense | $1,189,032 |
| *Total operating expense* | *$10,714,987* |
| Physician expense | $4,583,294 |
| *Total expense* | *$15,298,281* |
| *Net profit* | *($1,825,716)* |

**TABLE 12-10** Comparative Operating Norms for Waverly Health Care

| Indicator | WHC Value | State Survey Results |
|---|---|---|
| Operating expense per physician FTE | $446,457 | $473,639 |
| Revenue per physician FTE | $561,356 | $637,677 |
| Physician compensation per physician FTE | $190,970 | $269,024 |
| Support staff per physician FTE | 5.08 | 4.54 |
| Operating expenses to net revenue percent | 79.50% | 66.27% |
| RBRVS RVUs per physician FTE | 9,850 | 12,572 |

The Waverly Health Clinic is losing money because its physicians see fewer patients. On a positive note, operating expenses are well below the state average. It is doubtful that these same physicians practiced in this manner when they were in private practice. The critical factor for the long-term success of owning physician practices is directly related to the incentive structures used for physicians. Ideally, incentives should promote and not destroy physician entrepreneurial spirit.

*Learning Objective 5*

Describe alternative HMO organizational arrangements.

▸ **Health Plans**

Most individuals in the United States are covered by either public or private health insurance. In some cases, public and private coverage may be combined. For example, many Medicare beneficiaries have obtained private health insurance to pay for health expenses not covered by Medicare. At the end of 2015, most of the 55.5 million Medicare beneficiaries had

information for WHC can help shed some light on the most common reasons for lack of profitability. **TABLE 12-10** shows values for WHC expressed on a per physician full-time equivalent (FTE) basis, compared to some survey results for similar multispecialty clinics in WHC's state.

The Waverly Health Clinic has fewer operating expenses than does a typical medical group. The bottom line is that WHC spends $27,182 ($473,639 – $446,457) per physician FTE below what a typical medical group would spend for operating expenses. However, WHC generates $78,054 less revenue per physician FTE than the national norm. Therefore, it is clear that the real issue is related to low physician productivity. WHC physicians generated lower RBRVS RVUs than expected when compared to national averages—9,850 versus 12,572.

obtained Medicare supplemental insurance from private insurance companies. Because nearly all of the elderly are insured by Medicare, most uninsured Americans are nonelderly (under age 65). A majority of the nonelderly receives their health insurance as a job benefit, but not everyone has access to or can afford this type of coverage. The Affordable Care Act (ACA), which was passed in 2010, aimed to expand coverage by providing for an expansion of Medicaid for adults with incomes at or below 138% of poverty, building on employer-based coverage, and providing premium tax credits to make private insurance more affordable for many with incomes between 100 and 400% of poverty. Most of the major coverage provisions of the ACA went into effect in 2014, and millions of people have gained coverage under the law. However, many continue to lack coverage for a variety of reasons. For example, Medicaid eligibility for adults remains limited in states that have not adopted the expansion, some people remain ineligible for financial assistance for private coverage, and some still find coverage unaffordable even with financial assistance. The National Center for Health Statistics estimated that 36 million people were uninsured in 2014 compared to 44.8 million in 2013. While the number of uninsured has decreased, it is still a sizable population segment. This large pool of non-covered Americans creates costs of treatment that must be paid by someone. To date, it is not clear who will be responsible for paying for this group of people. Will it be the government, the health plans, or the providers?

The cost of private health insurance has been rapidly increasing during the last 20 years, as **TABLE 12-11** shows. Health insurance companies always have been big business, but the amount of money spent in selling, administration, reserve retention, and profit has increased greatly. In 2014, administrative costs accounted for approximately 14.1% of private health insurance payments. Table 12-11 shows that the cost of private health insurance in relation to administrative costs has generally been stable over the past three decades. It is this administrative cost that has caused much discussion among policy analysts. They have argued that most of the money spent for administration and profit are not necessary and add to the cost of health care in the United States.

The cost of private health insurance may not, however, be wasteful. The nature of risk and regulation in the industry may require these levels of expenditures. Insurance companies agree to provide a benefits package of services for some specified sum of money. If costs of services exceed this amount, the insurance company loses money. This is often referred to as underwriting risk. In addition, insurance companies are regulated and are required to maintain certain reserve balances to protect policyholders in the event of a financial catastrophe. The only alternative to private health insurance would be some type of government-financed and government-managed program. Government costs might be just as high or higher.

Healthcare insurance companies come in many different forms. The Health Insurance Association of America (HIAA, now known as America's Health Insurance Plans or AHIP) categorizes healthcare insurance firms as commercial, Blue Cross Blue Shield, and health maintenance organizations (HMOs). The trend toward managed care has blurred some of these distinctions. Commercial insurance companies often provide an HMO option, as do most Blue Cross Blue Shield plans. HMOs have broadened their coverage plans to include more traditional indemnity programs, and most provide some point-of-service (POS) option whereby enrollees can go outside the HMO network for care if they are willing to pay higher copayments or deductibles.

| **TABLE 12-11** Private Insurance Trends | | | | |
|---|---|---|---|---|
| Year | Personal Healthcare Expenditures (Billions) | Private Health Insurance Payments (Billions) | Administrative and Net Cost of Private Health Insurance (Billions) | Administrative Cost (%) |
| 2014 | 2,563.6 | 868.8 | 122.2 | 14.1% |
| 2010 | 2,194.1 | 754.8 | 108.3 | 14.3% |
| 2000 | 1,162.0 | 406.1 | 52.4 | 12.9% |
| 1990 | 615.3 | 204.8 | 29.1 | 14.2% |

Reproduced from the Center for Medicare and Medicaid Services

In their 1995 *Source Book of Health Insurance Data*, the HIAA defined managed care as a system that integrates the financing and delivery of appropriate healthcare services to covered individuals. The most common examples of managed-care organizations are HMOs and PPOs (preferred provider organizations). A PPO typically offers more flexibility than does an HMO by allowing more provider choice, but it attempts to direct patients to providers with whom it has negotiated special contracts.

The information in **TABLES 12-12** and **12-13** presents financial statements for a small hospital-owned HMO. It is important to point out that financial and operating information on any HMO is usually available publicly by contacting the Department of Insurance in the state where the HMO operates. In

**TABLE 12-12** Hospital HMO Balance Sheet

| | 2016 | 2015 |
|---|---|---|
| Assets | | |
| Current assets | | |
| Cash and cash equivalents | $1,363,932 | $1,719,453 |
| Short-term investments | 1,709,056 | 1,495,481 |
| Premiums receivable | 813,427 | 1,233,975 |
| Investment income receivables | 29,054 | 45,339 |
| Amounts due from affiliates | 7,727 | 2,588 |
| *Total current assets* | *$3,923,197* | *$4,496,836* |
| Other assets | | |
| Restricted cash and other assets | $177,966 | $139,059 |
| Long-term investments | 708,941 | 957,306 |
| *Total other assets* | *$886,907* | *$1,096,365* |
| Property and equipment | | |
| Total property and equipment | 397,842 | 247,047 |
| *Total assets* | *$5,207,946* | *$5,840,247* |
| Liabilities and net worth | | |
| Current liabilities | | |
| Accounts payable | $406,163 | $539,624 |
| Claims payable (reported and unreported) | 1,063,696 | 1,209,314 |
| Unearned premiums | 101,056 | 161,318 |

*(continues)*

**TABLE 12-12** Hospital HMO Balance Sheet    *(continued)*

|  | 2016 | 2015 |
|---|---|---|
| Aggregate write-ins for current liabilities | 10,300 | 13,390 |
| *Total current liabilities* | *1,581,216* | *1,923,646* |
| Other liabilities | | |
| Amounts due to affiliates (Schedule J) | 1,677,791 | 2,283,933 |
| *Total liabilities* | *3,259,007* | *4,207,579* |
| Net worth | | |
| Total net worth | 1,948,939 | 1,632,668 |
| *Total liabilities and net worth* | *$5,207,946* | *$5,840,247* |

**TABLE 12-13** Hospital HMO Statement of Revenue, Expenses, and Net Worth

|  | 2016 | 2015 |
|---|---|---|
| Member months | 174,967 | 191,465 |
| Revenues | | |
| Premium | $21,509,196 | $22,008,779 |
| Fee-for-service | 0 | 0 |
| Title XVIII-Medicare | 0 | 0 |
| Investment | 60,784 | 27,422 |
| Aggregate write-ins for other revenues | 47,038 | 76,537 |
| Total revenues | $21,617,019 | $22,112,738 |
| Expenses | | |
| Medical and hospital | | |
| Physician services | $1,582,006 | $1,689,578 |
| Other professional services | 1,835,226 | 1,788,844 |
| Outside referrals | 4,300,561 | 4,344,071 |
| Emergency room and out-of-area | 963,382 | 1,425,666 |

| | | |
|---|---|---|
| Inpatient | 7,865,005 | 7,462,942 |
| Aggregate write-ins for other medical and hospital expenses | 2,811,346 | 2,794,410 |
| Subtotal | $19,357,525 | $19,505,512 |
| Reinsurance expenses net of recoveries | 376,541 | 370,753 |
| Total medical and hospital | $19,734,067 | $19,876,264 |
| Administration | | |
| Compensation | $902,617 | $781,656 |
| Occupancy, depreciation, and amortization | 83,809 | 105,994 |
| Aggregate write-ins for other administration expenses | 688,055 | 540,625 |
| Total administration | $1,674,481 | $1,428,275 |
| Total expenses | 21,408,548 | 21,304,540 |
| Net income (loss) | $208,471 | $808,199 |

fact, this is the source of the financial information used in our example.

The data in Tables 12-12 and 12-13 reveal a lot about the structure of an HMO. First, you will note that a small percentage of the total assets of the HMO are invested in property, plant, and equipment—less than 8%. HMOs are not fixed-asset intensive; the bulk of their investment is in cash and investments. Our HMO has $1,948,939 in equity at the end of 2016, which represented about 37% of the total assets. This gives the appearance of a debt-laden organization relative to the financial standards listed in Table 12-1, but it should be noted that a loan due to an affiliate in the amount of $1,677,790 also exists. The sponsoring hospital granted this loan and, in some ways, reflects equity. A large portion of this loan was paid off during 2016, which can be seen from the decline in the loan balance from $2,283,933 in 2015 to $1,677,791 at the end of 2016.

The income statement in Table 12-13 depicts a large decrease in net income, from $808,199 in 2015 to $208,471 in 2016. One of the reasons for this decline is the drop in member months, from 191,465 in 2015 to 174,967 in 2016. TABLE 12-14 analyzes the expenses on a **per-member-per-month (PMPM)** basis.

The decline in net income for our HMO example is the direct result of premiums on a PMPM basis increasing less than expenses. Although not the largest increase, administration expenses increased sharply on both an absolute basis and a PMPM basis. Much of the cost in this area is fixed and cannot be reduced when volume declines. Inpatient expenses also sharply increased. It is not clear from this information whether the cause is higher rates per hospital visit or higher utilization. Additional information in the insurance filing that is not produced in our tables show that inpatient days in 2016 were 4,187, or 287 days per 1,000 members. In 2015, inpatient days per 1,000 members were 278, or 4,447 total days. The average price per inpatient day paid in 2016 was $1,878 ($7,865,005 / 4,187) compared with $1,678 ($7,462,942 / 4,447) in 2015. Therefore, both increased use and higher per diems paid to the hospitals contributed to the inpatient expense increase.

## ▶ SUMMARY

This chapter briefly examined the financial and operating characteristics of alternative healthcare firms. Although the concepts of financial analysis are the same across all firms, there are some industry specifics that will alter the interpretation of financial results. It is important to become familiar with the industry sector being analyzed before reaching general conclusions regarding the performance of any given firm.

**TABLE 12-14** PMPM Profitability

|  | 2016 | 2015 |
|---|---|---|
| Premiums | $122.93 | $114.9 |
| Expenses |  |  |
| Physicians services | $9.04 | $8.83 |
| Other professional services | 10.49 | 9.34 |
| Outside referrals | 24.58 | 22.68 |
| ER and out-of-area | 5.51 | 7.45 |
| Inpatient | 44.95 | 38.98 |
| Other medical and hospital | 16.07 | 14.60 |
| Reinsurance net of recoveries | 2.15 | 1.94 |
| *Total medical and hospital* | $112.79 | $103.80 |
| Administration | 9.57 | 7.46 |
| *Total expenses* | $122.35 | $111.26 |
| *Net income* | $0.58 | $3.64 |

## ASSIGNMENTS

1. Using the information provided in **TABLE 12-15** for United Healthcare Group, a major HMO, discuss some of the primary observations that you would conclude regarding the financial performance of the firm. Relate your discussion to the values presented in Table 12-1.

**TABLE 12-15** United Healthcare Group, Inc., 2015 (Data in Millions)

| Balance sheet data |  |
|---|---|
| Current assets |  |
| Cash and short-term investments | $12,911 |
| Net accounts receivable | 6,523 |
| Inventory | 0 |
| Other current assets | 12,205 |
| Total current assets | $31,639 |
| Net fixed assets | 4,861 |

| | |
|---|---|
| Long-term investments | 18,792 |
| Goodwill and other intangible assets | 52,844 |
| Other assets | 3,247 |
| Total assets | $111,383 |
| Liabilities and equity | |
| Total current liabilities | $42,898 |
| Long-term debt | 25,460 |
| Other liabilities | 9,300 |
| Equity | 33,725 |
| Total liabilities and equity | $111,383 |
| Income statement data | |
| Total revenue | $157,107 |
| Expenses | |
| Depreciation and amortization | $1,693 |
| Other operating expense | 144,393 |
| Total operating expense | $146,086 |
| Interest expense | 790 |
| Net income before taxes | $10,231 |
| Income tax | 4,363 |
| Net income after tax | $5,868 |

2. Using the information in **TABLE 12-16** for Kindred Healthcare, a major nursing home firm, discuss some of the primary observations that you would conclude regarding the financial performance of the firm.

**TABLE 12-16** Kindred Healthcare, Inc., 2015 (Data in Thousands)

**Balance Sheet Data**

| | 12/31/2015 | 12/31/2014 |
|---|---|---|
| Assets | | |
| Current assets | | |
| Cash and cash equivalents | $ 98,758 | $164,188 |

**TABLE 12-16** Kindred Healthcare, Inc., 2015 (Data in Thousands) *(continued)*

**Balance Sheet Data**

| | 12/31/2015 | 12/31/2014 |
|---|---|---|
| Net accounts receivable | $1,194,868 | $944,219 |
| Other current assets | $207,273 | $199,264 |
| Total current assets | $ 1,500,899 | $ 1,307,671 |
| Property, plant, and equipment, net | $ 971,996 | $ 902,104 |
| Goodwill | $ 2,669,810 | $ 997,597 |
| Intangible assets | $ 755,655 | $ 400,700 |
| Other assets | $ 620,576 | $ 2,044,892 |
| Total assets | $ 6,518,936 | $ 5,652,964 |
| Liabilities | | |
| Total current liabilities | $ 1,111,212 | $ 857,263 |
| Long-term debt | $ 3,137,025 | $ 2,852,531 |
| Other liabilities | $ 263,273 | $ 243,614 |
| Deferred long-term liability charges | $ 301,379 | $ 213,584 |
| Total liabilities | $ 4,812,889 | $ 4,166,992 |
| Total stockholders' equity | $ 1,706,047 | $ 1,485,972 |

**Income Statement Data**

| | 12/31/2015 | 12/31/2014 |
|---|---|---|
| Revenue | $ 7,054,907 | $ 5,027,599 |
| Expenses | | |
| Salaries, wages and benefits | $ 3,614,091 | $ 2,442,879 |
| Supplies | $ 384,354 | $ 289,043 |
| Rent | $ 382,609 | $ 313,039 |
| Depreciation and amortization | $ 157,251 | $ 155,570 |
| Interest expense | $ 232,395 | $ 17,044 |
| General and admin expenses | $ 1,395,288 | $ 973,223 |

| Income Statement Data | | |
|---|---|---|
| | **12/31/2015** | **12/31/2014** |
| Other operating expenses | $ 983,579 | $ 831,443 |
| Total operating expenses | $ 7,149,567 | $ 5,022,241 |
| Earnings before taxes | $ (94,660) | $ 5,358 |
| Income tax expense | $ (42,797) | $ 462 |
| Net income from continuing operations | $ (51,863) | $ 4,896 |
| Discontinued operations, net of income taxes | $ (41,521) | $ (84,733) |
| Net income | $ (93,384) | $ (79,837) |

## SOLUTIONS

1. **TABLE 12-17** provides financial ratio values for United Healthcare for 2015. United Healthcare is achieving values of profitability that are on par with industry averages. United Healthcare's high return on equity results from judicious use of debt in its capital structure relative to their profit margin. Their current liquidity position also appears adequate, with favorable days in receivables relative to industry averages. United also appears to be utilizing assets efficiency, although their fixed asset efficiency is low relative to industry averages.

**TABLE 12-17** Financial Ratios United Healthcare, 2015

| Financial Ratio | 2015 | Industry Average |
|---|---|---|
| Liquidity | | |
| Days in receivables | 15 | 31 |
| Days' cash-on-hand | 80 | 124 |
| Capital structure | | |
| Debt financing % | 70.0% | 41.0% |
| Long-term debt to capital % | 43.0% | 49.0% |
| Cash flow to debt % | 9.7% | 13.1% |
| Activity | | |
| Fixed asset turnover | 32.3 | 59.2 |
| Total asset turnover | 1.4 | 1.3 |

*(continues)*

**TABLE 12-17** Financial Ratios United Healthcare, 2015 *(continued)*

| Financial Ratio | 2015 | Industry Average |
|---|---|---|
| Profitability | | |
| Return on equity % | 17.4% | 14.5% |
| Total margin % | 3.7% | 3.6% |

2. **TABLE 12-18** provides financial ratios for Kindred Healthcare for the last 2 years. Kindred has not reported positive levels of profit in either of the 2 years. In addition, Kindred has high levels of debt in its capital structure. Coverage of existing debt obligations may be problematic with high levels of debt, negative margins, and low cash balances. Kindred has very high levels of goodwill and intangible assets that most likely arose from prior acquisitions.

**TABLE 12-18** Financial Ratios Kindred Healthcare, 2015

| Financial Ratio | 2015 | 2014 | Industry Average |
|---|---|---|---|
| Liquidity | | | |
| Current ratio | 1.35 | 1.53 | 1.4 |
| Days in receivables | 62 | 69 | 44.0 |
| Days' cash-on-hand | 5 | 12 | 44.0 |
| Capital structure | | | |
| Debt financing % | 74 | 74 | 53 |
| Long-term debt to capital % | 65 | 66 | 35 |
| Cash flow to debt % | 1.30 | 1.80 | 16.10 |
| Activity | | | |
| Current asset turnover | 4.70 | 3.84 | 4.17 |
| Fixed asset turnover | 7.26 | 5.57 | 4.47 |
| Total asset turnover | 1.08 | 0.89 | 1.25 |
| Profitability | | | |
| Return on equity % | −5.5% | −5.4% | 2.9% |
| Total margin % | −1.3% | −1.6% | 5.0% |

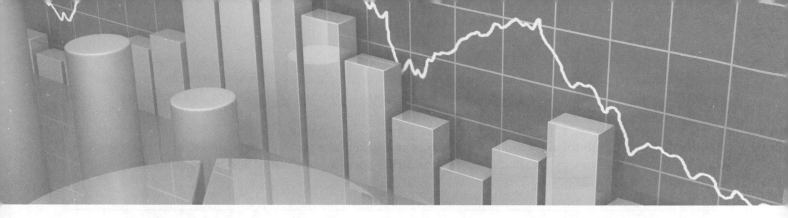

# CHAPTER 13

# Strategic Financial Planning

## LEARNING OBJECTIVES

After studying this chapter, you should be able to do the following:

1. Describe the relationship between financial planning and strategic planning.
2. List and describe the key financial policy targets for which the board is responsible.
3. List and describe the 10 requirements for effective financial planning and policymaking.
4. Explain the four steps involved in the development of a financial plan.
5. Explain how management control is used in conjunction with the financial plan.

## REAL-WORLD SCENARIO

Lydia Renee is the CEO of Golden Village, a large religious continuing care retirement community (CCRC) in an east coast metropolitan area. She is preparing materials for the upcoming board retreat to establish a clear direction for her firm in the years ahead. Her board is actively considering a number of strategies they believe are necessary to maintain the competitive position of the firm and to meet the needs of their constituency. All of the ideas for growth that board members currently support involve significant capital outlays followed by dramatic expansions in operating expenses.

One of the most controversial strategies calls for the complete relocation of the CCRC to a more suburban location. Many board members believe Golden must make major renovations to its plant to remain a competitive alternative to the large number of new CCRCs that have sprung up in suburban areas. The expected capital cost for this move is $50 million with a potential recovery of $12 million from the sale of the existing facility. It is not clear, however, if the sponsoring religious group would allow Golden to retain any of the $12 million from the expected sale of the land on which the present facility is located. Without any of the $12 million sale proceeds, Golden would be faced with a debt burden that may put the firm in default, which could lead to bankruptcy.

Margins at Golden Village have been dropping in the past few years for a variety of reasons. The increasing excess capacity in Golden's market has resulted in lower prices for both assisted living and independent housing units. This has hit Golden Village hard because their facility has exceptional services for residents, which are very costly to provide, but the actual units themselves are looking more and more dated. The nursing facility has also experienced a dramatic reduction in realized revenue as both Medicare and Medicaid have begun to ratchet back reimbursement levels.

Lydia believes that current financial projections show that Golden would find it very hard to pay for only modest capital renovations at the present site. Relocation would require a debt burden that simply could not be repaid without a change in current reimbursement trends. On the other hand, most board members believe that Golden Village is doomed if it stays at its present site. Most elderly people seeking CCRC accommodations want modern facilities in suburban locations, and the present marketplace provides ample low-cost alternatives. Lydia does not know what strategy she should recommend to the board at their retreat and is becoming more confused as she examines more data.

---

Is there a need to define corporate financial policy in a healthcare firm? If so, who should be responsible—the board of trustees, the chief executive officer, the chief financial officer, or some combination of these? How should the definition of financial policy be accomplished? What steps are required?

These kinds of questions are only now beginning to surface in the healthcare industry. Finance and financial management have long been areas of concern, but their orientation has recently shifted. Reimbursement and payment system management have given way to financial planning. Survival tomorrow is no longer guaranteed. Healthcare firms must establish realistic and achievable financial plans that are consistent with their strategic plans. The primary purpose of this chapter is to help provide a basis for the crucial task of forming financial policies in healthcare firms.

### Learning Objective 1

Describe the relationship between financial planning and strategic planning.

## ▶ Strategic Planning Process

Most observers probably would agree that financial policy and financial planning should be closely integrated within the strategic planning process. Thus, understanding the strategic planning process is a first step in defining and developing financial policy and financial planning. It would be ideal if there were agreement among leading experts regarding the definition of strategic planning, but this is not the case. The literature on strategic planning, which has largely been published since 1965, has been varied. Furthermore, the application of strategic planning principles to the healthcare industry, with most literature published since 1980, has reflected even more divergent perspectives.

One trend in healthcare strategic planning does appear clear, however: There is a definite movement away from "facilities planning" to a more market-oriented approach. Healthcare firms can no longer decide which services they want to deliver without assessing the economics of demand. This requirement appears consistent with the concept of strategic planning as it is used in general industry. Indeed, as the business environments of the healthcare industry and general industry become more alike, strategic planning in the two areas should become increasingly similar.

Much of the literature that deals with the **strategic planning** process in business organizations appears to be concerned with two basic decision outcomes. First, a statement of mission or goals (or both) is required to provide guidance to the organization. Second, a set of programs or activities to which the organization will commit resources during the planning period is defined.

**FIGURE 13-1** shows the integration of the financial planning process with the strategic planning process. *Financial planning* is fashioned by the definition of programs and services; it then assesses the financial feasibility of those programs and services. In many cases a desired set of programs and services may not be financially feasible. This may cause a redefinition of the organization's mission and its desired programs and services. For example, a hospital may decide to change from a full-scale hospital to a specialty hospital, or it may decide to eliminate specific clinical programs, such as pediatrics or obstetrics.

Three points concerning the integration of strategic and financial planning should be emphasized. First, both strategic planning and financial planning are the primary responsibility of the board of trustees. This does not exclude top management from the process, because they should be active and participating members of the board. Second, strategic planning should precede financial planning. In some situations the board may make strategic decisions based on the availability of funding. Although this may be fiscally conservative, it often can inhibit creative thinking. Third, the board should play an active, not a passive, role in the financial planning process. The board should not await word concerning the financial feasibility of its desired programs and services; it should actively provide guidelines for management or its consultants (or both) to use in developing the financial

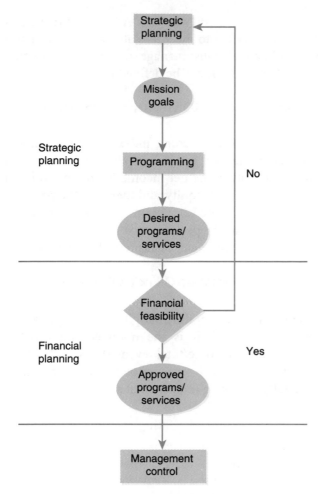

**FIGURE 13-1  Integration of Strategic and Financial Planning**

given certain key inputs. The validity of the projections depends on the reliability of the mathematical relationships, or model, and on the accuracy of the assumptions. Most financial feasibility studies developed in this way are never reviewed and never updated.

However conditions are changing—and changing rapidly. A large number of healthcare firms are now beginning to develop formal strategic plans. They are beginning to redefine, or at least reconsider, their basic mission and to identify future market areas. It is increasingly clear that their financial plans and financial strategies must be integral parts of their overall strategic plan.

Recognizing that healthcare board members and healthcare executives have an urgent need to understand financial policy and financial planning, can the requisite body of knowledge be conveyed in a manner that is capable of being understood? Must board members and executives remain passive observers in financial planning, or can they be given the means to establish key policy directives?

**FIGURE 13-2** identifies the critical financial planning relationships and the sequencing of the financial planning process. The premise on which the financial plan is built rests on some *projection of services* or levels of activity. The strategic plan usually provides this information by indicating which product lines the firm expects to provide during the next 5 years and at what level of expected activity. The first line in Figure 13-2 is from the income statement and shows

plan. Specifically, the board should establish key financial policy targets in the following three major areas:

1. Growth rate in assets
2. Debt policy
3. Profitability objective (return on equity)

List and describe the key financial policy targets for which the board is responsible.

## Financial Policy Targets

The term *financial feasibility* is often associated with an expensive study performed by a consulting firm in conjunction with the issue of debt. In such cases the financial projections are so incredibly complex that few people profess to understand them, and even fewer actually do. In many people's minds financial planning consists of a large number of mathematical relationships that can simulate future financial results,

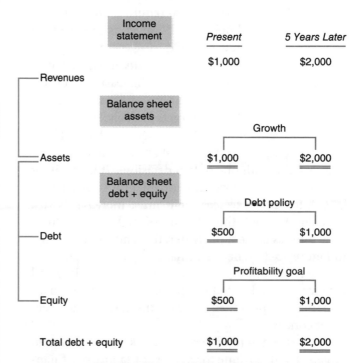

**FIGURE 13-2  Critical Financial Planning Relationships**

present and projected revenues. The projection of revenues can be directly related to the strategic plan. After all, revenue is merely the product of price multiplied by quantity. If the strategic plan specifies volume of services, then multiplying those volumes by expected price yields revenues.

Projected revenue serves as the basis for projecting the required level of investment or assets, which is the second step in the financial planning process set forth in Figure 13-2. In any business firm there are usually some specific relationships between investment required and production. For example, a healthcare firm with no existing clinic capacity that expected to provide 50,000 clinic visits per year 5 years from now would be required to invest heavily in physician practices to acquire this capacity. In the simple illustration of Figure 13-2, there appears to be a one-to-one relationship between revenue and investment: one dollar of investment in assets is required for every one dollar of revenue.

The third step is for the board to establish a **debt policy** for the organization. Stated simply, what percentage of the firm's investment will the board permit to be financed with debt? In Figure 13-2 the debt policy appears to be set at 50%. Fifty percent of the $2,000 investment in year 5 is financed with debt, which leaves the remaining 50% to be financed with equity.

The fourth and final step would appear to be the easiest stage in the planning process. If balance sheets balance, and they always do, the firm illustrated in Figure 13-2 will need to have $1,000 in equity at the end of year 5. A $1,000 equity balance when combined with the board-approved debt target of $1,000 will exactly finance the $2,000 required investment in assets. The critical question, however, is can the firm generate $500 in new equity during the next 5 years? Because most, if not all, of this equity must be generated from the profits of the firm, the feasibility of this increase in equity relates directly to the reasonableness of forecasted profitability targets or goals. If the firm is not able to generate $500 in new equity, what will happen? First, a balance sheet must always balance, so the firm is faced with one of two decisions. It must either reduce its level of investment, which of course translates into fewer services, or it must increase its risk exposure through the addition of higher debt limits. This process is most likely iterative and can be related to Figure 13-1. When the financial plan is feasible, an approved set of programs and services is in place and resources are allocated to accomplish the firm's goals. The financial plan then serves as the basis for management control.

It is essential to understand the key financial ratio targets that determine the success or failure of a financial plan. The most important relationship is the firm's growth rate in equity (GRIE). A firm that requires a 10% annual GRIE to meet its stated asset growth and debt policy goals must manage the critical drivers that define GRIE. GRIE can be defined as

Return on equity (ROE) ÷ Reported income index

The reported income index is simply current net income divided by current change in equity. In most usual situations net income for the period will equal the change in equity, and therefore the reported income index will be 1.0. This makes ROE the primary measure of financial performance. (This was discussed in Chapter 11.) ROE can be expressed as follows:

$$ROE = [OM + NOR] \times TAT \times (1/EF)$$

where OM is the operating margin (operating income/total revenue), NOR is the nonoperating revenue (nonoperating income/total revenue), TAT is the total asset turnover (total revenue/total assets), and EF is the equity financing (equity/total assets).

---

*Learning Objective 3*

List and describe the 10 requirements for effective financial planning and policymaking.

---

# Requirements for Effective Policymaking

The preceding discussion of the elements of financial planning and the three major target areas of financial policy suggest certain requirements for effective financial planning and policymaking. The following 10 requirements are of special importance.

1. *The accounting system should be capable of providing data on cost, revenue, and investment along program lines.* Programs, or "strategic business units," are the basic building blocks of any strategic plan. The financial plan must be developed on a basis consistent with the strategic plan. Unfortunately, present accounting systems are geared to provide data along responsibility center or departmental lines. For example, psychiatry may represent a program in the strategic plan, but the financial data on costs, investments, and revenues for the program may be intertwined with those of many departments, such as dietary, housekeeping, occupational therapy, and pharmacy. Still, this problem is not unique to healthcare firms. Many organizations have programs that cut across departmental lines. In such cases the financial data can be accumulated along programmatic lines, but some adjustments in cost and revenue assignments are necessary.

With the advent of the diagnosis-related group (DRG) payment system, the hospital industry has been making major advancements in the accumulation of financial data in terms of DRG categories. It is now possible to define major programs or product lines in a hospital as consisting of a specific set of DRGs. For example, if obstetrics was a program, it might be defined as MS-DRG 765 (Cesarean section with CC/MCC) to MS-DRG 795 (Normal newborns).

It is important to note that although problems exist in obtaining financial data along program lines, they are not insurmountable. The healthcare industry is, of course, different from the automotive industry, but the differences do not necessarily imply greater difficulties in costing.

2. *No growth does not imply a zero-growth rate in assets.* The fact that no growth does not necessarily imply zero growth in assets is so obvious that it is often overlooked by many planning committees. Inflation creates investment needs that exceed present levels, even though the organization's strategic plan may call for program stabilization or an actual retrenchment. An annual rate of inflation equal to 4% means a doubling of investment values every 18 years. For example, a nursing home with assets of $25 million today should plan on being a $50-million-asset firm 18 years from now. Just because the investment involved may not represent an increase in productive capacity does not negate the need for a financial plan that will generate $25 million in new equity and debt financing over the next 18 years.

Over time, of course, expectations about future rates of inflation may change. The financial plan should reflect the best current thinking in this area. This may necessitate periodic changes in the financial plan (Requirement 9). It is also important to recognize differences in investment inflation rates across programs. In some programs, such as oncology, in which dramatic technological changes are likely to occur, a greater relative inflation rate may have to be assigned.

3. *Working capital is a major element in computing total future asset needs.* In computing future investment needs, it is not uncommon to omit the working capital category. Most investment in any strategic plan is usually in bricks, mortar, and equipment. However, working capital can still be a rather sizable component, accounting for 20 to 30% of total investment in many healthcare firms.

The term *net working capital* is often used to describe the amount of permanent financing required to finance working capital or current assets. **Net working capital** is defined as current assets less current liabilities. It is important to remember this, because

some current liability financing is automatic or non-negotiated. Just as inflation increases the dollar value of outstanding accounts receivable, it also increases wages or salaries payable and accounts payable. It is the net amount of working capital that must be financed.

As an example, let's again consider the nursing home with $25 million in assets introduced in Requirement 2. Assume 30% of its assets are current assets, or $7.5 million ($25 million × 30%). If the firm has a prudent **current ratio** of 2.0, then the firm has $3.75 million in current liabilities (7.5 million ÷ 3.75 million = 2.0). Its net working capital is then $3.75 million ($7.5 million of current assets less $3.75 million of current liabilities). As the nursing home grows its total assets to $50 million over the next 18 years, its current assets will also grow at a 4% rate and will reach a value of $15 million. Assuming a stable current ratio of 2.0 implies that current liabilities would be $7.5 million. Thus, the firm's new net working capital will be $7.5 million, an increase in net working capital of $3.75 million.

Working capital requirements vary by program. New programs usually have significant working capital requirements, whereas existing programs may experience only modest increases resulting from inflation. One of the primary causes for failure in new business ventures is often an inadequate amount of available working capital. New programs also may have significantly different working capital requirements. For example, a home health program may require little fixed investment in plant and equipment, but significant amounts of working capital may be required to finance a long collection cycle and initial development costs. Many firms that rushed into the development of **home health agency** programs have become acutely aware of this problem.

If inadequate amounts of working capital are projected in the financial plan, the entire plan may be jeopardized. For example, an unanticipated $2 million increase in receivables requires an immediate source of funding, such as the liquidation of investments. If those investments are essential to provide needed equity in a larger financing program, certain key investments may be delayed or canceled in the future. A number of firms have had to reduce the scope of their strategic plans because of unanticipated demands for working capital.

4. *There should be some accumulation of funds for future investments critical to long-term solvency.* Saving for a rainy day has not been a policy practiced by many healthcare firms to any significant degree. As of 2016, Medicare data show that the average hospital had approximately 30 days of cash on hand. Given the way hospitals are required to report cash and

investments on the Medicare cost report this value is understated; however, audited financial information would only lift this average to about 120 days. Assuming that at least 20 days are needed to meet day-to-day transaction needs, only 10 to 100 days remain to meet capital replacement needs. This implies that the average hospital would likely need to borrow a sizable percentage of its replacement needs. This level of debt financing may no longer be feasible in the hospital industry as lenders reassess the relative degree of risk involved.

It is critical that healthcare boards and management establish formal policies for retention of funds for future investment. Healthcare firms can no longer expect to finance all their investment needs with debt. They must set aside funds for investment to meet future needs in the same manner that pension plans are funded. An actuarially determined pension funding requirement is analogous to a board policy of replacement reserve funding. Yet, few healthcare firms set aside sufficient replacement funds for future investment needs, which partially explains the dramatic growth in debt in the hospital industry.

5. *A formally defined debt capacity ceiling should be established.* Many healthcare firms have not formally defined their debt capacity or debt policy. This is in sharp contrast to most other industries. Without such a formally established debt policy, one of two unfavorable outcomes may result. First, debt may be viewed as the balancing variable in the financial plan. If a firm expects a $25 million increase in its investment and a $5 million increase in equity, $20 million of debt is required to make the strategic plan financially feasible. The firm will then try to arrange for $20 million of new debt financing. This is a situation in which many healthcare firms have found themselves.

Second, the balancing variable in the financial plan may shift to the investment side, but on an ex post facto basis. An approved financial plan may be unrealistic because the level of indebtedness required to finance the strategic plan exposes the firm to excessive risks. Management may not realize this until the actual financing is needed. At that point it may be required to scale down the programs specified in the strategic plan. If a realistic debt capacity ceiling had been established earlier, existing funded programs might have been canceled or cut back to make funds available for more desirable programs.

Debt capacity can be defined in a number of ways. It can be expressed as a ratio, such as a long-term debt to equity ratio, or it can be defined in terms of demonstrated **debt service coverage**. Whatever the method used, some limit on debt financing should

be established. That limit should represent a balance between the organization's desire to avoid financial risk exposure and the investment needs of its strategic plan. Debt policy should be clearly and concisely established before the fact; it should not be an ad hoc result. Historically, the U.S. hospital industry has financed 50% of its assets through debt.

6. *Return on investment (ROI) by program area should be an important criterion in program selection.* The principle that ROI by program area should govern program selection is related to the need for accounting data along product lines, as discussed previously. These ROI analyses by product line already are done outside the healthcare industry and need to be implemented in health care as well. To calculate ROI along program lines, financial data on revenues, expenses, and investment must be available along program lines. ROI should be used as part of an overall system of program evaluation and selection.

Portfolio analysis is a buzzword used lately to categorize programs in terms of market share and growth rate. Healthcare writers have applied the concept to the literature on healthcare planning and marketing. However, one difficulty with the application of portfolio analysis in the healthcare industry is the selection of the dimensions for developing the portfolio matrix. In most portfolio matrices the dimensions used are market share and growth. Market share and growth are assumed to have an explicit relationship to cash flow. High market share is associated with high profitability and thus with good cash flow. High market growth is assumed to require cash flow for investment. For example, a program with a high market share and low growth is regarded as a "cash cow." It produces high cash flow but requires little cash flow for reinvestment because of its low growth needs.

Here we use a slight modification of the portfolio analysis paradigm, incorporating the dimension of profitability. **FIGURE 13-3** illustrates the revised portfolio analysis matrix. Its two dimensions are ROI and community need. ROI is used as the measure of profitability because it is most directly related to strategic and financial planning. Profit is merely new equity that can be used to finance new investment. Absolute levels of profit or cash flow mean little unless they are related to the underlying investment. For example, if program A has a profit of $100,000 and an investment of $2,000,000, whereas program B has a profit of $50,000 and an investment of $100,000, which program is a better cash cow if both programs have low community need? In this example, B is clearly the better cash cow because it generates a much better return on its investment ($\text{ROI}_A = 5\%$ and $\text{ROI}_B = 50\%$).

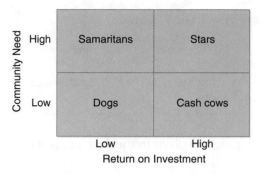

**FIGURE 13-3  Revised Portfolio Analysis Matrix**

In our revised portfolio analysis matrix, community need replaces the traditional marketing dimensions of growth and market share. Community need may be difficult to measure quantitatively, but the concept appears closely aligned to the missions of most voluntary healthcare firms—firms that usually were formed to provide healthcare services to some reasonably well-defined market.

Figure 13-3 categorizes programs as "dogs," "cash cows," "stars," and "Samaritans." With the exception of Samaritans, these terms are identical to those used in the existing literature. An example of a Samaritan program is one with a small or negative ROI but a high community need. For example, a hospital may provide a drug abuse program that loses money but meets a community need not met by any other healthcare provider. The program can continue if, and only if, the hospital has some stars or cash cows to subsidize the program's poor profitability. Dogs—programs with low community need and low profit—should be considered in light of the resources they draw from potential Samaritans. The new payment environment makes this kind of analysis mandatory.

7. *Nonoperating sources of equity should be included in the financial plan.* In the preceding discussion of ROI, we were concerned primarily with operating profitability. However, in many voluntary healthcare firms, nonoperating income also can be extremely important. In fact, in 2015 nonoperating revenue accounted for 15% of total reported net income in the hospital industry (Cleverley & Associates, 2016). If nonoperating income can be improved, a significant new source of funding will be available to help finance the strategic plan. This could mean either that a greater percentage of desired programs can be undertaken or that reduced levels of indebtedness are possible. The primary source of nonoperating income for most healthcare firms is investment income and gains.

The investment portfolio of many healthcare firms is large. Funds are available for retirement plans, professional liability self-insurance plans, funded depreciation, bond funds, endowments, and other purposes. Thus, small increases in investment yields can create sizable increases in income. For example, a 1% improvement in the yield on invested pension funds may reduce annual pension expense by as much as 10%. Clearly, management should formally establish and incorporate target investment yields in its financial plans.

New equity also can come from sources other than operating and nonoperating income. Corporate restructuring arrangements can create proprietary subsidiaries that can issue stock. Joint venture relationships with medical staff and others can be used to finance plant assets. It is important that both board members and executives have a clear understanding of the possible alternatives for raising new equity to finance the strategic plan. Raising new equity through stock or partnerships is no longer the exclusive domain of investor-owned firms.

8. *The financial plan must be integrated with the management control system.* The integration of the financial plan with the management control system is an obvious requirement, but it is often overlooked. Frequently, a large fee is paid to a consultant or enormous amounts of internal staff time are used to develop a financial plan that is never used.

Ideally, the financial plan should be the basis for the annual budget. The key link between the budget and the financial plan should be the ROI targets specified in the financial plan. These ROI targets are critical to the long-run fulfillment of the strategic plan. Failure to achieve the targeted levels of profit will require revisions in the strategic plan.

Healthcare board members would not need to be involved in pricing debates if approved financial plans were available. In such situations the profitability targets by program already would have been approved in the plans. The primary issues in the budgeting process should be the translation of profit targets by program lines to departmental lines via pricing allocations and the assessment of departmental operating efficiencies. Long, involved discussions about whether budgeted profit is too much or not enough should not be necessary.

9. *The financial plan should be updated at least annually.* Management should have the most recent financial "road map" available at all times. Few people would plan a drive to San Francisco from Boston with a 5-year-old road map, yet many organizations operate either with no long-range financial plan or with an outdated one. This can be especially dangerous for healthcare firms at the present time, because the business environment continues to change rapidly. Today,

financial plans based on yesterday's financial environment may be useless or even misleading. In all financial plans a careful reassessment of relative program profitability is periodically required, possibly prompting major revisions of the strategic plan. Knowing where you are going *and* how you expect to get there is critical to survival in a competitive environment.

10. *The financial plan is a board document and should be formally approved by the board.* In many firms the financial plan, if it exists, is regarded as a management document. The board may be only mildly interested in reviewing it and not at all interested in relating it to the strategic plan. This is rather strange behavior. Most boards would never dream of letting management operate without a board-approved annual budget for fear of failing to fulfill their board responsibilities. Yet planning for periods longer than 1 year is not regarded as important.

A recent hospital board meeting that followed a 2-day strategic planning retreat illustrates this traditional perspective. During the retreat strategic discussions about the future were held. The board and management agreed on a plan for the future that called for significant expansion into new market areas, such as long-term care. At the subsequent board meeting the chief executive officer and the chief financial officer presented the strategic plan and the related financial plan. The board members regarded approval of the financial plan as a waste of time. They did approve it, but in body only, not in spirit. Their rationale for apathy was clear. They could not foresee any problem with the financing. Most of them had been board members for a long time. Whenever money was needed in the past, they raised rates or borrowed, and they could not see any reason to change this policy in the future. This type of behavior in today's market is not only unwise but also suicidal.

Fortunately, this kind of reaction is becoming less common. Board members today are beginning to realize that the financial plan and the strategic plan are integrally related. It is impossible to develop one without the other, and both are ultimately the responsibility of the board.

## ▶ Developing the Financial Plan

In this section we describe in some detail the steps involved in preparing a financial plan using an actual case example. For our purposes, a *financial plan* may be defined as the bridge between two balance sheets. It is the income statement that provides the major connection between two balance sheets, and so we describe both balance sheet and income statement projection.

## Developmental Process

Explain the four steps involved in the development of a financial plan.

Four steps are involved in the development of a financial plan:

1. Assess financial position and prior growth patterns.
2. Define growth needs in total assets for the planning period.
3. Define acceptable level of debt for both current and long-term categories.
4. Assess reasonableness of required growth rate in equity.

## Assessment of Present Financial Position

The first step in the development of a financial plan is the assessment of present financial position. It is extremely important to determine the present financial health and position of the firm. Without such information, projections about future growth can be dangerous at best. In most situations past performance is usually a good basis for projecting future performance. For example, a financial plan may call for a future GRIE of 15% per year. If, however, the prior 5-year period showed an average annual GRIE of only 5%, there may be some doubt about the validity of the assumption of 15% and thus the reasonableness of the financial plan.

The following two categories of financial information need to be assembled to assess present financial position:

1. Financial statements for the past 3 to 5 years
2. Financial evaluation of the firm, using **ratio analysis**

To illustrate the application of this information in financial planning, the balance sheets presented in Table 13-1 are used. These balance sheets provide historical information for Omega Health Foundation (OHF) for the years 20X4 through 20X6.

**TABLES 13-1, 13-2,** and **13-3** present some useful historical data that will be helpful in assessing the present financial position and projecting asset growth rates. After a review of the three tables, the following summary may help to organize our thinking about OHF's 20X6 financial position.

- OHF has good levels of investment reserves. The present funded depreciation account has $55,794,000 in it and also has created a sizable

**TABLE 13-1** Balance Sheet for OHF as of June 30, 20X6, 20X5, and 20X4 (data in Thousands)

| | General Funds | | |
| --- | --- | --- | --- |
| | **20X6** | **20X5** | **20X4** |
| Assets current | | | |
| Cash and short-term investments | $9,692 | $9,456 | $11,388 |
| Accounts receivable | 24,324 | 25,597 | 23,381 |
| Due from third-party payers | 0 | 56 | 185 |
| Due from donor-restricted funds | 280 | 179 | 47 |
| Inventories | 1,763 | 2,251 | 2,252 |
| Prepaid expenses and other assets | 1,135 | 1,520 | 1,963 |
| Current portion of funds held by trustee | 990 | 925 | 1,580 |
| Current portion of self-insurance trust funds | 2,264 | 2,284 | 2,917 |
| Total current assets | $40,448 | $42,268 | $43,713 |
| Assets that have limited use | | | |
| Self-insurance trust funds, net of current portion | $9,321 | $9,013 | $9,962 |
| Board-designated funds and fund depreciation | 55,794 | 42,326 | 37,520 |
| Funds held by trustee, net of current portion | 338 | 726 | 1,037 |
| | $65,453 | $52,065 | $48,519 |
| Gross property, plant, and equipment | $146,794 | $137,631 | $130,404 |
| Less accumulated depreciation | 70,804 | 62,802 | 64,087 |
| Property, plant, and equipment, net | $75,990 | $74,829 | $66,317 |
| Investments in and advances to partnerships | 2,497 | 2,226 | 1,759 |
| Deferred financing costs, net | 1,139 | 1,306 | 1,394 |
| Deferred third-party reimbursement | — | 674 | 983 |
| Other assets | 1,067 | 654 | 575 |
| Total | $186,594 | $174,022 | $163,260 |

*(continues)*

**TABLE 13-1** Balance Sheet for OHF as of June 30, 20X6, 20X5, and 20X4 (data in Thousands) *(continued)*

| | General Funds | | |
|---|---|---|---|
| | **20X6** | **20X5** | **20X4** |
| Liabilities current | | | |
| Current portion of long-term debt | $1,401 | $1,506 | $1,784 |
| Notes payable | — | 250 | — |
| Accounts payable and accrued expenses | 11,087 | 7,215 | 6,791 |
| Accrued salaries, wages, and fees | 4,342 | 4,238 | 3,724 |
| Accrued restructuring costs | 2,078 | — | — |
| Accrued vacation | 3,288 | 3,331 | 3,223 |
| Accrued insurance costs | 2,234 | 2,284 | 2,917 |
| Advance from third-party payer | 1,205 | 1,142 | 941 |
| Due to third-party payers | 11,571 | 10,688 | 9,150 |
| Total current liabilities | $37,206 | $30,654 | $28,530 |
| Accrued retirement costs | $8,846 | $1,736 | $1,576 |
| Accrued insurance costs, net of current position | 4,636 | 3,450 | 2,124 |
| Deferred third-party reimbursement | 3,489 | 3,488 | 3,604 |
| Long-term debt, net of current position | 54,781 | 55,989 | 56,369 |
| Other liabilities | 238 | 2 | — |
| Total liabilities | $109,196 | $95,319 | $92,203 |
| Unrestricted net assets | 77,398 | 78,703 | 71,057 |
| Total | $186,594 | $174,022 | $163,260 |

amount of investment income. This value can be compared with the ending 20X6 accumulated depreciation value of $70,804,000. OHF has 78.8% of its accumulated depreciation in funded depreciation. This is a large percentage and implies that OHF could finance approximately 78.8% of its present replacement needs with existing funds. The actual percentage may be lower when the effects of inflation are considered.

■ Present operating profitability at OHF is not good, and an operating loss of $492,000 was experienced in 20X6. The primary cause for this poor operating position is an excessive cost structure. OHF took a restructuring charge of $5,110,000 in 20X6, which reflects its commitment to further cost reduction.

■ Age of plant at OHF is below the national average and might suggest lower levels of capital expenditures in the future. The board has, however,

| **TABLE 13-2** Statements of Revenue and Expenses of General Funds for OHF (data in Thousands) | | | |
|---|---|---|---|
| | **20X6** | **20X5** | **20X4** |
| Revenues | | | |
| Net patient service revenue | $160,574 | $162,323 | $147,596 |
| Equity in net income from partnership | 732 | 1,135 | 1,216 |
| Gifts and bequests | 258 | 435 | 296 |
| Other | 8,760 | 8,742 | 7,655 |
| Total revenues | $170,324 | $172,635 | $156,763 |
| Expenses | | | |
| Salaries and wages | $81,032 | $81,476 | $75,942 |
| Fringe benefits | 18,627 | 19,876 | 16,391 |
| Professional fees | 8,980 | 12,743 | 13,541 |
| Supplies and other | 39,607 | 38,539 | 30,658 |
| Interest | 4,364 | 4,369 | 4,421 |
| Bad-debt expense | 4,551 | 6,419 | 8,026 |
| Depreciation and amortization | 8,545 | 7,861 | 7,167 |
| Restructuring costs | 5,110 | — | — |
| Total expenses | $170,816 | $171,283 | $156,146 |
| Income (loss) from operations | $(492) | $1,352 | $617 |
| Nonoperating gains (losses) | | | |
| Income on investments | $4,717 | $4,658 | $3,837 |
| Gifts and bequests | 41 | 297 | — |
| Loss on disposal of assets | (84) | (601) | (150) |
| Nonoperating gains, net | $4,674 | $4,354 | $3,687 |
| Excess of revenues over expenses before cumulative effect of change in accounting principle | $4,182 | $5,706 | $4,304 |
| Cumulative effect of change in account principle | (5,086) | — | — |
| Excess of revenues over expenses | $(904) | $5,706 | $4,304 |

**TABLE 13-3** Historical Financial Ratios for OHF

| | 20X4 | 20X5 | 20X6 | U.S. Median* |
|---|---|---|---|---|
| Profitability | | | | |
| Total margin percentage | 2.7 | 3.2 | −0.5 | 5.0 |
| Operating margin percentage | 0.4 | 0.8 | −0.3 | 4.3 |
| ROE percentage | 6.1 | 7.3 | −1.2 | 8.5 |
| Liquidity | | | | |
| Current ratio | 1.53 | 1.38 | 1.09 | 1.92 |
| Days in accounts receivable | 57.8 | 57.6 | 55.3 | 53.0 |
| Days cash on hand | 119.8 | 115.7 | 147.3 | 33.0** |
| Capital structure | | | | |
| Debt financing percentage | 58.5 | 54.8 | 56.5 | 43.8 |
| Long-term debt to equity percentage | 79.4 | 71.1 | 70.8 | 23.6 |
| Cash flow to debt percentage | 13.5 | 15.7 | 8.3 | 16.0 |
| Times interest earned | 1.97 | 2.31 | 0.79 | 4.50 |
| Activity | | | | |
| Total asset turnover | 0.98 | 1.02 | 0.94 | 1.09 |
| Fixed asset turnover | 2.42 | 2.37 | 2.30 | 2.45 |
| Current asset turnover | 3.67 | 4.18 | 4.32 | 3.88 |
| Other ratios | | | | |
| Average age of plant | 7.5 | 8.0 | 8.3 | 11.1 |

*Median source: Cleverley & Associates. (2016). *State of the hospital industry. 2016 edition.* Worthington, OH: Cleverley & Associates.

**Days cash on hand based on Medicare Cost Report (Worksheet G) and may be understated.

approved capital expenditures of $10,000,000 per year during the next 5 years.

■ OHF has a capital structure that reflects more debt than national norms, but it has not issued any new debt in the last 3 years. The board's policy for future financing calls for no new long-term debt. Repayment of existing debt will continue using the existing debt principal schedule.

■ Present days in accounts receivable are 55.3 and it is expected that this present situation will continue.

## Defining Growth Rate in Assets

**TABLE 13-4** defines the assumptions used to develop the 5-year financial plan for OHF. As discussed earlier, it is impossible to forecast asset investment without first forecasting revenues as well as expenses. Revenue

**TABLE 13-4** Financial Planning Assumptions for OHF Years 20X3 to 20X7

| Account | Assumptions |
|---|---|
| Revenues | |
| Net patient revenue | 2% growth per year |
| Equity in partnerships | 5% growth per year |
| Gifts and bequests | 5% growth per year |
| Other | 5% growth per year |
| Expenses | |
| Interest expense | 7.5% of prior year long-term debt + current maturities of long-term debt |
| Salaries and wages | 1% growth per year |
| Fringe benefits | 23% of salaries and wages |
| Professional fees | 5% growth per year |
| Supplies | 5% growth per year |
| Restructuring costs | $2,078,000 in 20X7; zero thereafter |
| Depreciation expense | 5.8% of gross property and equipment |
| Bad debt expense | 2.8% of net patient revenue |
| Nonoperating gains | |
| Investment income | 8.3% of beginning balance in board-designated and funded depreciation |
| Gifts and bequests | $50,000 per year |
| Loss on disposals | $100,000 per year |
| Assets | |
| Cash and short-term investments | 20 days cash on hand |
| Accounts receivable | 15% of net patient revenue |
| Due from donor-restricted funds | $300,000 per year |
| Current portion held by trustee | Increasing by $65,000 per year |
| Current portion self-insurance | 5% growth per year |
| Inventory and prepaid expenses | 5% growth per year |

*(continues)*

**TABLE 13-4** Financial Planning Assumptions for OHF Years 20X3 to 20X7 *(continued)*

| Account | Assumptions |
|---|---|
| Total current assets | Subtotal of previous items |
| Gross property and equipment | Net new capital expenditures of $10,000,000 per year |
| Accumulated depreciation expense | Beginning balance + depreciation expense |
| Self-insurance trust | 5% growth per year |
| Board-designated and funded depreciation | Balancing account, all surplus cash flow will be invested here |
| Funds held by trustee | $338,000 per year |
| Investments in partnerships | 5% growth per year |
| Deferred financing costs | Schedule: $972,000 in 20X7, decreasing by $167,000 per year |
| Other assets | 10% growth per year |
| Liabilities | |
| Current maturities of long-term debt | Schedule based on debt principal due in Table 13-9 |
| Accounts payable | 5% growth per year |
| Accrued salaries and wages | 5.3% of salaries and wages expense |
| Accrued restructuring costs | Value goes to zero in 20X7 and remains at zero |
| Accrued vacation | Stable at $3,288,000 |
| Accrued insurance costs | 5% growth per year |
| Advances from third-party payers | 0.75% of net patient revenue |
| Due to third-party payers | 7.2% of net patient revenue |
| Total current liabilities | Subtotal of previous items |
| Long-term debt | Schedule based on payment of debt principal in Table 13-9 |
| Accrued retirement costs | 5% growth per year |
| Accrued insurance costs | 5% growth per year |
| Deferred third-party reimbursement | Stable at $3,489,000 |
| Other liabilities | 5% growth per year |
| Unrestricted net assets | Addition of net income to prior balance |

forecasts are an integral part of asset forecasts because the level of service drives the underlying required investment. For example, growth in property, plant, and equipment is directly related to the range and level of services expected to be provided in the planning period. Even items as mundane as accounts receivable are directly related to revenue forecasts. Projecting revenues leads to a forecast of expenses. When a firm defines its expected production levels, requirements for staffing, supplies, and other expense items are often directly tied to these forecasts. In addition, certain areas of asset investment are often directly related to expense levels. For example, short-term cash is often directly related to expense levels, and inventory investment is often tied to expected annual supplies expense.

In the remainder of this section we discuss some of the more significant assumptions used in the financial plan developed for OHF. The projected balance sheet, income statement, and financial ratios are presented in **TABLES 13-5**, **13-6**, and **13-7**, respectively.

**TABLE 13-5** Forecasted Balance Sheet for OHF as of June 30, 20X7, 20X8, 20X9, 20X0, and 20X1 (data in Thousands)

| | General Funds | | | | | |
| | 20X6 | 20X7 | 20X8 | 20X9 | 20X0 | 20X1 |
|---|---|---|---|---|---|---|
| Assets current | | | | | | |
| Cash and cash equivalents | $9,692 | $8,907 | $8,988 | $9,190 | $9,400 | $9,616 |
| Accounts receivable | 24,324 | 24,568 | 25,059 | 25,560 | 26,072 | 26,593 |
| Due from third-party payers | 0 | 0 | 0 | 0 | 0 | 0 |
| Due from donor-restricted funds | 280 | 300 | 300 | 300 | 300 | 300 |
| Inventories | 1,763 | 1,830 | 1,921 | 2,017 | 2,118 | 2,224 |
| Prepaid expenses and other assets | 1,135 | 1,192 | 1,251 | 1,314 | 1,380 | 1,449 |
| Current portion of funds held by trustee | 990 | 1,055 | 1,120 | 1,185 | 1,250 | 1,315 |
| Current portion of self-insurance trust funds | 2,264 | 2,377 | 2,496 | 2,621 | 2,752 | 2,890 |
| Total current assets | $40,448 | $40,229 | $41,135 | $42,187 | $43,272 | $44,387 |
| Other assets | | | | | | |
| Gross property, plant, and equipment | $146,794 | $156,794 | $166,794 | $176,794 | $186,794 | $196,794 |
| Less total accumulated depreciation | 70,804 | 79,898 | 89,572 | 99,826 | 110,660 | 122,074 |
| Net property, plant, and equipment | $75,990 | $76,896 | $77,222 | $76,968 | $76,134 | $74,720 |
| Self-Insurance trust funds, net of current portion | $9,321 | $9,787 | $10,276 | $10,790 | $11,330 | $11,896 |
| Board-designated funds and funded depreciation | 55,794 | 59,706 | 67,224 | 75,535 | 84,104 | 93,505 |
| Funds held by trustee, net of current position | 337 | 338 | 338 | 338 | 338 | 338 |

*(continues)*

**TABLE 13-5** Forecasted Balance Sheet for OHF as of June 30, 20X7, 20X8, 20X9, 20X0, and 20X1 (data in Thousands) *(continued)*

| | General Funds | | | | | |
| --- | --- | --- | --- | --- | --- | --- |
| | **20X6** | **20X7** | **20X8** | **20X9** | **20X0** | **20X1** |
| Investments in and advances to partnerships | 2,497 | 2,622 | 2,753 | 2,891 | 3,035 | 3,187 |
| Deferred financing costs, net | 1,139 | 972 | 805 | 638 | 471 | 304 |
| Deferred third-party reimbursement | 0 | 0 | 0 | 0 | 0 | 0 |
| Other assets | 1,067 | 1,174 | 1,292 | 1,420 | 1,562 | 1,718 |
| Total other assets | $70,155 | $74,619 | $82,710 | $91,638 | $100,867 | $110,981 |
| Total assets | $186,593 | $191,745 | $201,067 | $210,793 | $220,273 | $230,088 |
| Liabilities current | | | | | | |
| Current portion of long-term debt | $1,401 | $1,488 | $1,566 | $1,806 | $1,715 | $1,525 |
| Accounts payable and accrued expenses | 11,087 | 11,641 | 12,223 | 12,835 | 13,476 | 14,150 |
| Accrued salaries, wages, and fees | 4,342 | 4,338 | 4,381 | 4,425 | 4,469 | 4,514 |
| Accrued restructuring costs | 2,077 | 0 | 0 | 0 | 0 | 0 |
| Accrued vacation | 3,288 | 3,288 | 3,288 | 3,288 | 3,288 | 3,288 |
| Accrued insurance costs | 2,234 | 2,346 | 2,463 | 2,586 | 2,715 | 2,851 |
| Advance from third-party payer | 1,205 | 1,228 | 1,253 | 1,278 | 1,304 | 1,330 |
| Due to third-party payers | 11,571 | 11,793 | 12,028 | 12,269 | 12,514 | 12,765 |
| Total current liabilities | $37,205 | $36,122 | $37,202 | $38,487 | $39,481 | $40,423 |
| Accrued retirement costs | $8,846 | $9,288 | $9,753 | $10,240 | $10,752 | $11,290 |
| Accrued insurance costs, net of current position | 4,636 | 4,868 | 5,111 | 5,367 | 5,635 | 5,917 |
| Deferred third-party reimbursement | 3,489 | 3,489 | 3,489 | 3,489 | 3,489 | 3,489 |
| Long-term debt, net of current position | 54,781 | 53,380 | 51,892 | 50,326 | 48,520 | 46,805 |
| Other liabilities | 238 | 250 | 262 | 276 | 289 | 304 |
| Total liabilities | $109,195 | $107,397 | $107,709 | $108,185 | $108,166 | $108,228 |
| Unrestricted net assets | 77,398 | 84,348 | 93,358 | 102,608 | 112,107 | 121,860 |
| Total liabilities and unrestricted net assets | $186,593 | $199,745 | $201,067 | $210,793 | $220,273 | $230,088 |

**TABLE 13-6** Forecasted Income Statement for OHF (data in thousands)

| | 20X6 | 20X7 | 20X8 | 20X9 | 20X0 | 20X1 |
|---|---|---|---|---|---|---|
| Revenues | | | | | | |
| Net patient service revenue | $160,574 | $163,785 | $167,061 | $170,402 | $173,810 | $177,287 |
| Equity in net income from partnership | 732 | 769 | 807 | 847 | 890 | 934 |
| Gifts and bequests | 258 | 271 | 284 | 299 | 314 | 329 |
| Other | 8,760 | 9,198 | 9,658 | 10,141 | 10,648 | 11,180 |
| Total revenues | $170,324 | $174,023 | $177,810 | $181,689 | $185,662 | $189,730 |
| Expenses | | | | | | |
| Salaries and wages | $81,032 | $81,842 | $82,661 | $83,488 | $84,322 | $85,165 |
| Fringe benefits | 18,627 | 18,824 | 19,012 | 19,202 | 19,394 | 19,588 |
| Professional fees | 8,980 | 9,429 | 9,900 | 10,395 | 10,915 | 11,461 |
| Supplies and other | 39,607 | 41,587 | 43,667 | 45,851 | 48,143 | 50,550 |
| Interest | 4,364 | 4,214 | 4,115 | 4,009 | 3,910 | 3,768 |
| Bad debt expense | 4,551 | 4,586 | 4,678 | 4,771 | 4,867 | 4,964 |
| Depreciation and amortization | 8,545 | 9,094 | 9,674 | 10,254 | 10,834 | 11,414 |
| Restructuring costs | 5,110 | 2,078 | 0 | 0 | 0 | 0 |
| Total expenses | $170,816 | $171,654 | $173,707 | $177,970 | $182,385 | $186,910 |
| Income from operations | $(492) | $2,369 | $4,103 | $3,719 | $3,277 | $2,820 |
| Nonoperating gains (losses) | | | | | | |
| Income on investments | $4,717 | $4,631 | $4,957 | $5,581 | $6,272 | $6,983 |
| Gifts and bequests | 41 | 50 | 50 | 50 | 50 | 50 |
| Loss on disposal of assets | (84) | (100) | (100) | (100) | (100) | (100) |
| Nonoperating gains, net | $4,674 | $4,581 | $4,907 | $5,531 | $6,222 | $6,933 |
| Excess of revenues over expenses | $4,182 | $6,950 | $9,010 | $9,250 | $9,499 | $9,753 |

■ *Net patient revenues*: Net patient revenues were projected at an annual 2% growth rate. Net patient revenue actually decreased slightly in 20X6 but increased 9.4% in 20X5. What should we forecast?

Clearly, revenues should be set equal to volumes of services expected multiplied by expected net prices. At first, 2% might seem like a relatively small growth rate, but OHF presently has a very

**TABLE 13-7** Forecasted Financial Ratios for OHF

|  | 20X7 | 20X8 | 20X9 | 20X0 | 20X1 |
|---|---|---|---|---|---|
| Profitability |  |  |  |  |  |
| Total margin percentage | 3.9 | 4.9 | 4.9 | 5.0 | 5.0 |
| Operating margin percentage | 1.3 | 2.3 | 2.0 | 1.7 | 1.4 |
| Nonoperating revenue % | 2.6 | 2.9 | 3.0 | 3.2 | 3.5 |
| ROE percentage | 8.2 | 9.7 | 8.8 | 8.5 | 8.0 |
| Liquidity |  |  |  |  |  |
| Current | 1.11 | 1.11 | 1.09 | 1.09 | 1.09 |
| Days in accounts receivable | 54.8 | 54.8 | 54.8 | 54.8 | 54.8 |
| Days cash on hand (short term) | 20.0 | 20.0 | 20.0 | 20.0 | 20.0 |
| Capital structure |  |  |  |  |  |
| Equity financing percentage | 44.1 | 46.4 | 48.7 | 50.9 | 53.0 |
| Long-term debt to equity % | 63.3 | 55.6 | 49.1 | 43.2 | 38.4 |
| Cash flow to debt percentage | 14.9 | 17.4 | 18.0 | 18.8 | 19.6 |
| Times interest earned | 2.65 | 3.19 | 3.31 | 3.43 | 3.59 |
| Activity |  |  |  |  |  |
| Total asset turnover | 0.93 | 0.91 | 0.89 | 0.87 | 0.85 |
| Fixed asset turnover | 2.32 | 2.37 | 2.43 | 2.52 | 2.63 |
| Current asset turnover | 4.44 | 4.44 | 4.44 | 4.44 | 4.44 |
| Other ratios |  |  |  |  |  |
| Average age of plant | 8.8 | 9.3 | 9.7 | 10.2 | 10.7 |

high price structure, which it may not be able to maintain. A 2% growth rate is predicated on zero growth in net prices but a 2% growth in volume of services. A 2% growth in services seems reasonable given previous growth in outpatient and clinic services. The assumptions made about revenue growth (volume and price) are the most important variables in terms of impact on the financial plan. Small changes in these assumptions can have a sizable influence on projected financial results.

■ *Salaries and wages*: In the labor intensive healthcare industry the second most important assumption in any financial forecast is salaries and wages. Salary and wage cost are the product of three factors:

$$\text{Salary and wage costs} = \text{Volume of services} \\ \times \text{Staffing ratios} \times \text{Wage rates}$$

OHF has poor productivity and has undergone massive restructuring to try to reduce given staff levels and become more efficient. These staff reductions showed up as one-time restructuring costs in 20X6, and will be written off in 20X7. It is expected that future labor force reductions will be accomplished through attrition. It is therefore expected that salary and wages will increase only 1% per year over the next 5 years. Wage rates are expected to increase anywhere between 3% and 5% per year, but the reduction in staffing ratios resulting from attrition will keep the total increase to 1%. Any change in this assumption will have a dramatic effect on projected financial results.

■ *Fringe benefits*: Fringe benefits on average have constituted between 20 and 24% of salaries and wages. It is expected that future fringe benefit costs will constitute approximately 23% of salary and wage costs.

■ *Interest expense*: Projected average interest on existing long-term debt is expected to be 7.5%. This interest rate is applied to the beginning total of long-term debt plus current maturities of long-term debt.

■ *Restructuring costs*: Restructuring costs were $5,110,000 in 20X6, due in large part to costs associated with early retirement and layoffs. There are $2,078,000 of these costs still remaining as a current liability at the end of 20X6. These costs will be expensed in 20X7 and will be zero thereafter.

■ *Depreciation expense*: Depreciation expense was 5.8% of gross property, plant, and equipment in 20X6. This value is consistent with national averages and was used to forecast future depreciation.

■ *Bad-debt expense*: Bad-debt expense has been declining in recent years. In 20X6 bad-debt expense was 2.8% of net patient revenue. It is expected that future declines will be difficult to achieve and that present relationships will stabilize.

■ *Cash and short-term investments*: Cash balances in this account are needed to meet normal transaction needs for cash, such as salary, wages, and accounts payable. A typical transaction balance is approximately 20 days.

■ *Accounts receivable*: Accounts receivable have been approximately 15% of net patient revenue, or 55 days. It is expected that the present pattern of receivables will remain stable over the next 5 years.

■ *Gross property and equipment*: Gross property and equipment will increase each year by the amount of capital expenditures, less any assets that are sold or disposed. **TABLE 13-8** shows the board-approved capital expenditure plan.

## Definition of Debt Policy

Having defined the desired levels of investment for OHF, the next step is to define debt policy during the 5-year forecast period. Debt should not be viewed as the balancing variable in the financial plan. That is, the financial plan should not project assets and equity and then balance the equation with debt. Sound financial policy requires that the board and management define in advance what their position is regarding the assumption of debt. **TABLE 13-9** presents OHF's management and board policy on debt for the next 5 years.

**TABLE 13-8** Forecasted Property and Equipment for OHF

|  | 20X7 | 20X8 | 20X9 | 20X0 | 20X1 |
|---|---|---|---|---|---|
| Beginning gross property and equipment | $146,794 | $156,794 | $166,794 | $176,794 | $186,794 |
| Plus net capital expenditures | 10,000 | 10,000 | 10,000 | 10,000 | 10,000 |
| Ending gross property and equipment | $156,794 | $166,794 | $176,794 | $186,794 | $196,794 |

**TABLE 13-9** Forecasted Long-Term Debt for OHF

|  | 20X7 | 20X8 | 20X9 | 20X0 | 20X1 |
|---|---|---|---|---|---|
| Beginning long-term debt (LTD) | $54,781 | $53,380 | $51,892 | $50,326 | $48,520 |
| Less beginning current maturities of LTD | 1,401 | 1,488 | 1,566 | 1,806 | 1,715 |
| Ending long-term debt | $53,380 | $51,892 | $50,326 | $48,520 | $46,805 |

- *Long-term debt*: Board members at OHF have determined that they do not wish to borrow any additional money on a long-term basis over the next 5 years. They believe that their present capital structure has too much long-term debt, as evidenced by a high long-term debt to equity ratio. The present debt will therefore be repaid in accordance with existing debt amortization schedules. Table 13-9 summarizes OHF's long-term debt position over the next 5 years.
- *Accrued salaries and wages*: Although it may not be thought of as a form of debt, all current liabilities represent a form of financing. Accrued salaries and wages represent a form of financing from the firm's employees. The employees have contributed their labor before receiving their wages. Accrued salaries and wages, on average, have constituted about 5% of salaries and wages and constituted 5.3% in 20X6. This value is used in the forecast.
- *Due to third-party payers*: This current liability account represents overpayment by third-party payers during the course of the year and is a sizable account for OHF. In 20X6 the account balance was $11,571,000. OHF has consistently reported sizable values for this account, and this overpayment situation is expected to continue into the future. It is expected that the present relationship between net patient revenue and due to third-party payers will stabilize at approximately 7.2%. This is a critical relationship and represents interest-free financing that is currently being provided by OHF's third-party payers. Any change in this relationship would have a significant influence on OHF's financial projections.

## Assessing the Reasonableness of Required Equity Growth

At this stage in the development of the financial plan, we have projected balance sheets (Table 13-5), income statements (Table 13-6), and financial ratios (Table 13-7). The following two questions must be answered before our financial plan can be accepted:

1. Can we actually achieve the results currently projected, or are our assumptions realistic?
2. Are the financial results projected acceptable, or are we satisfied with the current projected financial performance?

Regarding the first question about the realistic nature of our assumptions, we already discussed these assumptions and the basis for them. This does not mean they are attainable, and we should review

again the critical assumptions on which the forecast is based. Especially important are the assumptions regarding revenue and expense growth.

One useful way to review the validity of a financial plan is to compare the projected financial ratios with historical values. Comparing the financial ratio values found in Tables 13-3 and 13-7 seems to indicate that the plan may be reasonable. The only major significant change appears in the area of profitability, especially margins. Operating income is projected to increase sharply from 20X6 levels. The basis for this increase is directly related to a modest 1% growth in salaries and wages. If we remain convinced that this goal is achievable because of scheduled productivity improvements, our initial forecast appears to be attainable.

Regarding the second question of acceptability, a comparison of historical and projected financial ratios is useful. In the initial forecast, there was no target set for board-designated and funded depreciation reserves. Surplus cash generated in the forecast was added to this balance, and any cash deficits would be subtracted from beginning balances. During the 5-year forecast OHF has added almost $38 million in new board-designated and funded depreciation reserves. The ending balance in 20X1 is projected to be $93,538,000. On the surface this seems like a healthy increase. But how does this compare with our replacement cost needs? In 20X1 our projected accumulated depreciation will be $122,074,000. The percentage of our projected funded depreciation to projected accumulated depreciation is 76.6%. This value is almost identical to the present 78.8% relationship, and we appear not to have compromised our replacement reserve integrity over the 5-year plan.

A further review of the financial ratios suggests only one area that may need some revision. The net plant and equipment actually declines during the 5-year financial planning period. Furthermore, OHF's average age of plant increases from 8.3 to 10.6 years. This may signal an underinvestment in plant and equipment. For the present time, however, we will assume that the projected level of capital expenditures is adequate, given the current surplus investment in inpatient facilities that will not require replacement. Most of the new capital will be deployed to fast-growing outpatient and clinic operations.

### Learning Objective 5

Explain how management control is used in conjunction with the financial plan.

## ► Integration of the Financial Plan with Management Control

The development of a financial plan is a useless exercise unless that plan is integrated into the management-control process. Management needs to know whether the plan is being realized and, if it is not, what corrective action can be taken. In some cases there may be little that management can do. For example, assume that the entity has experienced an unusually large reduction in its operating margins as a result of declining prices due to increased competition. In this case the only course of action open to management is perhaps to revise its plan to reflect more accurately the current situation or to cut expenses if possible. Indeed, it is important for management to assess the accuracy of its financial plan annually and to make appropriate changes as needed.

To integrate the financial plan with the management-control process, some structure is needed. Financial ratios provide that structure. The chart in **FIGURE 13-4** depicts detailed targets for OHF, reflecting its financial plan. In the chart specific ratio values are delineated. The primary targets involve the four major ratios that together determine the hospital's ROE. The secondary targets are concerned with additional data that can be used to monitor actual performance and detect possible problems.

To understand how the chart in Figure 13-4 might be used in management control, let us assume that the year 20X7 has just ended and the financial data essential to the calculation of the ratios are now available. OHF's actual ROE for 20X7 is assumed to be 7.6%, which represents an unfavorable variance from the required value of 8.4%.

Actual 20X7 values for the primary indicators are as follows:

Operating margin ratio percent, 1.0
Total asset turnover ratio, 0.93
Equity financing ratio percent, 44.0
Nonoperating revenue percent, 2.6

The major cause of the **unfavorable variance** in ROE deviates from the expected operating margin of 1.3 to 1.0%. In addition, the nonoperating revenue ratio also was below expectations, with an actual value of 2.6% compared with an expected value of 2.7%. All other ratio targets that determine equity growth were met. This narrows any corrective actions to the two areas of operating margins and nonoperating gains.

It is extremely important to remember the concept of sustainable growth. (This concept was introduced in Chapter 11.) Sustainable growth simply means that no organization can generate a growth rate in assets that exceeds its GRIE for a prolonged period. Ultimately, an organization is limited by the rate at which it can generate new equity.

ROE can be defined as follows:

$$\text{ROE} = \frac{[OM + NOR] \times TAT}{EF}$$

where OM is the operating margin ratio, NOR is the nonoperating revenue ratio, TAT is the total asset turnover ratio, and EF is the equity financing ratio. If top management and board members concentrate on this simple formula and the key relationships it represents, financial focus and direction will improve dramatically.

## ► SUMMARY

In the process of identifying the requirements for effective financial policy formulation in healthcare

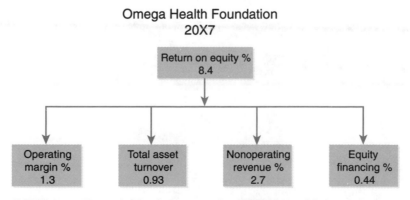

**Omega Health Foundation**
**20X7**

**FIGURE 13-4  Financial Ratio Targets for Omega Health Foundation**

firms, it is especially important to relate the strategic plan to the financial plan. The financial plan should not be developed in isolation from strategic planning, and the strategic plan should not be developed in isolation from the financial plan. Both plans need to be developed together, reflecting in that context their individual requirements and assumptions. A strategic plan is not valid if it is not financially feasible, and a financial plan is of little value if it does not reflect the strategic decisions reached by management and the board.

A financial plan should be updated at least annually, projecting a forecast period of 3 to 5 years. Financial plans that are not updated stand a good chance of becoming invalid. The environment of healthcare delivery is changing, and a healthcare entity's financial plan must reflect the changes. In fact, failure to update its financial plan can have disastrous consequences for an entity, leading perhaps to market share retrenchment or even financial failure.

Finally, financial plans should be integrated into the management-control process. Financial ratios can be useful in this regard. In particular, specific ratios can be usefully related to the key financial planning target of GRIE.

## ASSIGNMENTS

1. A financial plan may be thought of as a bridge between two balance sheets. What are the major categories of assumptions that must be specified to project a future balance sheet, given a current balance sheet?
2. What problems result from the present responsibility center or departmental orientation of most accounting systems in providing data for financial planning?
3. Your director of marketing is urging you to develop a new drug abuse treatment program. She has argued that there is no capital investment involved in the development of the new service. Do you believe this is an accurate statement?
4. Your hospital has a current funded depreciation to accumulated depreciation ratio of 0.20. What are the implications of this indicator for your hospital's financial planning?
5. Your controller has just provided you with ROI figures for your firm's major product lines. You have noticed that obstetrics has a very low ROI. What factors should be considered before you eliminate this service?
6. You are in the process of developing your firm's financial plan for the next 5 years. As an initial step you are analyzing financial ratios for the last 5 years. You notice that over the 5-year period, the average age of plant ratio has increased from 8.5 years to 12.2 years. What are the implications of this for your financial plan?
7. If current assets are expected to increase by $4 million over the next 5 years and you wish to increase your current ratio from 1.5 to 2.0, what additional amount of new equity must be generated to finance the increase in the current ratio on the incremental $4 million?
8. Beginning equity is $50 million and equity in 5 years is projected to be $100 million. What is the annual rate of growth implied by these values?
9. You are assessing the financial plan developed for you by a prestigious accounting firm. You are especially interested in the attainability of the projected GRIE. You know that if that growth rate is not realistic, the financial plan is not valid and you may have to scale back your projected increase in assets. TABLE 13-10 summarizes your findings. Does the accounting firm's plan appear to be reasonable?

### TABLE 13-10 Financial Plan Summary Values

|  | Historical Average | 5-Year Projections |
| --- | --- | --- |
| Reported income index ratio | 1.000 | 0.900 |
| Operating margin ratio | 0.025 | 0.027 |
| Total asset turnover ratio | 1.100 | 1.200 |

| Nonoperating revenue ratio | 0.011 | 0.011 |
|---|---|---|
| Equity financing ratio | 0.500 | 0.500 |
| Equity growth rate | 7.86% | 10.29% |

10. Using the data presented for OHF in this chapter, revise the existing financial plan. Assume that salaries and wages will increase 2% per year, not the original 1% used in the forecast. Prepare a revised forecasted balance sheet, income statement, and ratios for OHF.

## SOLUTIONS AND ANSWERS

1. Projection of a future balance sheet requires assumptions in the following three categories:

   a. Rates of growth for individual asset accounts
   b. Debt-financing policy for both current and long-term debt
   c. Realizable rate of growth in equity that is factored into five ratio areas:
      - Operating margins
      - Nonoperating revenue
      - Equity financing
      - Total asset turnover
      - Reported income index (defined as net income divided by the change in equity)

2. Strategic financial planning is usually done along program or product lines, not responsibility centers or departments. This requires the financial planner to transfer revenue, cost, and investment assignments from responsibility centers to product lines. This can be a difficult process.

3. Although some new investment in fixed assets may be required to start a drug abuse treatment program, the investment in working capital may be sizable. Some projection of the investment should be made to assess the potential ROI that is likely to result.

4. A funded depreciation to accumulated depreciation ratio of 0.20 implies that your hospital will need to borrow 80% of its replacement needs in the future. The percentage of debt financing is derived by the following formula:

   Debt financing = 100% − Funded depreciation to accumulated depreciation ratio

   This directly affects the debt policy assumptions that will be used in the financial plan. It also will have an impact on the firm's operating margins because of the potentially large increase in debt and the resulting increase in interest expense.

5. Eliminating a product line solely on the basis of an inadequate ROI may not be consistent with the firm's goals and objectives. Specifically, obstetrics may meet a community need and may be essential to the firm's mission; it may, in fact, be classified as a Samaritan (see Figure 13-3). Alternatively, a low ROI can sometimes be deceiving. The product line may have important externalities. For example, obstetrics may lose money, but gynecology may be very profitable. Eliminating obstetrics may mean that the firm's gynecology line, and its profits, would be reduced.

6. The current average age of plant ratio implies that the firm has a very old plant relative to industry norms. This will almost certainly mean that significant new investment is required in the planning period.

7. Use of a current ratio of 2.0 implies that the incremental investment of $4 million in current assets would be financed with $2 million of current liabilities. Use of a current ratio of 1.5 would imply current liability financing of $2.67 million. Therefore, the change in the current ratio implies that an additional equity requirement of $670,000 would be required.

8. The implied annual rate of growth is 14.86%.

9. The accounting firm's plan specifies a 30% increase in the annual GRIE, compared with the historical 5-year average (7.86% vs. 10.29%). The major changes are in the reported income index and total asset turnover ratios. In the past 5 years the firm has had no unreported income because the value for the reported income index is 1.0.

It is important to determine the expected source of the new equity. The increase in total asset turnover, although not large, does play an important role in the higher projected GRIE. Reasons for this increase should be verified.

10. **TABLES 13-11**, **13-12**, and **13-13** list the revised forecasts for OHF. Note the dramatic reduction in profit from a small change in one item. Also, OHF now will have $77,156,000 in board-designated funded depreciation in 20X1, not the original amount of $95,429,000. To understand the impact on board-designated funds, recognize that the increase in salary expense plus the associated increase in fringe benefits will reduce net income and therefore reduce the balance of cash available for investment. There is one other effect, however, and that is an increased requirement for holding nonincome-yielding cash and cash equivalents to meet the 20-day working capital requirement. For example, in 20X7 the increase in salary costs was $811,000 and the increased fringe benefits on this salary expense were 23%, or $186,000. The total increased expense is $997,000, which creates a demand to raise short-term cash balances by $55,000 [($997,000/365) × 20 days]. The total of the increased salary and benefit cost plus the increase in cash requirements is $1,052,000. This value is the difference between the original forecast value ($59,896,000) and the revised forecast value ($58,844,000). The reduction in the ending invested balance of $1,052,000 also cost the hospital $44,000 in reduced investment income, which will affect future year's investment and investment income levels. There is also a small financing advantage that results from the increased values for accrued salaries and wages. As the dollar amount of salaries and wages increases, there will be some benefit from the increased accrual.

**TABLE 13-11** Revised Forecasted Balance Sheet for OHF as of June 20X7, 20X8, 20X9, 20X0, and 20X1 (data in Thousands)

|  | General Funds | | | | |
|---|---|---|---|---|---|
|  | **20X7** | **20X8** | **20X9** | **20X0** | **20X1** |
| Assets current |  |  |  |  |  |
| Cash and cash equivalents | $8,962 | $9,099 | $9,359 | $9,628 | $9,906 |
| Accounts receivable | 24,568 | 25,059 | 25,560 | 26,072 | 26,593 |
| Due from third-party payers | 0 | 0 | 0 | 0 | 0 |
| Due from donor-restricted funds | 300 | 300 | 300 | 300 | 300 |
| Inventories | 1,851 | 1,944 | 2,041 | 2,143 | 2,250 |
| Prepaid expenses and other assets | 1,192 | 1,251 | 1,314 | 1,380 | 1,449 |
| Current portion of funds held by trustee | 1,055 | 1,120 | 1,185 | 1,250 | 1,315 |
| Current portion of self-insurance trust funds | 2,377 | 2,496 | 2,621 | 2,752 | 2,890 |
| Total current assets | $40,305 | $41,269 | $42,380 | $43,524 | $44,702 |
| Other assets |  |  |  |  |  |
| Gross property, plant, and equipment | $156,794 | $166,794 | $176,794 | $186,794 | $196,794 |
| Less total accumulated depreciation | 79,898 | 89,572 | 99,826 | 110,660 | 122,074 |
| Net property, plant, and equipment | $76,896 | $77,222 | $76,968 | $76,134 | $74,720 |

| | | | | | |
|---|---|---|---|---|---|
| Self-insurance trust funds, net of current portion | $9,787 | $10,276 | $10,790 | $11,330 | $11,896 |
| Board-designated funds | 58,697 | 64,096 | 69,055 | 72,905 | 76,074 |
| Funds held by trustee, net of current position | 338 | 338 | 338 | 338 | 338 |
| Investments in and advances to partnerships | 2,622 | 2,753 | 2,891 | 3,035 | 3,187 |
| Deferred financing costs, net | 972 | 805 | 638 | 471 | 304 |
| Deferred third-party reimbursement | 0 | 0 | 0 | 0 | 0 |
| Other assets | 1,174 | 1,291 | 1,420 | 1,562 | 1,718 |
| Total other assets | $73,611 | $79,584 | $85,160 | $89,672 | $93,552 |
| Total assets | $190,791 | $198,052 | $204,484 | $209,306 | $212,949 |
| Liabilities current | | | | | |
| Current portion of long-term debt | $1,488 | $1,566 | $1,806 | $1,715 | $1,525 |
| Accounts payable and accrued expenses | 11,641 | 12,223 | 12,835 | 13,476 | 14,150 |
| Accrued salaries, wages, and fees | 4,381 | 4,468 | 4,557 | 4,650 | 4,741 |
| Accrued restructuring costs | 0 | 0 | 0 | 0 | 0 |
| Accrued vacation | 3,288 | 3,288 | 3,288 | 3,288 | 3,288 |
| Accrued insurance costs | 2,346 | 2,463 | 2,586 | 2,715 | 2,851 |
| Advance from third-party payer | 1,228 | 1,253 | 1,278 | 1,304 | 1,330 |
| Due to third-party payers | 11,793 | 12,028 | 12,269 | 12,514 | 12,765 |
| Total current liabilities | $36,165 | $37,289 | $38,619 | $39,662 | $40,650 |
| Accrued retirement costs | $9,288 | $9,753 | $10,240 | $10,752 | $11,290 |
| Accrued insurance costs, net of current position | 4,868 | 5,111 | 5,367 | 5,635 | 5,917 |
| Deferred third-party reimbursement | 3,489 | 3,489 | 3,489 | 3,489 | 3,489 |
| Long-term debt, net of current position | 53,380 | 51,892 | 50,326 | 48,520 | 46,805 |
| Other liabilities | 250 | 262 | 276 | 289 | 304 |
| Total liabilities | $107,440 | $107,796 | $108,317 | $108,347 | $108,455 |
| Unrestricted net assets | 83,351 | 90,256 | 96,167 | 100,959 | 104,494 |
| Total liabilities and unrestricted net assets | $190,791 | $198,052 | $204,484 | $209,306 | $212,949 |

**TABLE 13-12** Revised Forecasted Income Statement for OHF (data in Thousands)

| | 20X7 | 20X8 | 20X9 | 20X0 | 20X1 |
|---|---|---|---|---|---|
| Revenues | | | | | |
| Net patient service revenue | $163,785 | $167,061 | $170,402 | $173,810 | $177,287 |
| Equity in net income from partnership | 769 | 807 | 847 | 890 | 934 |
| Gifts and bequests | 271 | 284 | 299 | 314 | 329 |
| Other | 9,198 | 9,658 | 10,141 | 10,548 | 11,180 |
| Total revenues | $174,023 | $177,810 | $181,689 | $185,662 | $189,730 |
| Expenses | | | | | |
| Salaries and wages | $82,653 | $84,306 | $85,992 | $87,712 | $89,466 |
| Fringe benefits | 19,010 | 19,390 | 19,779 | 20,174 | 20,577 |
| Professional fees | 9,429 | 9,900 | 10,395 | 10,915 | 11,461 |
| Supplies and other | 41,587 | 43,667 | 45,850 | 48,143 | 50,550 |
| Interest | 4,214 | 4,115 | 4,009 | 3,910 | 3,768 |
| Bad debt expense | 4,586 | 4,678 | 4,771 | 4,867 | 4,964 |
| Depreciation and amortization | 9,094 | 9,674 | 10,254 | 10,834 | 11,414 |
| Restructuring costs | 2,078 | 0 | 0 | 0 | 0 |
| Total expenses | $172,651 | $175,730 | $181,050 | $186,555 | $192,200 |
| Income from operations | $1,372 | $2,081 | $639 | $(892) | $(2,469) |
| Nonoperating gains (losses) | | | | | |
| Income on investments | $4,631 | $4,874 | $5,322 | $5,734 | $6,054 |
| Gifts and bequests | 50 | 50 | 50 | 50 | 50 |
| Loss on disposal of assets | (100) | (100) | (100) | (100) | (100) |
| Nonoperating gains, net | $4,581 | $4,824 | $5,272 | $5,684 | $6,004 |
| Excess of revenues over expenses | $5,953 | $6,905 | $5,911 | $4,792 | $3,535 |

| **TABLE 13-13** Revised Forecasted Financial Ratios for OHF | | | | | |
|---|---|---|---|---|---|
| | **20X7** | **20X8** | **20X9** | **20X0** | **20X1** |
| Profitability | | | | | |
| Total margin percentage | 3.5 | 4.0 | 3.4 | 2.7 | 1.9 |
| Operating margin percentage | 0.8 | 1.2 | 0.4 | −0.5 | −1.4 |
| Nonoperating revenue % | 2.7 | 2.8 | 3.0 | 3.2 | 3.3 |
| ROE percentage | 7.1 | 7.7 | 6.2 | 4.8 | 3.4 |
| Liquidity | | | | | |
| Current | 1.11 | 1.10 | 1.10 | 1.10 | 1.10 |
| Days in accounts receivable | 54.8 | 54.8 | 54.8 | 54.8 | 54.8 |
| Days cash on hand short term | 20.0 | 20.0 | 20.0 | 20.0 | 20.0 |
| Capital structure | | | | | |
| Equity financing percentage | 43.7 | 45.6 | 47.0 | 48.2 | 49.1 |
| Long-term debt to equity percentage | 64.0 | 57.5 | 52.3 | 48.1 | 44.8 |
| Cash flow to debt percentage | 14.0 | 15.4 | 14.9 | 14.4 | 13.8 |
| Times interest earned | 2.41 | 2.67 | 2.47 | 2.23 | 1.94 |
| Activity | | | | | |
| Total asset turnover | 0.88 | 0.87 | 0.86 | 0.86 | 0.86 |
| Fixed asset turnover | 2.19 | 2.23 | 2.25 | 2.36 | 2.40 |
| Current asset turnover | 4.18 | 4.17 | 4.15 | 4.13 | 4.10 |
| Other ratios | | | | | |
| Average age of plant | 8.8 | 9.3 | 9.7 | 10.2 | 10.7 |

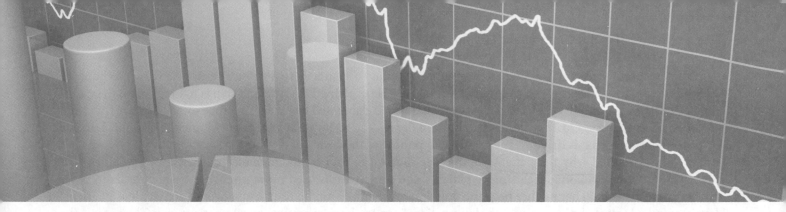

# CHAPTER 14

# Cost Concepts and Decision Making

## LEARNING OBJECTIVES

After studying this chapter, you should be able to do the following:

1. Discuss some of the ways to classify costs.
2. Discuss the four major categories of costs.
3. Explain what is meant by cost behavior, and differentiate between the five general types of cost behavior.
4. Explain the difference between controllable and noncontrollable costs.
5. Discuss the four types of costs that might be relevant when considering alternative projects.
6. Explain the role of direct and indirect costs in the costing process.
7. Describe the three methods of cost allocation.
8. Establish the importance of the semivariable cost function.
9. Calculate estimated fixed and variable costs using one of the described methods.
10. Calculate break-even and the volume necessary to achieve a desired net income.

## REAL-WORLD SCENARIO

Dr. Tim Martyn, the chief executive officer of Colonial Hospital, asked Stephen Carey, the chief financial officer of the hospital, to come to his office. Dr. Martyn wanted to talk to Carey about the hospital's maintenance expenses. Dr. Martyn, who generally had not paid much attention to such expenses, recently noticed that they varied considerably from month to month and wanted to know why.

As Carey sat down, Dr. Martyn mentioned that the maintenance expense report showed that over the last 6 months the maintenance expenses had been as low as $72,000 and as high as $96,000 per month. Not surprised, Carey responded that this amount of variation actually is quite normal. But Dr. Martyn knew that the hospital budgeted a constant $82,000 per month for those expenses. Why, he wondered, couldn't they do a better job of projecting those expenses? "With these kinds of fluctuations, how does management know if it has spent too much on maintenance expenses in a given month?" he said. He added, "What explains these fluctuations?"

Carey responded that his staff was in the process of trying to answer exactly those questions, in order to improve their budgeting for and control of maintenance expenses. He explained that the first step is to break all of the maintenance costs down into fixed and variable components. He elaborated by explaining that some costs are fixed and shouldn't change much. Other costs go up and down depending on how much patient volume the hospital has. The key is to figure out what is driving the variable component of the costs.

Dr. Martyn asked why the patient volume has such an impact on maintenance costs. Carey explained that he thinks that when Colonial treats more patients, the equipment is used more intensively, which leads to more maintenance expense. That further begs the question of what measure to use for the overall activity level. Patient-days seemed a logical choice, since each day a patient is in the hospital counts as one patient-day. The greater the number of patient-days in a month, the busier the hospital is.

Once the maintenance costs are broken down into its fixed and variable components, Carey said that they then would be able to predict what maintenance costs should be as a function of the number of patient-days. This information could be used for budgeting purposes and for benchmarking. Dr. Martyn was pleased to hear about the analysis being done by Carey's group and asked him to report when the analysis was complete.

---

So far we have focused on understanding and interpreting the financial information prepared through the financial accounting system and presented in general-purpose financial statements. This chapter focuses more on the use of cost information in decision making. Cost information is produced through an entity's cost accounting system. In most situations, cost information is shaped by the financial accounting system and the generally accepted principles of financial accounting on which financial accounting is based. However, cost information must be flexible, because it usually provides information for identifiable and specific decision-making groups, such as budgetary cost variance reports to department managers, cost reports to third-party payers, and forecasted project cost reports to planning agencies.

*Cost* is a noun that never really stands alone. In most situations, two additional pieces of information are added that enhance the meaning and relevance of the cost statistic. First, the object being costed is defined. For example, we might state that the cost of a clinic visit is $85. Objects of costing are usually of two types: (1) **products** (outputs or services) and (2) **responsibility centers** (departments or larger units). Often, we oversimplify this classification system and refer to cost information about products as *planning information* and cost information about responsibility centers as *control information*.

Second, usually an adjective is added to modify cost. For example, we might state that the direct cost of routine nursing care in a hospital is $400 per day. A number of major categories of modifiers refine the concept of cost; they are all used to improve the decision-making process by precisely defining cost to make it more relevant to decisions.

This chapter discusses some of the basic concepts of cost used in cost analysis. It is important to explain this jargon if decision makers are to use cost information correctly. Different concepts of cost are required for different decision purposes. In most situations, these concepts require specific, unique methodologies of cost measurement.

## ▶ Concepts of Cost

Cost may be categorized in a variety of ways to meet the specific needs of decision makers. See **TABLE 14-1** for examples of some of the ways to classify costs.

The far-left column lists the classification categories. Different ways to describe costs within these categories are shown in columns two, three, and, if applicable, four. For example, "direct" and "indirect" costs are different because of their traceability. **Direct costs** are directly linked and assigned to products or services. Direct costs would include things like direct labor and materials. **Indirect costs**, such as administrative overhead, are not easily traceable to a product or service. Indirect costs are traced to a product or service using some arbitrary allocation method.

Many of these classification systems will be covered in greater detail throughout this chapter. Regardless of the classification system, however, in most situations, the total value of the costs is the same. Using one cost concept in place of another simply slices the

**TABLE 14-1** Some of the Ways to Classify Costs

| Cost Classifications | Category 1 | Category 2 | Category 3 |
|---|---|---|---|
| Traceability | Direct costs | Indirect costs | — |
| Management control | Controllable | Noncontrollable | — |
| Relation to budget | Budgeted | Actual | — |
| Relation to time | Avoidable and sunk cost | Incremental cost | Opportunity cost |
| Relation to activity | Fixed costs | Variable costs | Mixed |

total cost pie differently. For example, in **TABLE 14-2**, the total cost of a laboratory for June 2017 is $21,360. Of that amount, $20,000 could be classified as direct

**TABLE 14-2** Cost Report, Laboratory, June 2017

| | Amount |
|---|---|
| Direct costs | |
| Salaries | $10,000 |
| Supplies | 5,000 |
| Other | 5,000 |
| Total direct costs | $20,000 |
| Allocated costs | |
| Employee benefits | $150 |
| Administration | 500 |
| Maintenance | 250 |
| Housekeeping | 200 |
| Laundry | 100 |
| Depreciation | 160 |
| Total indirect costs | $1,360 |
| Total costs | $21,360 |
| Relative value units (RVUs) | 10,000 |

cost and $1,360 as indirect cost. However, classifying costs by controllability might determine that $15,000 of the laboratory cost was controllable and $6,360 was not controllable, if the laboratory manager had no control over the $5,000 in other direct cost. The total cost, however, is the same in both cases.

This brings us to another important point. Because, in most cases, different concepts of cost simply slice total cost in different ways, there may be underlying relationships among the various concepts of costs. For example, direct costs and controllable costs may be related. In many situations, there are standard "rules of thumb" that may be used to relate cost measures.

The difference between **cost** and **expense** is another crucial definitional point. Accountants have traditionally defined cost in a way that leads one to think of cost as an expenditure. However, most people who are not accountants use the term *cost* to refer to expense. For example, in Table 14-2, depreciation is listed as a cost. However, depreciation is not an actual expenditure of cash but an amortization of prior cost. In the present context, unless otherwise indicated, when we are discussing cost statistics, the terms *costs* and *expenses* may be used interchangeably.

### Learning Objective 2

Discuss the four major categories of costs.

For purposes of discussion, we examine the following four major categories of costs:

1. Traceability to the object being costed
2. Behavior of cost to output or activity
3. Management responsibility for control
4. Future costs versus historical costs

## Traceability

Of all cost classifications, **traceability** is the most basic. Two major categories of costs classified by traceability are (1) direct costs and (2) indirect costs. A direct cost is specifically traceable to a given cost object. A **cost object** is an item for which the organization wishes to estimate the cost, such as a test, a visit, a patient or a patient-day. They fall into the following categories:

- Product
- Process
- Department
- Activity

For example, the salaries, supplies, and other costs in Table 14-2 are classified as direct costs of the laboratory. Indirect costs cannot be traced to a given cost object without resorting to some arbitrary method of assignment. In Table 14-2, depreciation, employee benefits, and costs of other departments would be classified as indirect costs.

Not all costs classified as indirect actually may be indirect, however. In some situations, they could be redefined as direct costs. For example, it might be possible to calculate employee benefits for specific employees; these costs then could be charged to the departments in which the employees work and thus become direct costs. However, the actual costs of performing these calculations might be prohibitive.

The classification of a cost as either direct or indirect depends on the given cost object. This is a simple observation, but one that is forgotten by many users of cost information. For example, the $20,000 of direct cost identified in Table 14-2 is a direct cost only regarding the laboratory department. If another cost object is specified, the cost may no longer be direct. For example, dividing the $20,000 of direct costs by the number of **relative value units (RVUs)**, 10,000, yields a direct cost per RVU of $2, but this is not a true figure. The direct cost of any given RVU may be higher or lower than the $2 calculated, which is the average value for all RVUs and not necessarily the cost for any specific unit.

Incorrect classification is a common problem in cost accounting. Costs are accumulated on a department or responsibility-center basis and may be direct or indirect regarding that department. However, it can be misleading to state that the same set of direct costs is also direct regarding the outputs of that department.

The major direct cost categories of most departments would include:

- Salaries
- Supplies

- Other (usually fees and purchased services such as dues, travel, and rent)

Indirect cost categories usually include:

- Depreciation
- Employee benefits
- Allocated costs of other departments

The concept of direct versus indirect cost may not seem to have much specific relevance to decision makers. To some extent, this is true; however, the concept of direct versus indirect costs is pervasive. It influences both the definition and measurement of other alternative cost concepts that do have specific relevance.

### Learning Objective 3

Explain what is meant by cost behavior, and differentiate between the five general types of cost behavior.

## Cost Behavior

Cost is also classified by the degree of variability in relation to output. The actual measurement of *cost behavior* is influenced by a department's classification of cost, which provides the basis for categorizing costs as direct or indirect.

For our purposes, we can identify five major categories of costs that are classified according to their relationship to output:

1. Variable
2. Fixed
3. Semi-fixed (or step fixed)
4. Semivariable
5. Curvilinear

Categories three, four, and five sometimes are referred to generally as mixed cost behavior. All three general cost behavior patterns—*variable, fixed,* and *mixed*—are found in most organizations. The relative proportion of each type of cost present in a firm is known as the firm's **cost structure**. For example, a firm might have many fixed costs but few variable or mixed costs. Alternatively, it might have many variable costs but few fixed or mixed costs. A firm's cost structure can have a significant impact on decisions.

**Variable costs** change as output or volume (or some other activity level) changes in a constant, proportional manner. That is, if output increases by 10%, costs also should increase by 10%; that is, there is some constant cost increment per unit of output. **FIGURE 14-1** illustrates, graphically and mathematically, the concept

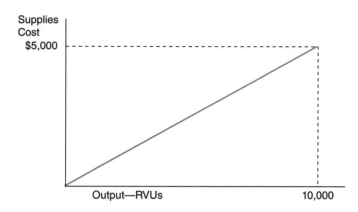

**FIGURE 14-1  Cost Behavior of Supplies Cost, Variable**

of variable cost for the laboratory example of Table 14-2. It is assumed that all supply costs in this case are variable. For each unit increase in RVUs, supply costs will increase by $0.50.

An activity is a measure of whatever causes the incurrence of variable cost. For this reason an activity base is sometimes referred to as a cost driver. Examples of common activity bases are direct labor hours, discharges, and patient visits. Other activity bases (cost drivers) might include the number of pounds of laundry processed by the laundry department, the number of medical records completed, and the number of occupied beds in a hospital or nursing home.

**Fixed costs** do not change in response to changes in volume. They are a function of the passage of time, not output. **FIGURE 14-2** illustrates fixed cost behavior patterns for the depreciation costs of the laboratory example. Each month, irrespective of output levels, depreciation cost will be $160.

**Semi-fixed** (also called "**step fixed**") costs do change as volume changes, but they are not proportional. A semi-fixed cost might be considered variable or fixed, depending on the size of the steps relative to the range of volume under consideration. For example,

in **FIGURE 14-3**, it is assumed that the salary cost of the laboratory is semi-fixed. If the volume of output under consideration were between 6,000 and 8,000 RVUs, salary costs could be considered fixed at $9,000. Some semi-fixed costs may be considered variable for cost analysis purposes. For example, if people could be employed other than as full-time equivalents (FTEs), such as by using overtime or part-time pools, the size of the steps might be significantly smaller than the 2,000 RVUs in our laboratory example. Presently, it is assumed that one additional FTE must be employed for every increment of 2,000 RVUs. In this situation treating salary costs as variable might not be bad practice (Figure 14-3).

**Semivariable** costs include elements of both fixed and variable costs. Utility costs are good examples. There may be some basic, fixed requirement per unit of time (e.g., month or year), regardless of volume—such as normal heating and lighting requirements. But there is also likely to be a direct, proportional relationship between volume and the amount of the utility cost. As volume increases, costs go up. **FIGURE 14-4** illustrates semivariable costs in our laboratory example.

Many costs that often are classified as variable actually behave in a *curvilinear* fashion. The behavior of a curvilinear cost is shown in **FIGURE 14-5**. Although many costs are not strictly linear when plotted as a function of volume, a curvilinear cost can be satisfactorily approximated with a straight line within a narrow band of activity known as the relevant range. The **relevant range** is that range of activity within which the assumptions made by the manager about cost behavior are valid. For example, note that the dashed line in Figure 14-5 can be used as an approximation to the curvilinear cost with very little loss of accuracy within the shaded relevant range. However, outside of the relevant range this particular straight line is a poor approximation to the curvilinear cost relationship. Managers should always keep in mind that a particular assumption made about cost behavior may be very inappropriate if activity falls outside of the relevant range.

In many situations, we do not focus on specific cost elements but aggregate several cost categories of interest. It is interesting to see what type of cost behavior pattern emerges when we do this. **FIGURE 14-6** aggregates four of the cost categories discussed earlier: variable, fixed, semi-fixed, and semivariable. A semivariable cost behavior pattern closely approximates the actual aggregated cost behavior pattern; this is true for many types of operations. In the next section, we discuss some simple but useful methods for approximating this cost function.

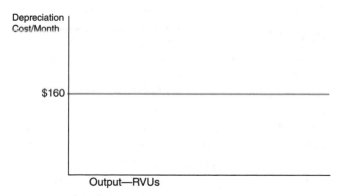

**FIGURE 14-2  Cost Behavior of Depreciation, Fixed**

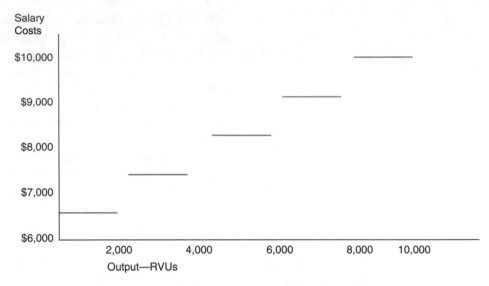

**FIGURE 14-3** **Cost Behavior of Salary Costs, Semi-Fixed**

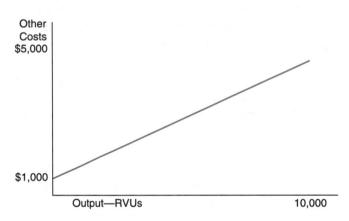

**FIGURE 14-4** **Cost Behavior of Other Costs, Semivariable**

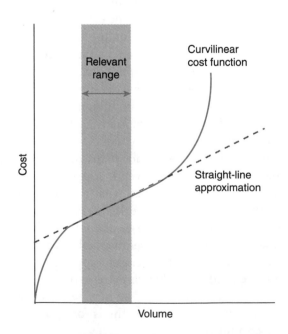

**FIGURE 14-5** **Curvilinear Costs and the Relevant Range**

Explain the difference between controllable and noncontrollable costs.

## Controllability

One of the primary purposes of gathering cost information is to aid the management control process. To facilitate evaluation of the management control process, costs must be assigned to individual responsibility centers, usually departments, where a designated manager is responsible for cost control. A natural question that arises is, for what proportion of the total costs charged to a department is the manager responsible? The answer to this question requires costs to be separated into two categories: controllable and non-controllable costs.

**Controllable costs** can be influenced by a designated responsibility center or departmental manager within a defined control period. It has been stated that all costs are controllable by someone at some time. For example, the chief executive officer of a healthcare facility, through the authority granted by the governing board, is ultimately responsible for all costs.

The matrix of costs shown in **FIGURE 14-7** categorizes the laboratory cost report data of Table 14-2. All costs must fall into one of the six cells of the matrix; however, it may be possible to categorize a cost that falls into several different categories into more than one cell of the matrix. In the laboratory example, other cost was viewed as semivariable, implying that part of the cost would be described as a direct variable cost ($4,000) and part as a direct fixed cost ($1,000).

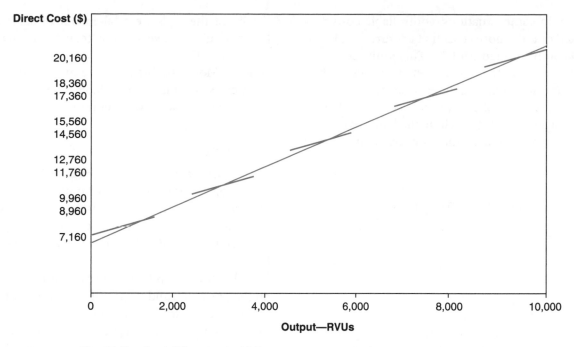

**FIGURE 14-6** **Cost Behavior of Aggregated Costs**

**Cost Behavior**

|  | | Variable | | Fixed | | Semi-Fixed | | Total |
|---|---|---|---|---|---|---|---|---|
| **Direct** | Other | $4,000 | Other | $1,000 | Salaries | $10,000 | $20,000 |
|  | Supplies | 5,000 | | | | | |
|  | | $9,000 | | $1,000 | | $10,000 | |
| **Indirect** | Employee Benefits | $150 | Depreciation | $160 | Maintenance | $250 | $1,360 |
|  | Housekeeping | 100 | Administration | 500 | Laundry | 100 | |
|  | | $250 | Housekeeping | 100 | | $350 | |
|  | | | | $760 | | | |
| **Totals** | | $9,250 | | $1,760 | | $10,350 | $21,360 |

*(Left axis label: **Traceables**)*

**FIGURE 14-7** **Laboratory Cost Behavior Organization**

There is a tendency in developing management control programs, especially in the healthcare industry, to use one of three approaches in designating controllable costs. First, controllable costs may be defined as the total costs charged to the department; the department manager would view all costs in the six cells of Figure 14-7. In our example, all $21,360 of cost would be viewed as controllable by the laboratory manager. In most normal situations, however, this grossly overstates the amount of cost actually controllable by a given department manager. The result of this overstatement has been negative in many situations. Department managers have rightfully viewed this basis of control as highly inequitable.

Second, controllable costs may be limited to those costs classified as direct. This system is also not without fault: specifically, there may be fixed costs attributed directly to the department that should not be considered controllable. Rent for pieces of equipment, for example, may not be under the department manager's control. There also may be indirect costs, especially costs that are variable that the department manager can control. For example, employee benefits may legitimately be the department manager's responsibility.

Third, in some situations, controllable costs may be defined as only those costs that are direct and variable ($9,000 from Figure 14-7). This limits costs that are controllable by the department manager to their lowest level. However, it excludes what could be a relatively large amount of cost influenced by the department manager. Failure to include the latter cost in the manager's control sphere may weaken management control.

## Future Costs

Decision making involves selection among alternatives; it is a forward-looking process. Actual historical cost may be useful as a basis for projecting future costs, but it should not be used without adjustment unless it can be assumed that future conditions will be identical to past conditions.

A variety of concepts and definitions have been used in the current discussion of costs for decision-making purposes. The following four types of costs seem to be basic to the process of selecting among alternative decisions:

1. Avoidable costs
2. Sunk costs
3. Incremental costs
4. Opportunity costs

## Avoidable Costs

Avoidable costs will be affected by the decision under consideration. Specifically, they are costs that can be eliminated or saved if an activity is discontinued; they will remain only if the activity continues. For example, if a hospital was considering curtailing its volume by 50% in response to cost-containment pressures, what would it save? The answer is those costs that are avoidable. In most situations, multiplication of current average cost per unit of output (patient-days or admissions) by the projected change in output would overstate avoidable costs because much of the cost might not be able to be reduced, at least in the short run. For example, depreciation and interest expenses might not change. Variable costs are almost always a subset of avoidable costs, but avoidable costs might include some fixed costs. For example, administrative staffing might be drastically reduced in a nursing home

if 50% of the beds were taken out of service. Most likely, administrative staffing costs would have been classified as fixed, given earlier expectations regarding volume. Most variable costs are avoidable, but some fixed costs also may be avoidable when large changes in volume are under consideration.

## Sunk Costs

Sunk costs are unaffected by the decision under consideration. In the previous example, large portions of cost—depreciation, administrative salaries, insurance, and others—are sunk or not avoidable in the proposed 50% reduction in volume in the nursing home.

The distinction between fixed and variable costs, on the one hand, and sunk and avoidable costs, on the other, is not perfect. Many costs classified as fixed also may be thought of as sunk, but some are not. For example, malpractice insurance premiums generally may be considered fixed cost, given an expected normal level of activity. However, if the institution is considering a drastic reduction in volume, malpractice premiums may not be entirely fixed. In summary, sunk costs are almost always a subset of fixed costs, but not all fixed costs need be sunk. In the evaluation of a decision to close a hospital, most of the hospital's costs (both fixed and variable) probably would be eliminated and therefore would be categorized as avoidable and not sunk regarding the closure decision.

## Incremental Costs

Incremental costs represent the change in cost that results from a specific management action. For example, someone might want to know the incremental cost of signing a managed-care contract that would generate 200 new admissions per year. There is a strong relationship between incremental and avoidable costs. They can be thought of as different sides of the same coin. We use the term *incremental costs* to reference the change in costs that results from a management action that increases volume. The term *avoidable costs* defines the change in cost that results from a management action that reduces volume. For decisions involving only modest changes in output, *incremental costs* and *variable costs* may be used interchangeably. In most situations, however, incremental costs are more comprehensive. A decision to construct a surgicenter adjacent to a hospital would involve fixed and variable costs. Depreciation of the facility would be a fixed cost, but it would be incremental to the decision if a new surgicenter were constructed.

## Opportunity Costs

Opportunity costs are values foregone by using a resource in a particular way instead of in its next best alternative way. Assume that a nursing home is considering expanding its facility and would use land acquired 20 years ago. If the land had a historical cost of $1 million but a present market value of $10 million, what is the opportunity cost of the land? Practically everyone would agree that if sale of the land constituted the next best alternative, the opportunity cost would be $10 million, not $1 million. Alternatively, a hospital might consider converting part of its acute care facility into a **skilled nursing facility** because of a reduction in demand or obsolescence in the facility. The question arises, what is the value, or what would be the cost of the facility, to the skilled nursing facility operation? If there is no way that the facility can be renovated or if the facility is not needed for the provision of acute care, its opportunity cost may be zero. This could contrast sharply to the recorded historical cost of the facility.

## ▶ Cost Measurement

In this section, we examine the methods of cost measurement for two cost categories: (1) direct and indirect cost and (2) variable and fixed cost. Both of these cost categories are useful in financial decisions, but the cost accounting system does not directly provide estimates for them.

### *Learning Objective 6*

Explain the role of direct and indirect costs in the costing process.

### Direct and Indirect Cost

In most cost accounting systems, costs are classified by department or responsibility center and by type of expenditure. Costs are charged to the departments to which they are traceable. Costs are also classified by object of expenditure; they may be identified as supplies, salaries, rent, insurance, or some other category.

Departments in a healthcare facility can be classified generally as direct or indirect departments, depending on whether they provide services directly to the patient. Sometimes the terms *revenue* and *nonrevenue* are substituted for direct and indirect. In the hospital industry, the breakdown in **TABLE 14-3** is used in general-purpose financial statements.

**TABLE 14-3** Operating Expense and Type of Department

| Operating Expense Area | Type of Department |
| --- | --- |
| Nursing services area | Direct/revenue |
| Other professional services | Direct/revenue |
| General services | Indirect/nonrevenue |
| Fiscal services | Indirect/nonrevenue |
| Administrative services | Indirect/nonrevenue |

Whatever the nomenclature used to describe the classification of departments, cost allocation is usually required. **Cost allocation** is the process of assigning pooled indirect costs to specific cost objects using an allocation base that represents a major function of a business. An **allocation base** (also called a "**cost driver**") is a volume metric that is used to allocate costs, based on its assumed relationship to why the costs occurred. The better the cause-and-effect relationship between why the cost occurred and the allocation basis, the more accurate the cost allocation. Some common allocation bases include square footage, the number of full-time equivalent employees (FTEs), and direct labor hours. For example, square footage is commonly used to allocate utility expenses, on the assumption that actual utility costs are proportional to the size of the space a service occupies.

The costs of the indirect, nonrevenue departments need to be allocated to the direct revenue departments for many decision-making purposes. For example, some payers reimburse on the basis of the full costs of direct departments and are interested in the costs of indirect departments only insofar as they affect the calculation of the departments' full costs (both direct and indirect). Pricing decisions need to be based on full costs, not just direct costs, if the costs of the indirect departments are to be covered equitably. It is also critical to include indirect costs when evaluating the financial return of specific programs or product lines. For example, some indirect costs would need to be assigned to an ambulatory surgery program to properly evaluate whether the program was financially viable.

Equity is a key concept in allocating indirect department costs to direct departments. Ideally, the allocation should reflect, as nearly as possible, the actual cost incurred by the indirect department to provide services for a direct department. Department managers who receive cost reports showing indirect allocations are vitally interested in this equity principle, and for good reason. Even if indirect costs are regarded as noncontrollable by the department manager, the allocation of costs to a given direct department can have an important effect on a variety of management decisions. Pricing, expansion or contraction of a department; the purchase of new equipment; and the salaries of department managers are all affected by the allocation of indirect costs. An outpatient surgery program that has unreasonable amounts of hospital overhead allocated to it may find itself noncompetitive.

Costs of indirect departments are in most cases not directly traceable to direct departments. If they were, they could be reassigned. In such cases, they must be allocated to the direct departments in some systematic and rational manner. In general, the following two allocation decisions must be made: (1) selection of the allocation basis and (2) selection of the method of cost apportionment.

**TABLE 14-4** provides sample data for a cost allocation. In this example, there are four departments: two are indirect (laundry/linen and housekeeping), and two are direct (radiology and nursing). How much the laundry weighs is the only allocation basis under consideration for the laundry and linen department. The housekeeping department can use one of two allocation bases, either square feet of area served or hours of service actually worked.

---

*Learning Objective 7*

Describe the three methods of cost allocation.

---

In general, there are only three acceptable methods of cost allocation:

1. Step-down method
2. Double-distribution method
3. Simultaneous-equations method

Most healthcare facilities still use the **step-down method** of cost allocation. In this method, the indirect department that receives the least amount of service from other indirect departments and provides the most service to other departments allocates its cost first. A similar analysis follows to determine the order of cost allocation for each of the remaining indirect departments. This determination can be subjective to allow some flexibility, as we shall observe shortly.

In the step-down allocation process illustrated in **TABLE 14-5**, the laundry and linen department allocates its cost first. Then, housekeeping allocates its direct cost, plus the allocated cost of laundry and linen, to the direct departments of radiology and nursing, based on the ratio of services provided to those departments. The numbers in parentheses represent the proportion of cost charged to that department.

The order of departmental allocation can be an important variable in a step-down method of cost allocation. **TABLE 14-6** depicts an alternative step-down cost allocation in which housekeeping allocates its cost first, preceding the laundry and linen department.

The **double-distribution** method of cost allocation is just a refinement of the step-down method. Instead of closing the individual department after allocating its costs, it is kept open and receives the costs of other indirect departments. After one complete allocation sequence, the former departments are then closed, using the normal step-down method.

The **simultaneous-equations** method of cost allocation is used in an attempt to calculate the exact

---

| **TABLE 14-4**  Cost Allocation Example | | | | |
|---|---|---|---|---|
| **Department** | **Direct Cost** | **Pounds of Laundry Used** | **Hours of Housekeeping** | **Square Feet** |
| Laundry/linen | $15,000 | — | 150 | 50,000 |
| Housekeeping | 30,000 | 5,000 | — | — |
| Radiology | 135,000 | 5,000 | 900 | 10,000 |
| Nursing | 270,000 | 90,000 | 1,950 | 140,000 |
| Total | $450,000 | $100,000 | 3,000 | 200,000 |

**TABLE 14-5** Step-Down Allocation Method—Alternative 1

|  | Direct Cost | Laundry/Linen | Housekeeping (Hours) | Total |
|---|---|---|---|---|
| Laundry/linen | $15,000 | $15,000 | | |
| Housekeeping | 30,000 | 750 (0.05) | $30,750 | |
| Radiology | 135,000 | 750 (0.05) | 9,711 (0.3158) | $145,461 |
| Nursing | 270,000 | 13,500 (0.90) | 21,039 (0.6842) | 304,539 |
| Total | $450,000 | $15,000 | $30,750 | $450,000 |

**TABLE 14-6** Step-Down Allocation Method—Alternative 2

|  | Direct Cost | Housekeeping (Hours) | Laundry/Linen | Total |
|---|---|---|---|---|
| Housekeeping | $30,000 | $30,000 | | |
| Laundry/linen | 15,000 | 1,500 (0.05) | $16,500 | |
| Radiology | 135,000 | 9,000 (0.30) | 868 (0.0526) | $144,868 |
| Nursing | 270,000 | 19,500 (0.65) | 15,632 (0.9474) | 305,132 |
| Total | $450,000 | $30,000 | $16,500 | 450,000 |

cost allocation amounts. A system of equations is established, and mathematically correct allocations are computed. In the previous example, if simultaneous equations had been used, the cost of radiology would be $145,075 and the cost of nursing would be $304,925, using the following system of equations:

$$\text{Laundry cost (LC)} = \$15,000 + 0.05\,\text{HC}$$
$$\text{Housekeeping cost (HC)} = \$30,000 + 0.05\,\text{LC}$$
$$\text{Radiology cost (RC)} = \$135,000 + 0.05\,\text{LC} + 0.30\,\text{HC}$$
$$\text{Nursing cost (NC)} = \$270,000 + 0.90\,\text{LC} + 0.65\,\text{HC}$$

Finally, it should be noted that using a different allocation base can create differences in cost allocation. For example, the use of square footage for housekeeping, instead of hours served, produces the pattern of cost allocation shown in **TABLE 14-7** when housekeeping allocates its cost first, using the step-down method.

The important point in this discussion is that total cost is not as objective and as exact of a figure as one might normally think. Indirect costs can be allocated in a variety of ways that can create significant differences in total costs for given departments. This flexibility should be remembered when examining and interpreting full-cost data.

*Learning Objective 8*

Establish the importance of the semivariable cost function.

## Variable and Fixed Cost

An important and widely used cost concept is variability regarding output. It is involved in determining a number of other costs, such as avoidable, sunk, incremental, and controllable costs. However, accounting records do not directly yield this type of

**TABLE 14-7** Step-Down Allocation Method—Alternative 3

| | Direct Cost | Housekeeping (Square Feet) | Laundry/Linen | Total |
|---|---|---|---|---|
| Housekeeping | $30,000 | $30,000 | | |
| Laundry/linen | 15,000 | 7,500 (0.25) | $22,500 | |
| Radiology | 135,000 | 1,500 (0.05) | 1,184 (0.0526) | $137,684 |
| Nursing | 270,000 | 21,000 (0.70) | 21,317 (0.9474) | 312,317 |
| Total | $450,000 | $30,000 | $22,500 | $450,000 |

cost information. Instead, the costs are classified by department and by object of expenditure. Thus, to develop estimates of variable and fixed costs, the relevant data must be analyzed in some way.

Our discussion of cost concepts classified by variability regarding output indicated that a semivariable cost pattern might be a good representation of many types of costs. A semivariable cost function has both a fixed and variable element. A semivariable cost function often results when various types of costs are aggregated together.

---

### *Learning Objective 9*

Calculate estimated fixed and variable costs using one of the described methods.

---

## Estimation Methods

Estimation of a semivariable cost function requires separation of the cost into variable and fixed components. A variety of methods, varying in complexity and accuracy, may be used. Four of the simplest methods are (1) visual-fit, (2) high–low, (3) semiaverages, and (4) regression.

To illustrate each of these methods, assume that we are trying to determine the labor cost function for the radiology department and we have the six biweekly payroll data points presented in **TABLE 14-8**.

In the **visual-fit method** of cost estimation, the previous individual data points are plotted on graph paper. A straight line is then drawn through the points to provide the best fit. Visual fitting of data is a good first step in any method of cost estimation. **FIGURE 14-8** shows a visual fitting of the previous radiology data.

**TABLE 14-8** Payroll Data

| Pay Period | No. of Films (x) | Hours Worked (y) | |
|---|---|---|---|
| 1 | 300 | 180 | (low) |
| 2 | 240 | 140 | (low) |
| 3 | 400 | 230 | (high) |
| 4 | 340 | 190 | (high) |
| 5 | 180 | 110 | (lowest) |
| 6 | 600 | 320 | (highest) |
| Total | 2,060 | 1,170 | |

The **high–low method** is a simple technique that can be used to estimate the variable and fixed-cost coefficients of a semivariable cost function. The variable cost parameter is solved first. It equals the change in cost from the highest to the lowest data point, divided by the change in output. In the previous radiology example, the variable hours worked would be calculated as follows:

$$\text{Variable labor hours/film} = \frac{320 - 110}{600 - 180} = \frac{210}{420} = 0.50$$

The fixed-cost parameter then may be solved by subtracting the estimated variable cost (determined by multiplying the variable cost parameter estimate by output at the high level) from total cost. In our

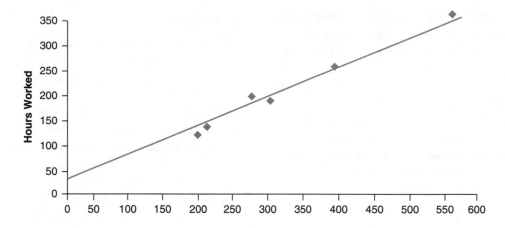

**FIGURE 14-8** **Visual Fitting of Radiology Data**

radiology example, fixed labor hours would equal the following:

$$\text{Fixed labor hours per pay period}$$
$$= 320 - (0.50 \times 600)$$
$$= 320 - 300 = 20$$

Alternatively, it is possible to plot the high and low points and then draw a straight line through them.

The **semiaverages method** is similar to the high–low method regarding its mathematical solution. To derive the estimate of variable cost, the difference between the mean of the high-cost points and the mean of the low-cost points is divided by the change in output from the mean of the high-cost points to the mean of the low-cost points. In the radiology example, variable cost would be calculated as follows:

$$\text{Variable labor hours/film} =$$
$$\dfrac{\dfrac{320 + 230 + 190}{3} - \dfrac{180 + 140 + 110}{3}}{\dfrac{600 + 400 + 340}{3} - \dfrac{300 + 240 + 180}{3}}$$
$$= \dfrac{246.67 - 143.33}{446.67 - 240.00} = 0.50$$

Fixed cost is solved in a manner identical to that used in the high–low method. In the radiology example, fixed labor hours would equal the following:

$$\text{Fixed labour hours per pay period}$$
$$= 246.67 - (0.50 \times 446.67)$$
$$= 23.34$$

The **simple linear regression method** (also called "**least-squares regression**") will produce estimates of variable cost (V) and fixed cost (F) that will minimize the variance between predicted and actual observations. In essence, linear regression is a more precise version of the visual-fit method. Rather than fitting a regression line through the scatter plot data by visual inspection, linear regression uses mathematical formulas to fit the regression line. Also, unlike the high–low and semiaverages methods, the least-squares regression method takes all of the data into account when estimating the cost formula.

A general regression would be:

$$\text{Total costs} = \text{Intercept} + (\text{Coefficient} \times \text{Volume})$$

Thus, the intercept estimates fixed costs and the regression coefficient estimates variable cost per member. Standard errors from the regression estimates are used to consider whether differences are statistically significant.

Because cost is usually plotted on the vertical axis, the vertical difference between the line and an actual data point is referred to as the estimation error. The regression line that is fitted to the data points is the one that minimizes the sum of the squared deviations between the estimated line and actual costs. Although the formulas that accomplish this are fairly complex (shown below), computers and many software programs, such as Excel, easily carry out these calculations. Each data point consists of the observed values of the activity level (or volume) as the X portion of the data point (the independent variable), and the cost associated with that volume level is the Y portion of each data point (the dependent variable). You simply enter the data points into the computer, and with an appropriate command, the computer and software do the rest.

In addition to estimates of the intercept (fixed cost) and slope (variable cost per unit), least-squares regression software ordinarily provides a number of other very useful statistics. One of these statistics is the adjusted $R^2$, called the coefficient of determination, which is a measure of the "goodness of fit." The adjusted $R^2$ tells us the percentage of the variation in the dependent variable (cost) that is explained by variation in the independent variable (activity). The adjusted $R^2$ varies from 0 to 100%, and the higher the percentage, the better (in terms of a change in the activity level explaining the change in cost).

The formulas for estimation are presented below, where $Q$ refers to output, $C$ refers to cost, and $N$ refers to the number of observations:

1. $$V = \frac{\Sigma Q - N \overline{Q}\overline{C}}{\Sigma Q^2 - N \overline{Q}^2}$$

2. $F = \overline{C} - V\overline{Q}$

Applying the previous formulas to the radiology data produces the following estimates:

1. $$V = \frac{456,000 - 401,696}{815,600 - 707,253} = 0.5012$$

2. $F = 195 - (0.5012 \times 343.33) = 22.92$

The four methods of estimating variable and fixed costs discussed thus far are relatively simplistic. They are useful in only limited ways to provide a basis for further discussion and analysis of what the true cost behavioral pattern might be. However, in most situations, a limited attempt, based on simplistic methods, to discover the underlying fixed and variable cost patterns is better than no attempt.

A slightly more sophisticated approach is *multiple regression*, which is an extension of the simple linear regression method. So far, we have assumed that a single factor such as patient-days drives the variable cost component of a mixed cost. This assumption is acceptable for many mixed costs, but in some situations there may be more than one causal factor driving the variable cost element. For example, shipping costs may depend on both the number of units shipped and the weight of the units. In a situation such as this, multiple regression is necessary. Multiple regression is an analytical method that is used when the dependent variable (i.e., cost) is impacted by more than one factor. Although adding more factors, or variables, makes the computations more complex, the principles involved are the same as in the simple least-squares regressions discussed above. Because of the complexity of the calculations, multiple regression is nearly always done with a computer and is easily done in Excel.

## Data Checks

When any of the previous methods are used, several data checks should be performed. First, the cost data being used to estimate the cost behavior pattern should be stated in a common dollar. If the wages paid for employees have changed dramatically from one year to the next, the use of unadjusted wage and salary data from the 2 years can create measurement problems. In our radiology example, we used a physical quantity measure of cost, namely, hours worked. A physical measure of cost should be used whenever possible.

Second, cost and output data should be matched; the figures for reported cost should relate to the activity of the period. In most situations, accounting records provide this type of relationship based on the accrual principle of accounting. However, in some situations, this may not happen; supply costs may be charged to a department when the items are purchased, not when they are used.

Third, the period during which a cost function is being estimated should include stable technology and a case mix. If the technology under consideration has changed dramatically during that period, there will be measurement problems. Estimating a cost function based on two different production technologies will produce a cost function that reflects neither.

---

*Learning Objective 10*

Calculate break-even and the volume necessary to achieve a desired net income.

---

## ▶ Break-Even Analysis

Certain techniques can be applied when analyzing the relationships among cost, volume, and profit. These techniques rely on categorizing costs as fixed and variable. They can serve as powerful management decision aids and may be valuable in a wide range of decisions. An understanding of these techniques is crucial for decision makers whose choices affect the financial results of healthcare facilities.

Profit in a healthcare facility is influenced by various factors:

- Rates or prices
- Volume
- Variable cost
- Fixed cost
- Payer mix
- Bad debts

The primary value of **break-even analysis**, or, as it is sometimes called, cost-volume-profit (CVP) analysis, is its ability to quantify the relationships among the previous factors and profit.

## Traditional Applications

Break-even analysis has been used in industry for decades with a high degree of satisfaction. Its name comes from the solution to an equation that sets profit equal to zero and revenue equal to costs. To illustrate, assume that a hospital has the following financial information:

| | |
|---|---|
| Variable cost per case | $1,000 |
| Fixed cost per period | $100,000 |
| Price per case | $2,400 |

The break-even volume can be solved by dividing fixed costs by the **contribution margin**, which is the difference between price and variable cost:

$$\text{Break-even volume in units} = \frac{\text{Fixed cost}}{\text{Price} - \text{Variable cost}}$$

Thus, in our hospital example, break-even volume is as follows:

$$\text{Break-even volume in units} = \frac{\$100,000}{\$2,400 - \$1,000}$$
$$= 71.4 \text{ cases}$$

If volume exceeds 72 cases, the hospital will make a profit; but if volume goes below 71 cases it will incur a loss. Sometimes, a revenue and cost relationship is put into graphic form to illustrate profit at various levels. Such a presentation is referred to as a break-even chart. For our hospital example, a break-even chart is shown in **FIGURE 14-9**.

In many cases, some targeted level of net income or profit is desired. The break-even model is easily adapted to this purpose; the new break-even point becomes the following:

$$\text{Break-even volume in units} =$$
$$\frac{\text{Fixed cost} + \text{Targeted net income}}{\text{Price} - \text{Variable cost}}$$

In our example, assuming that a profit of $6,000 was required, the new break-even point is as follows:

$$\text{Break-even volume in units} =$$
$$\frac{\$100,000 + \$6,000}{\$2,400 - \$1,000} = 75.7 \text{ cases}$$

## Multiple-Payer Model

Although break-even analysis is a powerful management tool, it cannot be used in the healthcare industry without adaptation. The major revision required relates to the revenue function. The preceding discussion of break-even analysis assumed that there was only one payer or purchaser of services. That payer was assumed to pay a fixed price per unit of product. However, this situation does not exist in the healthcare industry, where there may be three or more major categories of payers. For our purposes, we will assume that there are three categories of payers:

1. Cost payers (paying average cost of services provided)
2. Fixed-price payers (paying an established fee per unit of service, for example, a fixed price per diagnosis-related group [DRG])

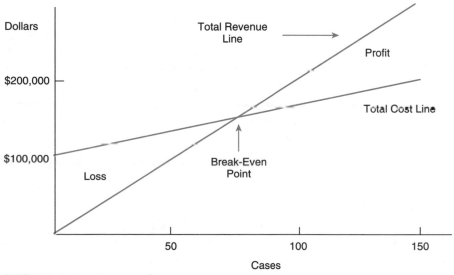

**FIGURE 14-9  Break-Even Chart**

3. Charge payers (paying on the basis of internally set prices, but maybe discounted)

The break-even formula in these three payer situations can be generalized as follows:

$$\text{Break-even volume in units} =$$
$$\frac{(1 - CO)F + NI}{(CH \times P_I) + (FP \times P_E) - (1 - CO)V}$$

This formula may look complex at first glance, but it is actually similar to the previous one-payer break-even formula. In fact, the previous equation can be used in the one-payer situation and provides an identical result. To aid in our understanding of the formula, we should first define the individual variables:

$V$ = Variable cost per unit of output
$F$ = Fixed cost per period
$NI$ = Targeted net income
$P_I$ = Internally set price that is paid by charge payers
$P_E$ = Externally set price paid by fixed-price payers
$CO$ = Proportion of cost payers
$CH$ = Proportion of charge payers
$FP$ = Proportion of fixed-price payers

Let us now examine each term in the equation:

- $(1 - CO)F$: This term represents the proportion of fixed costs ($F$) that is not paid by cost payers. Cost payers are assumed to pay their proportionate share of fixed costs. This leaves the residual portion $(1 - CO)$ unpaid; it is included in the numerator as a financial requirement that must be covered before break-even occurs. If there were no cost payers, $(1 - CO)$ would be 1, and all of the fixed costs would be included. This is the case in traditional break-even analysis. For example, a hospital designated as critical access by Medicare would be paid on a cost basis and the term $CO$ could be a large percentage of total business. For many other noncritical access hospitals, $CO$ would most likely be zero.
- $NI$: This term, targeted net income, is included as a financial requirement as in the traditional break-even formula. $NI$ is not reduced by the cost payer portion because it is assumed that cost payers are not contributing toward meeting the net income requirement. Cost payers pay cost—nothing less and nothing more.
- $CH \times P_I$: This term represents the weighted price paid by charge payers. When added to the next term ($FP \times P_E$), we have a measure of the price paid by the two price-paying categories of customers—charge payers and fixed-price payers.

It should be emphasized that $P_I$ represents the price received, not the charge made. For example, if 10% of the patients paid established charges of \$2,400 per case and 20% paid 90% of established charges of \$2,400 per case, the following values would result:

$$CH = 0.10 + 0.20 = 0.30$$
$$P_I = (1.0 \times \$2,400) \times 1/3 + (0.90 \times \$2,400) \times 2/3$$
$$= \$2,240$$

- $FP \times P_E$: This term represents the weighted price paid by fixed-price payers. The addition of this term to $CH \times P_I$ yields a measure of the price received for price-paying patients. The summation of the two terms can be compared with the price term used in the traditional break-even formula. Again, there may be circumstances when subweighting may be necessary. For example, assume that Medicare pays \$2,000 per case and that 40% of the cases are Medicare. Also assume that 10% of the cases are from a health maintenance organization (HMO) that pays \$2,200 per case. The following values would result:

$$FP = 0.40 + 0.10 = 0.50$$
$$P_E = [(0.40/0.50) \times \$2,000] + [(0.10/0.50) \times \$2,200] = \$2,040$$

- $(1 - CO)V$: This term represents the net variable cost that remains after reflecting the proportion paid by cost payers. Cost payers pay their share of both fixed and variable costs. If there were no cost payers, the entire value of the variable cost per unit would be subtracted to yield the contribution margin per unit.

To determine that the traditional break-even formula is actually derived from our more general three-payer model, let us compute the **break-even point** using the data from the case example developed in our discussion of traditional break-even analysis:

$$\text{Break-even volume in units} =$$
$$\frac{(1 - 0) \times \$100,000 + \$6,000}{(1.0 \times \$2,400) + (0 \times \$0) - (1 - 0)\$1,000}$$
$$= 75.7 \text{ cases}$$

Now, having tested the accuracy of the three-payer break-even formula in a one-payer situation, let us expand our initial case example to a more realistic multiple-payer situation. The data in **TABLE 14-9** are assumed.

**TABLE 14-9** Multiple Payer Case Example

| Payer Proportion | Payment Method |
|---|---|
| 0.20 | Pay average cost |
| 0.40 | Pay $2,000 per case (fixed-price payer) |
| 0.10 | Pay $2,200 per case (fixed-price payer) |
| 0.10 | Pay 100% of charges, $2,400 per case |
| 0.20 | Pay 90% of charges, $2,160 per case |

Also assume that the variable cost is $1,000 per case and fixed costs are $100,000 per period. In addition, the firm needs a profit of $6,000 to meet other financial requirements. The use of these data in our break-even model would produce the following result:

$$\text{Break-even volume in cases} =$$

$$\frac{\left(0.8 \times \$100,000\right) + \$6,000}{\left(0.3 \times \$2,240\right) + \left(0.5 \times \$2,040\right) - \left(0.8 \times \$1,000\right)}$$

$$= \frac{\$86,000}{\$892} = 96.413$$

To demonstrate the accuracy of the break-even formula, we can derive the following income statement for our case example, assuming 96.4 cases as the break-even volume:

| Patient revenue | |
|---|---|
| 0.20 × 96.4 × $2,037.34* | $39,279.92 |
| 0.40 × 96.4 × $2,000.00 | 77,120.00 |
| 0.10 × 96.4 × $2,200.00 | 21,208.00 |
| 0.10 × 96.4 × $2,400.00 | 23,136.00 |
| 0.20 × 96.4 × $2,160.00 | 41,644.80 |
| Net patient revenue | $202,388.72 |
| Less fixed cost | 100,000.00 |
| Less variable cost (96.4 × $1,000) | 96,400.00 |
| Net income | $5,988.72 |

\* Average cost = ($100,000 + 96,400)/96.4= $2,037.34

This income statement demonstrates that, at a volume of 96.4 patients, the firm's net income would be $5,988.72. This value does not exactly match the targeted net income level of $6,000 because of a small rounding error; the actual break-even volume was 96.413, not 96.4.

Before concluding this discussion of break-even analysis, it is useful to mention output determination. For the break-even model to be applicable, there must be one measure of output. It makes no difference whether the measure of activity is macro, such as a case, a patient-day, or a covered life, or whether the measure of activity is micro, such as a procedure or a laboratory test. The following two conditions, however, are necessary:

1.  It must be possible to define an average price paid for that unit for both fixed-price payers and charge payers. For example, both Medicare and Medicaid may pay a fixed rate per case, but all charge payers may pay some percentage of the billed charges. This would require someone to aggregate average charge-payer amounts for individual billed services to an expected price per case. This might also require an assignment of a per case amount paid by Medicare to an estimated amount for a specific service such as a physical therapy treatment if the focus of analysis was at the treatment level. In a situation of capitation, some transfer price must be established on a case, per diem, or procedure basis to apply break-even analysis if an output unit other than members or covered lives is used.
2.  A variable cost per unit of the defined output measure also must be established. This may mean aggregating across departments to create a variable cost value for an aggregated output measure such as a case or a patient-day. Disaggregation is not nearly as great a problem in variable cost measurement because costing systems usually provide reasonably good detail at the departmental level.

## Special Applications

The break-even formula has many applications other than that of computing break-even points. Two specific applications are (1) the computation of marginal profit of volume changes and (2) rate-setting analysis.

## Computation of Marginal Profit of Volume Changes

In most business situations, executives are concerned about the impact of volume changes on operating profitability. At the beginning of a budget period, management may not be sure what its actual volumes will be, but it still needs to know how sensitive profit will be to possible swings in volume. If the payer mix is expected to remain constant, the following simple formula can be used to calculate the marginal changes in profit associated with volume swings:

$$\text{Change in profit} = \text{Change in units} \times \text{Profitability index}$$

where

$$\text{Profitability index} = CH(P_I - V) + FP(P_E - V)$$

The profitability index remains constant and is simply multiplied by projected volume change to determine the profit change. Using our earlier case example, the profitability index would be

$$\text{Profitability index} = 0.3(\$2,240 - \$1,000)$$
$$+ 0.5(\$2,040 - \$1,000) = \$892$$

The value for the profitability index is actually the weighted contribution margin per unit of output. This fact is easily observed by comparing the value calculated previously with that from our three-payer break-even example. The values are the same, $892 in each case. This means that for every one unit change in output, the profit will increase on average by $892. An increase of one unit will increase profit by $892, and a decrease of one unit will decrease profit by $892. A useful question to ask at this point is, how large a reduction in volume can the firm experience before its profit decreases to $2,000? Using the preceding formula, the answer is as follows:

$$\text{Change in profit} = \text{Volume change} \times \text{Profitability index}$$
$$(\$6,000 - \$2,000) = \text{Volume change} \times \$892$$
$$\text{Volume change} = 4.48 \text{ cases}$$

If volume decreases by 4.48 cases, the firm's profit will decrease to $2,000. Further analysis could be used to portray other scenarios or to answer other "what-if" type questions. In each case, the resulting data could be displayed in a table or graph.

## Rate-Setting Analysis

Rate setting is an extremely important activity for most healthcare organizations. Until now we have briefly covered rate setting or pricing; we will now expand our discussion to incorporate the model parameters just referenced. (See Chapter 6 for a brief discussion of rate setting.) Usually, the objective of pricing is not profit maximization, but rather covering financial requirements. In general, pricing services can be stated in the following conceptual terms:

$$\text{Price} = \text{Average cost} + \text{Profit requirement}$$
$$+ \text{Loss on fixed-price patients}$$

If $Q$ represents total budgeted volume in units, we can use our earlier break-even model to develop the following pricing formula:

$$P_I = AC + \frac{NI}{CH \times Q} + \frac{(AC - P_E) \times (FP \times Q)}{CH \times Q}$$

where

$$AC = \text{Average cost per unit} = \frac{F}{Q} + V$$

Again, it is useful to examine the individual terms to understand their conceptual relationship.

- $AC$: This term represents the average cost per unit. Average cost is the basis on which the firm marks up to establish a price that can meet its financial requirements.
- $NI/(CH \times Q)$: This term divides the target net income ($NI$) by the number of charge-paying units ($CH \times Q$). This payment source generates the firm's profit. Internally set prices will not affect the amount of payment received from cost payers or fixed-price payers.
- $(AC - P_E) \times (FP \times Q)/(CH \times Q)$: This term is complex but has a simple interpretation. The difference between average cost ($AC$) and the fixed price ($P_E$) represents an additional requirement that must be covered by the firm's charge-paying units. This difference per unit is then multiplied by total fixed-price payer units ($FP \times Q$) to generate the total loss resulting from selling services to fixed-price payers. Dividing by the number of charge payers ($CH \times Q$) translates this loss into an additional pricing increment that must be recovered from the charge payers on a per unit basis. It is important to note that if the fixed price paid by fixed-price payers ($P_E$) exceeds average cost ($AC$), this term will be negative. Prices to the charge

payers then could be reduced because the fixed-price payers would be making a positive contribution to the firm's profit requirement.

To test the validity of the pricing formula, let us apply it to the data in our earlier three-payer break-even example. Assume that the volume is 96.4 cases.

$$P_I = \$2,037.34 + \frac{\$6,000}{0.3 \times 96.4}$$

$$+ \frac{(\$2,037.34 - \$2,040) \times (0.5 \times 96.4)}{0.3 \times 96.4}$$

$$\$2,037.34 + \$207.47 - 4.43 = \$2,240.38$$

The required price as determined previously, $2,240.38, is approximately equal to the price established for charge payers, $2,240. Again, a small discrepancy exists because of rounding errors.

It should be noted that $2,240 is not the actual charge or price set per case. The actual posted charge is $2,400. $P_I$ represents the net amount actually received. Because the firm had one category of charge payers who paid 90% of charges, the effective price realized was only $2,240. When using this pricing formula to define hospital charges, the defined price must be increased to reflect write-off due to discounts, bad debts, or charity care. The following general formula represents the mark-up requirement:

$$\text{Price} = P_I \div (1 - \text{Write-off proportion})$$

The write-off proportion is not based on total revenue; it is based only on the revenue from charge payers. For example, in our case example, the charge payers represented 30% of total cases. Of that 30%, 10% paid 100% of charges and 20% paid 90% of charges. The write-off percentage is thus the following:

$$(1/3) \times 0 + (2/3) \times 0.10 = 0.0667$$

Using this value to mark up the required net price of $2,240 would yield $2,400.

$$\$2,400 = \frac{\$2,240}{1 - 0.0667}$$

An important issue for many healthcare organizations concerns the maximization of profit per dollar of rate increase. In a number of states and regions, rate regulations impose restraints on a firm's ability to increase its rates. In addition, boards may wish to minimize rate increases in any given budgetary cycle.

The percentage of any price increase that will be realized as profit can be expressed as follows:

Percent price increase realized as profit =

(Percent charge payers) × (1 − Write-off proportion)

− Physician fee percent

Let us assume that a nursing home is interested in learning what effect a $5 increase in its per diem would have on its profitability. Its present payer mix and write-off proportions are presented in **TABLE 14-10**.

Thus, a $5 per diem increase would generate $2.25 per day in additional profit.

$$50\% \times (1 - 0.10) \times \$5.00 = \$2.25$$

## Evaluating Incremental Profit of New Business

One of the most common examples of the use of marginal analysis methods is evaluating the profitability of new business. Many healthcare providers are being approached on an almost daily basis with a proposal for a new block of patients. For example, a preferred provider organization (PPO) may present a hospital with the opportunity to be in the PPO's network if the hospital is willing to accept a discount from its present price structure. It is easy to define a conceptual model

| **TABLE 14-10** Nursing Home Pricing Data | | |
|---|---|---|
| **Payer Percentage** | **Payer Mode** | **Write-Off Proportion** |
| 10% | Medicare—pays fixed charge per diem | NA |
| 50% | Private payer—pays charges | 0.1 |
| 40% | Medicaid—pays fixed charge per diem | NA |

to organize the financial evaluation of this proposal or a similar one.

$$\text{Change in profit} =$$
$$\text{Change in volume} \times (\text{Price per unit} - \text{Incremental}$$
$$\text{cost per unit})$$
$$- (\text{Change in existing price} \times \text{Volume affected})$$

The terms are defined as follows:

- Change in volume: In many cases, there will be a reasonably good measure of what the new volume will be. For example, the PPO may be able to deliver 20 new cases per year. It is important to structure a contract that has a volume trigger related to the range of discounts. If high volumes are realized, then the full discount will be granted. However, if volumes are significantly lower than expected, the discount will get smaller. This provides an incentive for the contractor to send as much volume as possible to the provider firm.
- Price per unit: This variable is almost always known with some degree of precision. In many instances, it actually may be a given figure. Prices for services are established in the contract itself.
- Incremental cost per unit: This variable is often difficult to calculate, but not impossible. If the expected change in volume is relatively small, variable cost per unit would be a good approximation.
- Change in existing price: Once a contract is signed and new business is serviced, there may be

a negative effect on existing prices. If the organization has granted a discount to attract the client, it may find that its existing clients will demand similar discounts. The presence of cost payers also will create an automatic reduction in price. As more volume is delivered, the cost per unit will decrease as fixed costs are spread over more units. This means that cost payers will automatically benefit from increases in volume.

## ▶ SUMMARY

Cost accounting systems can be designed to provide different measures of cost for different decision-making purposes. This is a desirable characteristic, not an exercise in playing with numbers. To understand what measure of cost is needed for a specific purpose, the decision maker must have some knowledge of the variety of alternative concepts of cost. The terms covered in this chapter should be useful in helping decision makers define their needs more precisely.

Break-even analysis presents management with a set of simple analytical tools to provide information about the effects of costs, volume, and prices on profitability. In this chapter, we examined the application of several break-even models for healthcare providers with three categories of payers. These models should help analysts understand the conceptual framework for improving profitability in their healthcare organization.

## ASSIGNMENTS

1. What are the two major categories of decisions that use cost information?
2. What does it mean to state that a cost is direct?
3. Define the terms *variable costs* and *fixed costs*. Give some examples of each.
4. Is it true that indirect costs should never be included in the determination of controllable costs?
5. A hospital is considering using a vacant wing to set up a skilled nursing facility. What is the cost of the space?
6. A free-standing ambulatory care center averages $60 in charges per patient. Variable costs are approximately $10 per patient, and fixed costs are about $1.2 million per year. Using these data, how many patients must be seen each day, assuming a 365-day operation, to reach the break-even point?
7. You are attempting to develop a break-even for a capitation contract with a major HMO. Your hospital has agreed to provide all inpatient hospital services for 10,000 covered lives. You will receive $38 per-member-per-month (PMPM) to cover all inpatient services. It is anticipated that 93 admissions per 1,000 covered lives will be provided with an average length of stay equal to 5.0, or 465 days per 1,000.
   You anticipate that your hospital will incur fixed costs, or readiness to serve costs, of $1,860,000 for these 10,000 covered lives. Variable costs per patient-day are expected to be $600.
   Calculate the break-even point in patient-days under this contract.
8. Your hospital's board of trustees has just determined that the maximum revenue increase it will permit next year is 5%. It also has specified maximum and minimum rate increases by department. Data for the hospital's five departments are depicted in **TABLE 14-11**. Given the previous information, develop a rate change plan that will maximize the hospital's net income yet still adhere to the board's guidelines.

**TABLE 14-11** Rate Optimization Data

| | Current Charges | Budgeted Cost | Payer Composition Percentage | | | | | Rate Change Percentage | |
|---|---|---|---|---|---|---|---|---|---|
| | | | Cost | Fixed Price | Charge | Bad Debt | Physician Fee | Min. | Max. |
| Nursing | $2,000 | $2,200 | 30 | 30 | 40 | 10 | 0 | 5 | 20 |
| Emergency room | 200 | 190 | 70 | 10 | 20 | 10 | 0 | 0 | 10 |
| Operating room | 300 | 330 | 35 | 40 | 25 | 20 | 0 | 10 | 25 |
| Laboratory | 1,000 | 750 | 50 | 30 | 20 | 15 | 10 | −10 | 20 |
| Anesthesiology | 360 | 300 | 40 | 30 | 30 | 10 | 30 | 0 | 10 |
| Total | $3,860 | $3,770 | | | | | | | |

9. Develop an estimate of fixed and variable costs for labor expenses, based on the data presented in **TABLE 14-12**. Develop your estimates by using the high–low and semiaverages methods, and simple regression.

**TABLE 14-12** Data for Variable/Fixed Cost Example

| Period | Output in Units | Hours Worked |
|---|---|---|
| 1 | 16,156 | 3,525 |
| 2 | 19,160 | 4,151 |
| 3 | 17,846 | 3,829 |
| 4 | 20,238 | 4,454 |
| 5 | 21,198 | 4,657 |
| 6 | 14,640 | 3,406 |

10. An interdepartmental service structure and its direct costs are depicted in **TABLE 14-13**. Compute the total costs, direct and allocated, for each of the three revenue centers using the direct and step-down methods of cost apportionment. Assume that the order of allocation for the three service centers is 1 first, then 2, and finally 3.
11. Your hospital was denied a contract with an HMO last year. Legal counsel believes that there was a breach of contract and wishes to bring suit against the HMO for damages. The chief executive officer has asked you to work with the controller to develop a defensible measure of the damages experienced during the last year. Explain how you would organize your work to estimate the amount of damages.

**TABLE 14-13** Data for Cost Allocation Example

| Department | Direct Costs | Percentage of Service Consumed By | | | | | |
| --- | --- | --- | --- | --- | --- | --- | --- |
| | | S1 | S2 | S3 | R1 | R2 | R3 |
| Service center 1 | $10,000 | — | 10 | 10 | 40 | 20 | 20 |
| Service center 2 | 12,000 | 10 | — | 10 | 20 | 40 | 20 |
| Service center 3 | 10,000 | 10 | 10 | — | 20 | 20 | 40 |
| Revenue center 1 | 30,000 | | | | | | |
| Revenue center 2 | 25,000 | | | | | | |
| Revenue center 3 | 50,000 | | | | | | |

## SOLUTIONS AND ANSWERS

1. The two major categories of decisions that use cost data are planning and control. Planning decisions usually require costs that are accumulated by program or product line, whereas control decisions usually require costs that are accumulated by responsibility centers or departments.
2. A direct cost can be traced or associated with a specific cost object, usually related to a department or responsibility center.
3. A variable cost changes proportionately with volume. Common examples are materials and supplies. A fixed cost does not change with volume but remains constant. Common examples are rent, depreciation, and interest. Fixed costs are usually constant only for some "relevant range" of volume. For example, depreciation probably will increase if a facility experiences volume increases that exceed existing capacity.
4. It is not always true that indirect costs should never be included in the determination of controllable costs. There are some costs that may be classified as indirect but could be controlled by a manager. For example, housekeeping costs may be classified as an indirect cost to the physical therapy department. However, the actual amount of housekeeping services required by the physical therapy department may be affected by the actions of the physical therapy department manager.
5. The opportunity cost of the space—that is, its value in the next best alternative use—should be measured. Possible alternative uses might be as physician offices or as sleeping accommodations for patient families.
6. The number of patients that must be seen is 65.75 per day, based on the following calculation:

$$\text{Annual break-even volume} = \frac{1,200,000}{\$50} = 24,000 \text{ patients per year}$$

$$\text{Daily break-even volume} = \frac{24,000}{365} = 65.75$$

7. Fixed annual revenue = $10,000 \times \$38 \times 12 = \$4,560,000$

$$\text{Fixed costs} = \$1,860,000$$

$$\text{Variable cost per patient-day} = \$600$$

$$\text{Break-even point} = \frac{\$4,560,000 - \$1,860,000}{\$600} = 4,500 \text{ patient-days}$$

If utilization is above 4,500 patient-days, the hospital will lose money. **FIGURE 14-10** to illustrates this concept.

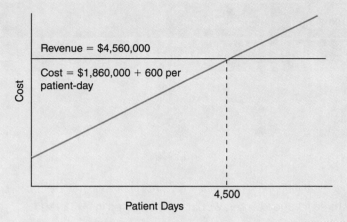

Revenue = $4,560,000

Cost = $1,860,000 + 600 per patient-day

4,500

Patient Days

**FIGURE 14-10**  Break-Even Point

8. The rate change plan could be developed in the manner depicted in **TABLE 14-14**. Results of loading as much of the rate increase as possible into nursing are depicted in **TABLE 14-15**.

**TABLE 14-14** Departmental Price Change Coefficients

| Department | Percentage of Price Realized as Profit |
|---|---|
| Nursing | 40.0% × 0.9 = 36.0% |
| Emergency room | 20.0% × 0.9 = 18.0% |
| Operating room | 25.0% × 0.8 = 20.0% |
| Laboratory | (20.0% × 0.85) − 10.0% = 7.0% |
| Anesthesiology | (30.0% × 0.9) − 30.0% = −3.0% |

**TABLE 14-15** Optimal Departmental Charges

| Department | Current Charges | Required Minimum | Additional Charges | Final Charges |
|---|---|---|---|---|
| Nursing | $2,000 | $100 | $163 | $2,263 |
| Emergency room | 200 | — | — | 200 |
| Operating room | 300 | 30 | — | 330 |
| Laboratory | 1,000 | (100) | — | 900 |
| Anesthesiology | 360 | — | — | 360 |
| | $3,860 | $30 | $163 | $4,053 |

9. **TABLE 14-16** depicts estimates of fixed and variable costs for labor expenses that could be developed.

**TABLE 14-16** Variable and Fixed Cost Estimates

|  | Variable Hours/Unit | Fixed Hours |
|---|---|---|
| High–low method | 0.1908 | 613 |
| Semiaverages method | 0.2093 | 193 |
| Simple regression | 0.1990 | 375 |

10. The total costs for the three revenue centers would be as depicted in **TABLE 14-17**.

**TABLE 14-17** Solution for Cost Allocation Example

| Department | Direct Costs | Direct Apportionment S1 | S2 | S3 | Total |
|---|---|---|---|---|---|
| Service center 1 | $10,000 | 10,000 | 12,000 | 10,000 |  |
| Service center 2 | 12,000 |  |  |  |  |
| Service center 3 | 10,000 |  |  |  |  |
| Revenue center 1 | 30,000 | 5,000 | 3,000 | 2,500 | 40,500 |
| Revenue center 2 | 25,000 | 2,500 | 6,000 | 2,500 | 36,000 |
| Revenue center 3 | 50,000 | 2,500 | 3,000 | 5,000 | 60,500 |
| Total | $137,000 |  |  |  | $137,000 |

| Department | Direct Costs | Step Down S1 | S2 | S3 | Total |
|---|---|---|---|---|---|
| Service center 1 | $10,000 | $10,000 |  |  |  |
| Service center 2 | $12,000 | $1,000 | $13,000 |  |  |
| Service center 3 | $10,000 | $1,000 | $1,444 | $12,444 |  |
| Revenue center 1 | $30,000 | $4,000 | $2,889 | $3,111 | $40,000 |
| Revenue center 2 | $25,000 | $2,000 | $5,778 | $6,222 | $39,000 |
| Revenue center 3 | $50,000 | $2,000 | $2,889 | $3,111 | $58,000 |
| Total | $137,000 |  |  |  | $137,000 |

11. A reasonable framework for the estimation of damages would be the equation introduced earlier in this chapter:

$$\text{Change in profit} =$$
$$\text{Change in volume} \times (\text{Price per unit} - \text{Incremental cost per unit})$$
$$- (\text{Change in existing price} \times \text{Volume affected})$$

The change in volume would be an estimate of the lost volume resulting from the breach of contract. Price per unit could be obtained from a price schedule used by the HMO to pay the hospital or other similar hospitals. Incremental cost per unit could be approximated by variable cost. Finally, if the hospital has cost payers, some recognition must be given to the higher levels of payment made by cost payers because of the lower volumes, which would have raised average cost per unit because of the presence of fixed costs. In short, the hospital would have experienced an increase in its existing price from its cost payers.

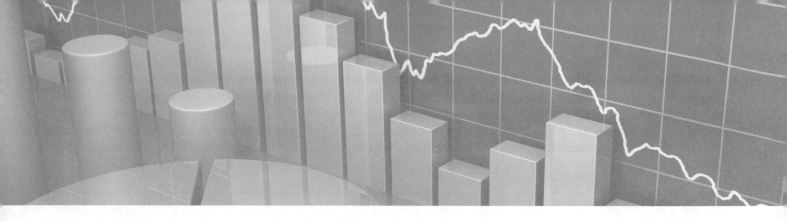

# CHAPTER 15

# Product Costing

## REAL-WORLD SCENARIO

Skylar Dean, CFO at Metro Regional Hospital, has been questioned by her CEO and Board with respect to cost and pricing for outpatient colonoscopy procedures. A newly formed physician-owned ambulatory surgery center has opened within the last 12 months and hospital volumes for selective outpatient procedures have dropped dramatically as outpatient surgery cases have migrated to the surgery center. Historically the hospital had been doing about 4,000 outpatient colonoscopy procedures per year but the volume has dropped to less than 2,000. The Board at Metro has asked the hospital to consider reducing their prices from approximately $3,500 per outpatient colonoscopy to $1,750, which is the current price at the surgery center.

Dean performed some simple revenue analysis and determined that 60% of the current volume is either Medicare or other payers that have a fixed-fee arrangement. A reduction in price would therefore not affect the ultimate level of profit because Metro's prices for colonoscopy procedures would not affect pricing. For the remaining 25% of their current book of business, payment is directly related to price. Ultimately, the key question that the Board wants answered is: What is the cost of an outpatient colonoscopy procedure performed at Metro Regional Hospital? If the cost of performing outpatient colonoscopy procedures is above $1,750—the surgery center's current price—perhaps Metro should consider dropping this procedure.

While Dean knows what information is required, obtaining the actual cost of performing an outpatient colonoscopy procedure is not an easy task. In some cases, different sets of individual procedures are performed for each colonoscopy. For example, about 50% of the time a biopsy is also performed during the colonoscopy, and that additional procedure does cost more. Dean realizes that she needs to know two specific pieces of information before she can cost outpatient colonoscopies or any procedure. First, she needs to know what specific intermediate procedures are required for each outpatient colonoscopy, such as biopsies, tissue exams, and anesthesia injections. Second, Dean also needs to know what each of the specific procedures required during an average colonoscopy cost. For example, what does anesthesia cost, what does a tissue exam cost, and what do other intermediate procedures cost? The current cost accounting system at Metro Regional Hospital does not provide the information that Dean needs and she is faced with the prospect of developing the required cost data from the existing cost system that exists.

---

Practically every healthcare provider expresses a strong and urgent interest in developing better cost accounting systems. The basis for this interest is easy to understand and relates to the nature of payment systems for healthcare providers. Before 1983, hospitals and many other healthcare providers were paid on the basis of actual cost. Hospitals, for example, were paid on a cost basis by Medicare, many Blue Cross plans, and most Medicaid programs. In this type of payment environment, costing was important, but allocation of costs to heavily cost reimbursed areas was emphasized, rather than accurate costing. Reimbursement maximization, not accurate costing, was the primary objective. With the advent of prospective payment systems in the early 1980s and the growing importance of managed care in the late 1980s, hospitals and other healthcare providers became concerned with the actual cost of service delivery. Providers wanted to know what the actual costs of producing a medical or surgical procedure were so they could compare these costs with the revenue received and make more intelligent decisions about products and product lines.

### Learning Objective 1

Describe the existing needs for cost information in healthcare firms.

## ▶ Healthcare Cost Accounting

While much attention has been given to costing in healthcare firms during the last two decades, there has been little real progress in the actual development and implementation of accurate costing systems. Many healthcare firms, especially hospitals, have spent large sums of money to implement sophisticated cost accounting systems, but most healthcare executives still believe the validity of the actual reported cost values are suspect. We believe that there are three basic questions that need to be answered before effective cost accounting systems for healthcare firms can become a reality:

1. What are we trying to cost?
2. For what time period is the cost information of value?

3. How do our needs for cost information relate to existing costing systems?

## What Are the Cost Objects?

Any costing system must first address the question of what are we trying to cost. Cost is not a neutral term but rather is always associated with some object. For example, if someone said the cost is $100 you would immediately ask the cost of what is $100? The same is true in healthcare firms. Because the title of this chapter is product costing, our focus is on healthcare firm products. Ultimately, the product of any firm is integrally linked to its customers or patients. In most situations firms in any industry want to know what their costs are for product that they are selling. For our purposes, we will define that product as the "unit of payment."

The unit of payment defines the collection of services that will be combined or bundled to trigger a payment. There are four payment unit categories. At the lowest combination level are *individual service arrangements*, where each specific service provided is paid separately. Traditionally, almost all healthcare services were paid on this basis. Even the original Medicare program for hospitals, which paid on a cost basis, used the services provided in the claim as the basis for payment.

The next level of combination is the *encounter level*. Here a payment is made for all of the services bundled into an encounter. In the hospital sector, this includes a case payment based on the MS-DRG for inpatients. The payment is still provider-specific, but there is a shifting of risk from payer to provider because the payment is the same regardless of the intensity of services provided during the encounter. For example, a hospital being paid at the encounter level receives no additional payment for larger amounts of ancillary services.

The next level of bundling is the *episode level*. At this level, payment is made for all encounters associated with a defined episode of care. The episode level shifts payment risk further to providers and away from payers because the provider is now responsible for not just the initial encounter, but any related encounters associated with that episode of care. At the episode level, the question arises about how to handle multiple providers involved in a single episode. The bundled payments for care improvement (BPCI) program was officially launched in January 2013. It is a program that tests alternative models for creating bundled payments for 48 clinical episodes of care that are defined by patients' Medicare DRG (MS-DRG). On July 9, 2015, CMS proposed a bundled payment model for hip and knee replacements—comprehensive care for joint replacement (CCJR)—that would require mandatory participation for most hospitals in 75 metropolitan areas in the United States. The proposal was implemented in 2016, and it continues CMS's trend to shift more risk to providers.

The final level of bundling is *capitation*. Risk is now fully shifted to the providers. A capitation plan may be limited to one area of service, such as hospital care, or may involve multiple areas of care.

Healthcare firms produce a large number and variety of different products, but many of these are bundled into a larger product that the patient actually purchases. For example, clean linen is one of many products produced in a hospital. A hospital inpatient expects that clean linen will be provided, but they do not expect nor do they receive a charge for clean linen. Hospitals include the cost of that intermediate product into other services such as a room charge.

At present the ultimate cost object for many healthcare firms is an encounter of care. An **encounter of care** encompasses all of the services and products that were provided to the patient during a specific treatment at the healthcare firm. For hospitals, an inpatient encounter of care may be a specific DRG such as MS-DRG 193 Simple Pneumonia and Pleurisy w/MCC. In an outpatient or ambulatory setting it may be a specific primary APC such as APC 5312 Level 2 Lower GI Procedures. Each of the possible encounter of care types may have different costs and different sets of intermediate products and services that are associated with them, but ultimately it is the encounter cost that is of interest to both patients and third-party payers. Because the healthcare firm's clients make purchase decisions based on the encounter of care, the healthcare firm has a vital interest in both knowing and controlling its encounter of care cost.

## What Time Period of Cost Information Is Relevant?

In some respects this is a very simple question to answer. Cost information can span only two periods of time. It will be either historical, and report what costs actually were in some prior time period, or it will reflect what costs will likely be in some future period. Cost data that are futuristic are linked to planning decisions. We want to know what the costs of specific encounters of care are so that we can establish pricing that will both cover our costs and provide for some return on our investment. If our required pricing does cover our expected future costs, then we have to determine whether we should continue to provide that type of medical service. Future costs are also used to establish standards in budgeting for which actual costs will be compared in some future time period.

Historical costs in and of themselves have little real value. Most executives want to know what costs will be and not what they have been. Historical costing is however the primary source of information regarding what future costs will be, and for this reason it is of critical importance. Historical cost data is also used in the management control phase to compare with budgeted or forecasted cost levels. Significant deviations of actual and forecast cost can be reviewed to assess whether there is some action that can be taken to correct an unfavorable variance from budget.

## How Do Our Needs for Cost Information Relate to Existing Costing Systems?

In a real-world situation, costing systems must be integrated with existing cost and reporting structures. It will make little sense to ignore what costing currently exists in healthcare firms and to start from scratch. Financial reporting still needs to be done, and Medicare cost reports must still be filed. This does not mean that new cost systems should rely on the existing structures if they cannot be modified to produce relevant information that is reliable and timely, but it also means that it is important to assess what currently exists.

At the present time, most people would agree that it is fairly easy to measure the total cost for a facility such as a hospital or nursing home. For example, few would question the validity of an audited total cost for a hospital of $100 million during the last fiscal year. While it is true that there are some costing issues that might cause variability in total reported facility costs, most of these issues can be resolved. For example, Medicare may deem that $5 million of the $100 million cost is not reimbursable, but management can base its cost on the total $100 million.

If we start with the premise that the facility-level cost is by and large valid, then the real issue is allocating that facility-level cost to individual products or encounters of care. We know that we have $100 million of total cost, but we are still a long way from agreeing on the cost of a specific DRG.

A second given in existing costing systems is the assignment of total costs to responsibility centers or departments. For example, the $100 million of total cost may be assigned to three departments: nursing, surgery, and administration. In most cases, the direct assignment of these expenses is also not hotly debated. The assignments of total costs are made to those departments where managers are held accountable for the level of costs that they incur. We now have our $100 million cost split into departments, but we still do not have specific DRG costs.

This is the dilemma that hospitals and other healthcare firms face in developing costing systems. They have reasonably sound measures of total cost and they also have good measures of departmental costs, but they do not have measures of cost by encounter of care. The real task is to either use the existing structure to develop encounter of care cost measures or to build a completely new system that will be capable of costing specific encounters of care.

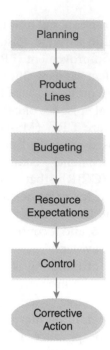

**FIGURE 15-1** **The Planning-Budgeting-Control Process**

### Learning Objective 2

Describe how cost information relates to the three key activities of management: planning, budgeting, and control.

## ▶ Relationship to Planning, Budgeting, and Control

Cost information is of value only as it aids in the management decision-making process. Management decision making is ultimately linked to three decision areas—planning, budgeting, and control. **FIGURE 15-1** presents a schematic that summarizes the planning-budgeting-control process in a business. Each decision phase has specific decision outcomes that answer critical business decisions.

- Planning answers the question of what shall be produced.
- Budgeting answers the question of how we shall produce it.
- Control answers the question of what we should do to realize our objectives.

## Products and Product Line

The terms *product* and *product line* are the direct result of the planning phase and seem easy to understand in most businesses. For example, a finished car is the product of an automobile company; individual types of cars then may be grouped to form product lines, such as the Chevrolet product line of General Motors.

Can this definition of a product be transposed to the healthcare sector? Many people think that products cannot be so easily defined in healthcare firms. The major dilemma seems to arise in the area of patients versus products. In short, is the product the patient or is it the individual services provided, such as laboratory tests, nursing care, and meals? In most situations, we believe that the treated patient is the basic product of a healthcare firm. As discussed earlier this leads to the definition of an encounter of care as the primary cost object in most healthcare firms. Even in situations where the unit of payment is an episode of care or a covered life, the individual encounters of care still form the building blocks that would be aggregated to produce cost estimates for an episode of care or a covered life.

This means that the wide range of services provided to patients, such as nursing, prescriptions, and tests, are to be viewed as intermediate products, not final products. There is, in fact, little difference between this interpretation and that applied in most manufacturing settings. For example, automobile fenders are, on one hand, a final product; on the other, they are only an intermediate product in preparation of the final product, the completed automobile. Ultimately, it is the automobile that is sold to the public, not the fenders. In the same vein, it is the treated patient who generates revenue, not the individual service provided in isolation. Indeed, a hospital that provided only laboratory tests would not be a hospital—it would be a laboratory. In short, patients must exist for an individual or an entity to be a healthcare provider.

Product lines represent an amalgamation of patients or encounters of care in a way that makes business sense. Sometimes people use the term **strategic business units** to refer to areas of activity that may stand alone. For our purpose, a product line is a unit of business activity that requires a go or no-go decision. For example, eliminating one diagnosis-related group (DRG) is probably not possible because that DRG may be linked to other DRGs within a clinical specialty area; it may be impossible to stop producing DRG 113 (Orbital Procedures) without also eliminating other DRGs, such as DRG 123 (Neurological Eye Disorders). Thus, in many cases, it is the clinical specialty, for example, ophthalmology, that defines the product line.

## Budgeting and Resource Expectations

The budgeting phase of operations involves a translation of the product-line decisions made earlier into a set of resource expectations. The primary purpose of this is twofold. First, management must assure itself that there will be sufficient funds to maintain financial solvency. Just as you and I must live within our financial means, so must any healthcare business entity. Second, the resulting budget serves as a basis for management control. If budget expectations are not realized, management must discover why not and take corrective actions. A budget or set of resource expectations can be thought of as a standard costing system. The budget represents management's expectations of how costs should behave, given a certain set of volume assumptions. It is important to remember that it is the forecasted or budgeted costs of a product that are of the greatest interest to management. Historical costs are useful, but only insofar as those costs indicate future costs.

The primary output of the budgeting process is a series of departmental or activity center budgets that explicate what costs should be during the coming budget period. Two separate sets of standards are involved in the development of these budgets. (These standards are described later in the chapter.)

## Control and Corrective Action

The control phase of business operations monitors actual cost experience and compares it with budgetary expectations. If there are deviations from expectations, management analyzes the causes of the deviation. If the deviation is favorable, management may seek to make whatever created the variance a permanent part of operations. If the variance is unfavorable, action will be taken in an attempt to prevent a recurrence. Much of the control phase centers around the topic of variance analysis. (This topic is explored in depth in Chapter 16.)

*Learning Objective 3*

Describe the three main phases of the costing process.

## ▶ The Costing Process

Most firms, whether they are hospitals, nursing homes, or steel manufacturers, have similar costing systems. In fact, in most cases, the similarities outweigh the differences. **FIGURE 15-2** presents a schematic of the cost-measurement process that exists in most businesses.

## Valuation

Valuation always has been a thorny issue for accountants—one that has not been satisfactorily resolved even today. We need only to consider the

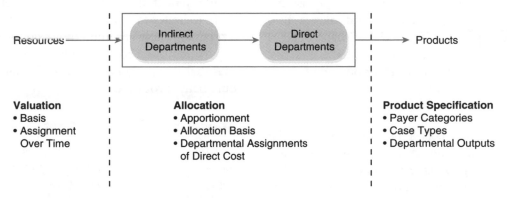

**FIGURE 15-2 The Cost Measurement Process**

current controversy over replacement costs versus historical costs to realize the full problem. For discussion purposes, we have chosen here to split the valuation process into two areas: (1) **cost basis** and (2) **assignment over time**. These two areas are not mutually exclusive, and to some degree, they overlap. However, both areas determine the total value or cost of a resource that is used to produce a final product.

The cost basis is the process by which a value is assigned to each and every resource transaction occurring between the entity being accounted for and another entity. For example, if a medical group acquires 500 doses of flu vaccine, what value or cost is placed on those doses of flu vaccine. In most situations, this value is historical cost and we will assume that this is true although some discussion has been given to using replacement cost measures.

Having determined that historical cost will be the valuation basis, there are two major types of situations when that cost will have to be assigned to a different time period than when it was acquired. First, the cost may be expended before the actual reporting of expense—the best example of this is depreciation. A firm may spend $1,000,000 today for a new piece of imaging equipment, but that cost will be assigned over the useful life of the equipment and not assigned to imaging procedures performed in the first year. Second, the cost may be recognized before an actual expenditure. Normal accruals such as wages and salaries are examples of this situation. Staff in a hospital may work for 2 weeks before they are actually paid. Services provided by the staff during that time period should be charged with the expected cost of staff time.

This brings us to a critical question in the costing process. For what period of time are we trying to develop cost measures? As the period being costed increases, the problems caused by assignment over time become less severe. For example, if the period being costed is 1 year, normal accruals for wages and salaries represent a very small percentage of total wage and salary costs. It may be perfectly acceptable to simply use the actual dollar amount paid for wages and salaries. But, if the period being costed is 1 week, estimates of costs or accruals must be made because no actual wages may have been paid during the 1-week period.

## Allocation

The end result of the cost-allocation process is the assignment of all costs determined during the valuation phase of costing to departments or responsibility centers. Departments in healthcare firms are usually categorized as either direct or indirect. A *direct*

*department* provides a service or product directly traceable to a patient encounter. For example, the laboratory is a direct department and provides specific laboratory procedures that are directly traced to an encounter of care. An **indirect department** may provide services, but they are usually not directly traceable to a specific patient encounter. For example, housekeeping cleans all areas in a hospital, but their services may not be directly traceable to a specific patient encounter.

Two phases of activity are involved in this assignment: First, all resource values to be recorded as expenses during a given period are assigned or allocated to the direct and indirect departments as direct expenses. Second, once the initial cost assignment to individual departments has been made, a further allocation is required. In this phase, the expenses of the indirect departments are assigned to the direct departments.

## Assigning Costs to Departments

In the first category, a situation may arise in which the departmental structure currently specified is not questioned, but some of the initial cost assignments are. For example, premiums paid for malpractice insurance might be charged to administration, or they may be charged directly to the nursing and professional departments that are involved. In the second category, a situation may arise in which the existing departmental structure has to be revised. For example, the administration department may be divided into several new departments, such as nonpatient telephone, data processing, purchasing, admitting, business office, and other. The analysis focuses on the discovery of activities that are related to the products being produced. For example, admitting activities may be a significant activity within the administration department that is clearly traceable to an individual patient. Dividing administration into admitting and other activity centers may greatly improve the accuracy of individual costing and permit management to better measure the actual costs of producing a product. There are numerous examples of overhead departments that could be split into component activities that then may be traced to the patient or procedure being produced.

## Allocation of Indirect Cost

During the second phase of cost allocation—the reassignment from indirect departments to direct departments—the following two primary decisions are involved: (1) selection of the cost-apportionment method and (2) selection of the appropriate allocation basis. Regarding the first category, cost-apportionment methods, such as **step-down**, **double-distribution**, and **simultaneous-equations** methods, are simply mathematical algorithms that redistribute cost from existing indirect departments to direct departments, given defined allocation bases. An example of an allocation basis decision is the selection of square feet or hours worked for housekeeping as an appropriate allocation basis for an indirect department. Sometimes the term **cost driver** is used to describe the selection of an appropriate allocation base. Ideally, the allocation basis selected should be that variable that has the most direct or causal relationship to cost. For example, square feet would not appear to be as accurate an allocation basis or cost driver for housekeeping as hours worked.

## Product Specification

In most healthcare firms, there are two phases in the production (or treatment) process. The schematic in **FIGURE 15-3** illustrates this process and also introduces a few new terms.

In Stage 1 of the production process, resources are acquired and consumed within departments or activity centers to produce a product or service. We define the services produced by a department as its **service units (SUs)**. Here, two points need to be emphasized.

First, all departments have SUs, but not all departments have the same number of SUs. For example, the nursing department may provide the following four levels of care: acuity levels 1, 2, 3, and 4. A laboratory, in contrast, may have 100 or more separate SUs that relate to the provision of specific tests. Second, not all SUs can be directly associated with the delivery of patient care; some of the SUs may be only indirectly associated with patient treatment. For example, housekeeping cleans laboratory areas, but there is no direct association between this function and patient treatment. However, the cleaning of a patient's room could be regarded as a service that is directly associated with a patient.

Stage 2 of the production process relates to the actual consumption of specific SUs during the treatment of a patient. Much of the production process is managed by the physician. This is true regardless of the setting (hospital, nursing home, home healthcare firm, or clinic). The physician prescribes the specific SUs that will be required to treat a given patient effectively. For example, the physician determines what imaging procedures are needed, what laboratory procedures are required, and many other critical resource decisions.

The lack of management authority in this area complicates management's efforts to budget and control its costs. This is not meant to be a criticism of

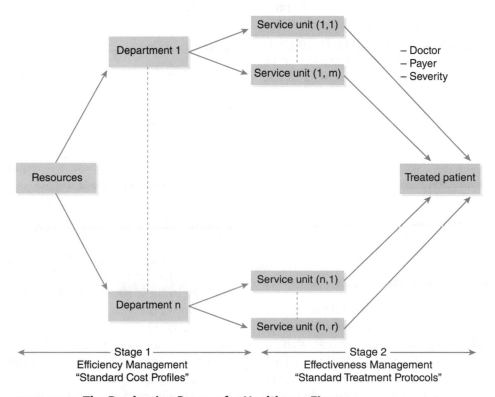

**FIGURE 15-3 The Production Process for Healthcare Firms**

current healthcare delivery systems; all of us would prefer to have a qualified physician rather than a lay healthcare executive direct our care. Yet this is perhaps the area of greatest difference between healthcare firms and other business entities. Management at General Motors can decide which automobiles will have factory-installed air conditioning and tinted glass and which will not. In contrast, a healthcare executive will have great difficulty in attempting to direct a physician to either prescribe or not prescribe a given procedure in the treatment of a patient.

Healthcare products to be costed may vary depending on the specific decision being considered. At one level, management may be interested in the cost of a specific SU or departmental output. Prices for some SUs (for example, radiograph procedures) may have to be established, and to do that, management must know their costs. In other situations, knowing the cost for one patient encounter or for a group of patient encounters may be desired. For example, management may wish to bid on a contract to provide home health services to a health maintenance organization (HMO). In this case, it is important for management to understand what the costs of treating HMO patients are likely to be. If the contract is signed, management then needs to determine the actual costs of treating the patients from the HMO to measure the overall profitability from that segment of the business. Alternatively, it may be necessary to group patients by specialty. A hospital may wish to know whether it is losing money from treating a particular DRG entity or some grouping of DRGs, such as obstetrics. This kind of cost information is especially critical to management decision making that involves expansion or contraction of specific clinical service areas and the recruitment of new medical staff.

---

*Learning Objective 4*

Explain the two systems necessary to accurately cost healthcare encounters of care.

---

▶ **Two Required Systems for Healthcare Costing**

Up to this point, we have learned that attaching cost values to a healthcare encounter of care requires an understanding of the production process that is involved in producing healthcare services. Figure 15-3 illustrates that all encounters of care require a set of specific healthcare services that are defined as SUs.

These SUs are produced in departments within the healthcare firm and a department can and often does have multiple types of services that it provides. Therefore in order to cost specific encounters of care we must be able to define the cost of specific SUs. For example, a patient encounter that required a specific surgical procedure, several lab tests, and some pharmacy items would require us to be able to determine what each of these SUs cost in order to establish a reliable cost for the patient encounter.

Not only must we be able to determine the cost of specific SUs, but we must also determine what SUs were used or required to produce a specific type of patient encounter. For example, we may be trying to determine what the average cost for an outpatient diagnostic cardiac catheterization either was in the past or will be in the future. We know that each catheterization will either be a left only, a right only, or a left and right procedure. Costs of these individual procedures are different. In addition, an electrocardiogram may also be required for some of the patients. We must know what the historical use patterns were or will be in the future if we are trying to establish meaningful cost measures for diagnostic cardiac catheterizations.

In order to accurately cost encounters of care on either a historical or future basis we need the following two systems: (1) a system of **standard cost profiles** and (2) a system of standard treatment protocols. The relationship between these two systems is shown in Figure 15-3. The "linchpin" between them is the SU concept.

## Standard Cost Profiles

The standard cost profile (SCP) is not a new concept; it has been used in manufacturing cost accounting systems for many years. For our purposes, there are two key elements in an SCP:

1. Definition of the SU being costed
2. Profile of resources required or actually used to produce the SU

As noted earlier, the number of SUs in a given department may vary; some departments may have 1, whereas others may have 100 or more. If the number of SUs is very large, however, there may be an unacceptable level of costing detail involved to make the system feasible. In these situations, it may be useful to aggregate some of the SUs. For example, the laboratory may perform 1,000 or more tests. In this situation, it may make sense to develop cost profiles for only the most commonly performed tests and to use some arbitrary assignment method for the remaining uncommon tests. An alternative approach in departmental areas with large numbers of SUs is to develop a **relative weighting system**. This topic will be explored at the end of the chapter.

The SU does not have to be a product or service that is directly provided or performed for a patient. Many indirect departments do not provide services or products to the patient; instead, other departments, both direct and indirect, consume their products or services. However, many indirect departments have SUs that are provided directly to the patient. For example, the dietary department, often regarded as an indirect department, may not have revenue billed for its product to the patient. However, a meal that the dietary department furnishes to a patient is an SU that is just as direct as a laboratory test or a chest radiograph. In a similar vein, housekeeping may provide cleaning for a patient's room that is, in effect, a direct service consumed by the patient.

Thus, SUs may be categorized as either direct or indirect. A direct SU is associated with a given patient. An indirect SU is provided to another department of the hospital, as opposed to a patient. The differentiation between direct and indirect SUs is important, not only in the development of SCPs but also in the development of standard treatment protocols. Direct SUs must be identified when standard treatment protocols are defined, whereas indirect SUs need not be specifically identified, although some estimate of allocated cost is often required.

In the development of an SCP for a given SU, the following resource expense categories are listed:

- Direct expenses (labor, materials, and departmental overhead)
- Allocated overhead

Ideally, the expense also should be categorized as variable or fixed. This distinction is particularly important in certain areas of management decision making. (See Chapter 14 for further discussion.) Specifically, the differentiation between **variable cost** and **fixed cost** is critical to many incremental pricing and volume decisions. It is also important in flexible budgeting systems and management control. These topics are explored in greater depth in Chapter 16.

**TABLE 15-1** presents an SCP for a regular patient meal in a dietary department. The total cost of providing one regular patient meal, or SU 181, is $5.80. The variable cost per meal is $3.00, and the average fixed cost per meal is $2.80.

In most situations, direct labor is the largest single expense category. In our dietary meal example, this is not true because the direct material cost, mostly raw food, is larger. It is possible, and in many cases desirable, to define direct labor costs by labor category. Thus, in our dietary meal example, we might provide separate listings for cooks, dietary aides, and dishwashers.

**TABLE 15-1** Standard Cost Profile for a Dietary/Regular Patient Meal SU 181

| Cost Category | Quantity | | Cost per Unit (column 3) | Average Variable Cost (1 x 3) | Average Fixed Cost (2 x 3) | Total Cost |
|---|---|---|---|---|---|---|
| | Variable (column 1) | Fixed (column 2) | | | | |
| Direct labor | 0.05 | 0.05 | $20.00 | $1.00 | $1.00 | $2.00 |
| Direct materials | 1.00 | 0.00 | 2.00 | $2.00 | $0.00 | $2.00 |
| Department overhead | 0.00 | 1.00 | 1.00 | $0.00 | $1.00 | $1.00 |
| Allocated costs | | | | | | |
| Housekeeping | 0.00 | 0.10 | 2.00 | $0.00 | $0.20 | $0.20 |
| Plant operation | 0.00 | 1.00 | 0.20 | $0.00 | $0.20 | $0.20 |
| Administration | 0.00 | 0.02 | 20.00 | $0.00 | $0.40 | $0.40 |
| Total | | | | $3.00 | $2.80 | $5.80 |

An important point here is the division of cost into fixed and variable quantities. Table 15-1 indicates that 0.05 units of variable labor time is required per meal, and 0.05 units of fixed labor is required per meal. (In Chapter 14, we discussed several methods for splitting costs into fixed and variable elements.) The fixed-cost assignment is an average based on some expected or actual level of volume. This is an important point to remember when developing SCPs; a decline in volume below expected levels will increase the average cost of production because the fixed cost is spread over fewer units of output.

The third column of Table 15-1 presents unit cost. This represents management's best guess regarding the cost or price of the resources to be used in the production process. Our dietary meal SCP indicates a price of $20 per unit of direct labor. This value reflects the expected wage per hour to be paid for direct labor in the dietary department. Again, it might be possible and desirable to divide direct labor further into specific job classifications. This usually permits better costing, but it also requires more effort.

Any fringe benefit cost associated with labor should be included in the unit cost. For example, the average direct hourly wage in our dietary meal example might be $16.00 per hour, but fringe benefits may average 25% of salaries or $4.00 per hour (0.25 × $16.00). In this case, the effective wage would be $20 per hour.

Departmental overhead consists of expenses that are charged directly to a department and do not represent either labor or materials. Common examples are equipment costs, travel allowances, expenses for outside-purchased services, and cost of publications. Usually, these items do not vary with level of activity or volume but remain fixed for the budgetary period. If this is the case, assignment to an SCP can be based on a simple average. For example, assume that our dietary department either expects or actually did provide 200,000 regular patient meals. Assume further that the department has either spent or been authorized to spend $200,000 in discretionary areas that constitute departmental overhead. The average cost per meal for these discretionary costs would be $1.00 and would be fixed.

Allocated costs are probably the most difficult to assign in most situations. In our dietary example, we include only three allocated cost areas. This is probably a low figure; a number of other departments most likely would provide service to the dietary department and should be properly included in the SCP.

There are two major alternatives to using estimates of allocated costs in an SCP. First, individual costing studies could be performed, and services from one department to another could be recorded. This process may be expensive, however, and not worth the effort. For example, if separate meters were installed, utility costs could be associated with each user department. However, the installation of such meters is probably not an effective expenditure of funds; costing accuracy would not be improved enough to justify the extra expenditure.

The second alternative would be a simple averaging method. All overhead costs might be aggregated and apportioned to other departments on the basis of direct expenses, FTEs, or some other criterion. This method is relatively simple, but its accuracy would be suspect if significant variation in departmental utilization exists.

We believe that the best approach to costing is to identify all possible direct SUs. These SUs, which can be directly associated with a patient, are much more numerous than one would expect. For example, a meal provided to a patient is a direct SU but is currently treated as an indirect product in most costing systems. Laundry and linen departments have certain SUs that are directly associated with a patient, such as clean sheets and gowns. Housekeeping provides direct services to patients when its personnel clean rooms. The administration and medical records departments also provide specific direct services to patients in the form of processed paperwork and insurance forms. If such costs, currently regarded as indirect, were reclassified as direct, there would be a substantially lower level of indirect costs that would require allocation. This would improve the costing of patients—the healthcare product—and make the allocation of indirect costs less critical. Currently, indirect costs in many healthcare settings are in excess of 50% of total cost. With better identification of services or SUs, we believe that level could be reduced to 25% or lower. This identification of services or activities is the heart of **activity-based costing (ABC)** systems. ABC systems mean many things to many people but the underlying core of ABC systems is "traceability." If there is an intermediate service or product that is directly linked to a final product, then charge that cost to the product directly—do not allocate it to overhead.

## Standard Treatment Protocols

There is an analogy between a standard treatment protocol (STP) and a job-order cost sheet used in industrial cost accounting. In a job-order cost system, a separate cost sheet is completed for each specific job. This is necessary because each job is different from jobs performed in the past and jobs to be performed in the future. Automobile repairs are an excellent example of a job-order cost system. A separate cost sheet is prepared for each job. That cost sheet then serves as the bill or invoice to the customer.

Healthcare firms also operate in a job-cost setting. Patient treatment may vary significantly across patients. The patient's bill may be thought of as a job-order cost sheet in that it reflects the actual services provided during the course of the patient's treatment. Of course, not all of the services provided are shown in the patient's bill. For example, meals provided are rarely charged as a separate item.

In a typical job-order cost setting, standards may not always be applied. When you leave your car at the dealership for servicing, the dealer does not prepare a standard job-order cost sheet. Dealers have no incentive to do this because they expect that customers will pay the actual costs of the service when they pick up their cars. If they do not, the dealer may take possession of the car as **collateral**.

In the past, a similar situation existed among healthcare firms; the client or patient would pay for the actual cost of services provided. Today, this is no longer true for the majority of healthcare products. Today, most healthcare firms are paid a fixed fee or price regardless of the range of services provided. Medicare's DRG payment system is an example of this type of payment philosophy. Healthcare providers that have accepted capitation have an additional dilemma because cost is now a function of both utilization and cost per episode. The provider must estimate the number of episodes of care as well as the cost per episode. It is similar to an automobile manufacturer providing a warranty. The manufacturer must determine both the frequency of claims and the average cost per claim.

In today's marketplace little revenue realized by a healthcare provider is derived from cost payers, and the majority of revenue is fixed price on either a case, per diem, procedure, or capitated basis. Because the revenue is fixed, understanding the cost of a treatment protocol is essential to effective management. **TABLE 15-2** shows a hypothetical STP for DRG 444 (Disorder of Biliary Tract w/MCC). (This STP is for illustrative purposes only; it should not be regarded as a realistic STP for DRG 444.)

In the STP depicted in Table 15-2, costs are split into fixed and variable components. Thus, the STP requires 25 patient meals at a variable cost of $3.00 per meal and a fixed cost of $2.80 per meal. The basis for these data is the SCP (see Table 15-1). As noted earlier, this division between fixed and variable costs may be valuable for management when it makes its

planning and control decisions. For example, if Medicare paid the hospital $2,800 for every DRG 444 patient treated, we would conclude that, at least in the short run, the hospital would be financially better off if it continued to treat DRG 444 cases, because the payment of $2,800 exceeds the variable cost of $2,039 and the hospital is therefore making a contribution to fixed costs.

Table 15-2 depicts two areas in which no actual quantity is specified: pharmacy prescriptions and other laboratory tests. In these instances, the total cost of the services is instead divided between fixed and variable costs. Because of the large number of products provided in each of these two areas, it would be impossible to develop an SCP for each product item. However, some of the heavier volume laboratory tests or pharmacy prescriptions may be separately identified and costed; for example, laboratory complete blood count is listed as a separate SU.

Some of the items shown in Table 15-2 may not be reflected in a patient's bill. For example, patient meals, linen changes, room preparation, and admission processing usually would not be listed in the bill. Also, separation of nursing care by acuity level may not be identified in the bill; many hospitals do not distinguish between levels of nursing care in their pricing structures.

A final point to emphasize is that not all SUs will show up in an STP. Only those SUs that are classified as direct are listed. A direct SU can be directly traced or associated with patient care. The costs associated with the provision of indirect SUs are allocated to the direct SUs. At the same time, the objective should be to create as many direct SUs as possible. The creation of traceable SUs is one of the objectives of ABC systems.

---

*Learning Objective 5*

Describe the concept of relative value units.

---

## ▶ Relative Value Costing

In a number of settings, the costing of individual products is difficult to accomplish and may not be worth the time and effort required. For example, medical groups often produce a large number of different medical procedures. Ancillary providers such as laboratories or imaging centers may produce hundreds of different procedures. Costing of any specific procedure is virtually impossible. Imagine for a moment the effort involved in costing a routine visit to a physician's

**TABLE 15-2** Standard Treatment for DRG 444 (Disorder of Biliary Tract)

| Service Unit No. | Service Unit Name | Quantity | Variable Cost/Unit | Fixed Cost/Unit | Total Cost/Unit | Total Variable Cost | Total Fixed Cost | Total Cost |
|---|---|---|---|---|---|---|---|---|
| 1 | Admission process | 1 | $96.00 | $104.00 | $200.00 | $96.00 | $104.00 | $200.00 |
| 7 | Nursing care level 1 | 1 | 160.00 | 80.00 | 240.00 | 160.00 | 80.00 | 240.00 |
| 8 | Nursing care level 2 | 7 | 170.00 | 90.00 | 260.00 | 1,190.00 | 630.00 | 1,820.00 |
| 9 | Nursing care level 3 | 1 | 220.00 | 90.00 | 310.00 | 220.00 | 90.00 | 310.00 |
| 29 | Pharmacy prescriptions | | 76.00 | 38.00 | 114.00 | 76.00 | 38.00 | 114.00 |
| 38 | Chest radiograph | 1 | 24.00 | 16.00 | 40.00 | 24.00 | 16.00 | 40.00 |
| 46 | Laboratory complete blood count | 1 | 8.00 | 7.00 | 15.00 | 8.00 | 7.00 | 15.00 |
| 49 | Other laboratory tests | | 170.00 | 110.00 | 280.00 | 170.00 | 110.00 | 280.00 |
| 57 | Patient meals | 25 | 3.00 | 2.80 | 5.80 | 75.00 | 70.00 | 145.00 |
| 65 | Linen changes | 5 | 1.20 | 1.00 | 2.20 | 6.00 | 5.00 | 11.00 |
| 93 | Room preparation | 1 | 14.00 | 6.00 | 20.00 | 14.00 | 6.00 | 20.00 |
| | Totals | | | | | $2,039.00 | $1,156.00 | $3,195.00 |

office. Once you identified the individual activities involved in the delivery of service and the indirect support costs associated with service delivery, it would be an accounting nightmare to assign those costs to 100 or more procedures routinely performed in the doctor's office.

One solution that is used in many settings is **relative value unit (RVU)** costing. In RVU costing, some relative weights are assigned for each of the commonly produced outputs. For medical groups, the most commonly accepted classification of outputs is **current procedural terminology (CPT) codes**. Medicare uses CPT codes in its resource-based relative value system. (This is discussed in Chapter 2.) These assigned weights can be used to cost individual procedures. For example, consider an ophthalmology practice that performs only two procedures (**TABLE 15-3**).

If we assume that the total expenses of the practice are presented as in **TABLE 15-4**, we then could develop a cost per procedure using the RVU concept.

The cost for each of the two procedures would then be calculated as shown in **TABLE 15-5**.

Various types of budgets then can be produced based on RVU weights. RVU-weighted office visits or procedures are ones that have been adjusted for the amount of resources they consume. It is necessary to

**TABLE 15-3** Relative Value Weights

| CPT No. | Number of Procedures | Physician Work Weight | Total Work Units | Practice Weight | Total Practice Units | Malpractice Weight | Total Malpractice Units |
|---|---|---|---|---|---|---|---|
| 67800 | 1,000 | 1.5 | 1,500 | 1.0 | 1,000 | 0.05 | 50 |
| 66985 | 500 | 8.5 | 4,250 | 14.0 | 7,000 | 0.75 | 375 |
| Total | 1,500 | | 5,750 | | 8,000 | | 425 |

**TABLE 15-4** Cost per Weighted Procedure

| | Total Expenses | Total Weighted Units | Cost per Weighted Unit |
|---|---|---|---|
| Physician compensation | $200,000 | 5,750 | $34.78 |
| Practice expenses | $450,000 | 8,000 | $56.25 |
| Malpractice expense | $7,500 | 425 | $17.65 |

**TABLE 15-5** Cost per Procedure

| | CPT 67800 | CPT 66985 |
|---|---|---|
| Physician work units x cost per unit | 1.50 $34.78 | 8.50 $34.78 |
| Physician cost per procedure | $52.17 | $295.63 |
| Practice work units x cost per unit | 1.00 $56.25 | 14.00 $56.25 |
| Malpractice cost per procedure | $56.25 | $787.50 |
| Malpractice work units x cost per unit | 0.05 $17.65 | 0.75 $17.65 |
| Malpractice cost per procedure | $0.88 | $13.24 |
| Total cost per procedure | $109.30 | $1,096.37 |

make these adjustments because various types of visits and procedures require different resources. Each organization must develop its own appropriate categorization scheme that applies to its services.

## SUMMARY

Product costing has become much more critical to healthcare executives today than it was before 1983. The emphasis on prospective prices and competitive discounting creates a real need to define costs. For healthcare purposes, the product is a treated patient or an encounter of care. Various aggregations of patients also may be useful. For example, we may want to develop cost data by DRG, by APCs, by clinical specialty, or by payer category.

To develop estimates of cost in a healthcare firm, two costing systems must be defined. First, a series of SCPs must be developed for all SUs. These SUs comprise the specific set of services that were or will be performed in the treatment of a specific patient encounter and represent intermediate departmental products produced by the firm. This part of costing is analogous to that of most manufacturing systems. Second, a set of STPs must be defined for major patient-treatment categories. These STPs must identify all the SUs that were or will be provided in the patient treatment. Physician involvement is critical in this area.

The purpose of costing is to make planning decisions, such as those involved in pricing and product mix, more precise and meaningful. Costing is also useful when making control decisions. Actual cost data can be compared to budgeted costs and corrective action taken when costs appear to be out of control.

## ASSIGNMENTS

1. An HMO has asked your hospital to provide all of its obstetric services. It has offered to pay your hospital $2,000 for a normal vaginal delivery, without complications (DRG 775). You have looked at the STP for this DRG and discovered that your hospital's cost is $2,400. What should you do?
2. Dr. Jones is scheduled to meet with you this afternoon. She has been an active admitter, but you would like to see her practice increase. After reviewing Dr. Jones's financial report, shown in **TABLE 15-6**, what recommendations would you make?
3. **TABLE 15-7** presents some summary cost data for MS-DRG 233 at your hospital compared to a national profile. Your hospital costs are almost $7,000 per case higher than U.S. averages and the largest areas are the two revenue codes presented here. From this data, what is the cause for the higher costs in these two areas?
4. The data in **TABLE 15-8** represent a cost accountant's effort to define the variable cost for DRG 216 (Cardiac Valve Procedures with Cardiac Catheter). Evaluate this method.

### TABLE 15-6 Dr. Jones's Financial Report

| DRG No. | Description | No. of Discharges | Actual LOS | Hospital Average LOS | Charges | Deductions | Net Revenue | Variable Cost | Gross Margin | Fixed Cost | Net Income |
|---|---|---|---|---|---|---|---|---|---|---|---|
| 0683 | Renal failure w/CC | 3 | 11.7 | 6.7 | $19,371 | $4,484 | $14,887 | $7,372 | $7,515 | $6,926 | $589 |
| 0674 | Other kidney and urinary tract procedures w/CC | 2 | 12.4 | 12.7 | 28,945 | 6,270 | 22,675 | 12,375 | 10,300 | 8,866 | 1,434 |
| 0981 | Extensive OR procedure unrelated to principal diagnosis | 3 | 32.2 | 11.3 | 87,309 | 12,739 | 74,570 | 33,421 | 41,149 | 30,955 | 10,194 |
| 0299 | Peripheral vascular disorders w MCC | 2 | 6.0 | 8.8 | 8,166 | 1,834 | 6,332 | 3,055 | 3,277 | 3,297 | (20) |
| | | 10 | | | $143,791 | $25,327 | $118,464 | $56,223 | $62,241 | $50,044 | $12,197 |

### TABLE 15-7 Cost Comparison MS-DRG 233 Coronary Bypass with Cardiac Cath with MCC

| | Hospital Average Cost per Case | National Average Cost per Case | Variance |
|---|---|---|---|
| Revenue codes | | | |
| Routine room (1xx) | $6,189 | $2,342 | $3,847 |
| Drugs requiring specific identification (63x) | $3,032 | $927 | $2,105 |
| | $9,221 | $3,269 | $5,952 |

| Routine room analysis | | | |
|---|---|---|---|
| Routine length of stay | 6.94 | 3.01 | 3.93 |
| Routine cost per day | $891.21 | $778.93 | $112.28 |
| Pharmacy analysis | | | |
| Epoetin alfa, non-ESRD, inj, units | 59.83 | 7.78 | 52.05 |
| Epoetin alfa, non-ESRD, inj, price per unit | $20.51 | $24.61 | $(4.10) |

**TABLE 15-8** Format for Defining Variable Cost for DRG 216 (Cardiac Valve Procedures with Cardiac Catheter)

| Department | Average Charges | Ratio of Direct Costs to Charges | Estimated Costs | Estimated Variable Costs (as Percentage of Total Estimated Costs) | Estimated Variable Costs |
|---|---|---|---|---|---|
| General nursing | $1,240 | 0.71 | $880 | 70 | $616 |
| Special care unit | 1,810 | 0.68 | $1,231 | 70 | $862 |
| Central supply | 180 | 0.28 | $50 | 75 | $38 |
| Laboratory | 270 | 0.47 | $127 | 10 | $13 |
| ECG | 50 | 0.37 | $19 | 20 | $4 |
| EEG | 60 | 0.38 | $23 | 20 | $5 |
| Nuclear medicine | 190 | 0.37 | $70 | 30 | $21 |
| Diagnostic radiology | 95 | 0.38 | $36 | 25 | $9 |
| Operating room | 650 | 0.47 | $306 | 65 | $199 |
| Emergency department | 105 | 0.49 | $51 | 40 | $21 |
| Transfusion | 405 | 0.63 | $255 | 70 | $179 |
| Pharmacy | 320 | 0.28 | $90 | 75 | $67 |
| Anesthesiology | 180 | 0.44 | $79 | 30 | $24 |
| Respiratory therapy | 295 | 0.35 | $103 | 25 | $26 |
| Physical therapy | 85 | 0.61 | $52 | 25 | $13 |
| Clinic | 110 | 0.53 | $58 | 30 | $17 |
| Totals | $6,045 | | $3,431 | | $2,112 |

ECG, electocardiogram; EEG, electroencephalogram.

## SOLUTIONS AND ANSWERS

1. Hopefully, the STP for DRG 775 separates the costs into variable and fixed elements. If the variable cost is less than $2,000, your hospital may earn some marginal profit from the additional business. However, the HMO physicians should closely examine the STP. There may be some patient management differences, especially regarding length of stay, which could result in more or less cost. An agreement on the STP with the HMO physicians should be negotiated. For example, what is the expected length of stay (LOS)? If the HMO physicians anticipate a 3-day LOS and your cost estimates anticipate a 2-day LOS there could be a problem.

2. Most of the income generated by Dr. Jones is in areas where her LOS is well above hospital averages. This may be a reflection of the severity of patients that she is treating. The highest area of profit is DRG 981 where her LOS is well above the hospital average. Most likely this reflects either extensive outlier payments, or patients who paid on a per day or billed charge basis. Before encouraging greater admissions from Dr. Jones it will be critical to address present LOS issues and determine what the causal factors for the higher LOS are.

3. In the routine cost area our hospital has a longer LOS (6.94 versus a 3.01 U.S. average). The actual cost of production of a routine day is also higher at our hospital ($891.21 versus $778.93). In the pharmaceutical area our hospital is using a much higher quantity of epoetin than the U.S. average (59.83 versus 7.78), but our cost per unit for this drug is actually lower ($20.51 versus $24.61).

4. The first potential weakness in the cost accountant's method is the use of a cost-to-charge ratio. There is no guarantee that charges for departmental services always will be related to costs. Some specific procedures within the department may be priced at different markups to take advantage of third-party payer contracts. A second weakness is the failure to incorporate any indirect costs, of which some might be variable. For example, there may be actual housekeeping costs that are traceable to each specific patient encounter, such as room cleaning, that are completely ignored in this approach. The method simply does not relate well to the two-stage definition of costs involving SCPs and STPs, as discussed in this chapter. In fairness, it must be noted that the cost accountant's method would cost significantly less than other methods. Also, it is not clear whether the improved accuracy that might result from some other, more sophisticated system would be worth the extra cost.

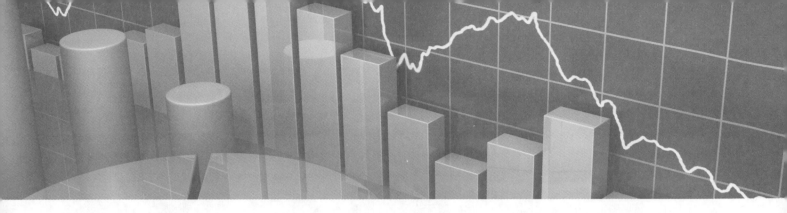

# CHAPTER 16

# The Management Control Process

## REAL-WORLD SCENARIO

James Olin has been recently named as supervisor of the Endoscopy Lab and has been reviewing recent cost reports for his department compared to budget. He is especially interested in his labor costs over the last three biweekly cost periods, which he has noticed have shown increasing unfavorable variances. **TABLE 16-1** summarizes the data Olin is reviewing.

The budgeted value for worked hours per procedure is 13.0 and Olin can see that his labor hours utilization variance is increasing and becoming more unfavorable. The CFO has noticed the unfavorable variation in Olin's area and has asked for an explanation and a plan to bring his actual costs in line with budgeted values. While Olin is new to his role as supervisor, he has been involved in the department for 5 years as a nurse and is very familiar with the operation. It is his opinion that there is no excess labor and that his employees are stretched to their limits already. A reduction in staff of 293 hours during the last biweekly pay period to meet budget would have removed 3.66 FTEs and put a tremendous strain on the department's ability to provide quality care on a timely basis. Olin is further confused because he has already cut his work force by 117 hours or nearly 1.5 FTEs since the first payroll period to reflect a decrease in the number of procedures being performed.

| **TABLE 16-1** Olin's Data | Period 1 | Period 2 | Period 3 |
|---|---|---|---|
| Procedures | 330 | 315 | 300 |
| Actual hours worked | 4,310 | 4,251 | 4,193 |
| Budgeted hours | 4,290 | 4,095 | 3,900 |
| Difference | 20 Unfavorable | 156 Unfavorable | 293 Unfavorable |
| Budgeted hours per procedure | 13 | 13 | 13 |
| Hours worked per procedure | 13.1 | 13.5 | 14 |

The more that Olin thinks about this issue the more he becomes convinced that the problem must be related to the decrease in volume, which he has experienced. He reasons that some of his staff must be available irrespective of the actual volume of procedures performed. A review of current staff positions leads him to believe that approximately 38 FTE staff members must be in place to adequately provide services given the current delivery structure of his department. With 38 required staff, Olin figures that 3,040 hours (38 × 80 hours per payroll period) of staff time are required irrespective of actual volume. Most of his staffing budget is therefore fixed and would not decline with volume reductions.

Olin has recently read something about a concept of budgeting referred to as "flexible budgeting" that is appropriate when costs in a department are composed of both fixed and variable elements. Olin is preparing to develop a flexible budget for his department and present this information to the CFO.

---

Thirty years ago, the word *budgeting* would not have been found in the vocabularies of many healthcare executives. Today, this is no longer true. Most hospitals and other healthcare firms now develop and use budgets as an integral part of their overall management control process.

To a large extent, the attention healthcare providers pay to budgeting is attributable to changes in the environment. Over the last 30 years, the healthcare industry has experienced a dramatic shift in its revenue function from cost-related to fixed prices on either a procedure, case, or covered-life basis. Firms that sell products or services in markets where prices are fixed must control their costs. Budgeting is, of course, a logical way for any business organization to control its costs.

External market forces thus certainly have stimulated the development of budgets in the healthcare industry; but most likely, such budgets would have been developed in any case. Hospitals and healthcare

firms have grown larger and more complex, in both organization and finances. And budgeting is imperative in organizations in which management authority is delegated to many individuals.

### Learning Objective 1

Define a budget and describe how management uses them.

▶ **Essential Elements**

For our purposes, a **budget** is defined as a quantitative expression of a plan of action. It is an integral part of the overall management control process of an organization. Management control is a process by which managers ensure that resources are obtained and used effectively and efficiently while accomplishing an organization's objectives.

## Efficiency and Effectiveness

In the previous definition, special emphasis is placed on attaining *efficiency* and *effectiveness*. In short, they determine the success or failure of management control.

These two terms have precise meanings. Often, people talk about the relative efficiency and effectiveness of their operations as if efficiency and effectiveness were identical, or at least highly correlated. They are not identical, nor are they necessarily correlated. An operation may be effective without being efficient, and vice versa. A well-managed operation ideally should be both effective and efficient. Efficiency is easier to measure and its meaning is fairly well understood; efficiency is simply a relationship between outputs and inputs. For example, a cost per patient-day of $1,100 is a measure of efficiency; it tells how many resources, or inputs, were used to provide one day of care, the measure of output.

Managers and other people wishing to assess performance in the healthcare industry are increasing their use of efficiency measures. In most situations, efficiency is measured by comparison with some standard. Several basic considerations should be understood if efficiency measures are to be used intelligently. First, output measures may not always be comparable. For example, comparing the costs per patient-day of care in a 50-bed rural hospital with those in a 1,000-bed teaching hospital is not likely to be meaningful. A day of care in a teaching hospital typically entails more service. Second, cost measures may not be comparable or useful for the specific decision being considered. For example, two operations may be identical, but one may be in a newer facility and thus would have a higher depreciation charge; or the two operations may account for costs differently. One hospital may use an accelerated depreciation method, such as the sum of the year's digits, whereas the other may use straight-line depreciation. Third, the cost concepts used may not be relevant to the decision being considered. For example, a certificate-of-need review to decide which of two hospitals should be permitted to develop a cardiac catheterization lab obviously will consider cost. However, comparing the full costs of a procedure in each institution and selecting the least expensive one could produce a bad decision. For this specific decision, the full-cost concept is wrong and incremental or variable cost would be the relevant cost concept. Chapter 14 discusses these cost concepts in greater detail. The focus of interest is on what the future additional cost would be, not what the historical average cost was.

**Effectiveness** is concerned with the relationship between an organization's outputs and its objectives or goals. A healthcare firm's typical goals might include solvency, high quality of care, low cost of patient care, community healthcare access, and growth. Measuring effectiveness is more difficult than measuring efficiency for at least two reasons. First, defining the relationship between outputs and some goals may be difficult because many firms' goals or objectives are not likely to be quantified. For example, exactly how does an alcoholism program contribute to quality of care? Still, objectives and goals usually can be stated more precisely in quantitative terms. In fact, they should be quantified to the greatest extent possible. In the alcoholism program example, quality scales, such as frequency of repeat visits or new patients treated, might be developed. Second, the output usually must be related to more than one organization goal or objective. For example, both solvency and community access are legitimate objectives for a hospital. Yet, continuing an alcoholism program might affect solvency negatively and but meet a community healthcare need. How should decision makers weigh these two criteria to determine an overall measure of effectiveness?

## Control Unit

In most healthcare facilities, management control is exercised through specific organizational units or responsibility centers. These centers are generally referred to as departments. **FIGURE 16-1** presents an organizational chart of a hospital and its departments.

Usually, the departments perform special functions that contribute to overall organization goals, directly or indirectly. They receive resources or inputs and produce services or outputs. **FIGURE 16-2** illustrates this relationship.

**Responsibility centers** are the focus of management control efforts. Emphasis is placed on both the efficiency and effectiveness of their operations. Measurement problems occur when the responsibility structure is not identical to the program structure. Decision makers are frequently interested in a program's total cost. Yet, in the case of a burn-care program, for example, it is unlikely that all of the resources used in the program will be assigned to it directly; the costs of medical support services (such as physical therapy, laboratory, and radiology services, as well as other general and administrative services) will not likely be contained in the burn-care unit. Program lines typically run across responsibility center or

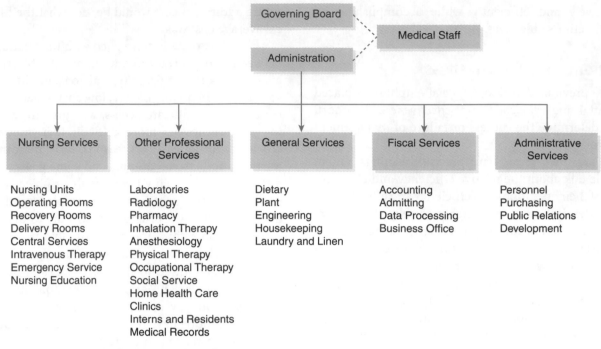

**FIGURE 16-1 Hospital Organization Chart**

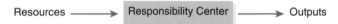

**FIGURE 16-2 Responsibility Center Production Relationship**

departmental lines. This necessitates cost allocations for decisions that require program cost information. It should be remembered that when cost allocations are involved, the accuracy of the information as well as its comparability may be suspect. For example, one may be interested in the specific costs of a burn-care program, but then find that those costs must be allocated from various departments or responsibility centers, such as laboratory, radiology, and housekeeping departments.

Responsibility centers vary greatly, depending on the controlling organization. For a regulatory agency, the responsibility center might be an entire healthcare firm; for a healthcare firm manager, it may be an individual department; for a department manager, it may be a unit within the department. The only requirement is that a designated person be in charge of the identified responsibility center.

---

*Learning Objective 2*

Explain the concept of management control and how budgeting is used as part of it.

---

## Phases of Management Control

**FIGURE 16-3** illustrates the relationship of various phases of the management control process to each other and to the planning process. Management control relies on the existence of goals and objectives; without them, the structure and evaluation of the management control process is incomplete. Poor or no planning usually limits the value of management control. Effectiveness becomes impossible to assess without stated goals and objectives; in such cases, one can focus only on measuring and attaining efficiency. The organization can assess only whether it has produced outputs efficiently; it cannot evaluate the desirability of those outputs.

For the purposes of this discussion, we are concerned with the four phases of management control:

1. Programming
2. Budgeting
3. Accounting
4. Analysis and reporting

## Programming

**Programming** is the phase of management control that determines the nature and size of programs an organization will provide to accomplish its stated goals and objectives. It is the first phase of the management control process, and it interrelates with planning. In some cases, the boundary dividing the two activities may in fact be difficult to establish. Programming

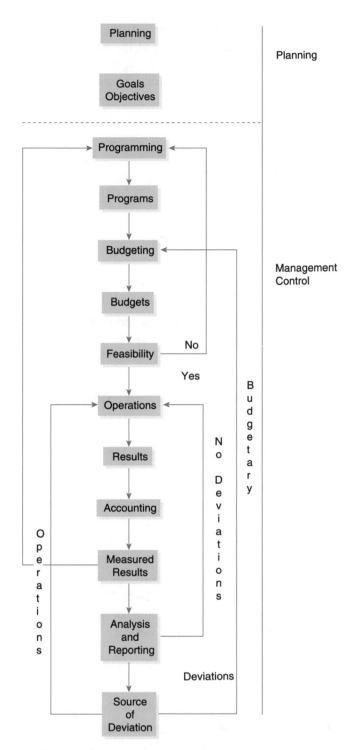

**FIGURE 16-3** **The Management Control Process**

usually lasts 3 to 5 years—longer than budgeting, but shorter than planning.

Programming decisions deal with new and existing programs. The methodology for programming is different in these two areas. Programming decisions for new programs involve capital investment or capital budget decision making. (This process is examined more extensively in Chapter 19.) The method for making programming decisions for existing programs is

often referred to as zero-base review, or zero-base budgeting (this method is discussed later in this chapter).

To illustrate the programming process, assume that a stated objective of a hospital organization is to develop and implement an ambulatory care program in the community. The decision makers in the programming phase of management control would take this stated objective and evaluate alternative programs to accomplish it, such as a surgicenter, an outpatient clinic, or a mobile health-screening unit. After this analysis, a decision might be made to construct a 10-room surgicenter on a lot adjacent to the hospital. This would be a program decision.

## Budgeting

Budgeting is the management control phase of primary interest. It was defined earlier as a quantitative expression of a plan of action. Budgets are usually stated in monetary terms and cover a period of 1 year.

The budgetary phase of management control follows the determination of programs in the programming phase. In many cases, no real review of existing programs is undertaken; the budgeting phase then may be based on a prior year's budget or on the actual results of existing programs. Proponents of zero-base budgeting (discussed later in this chapter) have identified this practice as a major shortcoming.

The budgeting phase primarily translates program decisions into terms that are meaningful for responsibility centers. The decision to construct a 10-room surgicenter will affect the revenues and costs of other responsibility centers, such as the laboratory, radiology, and anesthesiology departments, and the business office. The effects of program decisions thus must be carefully and accurately reflected in the budgets of each of the relevant responsibility centers.

Budgeting also may change programs. A more careful and accurate estimation of revenues and costs may prompt one to reevaluate prior programming decisions as financially unfeasible. For example, the proposed 10-room surgicenter may be shown, through budget analysis, to produce a significant operating loss. If the hospital cannot or will not subsidize this loss from other sources, the programming decision must be changed. The size of the surgicenter may be reduced from 10 rooms to 5 to make the operation "break even."

## Accounting

**Accounting** is the third phase of the management control process. Once the decision about which programs to implement has been made and budgets have been developed for them along responsibility center lines, the operations phase begins. The accounting department accumulates and records information on both outputs and inputs during the operating phase.

It is important to note that cost information is provided along both program and responsibility center lines. Responsibility center cost information is used in the reporting and analysis phase to determine the degree of compliance with budget projections. Programmatic cost information is used to assess the desirability of continuing a given program at its present size and scope in the programming phase of management control.

## Analysis and Reporting

The last phase of management control is analysis and reporting. In this phase, differences between actual costs and budgeted costs are analyzed to determine the probable cause of the deviations and are then reported to the individuals who can take corrective action. The method used in this phase is often referred to as variance analysis. This concept is discussed in greater detail in Chapter 17. Those doing the analysis and reporting rely heavily on the information provided from the accounting phase to break down the reported deviations into categories that suggest causes.

### Learning Objective 3

List sources of differences between budgeted and actual amounts.

In general, there are three primary causes for differences between budgeted and actual costs:

1. Prices paid for inputs were different from budgeted prices.
2. Output level was higher or lower than budgeted.
3. Actual quantities of inputs used were different from budgeted levels.

Within each of these causal areas, the problem may arise from either budgeting or operations. A budgetary problem is usually not controllable; no operating action can be taken to correct the situation. For example, the surgicenter may have budgeted for 10 registered nurses (RNs) at $4,000 each per month. However, if there was no way to employ 10 RNs at an average wage less than $4,200 per month, the budget would have to be adjusted to reflect the change in expectations. Alternatively, the problem may arise

from operations and be controllable. Perhaps the use of overtime nurse staffing at the surgicenter has increased the actual nursing cost. If this is true, some action should be taken to reduce the use of overtime in the upcoming periods.

### Learning Objective 4

Explain the budgeting process.

## ▶ The Budgeting Process

### Elements and Participants

Budgeting is regarded by many as the primary tool that healthcare managers can use to control costs in their organizations. The objectives of budgetary programs, as defined by the American Hospital Association, are fourfold:

1. To provide a written expression, in quantitative terms, of the policies and plans of the hospital
2. To provide a basis for the evaluation of financial performance in accordance with the plans
3. To provide a useful tool for the control of costs
4. To create cost awareness throughout the organization

The budgetary process encompasses a number of interrelated but separate budgets. **FIGURE 16-4** provides a schematic representation of the budgetary process and the relationships between specific types of budgets.

The individuals and roles involved in the budgetary process may vary. In general, the following individuals or parties may be involved:

- Governing board
- Chief executive officer (CEO)
- Controller
- Responsibility center managers
- Budgetary committee

Involvement of the **governing board** in the budgetary process is usually indirect. The board provides the goals, objectives, and approved programs that are used as the basis for budgetary development. In many cases, it formally approves the finalized budget, especially the cash budget and budgeted financial statements; these are critical when assessing financial condition, which is a primary responsibility of the board.

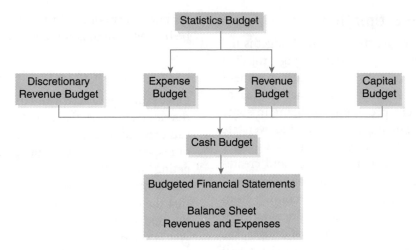

**FIGURE 16-4** **Integration of the Budgetary Process**

The *CEO* or administrator of the healthcare facility has overall responsibility for budgetary development. The budget is the administrator's tool in the overall program of management by exception, which enables the CEO to focus only on those areas where problems exist.

*Controllers* often serve as budget directors. Their primary function is facilitation: they are responsible for providing relevant data on costs and outputs and for providing budgetary forms that may be used in budget development. They are not responsible for either making or enforcing the budget.

Responsibility centers are the focal points of control. Managers of departments should be actively involved in developing budgets for their assigned areas of responsibility and are responsible for meeting the budgets developed for their areas.

Many large healthcare firms use a special **budgetary committee** to aid in budget development and approval. Typically, this committee is composed of several department managers, headed by the controller. A committee structure such as this can help legitimize budgetary decisions that might appear arbitrary and capricious if made unilaterally by management.

### Learning Objective 5

List the major types of budgets and describe how they are used.

## Statistics Budget

Development of the **statistics budget** is the first step in budgeting. It provides the basis for subsequent development of the revenue budget and the expense budget. Together, these three budgets are sometimes referred to as the **operating budget**.

The objective of the statistics budget is to provide measures of workload or activity in each department or responsibility center for the next budget period. The following three issues are involved in this task:

1. Output expectations
2. Responsibility for estimation
3. Estimation methodology

## Output Expectation

Sales forecasts in many businesses reflect management's output expectations—how much of the business's product can be sold, given certain promotional efforts. There is some question about the extent to which healthcare firms can determine their volume of service, at least within the usual budgetary period. Although, in the long run, through the development or discontinuation of certain programs, volume may be changed, most healthcare firms implicitly assume while developing their statistics budget that they cannot affect their overall volume during the next budgetary period. Instead, they assume that they will provide services to meet their actual demand. This leads to a reliance on past-period service levels to forecast demand. Demand patterns in the budget period, however, may not be similar to prior periods and can cause problems. First, foreseeable but uncontrollable forces may dramatically alter service patterns. For example, retirement of key medical staff with no replacement could drastically reduce admissions. Second, the healthcare facility may in fact control service levels in the short run and do so in a way that reduces costs. For example, a hospital may decide to develop clinical pathways in conjunction with its physicians, thus reducing total volume and total cost.

## Responsibility for Estimation

The second issue regarding the statistics budget is the assignment of responsibility for developing projected output or workload indicators. Should department managers provide this information themselves, or should top management provide it to them? In some situations, department managers may tend to overstate demand. Overstatement of demand implies a greater need for resources within their own area and creates potential budgetary slack if anticipated volumes are not realized. The result of the information coming from top management may be the converse: understatement of demand may result in a lower total cost budget that might not provide adequate resources to meet actual output levels. Negotiation thus often becomes necessary when determining demand for budgetary purposes.

## Estimation Methodology

The last area of statistics budget development concerns problems of estimation. In most healthcare facilities, department activity depends on a limited number of key indicators, such as patient-days, outpatient visits, or covered lives.

Prior values for these indicators can be related to departmental volume through statistical analysis. The major problem becomes one of accurately forecasting values for the indicators.

The use of seasonal, weekly, and daily variations in volume poses an important estimation problem. Too often, yearly volume is assumed to be divided equally between the monthly periods throughout the year, even when that is clearly not the case. Recognition of seasonal, weekly, and daily patterns of variation in volume can in fact create significant opportunities for cost reduction, especially in labor staffing.

Finally, output at the departmental level is often multiple in nature. In fact, a department normally produces more than one type of output; for example, a laboratory may provide hundreds of different tests. In such situations, a weighted unit of service is needed, such as the relative value units (RVUs) used in areas such as laboratory and radiology. Using weighted unit measures in the statistics budget is especially important when the mix of services is expected to change. Assume that a hospital is rapidly increasing its volume in outpatient clinics. This expansion in volume will increase activity in many other departments, including the pharmacy department. If, in such a situation, the filling of an outpatient prescription requires significantly more effort than the filling of an inpatient prescription, the use of an unweighted activity measure for prescriptions could provide misleading information

for budgetary control purposes. Much less labor might be budgeted than is actually needed.

## Expense Budget

Once estimates of activity for individual departments are developed in the statistics budget, department managers can proceed to develop expense budgets for their areas of responsibility. Expense budgeting is the area of budgeting "where the rubber meets the road." Management cost control efforts are finally reflected in hard numbers that the departments must live with, in most cases, for the budget period. Major categories of expense budgets at the departmental level include payroll, supplies, and other. In some situations, a budget for allocated costs from indirect departments also may be included, although departmental managers usually do not do this.

In our discussion of expense budgeting, we focus on the following four issues of budgeting that are of general interest:

1. Length of the budget period
2. Flexible or forecast budgets
3. Standards for price and quantity
4. Allocation of indirect costs

## Length of the Budget Period

Generally speaking, there are two alternative budget periods that may be used—fixed and rolling. Of the two, a **fixed budget period** is much more frequently used in the healthcare industry. A fixed budget covers some defined time from a given budget date, usually 1 year. This contrasts with a rolling budget, in which the budget is periodically extended on a frequent basis, usually by 1 month or a 3-month quarter. For example, in a **rolling budget** period with a monthly update, the entity always would have a budget that projected at least 11 more months. The same is not true in a fixed budget, in which, at fiscal year end, there may be only 1 week or 1 month remaining.

A rolling budget has many advantages, but it requires more time and effort and therefore more cost. Among its major advantages are the following:

- More realistic forecasts, which should improve management planning and control
- Equalization of the workload of budget development during the entire year
- Improved familiarity and understanding of budgets by department managers

## Flexible or Forecast Budgets

The use of a flexible budget versus a forecast budget has been discussed heavily by healthcare financial people. Presently, few healthcare firms use a formal system of flexible budgeting. However, flexible budgeting is a more sophisticated method of budgeting than typical forecast budgeting and is being adopted by more and more healthcare firms as they become experienced in the budgetary process.

A **flexible budget** adjusts targeted levels of costs for changes in volume. For example, the budget for a nursing unit operating at 95% occupancy would be different from the budget for that same unit operating at 80% occupancy. A *forecast budget*, in contrast, would make no formal differentiation in the allowed budget between these two levels.

The difference between a forecast and a flexible budget is illustrated by the historical data and projected use levels for the laboratory presented in **TABLE 16-2**. The forecast levels of volume in RVUs for 2017 are identical to the actual volumes of 2016, except that a 10% growth factor is assumed. The department manager using this statistics budget must develop a budget for hours worked in 2017. A common approach to this task is to assume that past work experience indicates future requirements. In this case, the average value for hours of work required per RVU in 2016 was 0.5061. A common method for developing a forecast budget is to multiply this value of 0.5061 by the estimated total workload for the budget period, which is expected to be 72,160, and spread the total product equally over each of the 12 months. This is the forecast budget depicted in **TABLE 16-3**.

A major difference between a flexible budget and a forecast budget is that a flexible budget must recognize and incorporate underlying cost behavioral patterns. In this laboratory example, hours worked might be written as a function of RVUs as follows:

$$\text{Hours worked} = (1,400 \text{ hours per month}) + (0.25 \times \text{RVUs})$$

Application of this formula to the budgeted RVUs expected in 2017 yields the flexible budget presented in Table 16-3.

### TABLE 16-2 Laboratory Productivity Data

| | 2016 Actual | | 2017 Budgeted |
| --- | --- | --- | --- |
| | **Hours Worked** | **RVUs** | **RVUs** |
| January | 2,825 | 5,700 | 6,270 |
| February | 2,700 | 5,200 | 5,720 |
| March | 2,900 | 6,000 | 6,600 |
| April | 2,875 | 5,900 | 6,490 |
| May | 2,825 | 5,700 | 6,270 |
| June | 2,700 | 5,200 | 5,720 |
| July | 2,750 | 5,400 | 5,940 |
| August | 2,625 | 4,900 | 5,390 |
| September | 2,725 | 5,300 | 5,830 |
| October | 2,750 | 5,400 | 5,940 |
| November | 2,750 | 5,400 | 5,940 |
| December | 2,775 | 5,500 | 6,050 |
| Total | 33,200 | 65,600 | 72,160 |

Note: 2016 average hours/RVU = 33,200/65,600 = 0.5061

**TABLE 16-3** Alternative Hours-Worked Budget for Laboratory

|  | Forecast Budget* | Flexible Budget** |
|---|---|---|
| January | 3,043 | 2,967 |
| February | 3,043 | 2,830 |
| March | 3,043 | 3,050 |
| April | 3,043 | 3,022 |
| May | 3,043 | 2,967 |
| June | 3,043 | 2,830 |
| July | 3,043 | 2,885 |
| August | 3,043 | 2,747 |
| September | 3,043 | 2,857 |
| October | 3,043 | 2,885 |
| November | 3,043 | 2,885 |
| December | 3,043 | 2,912 |
| Total | 36,516 | 34,837 |

*$(0.5061 \times 72,160)/12 = 3,043.35$

**January value $= 1,400 + (0.25 \times 6,270)$

Two points should be made before concluding our discussion of flexible budgeting versus forecast budgeting. First, a flexible budget may be represented as a forecast budget for planning purposes. For example, in the laboratory problem of Table 16-3, the flexible budget would provide an estimated hours-worked requirement of 34,837 hours for 2017. However, in an actual control period evaluation, the flexible budget formula would be used. To illustrate, assume that the actual RVUs provided in January 2017 amounted to 6,500 instead of the forecasted 6,270. Budgeted hours in the flexible budget then would not total 2,967 but 3,025:

$$1,400 + (0.25 \times 6,500) = 3,025$$

This value would be compared with the actual hours worked, not the initially forecasted 2,967.

Second, dramatic differences in approved costs can result from the two methods. Recognizing the underlying cost behavioral patterns can change the estimated resource requirements approved in the budgetary process. In our laboratory example in Table 16-3, the forecast budget calls for 36,516 hours versus the flexible budget hours requirement of 34,837. The difference results from the method used to estimate hours worked. In a forecast budget method, the prior average hours per RVU relationship is used. In most situations, average hours or average cost should be greater than variable hours or variable cost. In departments with expanding volume, the estimated requirements for resources could be overstated. This is the situation in our laboratory example where volume increased 10% from the prior year. Because some of the labor cost was fixed (1,400 hours per month), the increase in total labor costs was not proportional. The converse may be true in departments with declining volume. In many cases, use of forecast budgeting methods is based on the incorporation of prior average cost relationships. This error is not made with flexible budgeting methods because their use depends on explicit incorporation of cost behavioral patterns that distinctly recognize variable and fixed costs.

A flexible budget makes sense when there are expenses that could vary with small changes in volume. Expense categories such as supplies are usually variable in nature. Labor costs may or may not be variable. The use of part-time labor, overtime, and outside pools all tend to make labor costs variable. In general, greater variability or uncertainty in volume forecasts should lead management to adopt more flexible staffing policies.

## Standards for Price and Quantity

Earlier, three factors were identified that can create differences between budgeted and actual costs: volume, prices, and usage or efficiency. The use of flexible budgeting is an attempt to improve the recognition of deviations caused by changes in volume. The use of standards for prices and wage rates, coupled with standards for physical quantities, is an attempt to improve the recognition of deviations from budgets that result from prices and usage.

For example, assume that the flexible budget-hours requirement for the laboratory example is still hours worked $= 1,400 + (0.25 \times$ RVUs). Assume further that the budgeted wage rate is $20 per hour and the actual RVUs for January 2017 amounted to 6,500. Actual payroll cost for hours worked in January was $68,200 and actual hours worked was 3,100. This would mean that the actual wage rate per hour would be $22.00 ($68,200/3,100). The variance analysis report presented in **TABLE 16-4** summarizes the computation of price and efficiency variances applicable to the laboratory department.

**TABLE 16-4** Standard Cost Variance Analysis for Labor Costs, Laboratory, January 2017

| | |
|---|---|
| 1. Price variance | = (Actual hours worked) × (Actual wage rate) – (Actual hours worked) × (Budgeted wage rate) |
| | = (3,100 × $22.00) – (3,100 × 20.00) |
| | = $6,200 [Unfavorable] |
| 2. Efficiency variance | = (Actual hours worked) × (Budgeted wage rate) – (Budgeted hours worked) × (Budgeted wage rate) |
| | = (3,100 × $20.00) – (3,025 × $20.00) |
| | = $1,500 [Unfavorable] |
| 3. Total variance | = $6,200 + $1,500 = $7,700 [Unfavorable] |

Note: Actual wage rate = $68,200/3,100 = $22.00
Budgeted wage rate = $20.00
Actual hours worked = 3,100
Budgeted hours worked = (1,400) + (0.25 × 6,500) = 3,025

The total unfavorable variance of $7,700 results from a $6,200 unfavorable price variance and a $1,500 unfavorable efficiency variance. Splitting the variance in this manner helps management quickly identify possible causes. For example, the $6,200 price variance may be due to a negotiated wage increase of $2 per hour. If this is the case, the department manager is clearly not responsible for the variance. If, however, the difference is due to an excessive use of overtime personnel or a more costly mix of labor, then the manager may be held responsible for the difference and should attempt to prevent the problem from occurring again. The unfavorable efficiency variance of $1,500 reflects excessive use of labor during the month in the amount of 75 hours. An explanation for this difference should be sought and steps taken to prevent its recurrence.

Standard costing techniques have been used in industry for many years as an integral part of management control. Although it is true that input and output relationships may not be as objective in the healthcare industry as they are in general industry, this does not imply that standard costing cannot be used. In fact, there are many areas of activity within a healthcare facility that have fairly precise input–output relationships—housekeeping, laundry and linen, laboratory, radiology, and many others. Standard costing can prove to be a valuable tool for cost control in the healthcare industry, if properly applied. (This topic is explored in greater detail in Chapter 17.)

## Allocation of Indirect Costs

There probably has been more internal strife in organizations over the allocation of indirect costs than over any other single budgetary issue. A comment often heard is, "Why was I charged $10,000 for housekeeping services last month when my department didn't use anywhere near that level of service?"

A strong case can in fact be made for not allocating indirect costs in **budget variance** reports. In most normal situations, the receiving department has little or no control over the costs of the servicing department. Allocation may thus raise questions that should not be raised. Although it is true that indirect costs need to be allocated for some decision-making purposes, such as pricing, they are generally not needed for evaluating individual responsibility center management.

However, an equally strong argument can be made for including indirect costs in the budgets of benefiting departments. They are legitimate costs of the total operation, and department managers should be aware of them. If the decisions of department managers can influence costs in indirect areas, these managers should be held accountable for those costs. For example, maintenance, housekeeping, and other indirect costs can be influenced by the decisions of benefiting departments. Ideally, a charge for these indirect services should be established and levied against the using departments, based on their use. Labeling the cost of indirect areas as totally uncontrollable can stimulate excessive and unnecessary use of indirect services and thus have a negative impact on the total cost control program in an organization.

## Revenue Budget

The **revenue budget** can be set effectively only after the expense budget and the statistics budget have been developed. Revenues must be set at levels that cover all associated expenses plus provide a return on invested capital. This is a fundamental rule of finance and is equally valid for both voluntary not-for-profit firms and investor-owned firms. Moreover, because of the presence of cost-reimbursement formulas, some of the total revenue actually realized by a healthcare facility is directly determined by expenses.

## Rate Setting

In this discussion of the revenue budget, we focus on only one aspect of revenue budget development—pricing or rate setting. Specifically, we illustrate the rate-setting model through an additional example. This model is discussed further in Chapters 6 and 14.

**FIGURE 16-5** illustrates the rate-setting model. Sources of information to define the variables of the model are identified. However, the following three parameters have no identified source:

1. Desired profit
2. Proportion of charge-paying patients
3. Proportion of charge-paying patient revenue not collected

In most situations, separate figures for the percentage of write-offs on charge-paying patients and the percentage of charge-paying patients are not available on a departmental basis. Sometimes the best information available may be the percentage of bad-debt write-offs on total revenue for the institution as a whole. Using the example data for Department 1 in **TABLE 16-5**, a 1% write-off on 20% of the patients who paid charges in the department implies that 5% of the charge-paying patient revenue in that department is written off.

The corresponding figure for Department 2 is 50%. Using these data, and substituting the total or aggregate values for the percentage write-offs on charge-paying patients and the percentage of charge-paying patients, the following rates are established:

$$\text{Department 1 price} = \frac{\dfrac{\$10,000}{100} + \dfrac{\$500}{100 \times 0.4}}{1 - 0.3875} = \$183.67$$

$$\text{Department 2 price} = \frac{\dfrac{\$10,000}{100} + \dfrac{\$500}{100 \times 0.4}}{1 - 0.3875} = \$183.67$$

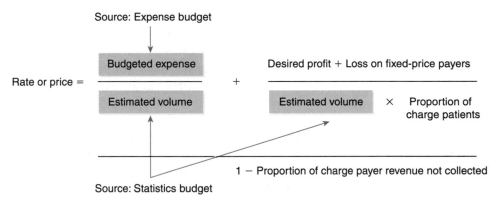

$$\text{Rate or price} = \frac{\text{Budgeted expense}}{\text{Estimated volume}} + \frac{\text{Desired profit} + \text{Loss on fixed-price payers}}{\text{Estimated volume} \times \text{Proportion of charge patients}}$$

Source: Expense budget
Source: Statistics budget
1 − Proportion of charge payer revenue not collected

**FIGURE 16-5** **Rate Setting in the Revenue Budget**

| **TABLE 16-5** Rate-Setting Example Data | | | |
|---|---|---|---|
| | **Department 1** | **Department 2** | **Total** |
| Loss on fixed price payers | – | – | – |
| Desired profit | $500 | $500 | $1,000 |
| Budgeted expense | $10,000 | $10,000 | $20,000 |
| Estimated volume | 100 | 100 | – |
| Percentage bad debt | 1% | 30% | 15.5% |
| Percentage charge-paying patients | 20% | 60% | 40% |
| Percentage bad debt on charge-paying patients | 5% | 50% | 38.75% |

Proper reflection of the departmental values, however, produces the following rates:

$$\text{Department 1 price} = \frac{\dfrac{\$10,000}{100} + \dfrac{\$500}{100 \times 0.2}}{1 - 0.05} = \$131.58$$

$$\text{Department 2 price} = \frac{\dfrac{\$10,000}{100} + \dfrac{\$500}{100 \times 0.6}}{1 - 0.50} = \$216.67$$

In the former case, the use of aggregate or average values produces an inequitable pricing structure. The price for Department 1 was initially overstated, whereas the price for Department 2 was initially understated. If equity in rate setting is an objective, reliance on average values can prevent the development of an equitable rate structure along departmental lines. In many cases, the errors may be significant.

## Desired Profit Levels

Determining a desired level of profit is not easy. In many cases, it is a subjective process, made to appear objective through the application of a quantitative profit requirement. For example, desired profit may be arbitrarily set at some percentage of budgeted expenses, such as 10% above expenses, or as a certain percentage of total investment. However, desired levels of profit can, in general, be stated as the difference between financial requirements and expenses as follows:

Desired profit = Budgeted financial requirements

− Budgeted expenses

Budgeted financial requirements are cash requirements that an entity must meet during the budget period. Four elements usually constitute total budgeted financial requirements:

1. Budgeted expenses, excluding depreciation
2. Requirements for debt principal payment
3. Requirements for increases in working capital
4. Requirements for capital expenditures not financed with debt

Budgeted expenses at the departmental level should include both direct and indirect (or allocated) expenses. Depreciation charges are excluded because depreciation is a noncash requirement expense.

Debt principal payments include only the principal portion of debt service due. In some cases, additional reserve requirements may be established, which may require additional funding. Interest expense is already included in budgeted expenses and should not be included in debt principal payments.

Working capital requirements were discussed earlier. The maintenance of necessary levels of inventory, accounts receivable, and precautionary cash balances requires an investment. Changes in the total level of this investment must be funded from cash, additional indebtedness, or a combination of the two. Planned financing of increases in working capital is a legitimate financial requirement.

Capital expenditure requirements may be of two types. First, actual capital expenditures may be made for approved projects. Those projects not financed with indebtedness require a cash investment. Second, prudent fiscal management requires that funds be set aside and invested to meet reasonable requirements for future capital expenditures. This amount should be related to the replacement cost depreciation of existing fixed assets.

Any loss incurred on fixed-price payers, such as Medicare, must be added to the desired profit target, as Figure 16-5 shows. The amount of the loss would represent the projected difference between allocated costs or expenses and net revenue received from fixed-price payers. If revenues from fixed-price payers exceed costs, the difference would be subtracted from the profit target. For example, if a firm received $5,000,000 in revenue from Medicare and incurred $4,800,000 in costs to provide care to Medicare patients, the difference of $200,000 would be subtracted from the desired profit target. The effect would be lower required rates or prices. (Chapter 14 provides more detail on price setting.)

A logical question is, "How is the desired profit requirement allocated to individual departments?" Usually, it is just assigned on the basis of some percentage of budgeted expenses. If a nursing home budgets $5 million in expenses and determines that $500,000 profit is required, each department might set its rates to recover 10% above its expenses. However, the importance of cost reimbursement and bad debts at the departmental level also should be considered. As was seen previously in our departmental pricing example, variances in bad-debt percentages or payer-mix differences by department can create inequitable and inaccurate pricing values.

## Discretionary Revenue Budget and Capital Budget

Discretionary revenue may be important, especially for institutions with large investment portfolios. A good management control system will have a budget for expected return on investments. Variations from the expected level then would be investigated. In some cases, changes in investment management may be necessary.

Capital budgeting can give many healthcare managers a major control tool. It can significantly affect the level of cost. This is especially true when not only the initial capital costs associated with given capital expenditures are considered but also the associated operating costs for salaries and supplies. (The capital budgeting process is examined in detail in Chapter 19.)

## The Cash Budget and Budgeted Financial Statements

The cash budget is management's best indicator of the organization's expected short-run solvency. It translates all of the previous budgets into a statement of cash inflows and outflows. The cash budget is usually broken down by periods, such as months or quarters, within the total budget period. An example of a cash budget is shown in TABLE 16-6.

| **TABLE 16-6** Cash Budget, Budget Year 2017 | | | | | | |
|---|---|---|---|---|---|---|
| | **1st Quarter** | | | | | |
| | **January** | **February** | **March** | **2nd Quarter** | **3rd Quarter** | **4th Quarter** |
| Receipts from operations | $300,000 | $310,000 | $320,000 | $1,000,000 | $1,100,000 | $1,100,000 |
| Disbursements from operations | 280,000 | 280,000 | 300,000 | 940,000 | 1,000,000 | 1,000,000 |
| Cash available from operations | $20,000 | $30,000 | $20,000 | $60,000 | $100,000 | $100,000 |
| Other receipts | | | | | | |
| Increase in mortgage payable | | | | 500,000 | | |
| Sale of fixed assets | | 20,000 | | | | |
| Unrestricted income endowment | | | 40,000 | 40,000 | 40,000 | 40,000 |
| Total other receipts | $- | $20,000 | $40,000 | $540,000 | $40,000 | $40,000 |
| Other disbursements | | | | | | |
| Mortgage payments | | | 150,000 | | 150,000 | |
| Fixed-asset purchase | | | | 480,000 | | |
| Funded depreciation | | | 30,000 | 130,000 | 30,000 | 30,000 |
| Total other disbursements | $0 | $0 | $180,000 | $610,000 | $180,000 | $30,000 |
| Net cash gain (loss) | 20,000 | 50,000 | (120,000) | (10,000) | (40,000) | 110,000 |
| Beginning cash balance | 100,000 | 120,000 | 170,000 | 50,000 | 40,000 | 0 |
| Cumulative cash | $120,000 | $170,000 | $50,000 | $40,000 | $- | $110,000 |
| Desired level of cash | 100,000 | 100,000 | 100,000 | 100,000 | 100,000 | 100,000 |
| Cash above minimum needs (financing needs) | $20,000 | $70,000 | $(50,000) | $(60,000) | $(100,000) | $10,000 |

Departmental expense budgets, departmental revenue budgets, a discretionary revenue budget, and a capital budget that do not provide a sufficient cash flow can necessitate major revisions. If the organization cannot or will not finance the deficits, the budgets must be changed to maintain the solvency of the organization. A poor cash budget could cause an increase in rates, a reduction in expenses, a reduction in capital expenditures, or many other changes. These changes and revisions must be made until the cash budget reflects a position of short-run solvency.

The two major financial statements that are developed on a budgetary basis are the balance sheet and the statement of revenue and expense. These two statements are indicators of both short- and long-run solvency; however, they are more important in assessing long-run solvency. Changing projections in either statement might cause changes in any of the other budgets.

In short, the budgeted financial statements and the cash budget test the adequacy of the entire budgetary process. Budgets that result in an unfavorable financial position, as reflected by the budgeted financial statements and the cash budget, must be adjusted. Solvency is a goal that most organizations cannot sacrifice. Cash budgeting is explored in greater detail in Chapter 23.

---

### Learning Objective 6

Describe the concept of zero-base budgeting.

---

## ▶ Zero-Base Budgeting

**Zero-base budgeting** is a term that has gained much publicity. It has been touted as management's most effective cost-containment tool. It also has been described as the biggest hoax of the century. The truth lies somewhere in the middle.

Zero-base budgeting, or zero-base review as some prefer to call it, is a way of looking at existing programs. It is part of programming, but it focuses on existing programs instead of new programs. Zero-base budgeting assumes that no existing program is entitled to automatic approval. Many individuals have identified automatic approval with existing budgetary systems that are based on prior-year expenditure levels.

Zero-base budgeting looks at the entire budget and determines the efficacy of the entire expenditure. It thus requires a tremendous effort and investment of time. It cannot be done well on an annual basis. This is why many refer to it as zero-base review instead of zero-base budgeting. Some have suggested that a zero-base review of a given activity would be appropriate every 5 years.

Zero-base budgeting is a process of periodically reevaluating all programs and their associated levels of expenditures. Management decides the frequency of this reevaluation and may vary it from every year to every 5 years.

Although most decision makers agree with the concept of zero-base budgeting, in practice it poses the following two significant questions:

1. What evaluation methodology should be used in zero-base budgeting?
2. Who should be involved in the actual decision-making process?

In each case, the answers are important to the success or failure of the zero-base budget program. Yet, there still is not complete agreement among experts regarding the answers.

Nearly everyone would agree that cost-benefit analysis should be the evaluation methodology of zero-base budgeting. There are two important issues involved in the application of cost-benefit analysis to zero-base budgeting programs: (1) Are the services that are presently provided being delivered in an efficient manner? (2) Are these services being delivered in an effective manner in terms of the organization's goals and objectives? A procedure for quantitatively answering these two questions involves the following seven sequential steps:

1. Define the outputs or services provided by the program or departmental area.
2. Determine the costs of these services or outputs.
3. Identify options for reducing the cost through changes in outputs or services.
4. Identify options for producing the services and outputs more efficiently.
5. Determine the cost savings associated with options identified in Steps 3 and 4.
6. Assess the risks, both qualitative and quantitative, associated with the identified options of Steps 3 and 4.
7. Select and implement those options with an acceptable cost-to-risk relationship.

---

### Learning Objective 7

Explain how benchmarking is performed at the departmental level.

---

# ▶ Benchmarking at the Departmental Level

One of the critical aspects to management control at the departmental or responsibility center level is access to relevant productivity standards. How much labor should be used to produce a certain level of output? In general, there are three sources of productivity standards:

- Internally developed historical standards
- Engineered standards
- Comparative group standards

Internally developed standards based on historical performance are the easiest and least costly method of productivity standard development. It is also the most commonly used method. For example, a hospital laundry and linen department may have a historical average of 20 hours of labor per 1,000 pounds of laundry. That historical average could be used to budget labor hours for the coming year. The biggest disadvantage of using this method is that historical averages do not provide information about relative efficiency. Is

20 hours of labor per 1,000 pounds of laundry an efficient level of productivity or not?

Engineered standards can be developed with internal staff, or they can be developed with the help of outside consultants. The key aspect to this method is an exhaustive study of the work setting and the definition of normative standards of productivity. For example, a consultant might determine that only 14 hours of labor is required per 1,000 pounds of laundry. Significant opportunities for cost reduction may result because of this engineered standard. The management problem of achieving this standard still remains; however, and there is no guarantee that the projected savings can be realized soon, if ever. Management must act on the information that it was given if it is to realize savings. The primary disadvantage of engineered standards is cost. The use of specialized internal staff or outside consultants can be costly.

Comparative group productivity standards are available in most healthcare industry sectors. Sometimes associations that represent healthcare firms collect data and distribute them to members, or private firms may provide comparative group standards from survey data they have collected. **TABLE 16-7** provides

**TABLE 16-7** Productivity and Cost Standards for Selected Hospital Departments

| Department | Output Unit | Direct Cost per Output Unit |
|---|---|---|
| Nursing | | |
| Intensive care unit | Patient-days | $757.94 |
| General routine care | Patient-days | 377.52 |
| Nursery | Patient-days | 292.96 |
| Professional services | | |
| Operating room | Weighted procedures | $16.52 |
| Radiology-diagnostic | Weighted procedures | 27.56 |
| Laboratory | Weighted procedures | 53.97 |
| Physical therapy | Weighted procedures | 47.11 |
| General services | | |
| Laundry and linen | 1,000 pounds | $630.00 |
| Housekeeping | 100 square feet | 696.00 |
| Food services | Meals | 11.12 |

Cleverley & Associates. (2015). Departmental benchmarking report, U.S. average for hospital between 150 to 250 beds.

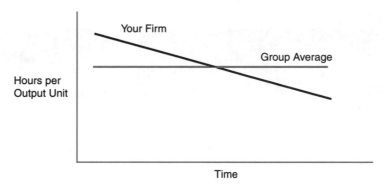

**FIGURE 16-6** **Closing the Performance Gap**

some hospital departmental standards from Cleverley & Associates in Worthington, Ohio. The data indicate that the average direct cost in hospitals between 150 and 250 beds for laundry departments was $630.00 per 1,000 pounds.

Comparative group data are usually less expensive to obtain than engineered standards, but there are several drawbacks. First, is the productivity standard comparable across all departments in the group? To be comparable, both the measure of cost and output must be defined in the same manner by all reporting members. For example, is the number of pounds of laundry measured wet or dry? Does the measure of labor hours include vacation and sick time? Second, knowing there is a difference between a group average and your department's performance does not tell you *why* the difference exists. Your laundry may require 20 hours per 1,000 pounds, and the national average may be 12 hours, but how can you achieve that standard? Perhaps the equipment used is old and requires more labor costs. The difference does imply that something is wrong and that change is needed, but communication with other group members may be necessary to realize savings. Many

of the comparative group reporting services provide mechanisms for interfirm communication to learn and adopt best practices. Ultimately, the objective is to achieve superior performance, as **FIGURE 16-6** illustrates.

## ▶ SUMMARY

This chapter has focused on the process of management control that is used in organizations. Most management control processes involve the following four phases of activity: programming, budgeting, accounting, and analysis and reporting. Budgeting is an activity that many department managers view as the primary focus of management control because of its direct focus on resource allocation and emphasis on efficiency. Efficiency standards are primary inputs into the budgeting process and are often provided through comparative benchmarking data.

### Reference

Anthony, R., & Young, D. (2003). *Management control in nonprofit organizations.* New York: McGraw-Hill.

## ASSIGNMENTS

1. Under what conditions is a flexible budget likely to be more effective than a forecast budget?
2. Can an organization be efficient but not effective? Discuss the circumstances in which this could be true.
3. The first step in the budgeting process is to develop the statistics budget. Why is this true?
4. Ann Walker, CPA, is the controller for your hospital. For a long time, Walker has been concerned about management control in the hospital, and she finally has developed a new departmental labor control system. It is based on the data in **TABLE 16-8** for the obstetrics nursing unit.

   Using these data, Walker developed a two-factor variance model for labor costs in the obstetrics department. In Period 1, the variances in this model would be as follows:

   Labor rate variance = (Actual rate − Budgeted rate) × Actual hours

   = ($27.00 − $27.28) × 1,550 = $434.00 (Favorable)

**TABLE 16-8** Budget Data for OB Example

| Period | Patient-Days | Hours Worked | Rate | Total Cost |
|--------|-------------|--------------|-------|-----------|
| 1 | 350 | 1,550 | $27.00 | $41,850 |
| 2 | 400 | 1,700 | 27.60 | 46,920 |
| 3 | 300 | 1,400 | 26.40 | 36,960 |
| 4 | 375 | 1,625 | 27.60 | 44,850 |
| 5 | 450 | 1,850 | 27.60 | 51,060 |
| Total | 1,875 | 8,125 | | $221,640 |

Average rate = $27.28 = $221,640/8,125
Average hours/Patient-day = 4.33 = 8,125/1,875

$$\text{Labor usage variance} = (\text{Actual labor used} - \text{Budgeted labor}) \times \text{Budgeted rate}$$
$$= (1,550 - 4.33 \times 350) \times \$27.28 = \$941.16 \text{ (Unfavorable)}$$

A similar model for labor control has been adopted in all other departments. As the chief executive officer of the hospital, are you satisfied with this labor control system? What suggestions for revisions would you make?

5. Floyd Farley is the maintenance department head. His department is participating in a wage-incentive program in which he and his staff receive 20% of the department's income as supplemental income. Net income is defined as $25 multiplied by maintenance staff hours charged, less direct departmental expense. Do you see any problems with this system? If so, how might they be solved?

6. You have been asked to prepare a flexible budget for a 40-bed nursing unit. A schedule of staffing requirements by occupancy is presented in **TABLE 16-9**. Prepare a budget for management that shows expected personnel costs for this nursing unit by occupancy level.

7. You must establish a pricing schedule for laboratory procedures. From a total hospital perspective, management has decided that the hospital must earn 5% above costs. The hospital has established that it loses 10% on each fixed-price payer (Medicare). That is, for every $100 of cost incurred to treat a fixed-price payer, the hospital receives only $90 in payment. You must build both the required profit and the expected loss on fixed-price payers into your rate structure. Payer mix for the laboratory is expected to be as presented in **TABLE 16-10**.

   Medicare pays on a fixed price per diagnosis-related group for all inpatients. There is thus no separate payment for laboratory tests. Medicaid pays average costs for both inpatient and outpatient tests. Medicare also pays on a fee schedule for outpatient tests. On average Medicare pays 80% of cost for outpatient lab tests. Blue Cross pays 95% of charges for both inpatient and outpatient procedures. All other commercial insurance and health maintenance organization (HMO) patients pay 100% of charges. If budgeted expenses are $1,000,000 ($2.00 per RVU), what price must be set to meet management's profit expectations?

8. How would you calculate the amount of revenue to be realized as cash from patient sources in a fiscal period?

9. What is the major conceptual difference between zero-base budgeting and conventional budgeting?

10. In a hospital operation, what key variables are important when projecting volume at departmental levels?

**TABLE 16-9** Staffing Budget for Nursing Unit

| | Below 60% Occupancy | 60 to 80% Occupancy | 80 to 100% Occupancy |
|---|---|---|---|
| First shift | | | |
| Head nurse | 1 | 1 | 1 |
| Registered nurse | 1 | 1 | 2 |
| Licensed practical nurse | 1 | 1 | 1 |
| Aides | 1 | 2 | 2 |
| Second shift | | | |
| Registered nurse | 2 | 2 | 2 |
| Licensed practical nurse | 1 | 1 | 1 |
| Aides | 2 | 3 | 3 |
| Third shift | | | |
| Registered nurse | 1 | 1 | 1 |
| Licensed practical nurse | 1 | 1 | 1 |
| Aides | 0 | 1 | 2 |
| Daily personnel costs by job title and shift | | | |
| Head nurse | $175 | | |
| Registered nurse-first shift | 135 | | |
| Second and third shifts | 155 | | |
| Licensed practical nurse first shift | 85 | | |
| Second and third shifts | 100 | | |
| Aides-first shift | 70 | | |
| Second and third shifts | 75 | | |

**TABLE 16-10** Laboratory Pricing Data

| | Budgeted RVUs | | |
|---|---|---|---|
| | **Inpatient** | **Outpatient** | **Total** |
| Medicare | 200,000 | 50,000 | 250,000 |
| Medicaid | 40,000 | 10,000 | 50,000 |
| Blue Cross | 80,000 | 20,000 | 100,000 |
| Commercial insurance and HMOs | 60,000 | 10,000 | 70,000 |
| Bad debt and charity | 15,000 | 15,000 | 30,000 |
| Total RVUs | 395,000 | 105,000 | 500,000 |

## SOLUTIONS AND ANSWERS

1. Two conditions are necessary for a flexible budget to be more useful than a forecast budget. First, there must be some indication that costs are variable, at least in part. Second, there must be some variability in activity levels, that is, volume is not expected to be constant in each period.
2. Efficiency relates to the costs per unit of output produced. Effectiveness relates to the attainment of organizational objectives given its outputs. It is possible for a firm to be efficient but not effective. For example, a hospital might provide inpatient care at an extremely low cost. However, this might not be effective if the provision of the inpatient' care is accomplished at rates that threaten the hospital's goal of financial solvency.
3. Figure 16-4 indicates that the statistics budget provides input for the development of the expense budget and the revenue budget. Projection of both expenses and revenues is a function of expected volume and variability of volume over the budget period. In cases when volume is expected to vary significantly, management may try to make more of their costs variable to maximize their ability to control costs, given volume changes. For example, more variable staffing may be used through the use of part-time employees, nursing pools, or overtime.
4. The primary weakness of Walker's model is its failure to incorporate fixed labor requirements. A flexible budgeting system should be put into effect instead. Using a high–low method to estimate costs (Chapter 14), the following budget parameters for hours required can be estimated:

$$\text{Variable hours} = \frac{1,850 - 1,400}{450 - 300} = 3.0 \text{ hours per patient-day}$$

$$\text{Fixed hours per period} = 1,850 - (3.0 \times 450) = 500 \text{ hours per period}$$

   The deviation in hours worked per period is removed when the fixed labor requirement is recognized (**TABLE 16-11**).
5. Farley has an incentive to engage his staff in what might be needless maintenance. This could be controlled by setting limits on the absolute level of incentive payment that could be earned, for example, by basing the incentive payments on the difference between actual and budgeted costs or by establishing control systems for authorizing maintenance work.
6. The budget in **TABLE 16-12** could be developed to show daily standard personnel costs by occupancy level for the nursing unit.

**TABLE 16-11**  Flexible Budget Comparison of Actual Versus Budgeted Hours

| Period | Patient-Days | Actual Hours | Budgeted Hours (500 + 3.0 × Patient-Day) | Difference |
|---|---|---|---|---|
| 1 | 350 | 1,550 | 1,550 | 0 |
| 2 | 400 | 1,700 | 1,700 | 0 |
| 3 | 300 | 1,400 | 1,400 | 0 |
| 4 | 375 | 1,625 | 1,625 | 0 |
| 5 | 450 | 1,850 | 1,850 | 0 |

**TABLE 16-12**  Nursing Unit Budget

| | Occupancy | | |
|---|---|---|---|
| | Below 60% | 60 to 80% | 80 to 100% |
| First shift | | | |
| Head nurse | $175 | $175 | $175 |
| Registered nurse | 135 | 135 | 270 |
| Licensed practical nurse | 85 | 85 | 85 |
| Aides | 70 | 140 | 140 |
| Second shift | | | |
| Registered nurse | 310 | 310 | 310 |
| Licensed practical nurse | 100 | 100 | 100 |
| Aides | 150 | 225 | 225 |
| Third shift | | | |
| Registered nurse | 155 | 155 | 155 |
| Licensed practical nurse | 100 | 100 | 100 |
| Aides | 0 | 75 | 150 |
| Total standard personnel costs | $1,280 | $1,500 | $1,710 |

**TABLE 16-13** Budgeted Income

|  | Revenue |
|---|---|
| Medicare inpatient (0.4 × $1,000,000 × 0.9) | $360,000 |
| Medicare outpatient (0.1 × $1,000,000 × 0.8) | 80,000 |
| Medicaid (0.1 × $1,000,000) | 100,000 |
| Blue Cross (100,000 × $3.0909 × 0.95) | 293,636 |
| Commercial insurance and HMO (70,000 × $3.0909) | 216,364 |
| Bad debt and charity | 0 |
| Total revenue | $1,050,000 |
| Less expenses | 1,000,000 |
| Budget profit | $50,000 |

Medicare IP = % of business × Expenses × Payment % of cost
Medicare OP = % of business × Expenses × Payment % of cost
Medicaid revenue = % of business × Expenses
Blue Cross revenue = Number of RVUs × Charge per RVU × Payment%
Commercial revenue = Number of RVUs × Charge per RVU

7. Using the formula in Figure 16-5 and **TABLE 16-13**, the following rate structure can be established to meet management's profit expectations:

$$\text{Price} = \frac{\dfrac{\$1,000,000}{500,000} + \dfrac{(\$50,000 + \$60,000)}{500,000 \times 0.40}}{1 - 0.175} = \$3.0909$$

$$\text{Desired profit} = 0.05 \times \$1,000,000 = \$50,000$$

Loss on Medicare IP = Medicare IP volume × Average cost × Loss on Medicare IP business

$$= 200,000 \times \$2.00 \times 10\% = \$40,000$$

Loss on Medicare OP = Medicare OP volume × Average cost × Loss on Medicare OP business

$$= 50,000 \times \$2.00 \times 20\% = \$20,000$$

$$\text{Total loss on Medicare} = \$40,000 + \$20,000 = \$60,000$$

Total charge volume in RVUs = Blue Cross (100,000) + Bad debt (30,000)

$$+ \text{Commercial} (70,000) = 200,000$$

$$\text{Proportion of charge payers} = (100,000 + 70,000 + 30,000)/500,000 = 0.40$$

Total charge volume not paid = Blue Cross 5% discount (5,000) +

$$\text{Bad debt} (30,000) + \text{Commercial} (0) = 35,000$$

$$\text{Proportion of charge payer revenue not collected} = 35,000/200,000 = 0.175$$

8. Cash realized from patient sources could be expressed as follows:

$$\text{Cash flow} = \text{Net patient revenue} + \text{Beginning patient accounts receivable} - \text{Ending patient accounts receivable}$$

9. Zero-base budgeting starts from a zero base. That is, all expenditures must be justified in the budgeting review. Conventional budgeting looks primarily at expenditures that are above prior levels.

10. The volume of actual cases treated (discharges or admissions) and outpatient activity are the key variables that affect departmental volumes. For example, laboratory tests are usually related to discharges and outpatient visits. Patient-days are derived from discharges by assuming an average length of stay. Refinements in forecasting can be achieved by projecting case mix. Finally, more or fewer ancillary services per discharge may be required, depending on the type of case.

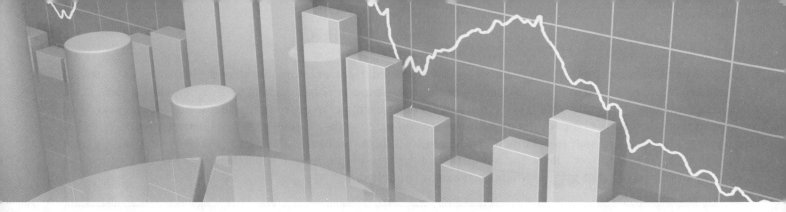

# CHAPTER 17
# Cost Variance Analysis

## LEARNING OBJECTIVES

After studying this chapter, you should be able to do the following:

1. Describe what is meant by cost control.
2. Describe the two major theories used for the detection of out-of-control costs.
3. Define variance analysis and how it is used by management.
4. Calculate the various types of cost variances.
5. Explain and calculate price, efficiency, and volume variances.

## REAL-WORLD SCENARIO

Linda Wills, CEO at Buckeye Valley Community Hospital, is preparing for the monthly board meeting. She was contacted earlier in the day by one of the board members, Doug Marshall, who was very upset by the plunge in hospital profit. Preliminary projections show the hospital closing the year with a loss of $7.5 million. As a banker, Marshall is concerned about the pressure that puts on the hospital and questions whether the hospital will be in compliance with its debt service coverage covenants. Marshall has always questioned the management ability of Wills's staff, and especially their ability to control costs. The data clearly show that the hospital's primary problem is related to cost. Revenues have been increasing slowly because of restricted government payments and deeply discounted managed-care contracts while costs have been escalating.

Data presented at the last board meeting showed hospital costs per adjusted discharge increasing by 8% last year. This fact just irritated Marshall and sent him off on a 30-minute tirade about how his business wouldn't survive if he let his costs increase at that magnitude. Wills and her CFO tried to explain the issues involved in dealing with healthcare costs in general and hospital costs in particular. All these arguments fell on Marshall's deaf ears. He closed the meeting with a challenge to Wills and her staff. He asked them to explain why costs changed 8% with specific details, not generalities. Wills has tried to do this and thought a couple of specific procedures might help drive some of these issues home.

She chose Single Vessel PTCA, which experienced an increase in costs of 21.7%, from $7,605 to $9,254. The increase in cost had puzzled most of Wills's management staff because length of stay actually dropped from 4.9 days to 4.3 days. Nursing costs fell, but ancillary costs skyrocketed. Upon examination, all of the increase was tracked to medical supplies. Most of the cardiologists performing this procedure had decided to use a new closure device that improves the quality of care but is very costly. Many other examples in different product segment areas also could be explained when the costs of the procedure were compared at the revenue code level between years. Wills has directed her financial staff to document changes in costs for major procedures during the last year using variance analysis at the revenue code level. She is hopeful that this type of information will help answer Marshall's questions as well as direct her staff to areas where costs can be controlled.

---

**Cost variance analysis** is of great potential importance to the healthcare industry. Successful use of cost variance analysis requires a sound system of standard setting, or budgeting, and a related system of cost accounting. Perhaps the major factor impeding the widespread adoption of more effective cost variance analysis in the healthcare industry has been the lack of interaction between it and existing systems of cost accounting.

Cost accounting systems usually serve two basic informational needs. First, they supply data essential for product or service costing. Second, they provide information for managerial cost control activity. This second role is the major topic of this chapter.

## ▶ Cost Control

The following conceptual model in **FIGURE 17-1** is used to discuss the major alternatives to cost control in organizations. In general, there are three distinct time phases in an out-of-control situation or a situation where some problem has occurred that needs correction:

1.  Recognition of problem (0 to $t_1$)
2.  Determination of problem or cause ($t_1$ to $t_2$)
3.  Correction of problem ($t_2$ to $T$)

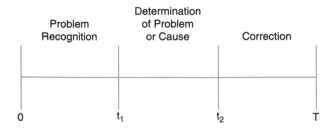

**FIGURE 17-1  Out-of-Control Timing**

The unit of time used in the previous representation may be minutes, hours, days, weeks, or even months. The important point is that the longer the problem remains uncorrected (0 to $T$), the greater the cost to the organization.

The term *efficiency cost* is sometimes used to describe the total cost incurred by an organization as a result of an out-of-control situation. Efficiency cost may be represented as follows:

$$\text{Efficiency cost} = T \times R \times P$$

where $T$ is the total time units that the problem remains uncorrected, $R$ is the loss or cost per time unit, and $P$ is the probability that the problem occurrence is correctable.

The objective of management should be to minimize the efficiency cost in any given situation. While accomplishing this objective, two major alternatives are available to management: the preventive approach and the detection–correction (DC) approach.

In the *preventive approach*, management attempts to minimize the efficiency cost by minimizing the probability that a problem will occur ($P$). One of the major methods for reducing the value of $P$ centers on staffing. Management attempts not only to hire the most competent individuals available but also to provide them with relevant training programs and materials to ensure consistently high levels of performance. The nature of the reward structure, both monetary and nonmonetary, also enters into this management strategy. The preventive approach is obviously used by most organizations, but the emphasis on it is usually greater in small organizations. In these organizations, the number of people supervised by one manager is usually smaller and the evaluation of individual performance is more direct.

The *DC approach* seeks to minimize efficiency cost by minimizing the time that a problem remains uncorrected ($T$). This method is directly related to the effectiveness of variance analysis. Effective variance analysis should result in a reduction of both the recognition of problem phase (0 to $t_1$) and the determination of cause phase ($t_1$ to $t_2$). The actual correction phase ($t_2$ to $T$) relies primarily on the effective motivation of management.

The development of cost variance analysis systems to reduce the recognition and determination phases usually involves the expenditure of funds. Prudent management dictates that the marginal expenditures of funds for system improvements be evaluated by their expected reductions in efficiency cost. For example, the frequency of reporting could be increased to reduce the problem recognition phase, or the number of cost areas reported could be increased to improve both recognition and determination times. However, these improvements are likely to result in increased cost and may not be justified. Areas of relatively small dollar expenditure or uncontrollable costs thus are not prime candidates for major system improvements.

## ▶ Investigation of Variances

In the DC approach to cost control, cost variances are the clues that both signal that a potential problem exists and suggest a possible cause. These variances are usually an integral part of any management-by-exception plan of operations. A decision to investigate a given variance is not an automatic occurrence. It involves some financial commitment by the organization and thus should be weighed carefully against the expected benefits. Unfortunately, management rarely knows whether any given variance is due to a random or noncontrollable cause or to an underlying problem that is correctable or controllable.

Many organizations have developed rules to determine what variances will be investigated. Common examples of such rules are to investigate the following:

- All variances that exceed an absolute dollar size (for example, $500)
- All variances that exceed budgeted or standard values by some fixed percentage (for example, 10%)
- All variances that have been unfavorable for a defined number of periods (for example, three periods)
- Some combination of the previous rules

Actual specification of criteria values in the previous rules is highly dependent on management judgment and experience. A variance of $1,000 may be considered normal in some circumstances and abnormal in others.

| *Learning Objective 2* |
|---|

Describe the two major theories used for the detection of out-of-control costs.

At some point, management may wish to determine whether the historical criteria for determining when a variance needs investigation should be changed. In that case, some method of testing whether the historical values are acceptable or not acceptable must be developed. In general, there are two possible theories that may be used to develop this information: classical statistical theory and decision theory.

## Classical Statistical Theory

One of the most commonly used means to determine which cost variances to investigate is the control chart. The **control chart** is often used to monitor a physical process by comparing output observations with predetermined tolerance limits. If actual observations fall between predetermined upper and lower control limits on the chart, the process is assumed to be in control.

Control charts can be established for determining when a cost variance should be investigated. The major assumption underlying the traditional development of control charts is that observed cost variances are distributed in accordance with a normal probability distribution. In a normal distribution, it can be anticipated that approximately 68.3% of the observations will fall within one standard deviation ($\sigma$) of the mean ($\bar{x}$), 95.5% will fall within two standard deviations ($\bar{x} \pm 2\sigma$), and 99.7% will fall within three standard deviations ($\bar{x} \pm 3\sigma$).

The control limits for any given variance will then be set at the following:

$$\bar{x} \pm K\sigma$$

If the costs of investigation are high relative to the benefits in a given situation, then $K$ may be set to a high value (for example, 3.0). This will ensure that few investigations will be made and that some out-of-control situations may continue. Conversely, if benefits are high relative to the costs of investigation, then lower values of $K$ may be selected that will ensure that more investigations will be performed and that some situations that are not out of control will be investigated. The **coefficient of variation** is the ratio of the standard deviation divided by the mean. Large values for a coefficient of variation in a budgeting context would imply large control limit corridors.

To develop the control chart, the underlying distribution must be specified. An assumption that the distribution is normal means that the analyst must define both the mean ($\bar{x}$) and the standard deviation ($\sigma$). In most situations, this specification will result from an analysis of prior observations.

**TABLE 17-1** Labor Variances by Pay Period

| Pay Period | Variances ($x_i$) |
|:---:|:---:|
| 1 | 800 |
| 2 | 400 |
| 3 | −500 |
| 4 | −100 |
| 5 | 200 |
| 6 | −700 |
| 7 | 500 |
| 8 | −300 |
| 9 | −200 |
| 10 | 300 |
| 11 | 200 |
| 12 | −200 |
| 13 | −400 |
| | 0 |

To illustrate this process, assume that the pattern of labor variances in TABLE 17-1 occurred during the 13 biweekly pay periods. The mean ($\bar{x}$) of these observations is calculated as follows:

$$\bar{x} = \frac{\sum x_i}{n} = \frac{0}{13} = 0$$

An estimate of the standard deviation ($\sigma$) is calculated as follows:

$$\sigma = \sqrt{\frac{\sum (x_i - \bar{x})^2}{n-1}} = 437.80$$

If the labor cost variances in this example are expected to follow a normal distribution in the future with $\bar{x} = 0$ and $\sigma = \$437.80$, control limits for investigation at the 95% level could be defined by multiplying the estimated standard deviation by 2. The following control chart would result:

$$\bar{x} + 2\sigma = 875.60$$
$$\bar{x} = 0$$
$$\bar{x} - 2\sigma = -875.60$$

Any observation falling within the control limits would not be investigated, whereas variances falling outside the established limits would be investigated.

The major deficiency in the classical statistical approach is that it does not relate the expected costs of investigation and benefits with the probability that the variance signals are out of control. The control chart can signal when a situation is likely to be out of control, but it cannot directly evaluate whether an investigation is warranted.

## Decision Theory

Decision theory provides a framework for directly integrating the probability of the system being out of control and the costs and benefits of investigation into a definite decision rule. Central to this approach is the payoff table, which specifically considers costs and benefits. TABLE 17-2 provides an example of a payoff table, where $I$ equals the cost of investigation and $L$ equals the cost of letting an out-of-control situation continue (expected loss).

The payoff table is a conceptualization of the actual decision evaluation process. It can be applied to any cost variance situation. The objective is to minimize the actual cost for a given situation. To accomplish this, estimates of the probabilities for the two states, in control and out of control, are required.

Assume that $P$ denotes the probability that the system is in control and that $(1 - P)$ represents the probability that the system is out of control. The expected cost of the two courses of action can be defined as follows:

Expected cost of investigating $= (P \times I) + (1 - P)I = I$

Expected cost of not investigating $= (P \times O) + (1 - P)L = (1 - P)L$

By setting the two expected costs equal to each other, we can determine the value of $P$ to which the decision maker is indifferent. This break-even probability would be calculated as follows:

$$P^* = 1 - (I/L)$$

Evaluation of this formula provides a nice summarization of earlier comments concerning the costs and benefits of investigating variances. In situations of

**TABLE 17-2** Variance Investigation Payoff Table

| | State | |
|---|---|---|
| **Action** | **In Control** | **Out of Control** |
| Investigate | *I* | *I* |
| Do not investigate | *O* | *L* |

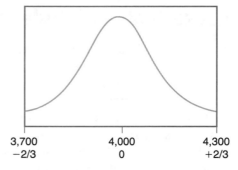

| 3,700 | 4,000 | 4,300 |
|---|---|---|
| −2/3 | 0 | +2/3 |

**FIGURE 17-2 Normal Distribution of Labor Cost Utilization**

high investigation costs (*I*) and low net benefits (*L*), the critical value of *P* (*P**) becomes low. This, of course, means that to justify an investigation, the probability that the system is actually in control (*P*) must be very low, or, alternatively, the probability that the system is actually out of control (1 − *P*) must be large.

To use the decision theory model just described, the analyst must have estimates of *I*, *L*, and *P*. In most situations, there is a reasonable expectation that *I* will be relatively constant. These costs are usually directly related to the labor involved in the analysis. *L*, however, usually varies, depending on the size of the cost variance. In short, the loss depends on the proportion of the variance to be saved in future periods and the number of periods over which the loss is expected to occur if the situation is not corrected.

The value of *P* is, in many respects, the most difficult of the parameter values to specify. Either objective or subjective approaches may be used. An objective method may be used to develop an estimated probability distribution for the system. If the underlying distribution is assumed to be normal, estimating the mean and standard deviation from prior observations will enable the analyst to specify the distribution from this estimated distribution. The probability that any given system is under control (*P*) then can be defined.

Subjective estimates of *P* are possible on both a prior basis and an ex post facto basis. A subjective normalized distribution of variances can be built in advance as a basis for the estimate. The analyst might ask department managers between which two values they would expect 50% of actual observations to fall. In a normal distribution, 50% of the observations will fall within plus or minus two-thirds of one standard deviation. If the budget cost for labor in a department is $4,000 per pay period, the department manager might specify that he or she expects actual observations to fall between $3,700 and $4,300 50% of the time. Using this information, a normalized distribution could be defined as presented in **FIGURE 17-2**.

Subjective estimates of *P* also may be made after an actual variance occurred and then related directly to the actual size of the cost variance. This assessment then can be related to a table of critical values of *P* necessary for an investigation decision of a given variance. This permits analysts to directly use sensitivity analysis in their decisions. For example, assume that *I* is $200. Assume further that *L* is equal to two times the absolute size of the variance. **TABLE 17-3** defines the critical values of *P* based on the previous information. For example, if the variance was $200, the critical value of *P* would be 0.50 (1 − [200/400]).

This table is relatively straightforward. As the dollar size of the variance increases, the probability that the system is under control must increase to justify a "do not investigate" decision. For example, if a variance of $600 occurred, the analyst must believe that there is at least a 83.3% probability that the system is under control.

---

*Learning Objective 3*

Define variance analysis and how it is used by management.

---

**TABLE 17-3** Relationship of *P** to Variance Size

| Critical Value of P (*P**) | Size of Variance |
|---|---|
| 50.0% | $200 |
| 66.7% | $300 |
| 75.0% | $400 |
| 80.0% | $500 |
| 83.3% | $600 |

# ▶ Variance Analysis Calculations

Variance analysis is simply an examination of the deviation of an actual observation from a standard. For the purposes of this chapter, the following two types of standards for comparative purposes are used: *prior-period values* and *budgeted values*. In each case the objective of cost variance analysis is to explain why actual costs are different, either from budgeted values or from prior-period actual values. This objective is an important element in the cost-control process of the organization.

## Prior-Period Comparisons

### Relevant Factors

An evaluation of the difference between current levels of cost and prior costs should suggest to management which factors have contributed to the change. In general, the following four major factors influence costs: (1) input prices, (2) **productivity of inputs**, (3) **service intensity**, and (4) **output levels**.

Input prices usually are expected to increase over time. It is important, however, from management's perspective, to evaluate what portion, if any, of that increase was controllable or avoidable. Rapidly increasing prices for some commodities may signal opportunities for resource substitutions, for example, by switching to a less expensive mix of labor or substituting one supply item for another. Measuring productivity has, in fact, become increasingly important in the healthcare industry as a result of the emphasis on cost containment. One of the major difficulties in evaluating productivity, however, has been the changing nature of healthcare services. Comparison of productivity within a hospital for two periods requires that the services in each period be identical. For example, a comparison of full-time equivalents (FTEs) per patient-day in 2017 with FTEs per patient-day of care in 2014 is meaningless unless a patient-day of care in 2017 is identical to a patient-day of care in 2014. Finally, changes in output levels also influence the level of costs. This influence may occur in two ways. First, the absolute level of output provided may affect the quantity of resources necessary to produce the output level. For example, average cost per unit may increase if actual volumes declined given the existence of fixed costs. Second, service intensity may affect resource requirements. Any increase in the number of services required per unit of output will directly affect costs. For example, a change in the number of laboratory procedures performed per patient-day of care probably will affect the total cost per patient-day of care.

This discussion can be summarized in the following cost function:

$$\text{Total cost} = P \times \frac{1}{X} \times \frac{X}{Q} \times Q$$

where $P$ is the input prices, $I$ is the physical quantities of inputs, $X$ is the services required per unit of output, and $Q$ is the output level.

In the previous cost equation, $P$ represents the effect of input prices, $I/X$ represents the effect of productivity, $X/Q$ represents the effect of service intensity, and $Q$ represents the influence of output. Changes in cost can result from changes in any one of these four terms.

---

### *Learning Objective 4*

Calculate the various types of cost variances.

---

## Facility Level Analysis

There are many occasions when it is important to discover and communicate the causes for cost increases at the facility level, whether that organization is a hospital, nursing home, or surgicenter. For example, your board may want to know why your total costs have increased 60% in the last 3 years. A useful framework can be developed to provide answers to questions such as this, provided that some critical pieces of information can be defined.

- There must be one measure of activity or output for the entire organization. This might be an adjusted discharge, patient-day, visit, or other measure.
- It must be possible to define a measure of activity for each department within the organization and to define a cost per unit for that measure. It may not be necessary to define an output unit for indirect departments—those departments that do not directly provide a product or service to the patient—provided that the costs of the indirect departments have been allocated to the direct departments.

We will now develop a model and example for a hospital to illustrate the use of this facility-level analysis. First, we will assume that our measure of activity is an adjusted discharge. The term *adjusted* simply reflects that outpatient activity has been recognized. This recognition may have occurred through a simple ratio of inpatient revenue to total patient revenue at the organization-wide level or at the individual departmental level.

The general cost per adjusted discharge (CPD) can be defined in the following equation:

$$CPD^t = C^t \times Q^t$$

where $C^t$ is the cost (direct and indirect) per unit, of output in each department and $Q^t$ is the units of output in each department required per adjusted discharge.

The following example is presented to help clarify the previous concepts. The data in TABLE 17-4 represent cost and volume information for the year 2017. These data are compared with cost and volume data for 2015.

In this example, the CPD increased 31.6% from 2015 to 2017($3,275 in 2015 to $4,310.34 in 2017). Causes for the increase could be partitioned into the following two possible areas:

1. *Intensity of service*—More units of intermediate services are required per discharge, such as laboratory tests and days in intensive care unit.
2. *Cost*—Cost increases could have resulted from higher prices paid for inputs such as wage and salary.

**TABLE 17-4** Summary of Cost per Discharge (2017 and 2015)

| | | 2017 Cost Summary 11,600 Discharges | | | |
|---|---|---|---|---|---|
| Department | Volume | Cost (000s) | Cost/Unit ($C^t$) | Units/Discharge ($Q^t$) | |
| Intensive care unit | 5,600 | $4,000 | $714.29 | 0.4828 | $285.72 |
| Routine nursing | 71,400 | 22,000 | 308.12 | 6.1552 | $2,033.59 |
| Operating room | 20,000 | 10,000 | 500.00 | 1.7241 | $750.00 |
| Laboratory | 70,000 | 6,000 | 85.71 | 6.0345 | $428.55 |
| Radiology | 28,000 | 8,000 | 285.71 | 2.4138 | $571.42 |
| | | $50,000 | | | $4,069.28 |
| | | | | | $1.24 |

CPD = $50,000,000/11,600 = $4,310.34

| | | 2015 Cost Summary 12,000 Discharges | | | |
|---|---|---|---|---|---|
| Department | Volume | Cost (000s) | Cost/Unit ($C^t$) | Units/Discharge ($Q^t$) | |
| Intensive care unit | 4,800 | $2,700 | $562.50 | 0.40000 | $271.55 |
| Routine nursing | 79,200 | 20,000 | 252.52 | 6.60000 | $1,554.31 |
| Operating room | 18,000 | 8,500 | 472.22 | 1.50000 | $814.15 |
| Laboratory | 60,000 | 4,500 | 75.00 | 5.00000 | $452.59 |
| Radiology | 24,000 | 3,600 | 150.00 | 2.00000 | $362.07 |
| | | $39,300 | | | $3,454.67 |

CPD = $39,300/12,000 = $3,275.00

The following two indices capture the impact of each of these two areas.

$$\frac{\text{CPD}^t}{\text{CPD}^0} = \frac{C^tQ^t}{C^0Q^0} = \text{HCI} \times \text{HII}$$

The hospital cost index (HCI) is defined as the following:

$$\text{HCI} = \frac{C^tQ^0}{C^0Q^0}$$

The HCI measures the change in cost attributed to both price increases and productivity changes. The other index, the hospital intensity index (HII) is defined as follows:

$$\text{HII} = \frac{C^0Q^t}{C^0Q^0}$$

The HII measures the change in cost due to changes in service intensity.

Using this framework in our example data yields the following values:

$$\text{HCI} = \frac{\begin{array}{c}(\$714.29 \times 0.4000)+ \\ (\$308.12 \times 6.6000)+ \\ (\$500.00 \times 1.5000)+ \\ (\$85.71 \times 5.0000)+ \\ (\$285.71 \times 2.0000)\end{array}}{\begin{array}{c}(\$562.50 \times 0.4000)+ \\ (\$252.52 \times 6.6000)+ \\ (\$472.22 \times 1.5000)+ \\ (\$75.00 \times 5.000)+ \\ (\$150.00 \times 2.0000)\end{array}} =$$

$$\frac{\$4,069}{\$3,275} = 1.242 \quad \begin{array}{l}(24.2\% \text{ of the increase in cost is} \\ \text{attributable to cost of service increases})\end{array}$$

$$\text{HII} = \frac{\begin{array}{c}(\$562.50 \times 0.4828)+ \\ (\$252.52 \times 6.1552)+ \\ (\$472.22 \times 1.7241)+ \\ (\$75.00 \times 6.0345)+ \\ (\$150.00 \times 2.4138)\end{array}}{\begin{array}{c}(\$562.50 \times 0.4000)+ \\ (\$252.52 \times 6.6000)+ \\ (\$472.22 \times 1.5000)+ \\ (\$75.00 \times 5.0000)+ \\ (\$150.00 \times 2.0000)\end{array}} =$$

$$\frac{\$3,455}{\$3,275} = 1.055 \quad \begin{array}{l}(5.5\% \text{ of the increase is attributable} \\ \text{to intensity of service increases})\end{array}$$

The previous calculations show that the increase in CPD from 2015 to 2017 could be broken down as follows:

| | |
|---|---|
| Percentage increase due to cost increases | 24.2% |
| Percentage increase due to intensity | 5.5 |
| Joint cost and intensity | 1.9 |
| Total increase | 31.6% |

The previous analysis shows that 76.5% (24.2/31.6) of the 2-year increase in cost per discharge is directly attributable to increases in the cost of specific services. For example, all five of the departmental services reported experienced increases in cost per unit from 2015 to 2017. While intensity of services per discharge increased, the magnitudes were not nearly as large.

## Departmental Analysis of Variance

The preceding indices are useful for analyzing cost changes at the total facility level. In such situations, a measure of output for the facility as a whole, such as patient-days, admissions, discharges, visits, or enrollees, would be used. However, although this type of analysis may be useful, it is also often desirable to analyze the reasons for cost changes at the departmental level. In general, the primary reason for a cost change at the departmental level between two periods can be stated as a function of the following three factors:

1. Changes in input prices
2. Changes in input productivity (efficiency)
3. Changes in departmental volume

> ### Learning Objective 5
>
> Explain and calculate price, efficiency, and volume variances.

The following variances can be calculated to compute the effects of these three factors:

Price variance = (Present price − Old price) × Present quantity

Efficiency variance = (Present quantity − Expected quantity at old productivity) × Old price

Volume variance = (Present volume − Old volume) × Old cost per unit

These formulas may be applied to the laundry example found in **TABLE 17-5**. It is assumed that the laundry has only two inputs: soap and labor.

**TABLE 17-5** Cost Data for Linen/Linen Department

| | 2015 | 2017 |
|---|---|---|
| Pounds of laundry | 140,000 | 180,000 |
| Units of soap | 1,400 | 1,800 |
| Soap units per pound of laundry | 0.01 | 0.01 |
| Price per soap unit | $40.00 | $50.00 |
| Productive hours worked | 19,600 | 27,000 |
| Productive hours per pound of laundry | 0.14 | 0.15 |
| Wage rate per productive hour | 10.50 | 12.00 |
| Total cost | $261,800 | $414,000 |
| Cost per pound | $1.870 | $2.300 |
| Patient-days | 70,000 | 80,000 |
| Pound of laundry per patient-day | 2.00 | 2.25 |
| **Price variances** | | |
| Soap = ($50.00 − $40.00) × 1,800 = $18,000 (unfavorable) | | |
| Labor = ($12.00 − $10.50) × 27,000 = $40,500 (unfavorable) | | |
| **Efficiency variances** | | |
| Soap = (1,800 − [0.01 × 180,000]) × $40.00 = 0 | | |
| Labor = (27,000 − [0.14 × 180,000]) × $10.50 = $18,900 (unfavorable) | | |
| **Volume variances** | | |
| Volume variance = (180,000 − 140,000) × $1.870 = 74,800 (unfavorable) | | |
| Total cost | 261,800 | 414,000 |

With these calculations, **TABLE 17-6** summarizes the factors that created cost changes in the laundry department. Table 17-6 indicates that increased volume was the largest source of the total change in cost. It is often useful to factor this volume variance into two areas:

1. Intensity = (Change in volume due to intensity difference) × Old cost per unit

2. Pure volume = (Change in volume due to change in overall service) × Old cost per unit

Here, the intensity variance represents the change in volume due to increased intensity of service. For example, in 2017, 2.25 pounds of laundry were provided per patient-day (180,000/80,000). The corresponding value for 2015 was 2.00 pounds per patient

**TABLE 17-6** Variance Analysis Summary

|  | Causes of Laundry Department Cost Change—2015 to 2017 | |
| --- | --- | --- |
|  | Dollars | % Change |
| Increase in wages | $40,500 | 26.6% |
| Increase in soap price | 18,000 | 11.8% |
| Decline in labor efficiency | 18,900 | 12.4% |
| Increase in volume | 74,800 | 49.1% |
| Total change in cost | $152,200 | 100.0% |

day (140,000/70,000). The two volume variances are as follows:

$$\text{Intensity variance} = ([2.25 - 2.00] \times 80,000) \times \$1.870 = \$37,400$$

$$\text{Pure volume} = 2.00 \times (80,000 - 70,000) \times \$1.870 = \$37,400$$

The system of cost variance analysis described previously should be a useful framework in which to discuss factors causing changes in departmental costs. Aggregation of some resource categories is probably both necessary and desirable. There would be little point in calculating price and efficiency variances for each of 100 or more supply items. Only major supply categories should be examined. The supply items that are aggregated together could not be broken down in terms of individual price and efficiency variances because there would be no common input quantity measure. For example, the addition of pencils, sheets of paper, and boxes of paper clips would not produce a comparable unit of measure. For these smaller areas of supply or material costs, a simple change in cost per unit of departmental output may be just as informative as detailed price and efficiency variances.

## ▶ Variance Analysis in Budgetary Settings

A final area in which variance analysis can be applied is the operation of a formalized budgeting system. The presentation that follows assumes a budgeting system that is based on a flexible model. This means that the management must have identified those elements of cost presumed to be fixed and those presumed to be variable in the budgetary process. Although relatively few healthcare organizations use flexible budgeting models at the present time, a trend toward their adoption is clearly visible. In this context, the variance analysis models examined here may be applied to any budgetary situation, fixed or flexible.

The cost equation for any given department may be represented as follows:

$$\text{Cost} = F + (V \times Q)$$

where $F$ is the fixed cost, $V$ is the variable cost per unit of output, and $Q$ is the output in units.

The fixed and variable cost coefficients are the sum of many individual resource quantity and unit price products. These terms can be represented as follows:

$$F = I_f \times P_f$$

$$V = I_v \times P_v$$

where $I_f$ is the physical unit of fixed resources, $P_f$ is the price per unit of fixed resources, $I_v$ is the physical unit of variable resources per unit of output, and $P_v$ is the price per unit of variable resources.

In most budgeting situations, there are three levels of output or volume that are critical in cost variance analysis. The first is the **actual level of volume** produced in the budget-reporting period. This level of activity is critical because, if management has established a set of expectations concerning how costs should behave, given changes in volume from budgeted levels, an adjustment to budgeted cost can be made for a change in volume.

The second critical level is that of **budgeted or expected volume**. It is on this expected volume level that management establishes its commitments for resources, and therefore incurs cost. An unjustified faith in volume forecasts can lock management into a sizable fixed-cost position, especially regarding labor costs.

The third critical level is that of **standard volume**. Standard volume is equal to actual volume, unless there is some indication that not all of the output was necessary. For example, a utilization review committee may determine that a certain number of patient-days were medically unnecessary or that some surgical procedures were not warranted. Alternatively, in some indirect departments, such as maintenance, it may be important to identify the difference between actual and standard, or necessary, output. The cost effect of these output decisions needs to be isolated, and control should be directed to the individual(s) responsible.

The expected level of costs to be incurred at each of the three levels of volume (actual, budgeted, and standard) may be expressed as follows:

$$FB^a = F + (V \times Q^a)$$

$$FB^b = F + (V \times Q^b)$$

$$FB^s = F + (V \times Q^s)$$

where $FB^a$ is the flexible budget at actual output level, $FB^b$ is the flexible budget at budgeted output level, $FB^s$ is the flexible budget at standard output level, $Q^a$ is the actual output, $Q^b$ is the budgeted output, and $Q^s$ is the standard output.

The major categories of variances now can be defined to explain the difference between actual cost ($AC$) and applied cost ($Q^s \times FB^b/Q^b$). See **TABLE 17-7**.

**TABLE 17-7** Categories of Budgetary Variances

| Variance Name | Definition | Cause |
|---|---|---|
| Spending | $(AC - FB^a)$ | Price and efficiency |
| Utilization | $(Q^a - Q^s) \times (FB^b/Q^b)$ | Excessive services |
| Volume | $(Q^b - Q^a) \times (F/Q^b)$ | Difference from budgeted volume |

For control purposes, it is important to further break down the spending variance into individual resource categories, and also to isolate the change due to price and efficiency factors. This will not only better isolate control for budget deviations but also improve the problem definition and determination phase times discussed earlier in the detection-correction approach to cost control. The spending variances are broken down as follows:

$$\text{Efficiency} = (I^a - I^b)P^b$$

$$\text{Price} = (P^a - P^b)I^a$$

where $I^a$ is the actual physical units of resource, $I^b$ is the budgeted physical units of resource, $P^a$ is the actual price per unit of resource, and $P^b$ is the budgeted price per unit of resource.

With this background, we must now relate the structure we developed for standard costing to our analyses of budgetary variances. (See Chapter 15.) The following two sets of standards are involved: standard cost profiles (SCPs) and standard treatment protocols (STPs). SCPs are developed at the departmental level. They reflect the quantity of resources that should be used and the prices that should be paid for those resources to produce a specific departmental output unit, defined as a service unit (SU). **TABLE 17-8** provides an SCP for a nursing unit, with the SU defined as a patient-day.

Using Table 17-8, a standard variance analysis could be performed for any period. For example, the

**TABLE 17-8** Standard Cost Profile for Nursing Unit

| Resource | Fixed Hours | Quantity Variable | Quantity Fixed | Unit Cost | Variable Cost | Average Fixed Cost | Average Total Cost |
|---|---|---|---|---|---|---|---|
| | | | Standard Cost Profile Nursing Unit Number 6 Patient-Day = Service Unit Expected Patient-Days = 630 | | | | |
| Head nurse | 189 | 0.00 | 0.30 | $30.00 | $0.00 | $9.00 | $9.00 |
| Registered nurse (RN) | 630 | 2.00 | 1.00 | 24.00 | $48.00 | $24.00 | $72.00 |
| Licensed practical nurse (LPN) | 0 | 2.00 | 0.00 | 16.00 | $32.00 | $0.00 | $32.00 |
| Aides | 630 | 3.00 | 1.00 | 10.00 | $30.00 | $10.00 | $40.00 |
| Supplies | 0 | 2.00 | 0.00 | 4.40 | $8.80 | $0.00 | $8.80 |
| Total | | | | | $118.80 | $43.00 | $161.80 |

data in **TABLE 17-9** reflect actual experience in the most recent month.

In this example, the nursing unit would have incurred actual expenditures of $99,300 during the month. It would have charged its standard cost ($161.80) times the number of actual patient-days (600).

Cost charged to patients = $97,080 = $161.80 × 600

The total variance to be accounted for would be the difference ($99,300 − $97,080), or $2,220, which is an unfavorable variance. The individual variances that constitute this total are shown in the following calculations:

1.  Spending variances
    ▪ Efficiency variances ($[I^a - I^b] \times P^b$) (Actual quantity − Budgeted quantity) × Budgeted price
        a.  Head nurse = (180 − 189) × $30.00 = $270.00 (favorable)
        b.  RN = (1,800 − 1,830) × $24.00 = $720.00 (favorable)
        c.  LPN = (1,200 −1,200) × $16.00 = 0
        d.  Aides = (2,400 − 2,430) × $10.00 = $300.00 (favorable)
        e.  Supplies = (1,300 − 1,200) × $4.40 = $440.00 (unfavorable)
    ▪ Price variances ($[P^a - P^b] \times I^a$) (Actual price − Budgeted price) × Actual quantity
        a.  Head nurse = ($31.00 − $30.00) × 180 = $180.00 (unfavorable)
        b.  RN = ($25.00 − $24.00) × 1,800 = $1,800.00 (unfavorable)

        c.  LPN = ($16.20 − $16.00) × 1,200 = $240.00 (unfavorable)
        d.  Aides = ($9.60 − $10.00) × 2,400 = $960.00 (favorable)
        e.  Supplies = ($4.80 − $4.40) × 1,300 = $520.00 (unfavorable)
2.  Volume variance ($[Q^b - Q^a] [F/Q^b]$) (Budgeted volume − Actual volume) × Budgeted fixed cost per unit
    ▪ Volume variance = (630 − 600) × $43.00 = $1,290.00 (unfavorable)

| | | |
|---|---:|---|
| Efficiency—Head nurse | $ −270 | (favorable) |
| Efficiency—RN | −720 | (favorable) |
| Efficiency—LPN | 0 | |
| Efficiency—Aides | −300 | (favorable) |
| Efficiency—Supplies | 440 | (unfavorable) |
| **Total efficiency variance** | **−850** | **(favorable)** |
| Price—Head nurse | 180 | (unfavorable) |
| Price—RN | 1,800 | (unfavorable) |
| Price—LPN | 240 | (unfavorable) |
| Price—Aides | −960 | (favorable) |
| Price—Supplies | 520 | (unfavorable) |
| **Total price variance** | **1,780** | **(unfavorable)** |
| **Volume** | **1,290.00** | **(unfavorable)** |
| Total | $2,220.00 | (unfavorable) |

A few additional statements about the calculation of the **efficiency variances** may be necessary. The formula states that the difference between actual quantity ($I^a$) and budgeted quantity ($I^b$) is multiplied by budgeted price ($P^b$). The most difficult calculation is that for budgeted quantity. It represents the quantity of resource that should have been used at the actual level of output, or the sum of the budgeted fixed requirement plus the variable requirement at actual output (600 patient-days). **TABLE 17-10** shows the calculation of fixed and variable requirements for the individual resource categories. For example, the budgeted level of hours for the RN category is 1,830 hours. That budgeted total is equal to:

Fixed hours (630) + Variable hours per patient-day

(2.00) × Actual patient-day (600)

or

630 + 2.00 × 600 = 1,830 hours

The calculation for **volume variance** also may require some further explanation. This variance is simply the product of the difference between budgeted and actual volume ($Q^a - Q^b$) and the average fixed cost budgeted ($F/Q^b$). The average fixed cost, as calculated in Table 17-8, amounted to $43.00. Note that in our

**TABLE 17-9** Actual Cost for Nursing Unit

| Resource | Quantity Used | Unit Cost | Total Cost |
|---|---|---|---|
| | **Actual Month's Cost Nursing Unit Number 6 Actual Patient-Days = 600** | | |
| Head nurse | 180 | $31.00 | $5,580 |
| RN | 1,800 | 25.00 | 45,000 |
| LPN | 1,200 | 16.20 | 19,440 |
| Aides | 2,400 | 9.60 | 23,040 |
| Supplies | 1,300 | 4.80 | 6,240 |
| Total | | | $99,300 |

**TABLE 17-10** Calculation of Budgeted Resource Requirements

| 1<br>Resource<br>Category | 2<br>Average Fixed<br>Requirement/Unit | 3<br>Budgeted Fixed<br>Requirement<br>(Col. 2 x 630) | 4<br>Average Variable<br>Requirement/Unit | 5<br>Budgeted Variable<br>Requirement<br>(Col. 4 x 600) | 6<br>Budgeted<br>Requirement<br>(Col. 3 + Col. 5) |
|---|---|---|---|---|---|
| Head nurse | 0.30 | 189 | 0.00 | 0 | 189 |
| RN | 1.00 | 630 | 2.00 | 1,200 | 1,830 |
| LPN | 0.00 | 0 | 2.00 | 1,200 | 1,200 |
| Aides | 1.00 | 630 | 3.00 | 1,800 | 2,430 |
| Supplies | 0.00 | 0 | 2.00 | 1,200 | 1,200 |

example volume variance is unfavorable because actual volume of patient-days (600) was less than budgeted patient-days (630). Because actual volume was less than budgeted, the average fixed cost per unit will increase. The reverse situation would have existed if actual volume had exceeded budgeted volume. In that situation, the volume variance would have been favorable.

The third type of variance, **utilization variance**, results from a difference between actual volume and standard volume, or the quantity of volume actually needed. The measure of standard volume is generated from STPs, which define how much output or how many specific SUs are required per treated patient type. These concepts were introduced in Chapter 15.

Let us now generate a hypothetical set of data to apply to our nursing unit example. Assume that the patients treated in Nursing Unit Number 6 are all in diagnosis-related group (MS-DRG) 470 (major joint procedures) and associated with one physician, Dr. Mallard. Our STP for MS-DRG 470 calls for a 7-day length of stay. A review of Dr. Mallard's patient records reveals that only 560 patient-days of care should have been used (80 cases at 7 days per case). Dr. Mallard had 40 patients with lengths of stay greater than 7 days. These 40 patients accounted for an excess of 80 patient-days. Dr. Mallard also had 20 patients with shorter lengths of stay. These patients offset 40 days of the 80-day surplus. Thus, although 600 patient-days of care were provided, only 560 should have been used given the expected length of stay. This creates an unfavorable utilization variance, calculated as the product of budgeted cost per unit and the difference between actual and standard volume. In our example of Nursing Unit Number 6, the utilization variance would be as follows:

$$\text{Utilization variance} = (\text{Actual patient-days} - \text{Expected}$$
$$\text{patient-days}) \times \text{Budgeted cost}$$
$$\text{per patient-day} = (600 - 560) \times$$
$$\$161.80 = \$6,472.00 \text{ (unfavorable)}$$

This variance is not charged to the nursing department. It is charged to the manager of patient treatment, in this case Dr. Mallard.

**FIGURE 17-3** depicts the flow of costs and the variances associated with each account. This delineation of variances represents a powerful analytical tool for analyzing cost variances from budgeted cost levels. The existence of a flexible budget model is not a prerequisite to its use. The only real prerequisite is that major resource cost categories be separated into price and utilization components. Because effective cost control appears to be predicated on a separate analysis of price and utilization decisions, this does not seem too difficult a task, considering the potential payoff. Finally, it should be noted that there is no requirement to formally include these variances into the budget-reporting models. They can be calculated on an ad hoc basis to investigate and explain large cost variances.

# ▶ Variance Analysis in Managed-Care or Bundled Payment Settings

Variance analysis is an important analytical tool that has become useful to managed-care firms that are seeking to monitor and control their costs. Because

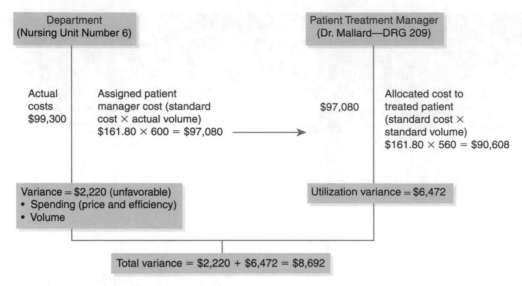

**FIGURE 17-3 Variance Analysis Summary**

most managed-care firms operate with relatively small margins, and because most of their cost is variable, changes in budgetary assumptions can have a sizable influence on costs and, therefore, profitability. As more providers enter into either capitated or bundled care payment arrangements variance analysis will also become a key tool for cost management.

The following relationships will help us to formulate a variance analysis model that will separate cost variations into factors that are suggestive of cause and should lead to corrective actions more quickly.

- **Total cost = Inpatient cost + Outpatient cost**
- **Inpatient cost (IPC)**
  - IPC = Admissions × Cost per admission
    - Admissions = [Enrollees (E)] × [Admissions per member (APM)]
    - Cost per admission = [Cost per admission at case mix of 1.0 (CPA)] × [Admission case-mix index (ACMI)]
  - **IPC = E × APM × CPA × ACMI**
- **Outpatient Cost (OPC)**
  - OPC = Visits × Cost per visit
    - Visits = [Enrollees (E)] × [Visits per member (VPM)]
    - Cost per visit = [Cost per visit at case mix of 1.0 (CPV)] × [Visit case-mix index (VCMI)]
- **OPC = E × VPM × CPV × VCMI**

The previous formulas define the following primary cost drivers:

- Enrollment (E)
- Utilization (APM or VPM)
- Efficiency (CPA or CPV)
- Patient mix (ACMI or VCMI)

Costs in a managed-care setting can increase due to changes in any one of these four factors. An increase in enrollment most likely will lead to an increase in costs, but this increase in costs may be offset by an increase in revenues, and profits may actually improve. Increases in utilization most likely will lead to an increase in costs because more units of service, either more admissions or more visits, are being provided per member. An increase in costs per unit (CPA or CPV) might signal a move by subscribers to more costly providers. Finally, changes in patient mix, ACMI or VCMI, can adversely affect costs. Utilization of more costly procedures can have a negative effect on profits. To illustrate the use of this framework, a case example is presented in **TABLE 17-11**. The total variance to account for in the case presented in Table 17-11 is shown in **TABLE 17-12**.

The numbers indicate that costs were much higher than expected, but they do not explain the cause of the variance. The definition of individual variances can help explain causes for the total variance and suggest possible solutions. We know from the data in Table 17-11 that there were 880 actual inpatient admissions and that the actual cost per case was $5,304, which generated actual inpatient costs of $4,667,520 (880 × $5,304). There were 750 budgeted inpatient admissions, and budgeted costs per case were $5,000, which generated an expected or budgeted cost of $3,750,000 (750 × $5,000). Costs were higher than budgeted because we admitted more patients and the cost to treat them was higher than expected. Let's use the framework described previously to partition the total variance into areas that might suggest possible causes and solutions.

**TABLE 17-11** Managed-Care Budget to Actual Comparison

| | Budget | Actual |
|---|---|---|
| Enrollees (E) | 10,000 | 11,000 |
| Admissions per member (APM) | 0.075 | 0.080 |
| Admissions (E × APM) | 750 | 880 |
| Visits per member (VPM) | 4.5 | 5.0 |
| Visits (E × VPM) | 45,000 | 55,000 |
| Cost per admission at CMI of 1.0 (CPA) | $5,000 | $5,200 |
| Admission case-mix index (ACMI) | 1.0 | 1.02 |
| Cost per admission (CPA × ACMI) | $5,000 | $5,304 |
| Cost per visit at CMI of 1.0 (CPV) | $75 | $80 |
| Visit case-mix index (VCMI) | 1.10 | 1.15 |
| Actual cost per visit (CPV × VCMI) | $82.50 | $92.00 |
| Inpatient costs | $3,750,000 | $4,667,520 |
| Outpatient costs | $3,712,500 | $5,060,000 |
| **Total costs** | **$7,462,500** | **$9,727,520** |

**TABLE 17-12** Summary of Cost Variance

| | Inpatient Costs | Outpatient Costs | Total Costs |
|---|---|---|---|
| Actual costs | $4,667,520 | $5,060,000 | $9,727,520 |
| Less budgeted costs | 3,750,000 | 3,712,500 | 7,462,500 |
| Variance | $917,520 | $1,347,500 | $2,265,020 |

## Volume-Related Variances

We know that we admitted 130 more patients than expected (880 – 750) and experienced 10,000 more outpatient visits than expected (55,000 – 45,000). This deviation in volume can result from two possible causes:

1. Changes in enrollees
2. Changes in utilization rates

## Enrollment Variances

Enrollment variances are simply the product of budgeted cost per unit times the change in enrollment times budgeted utilization. The formulas for these variances are presented in **TABLE 17-13**.

There were 1,000 more enrollees than budgeted; this would generate more expected volume. The budgeted rate for inpatient admissions was 0.075, which

**TABLE 17-13** Variance Definitions—Enrollment

| Variance Formula | Calculation | Variance |
|---|---|---|
| Inpatient = $(E^a - E^b) \times APM^b \times CPA^b \times ACMI^b$ | $(11,000 - 10,000) \times 0.075 \times \$5,000 \times 1.0$ | \$375,000 |
| Outpatient = $(E^a - E^b) \times VPM^b \times CPV^b \times VCMI^b$ | $(11,000 - 10,000) \times 4.5 \times \$75 \times 1.1$ | \$371,250 |
| Total enrollment variance | | \$746,250 |

means that 0.075 times 1,000 or 75 more admissions would have been expected resulting in a cost variance of \$375,000 at the budgeted cost per case of \$5,000. The budgeted rate for outpatient visits was 4.5 which means that 4.5 times 1,000 or 4,500 more visits would have been expected resulting in a cost variance of \$375,000 at the budgeted cost per case of \$82.50.

## Utilization Variances

Utilization variances are simply the product of the change in volume due to the change in usage rates calculated at the actual number of enrollees times budgeted cost per unit (TABLE 17-14).

The inpatient admission rate increased in the period to 0.080, which was above the budgeted rate of 0.075. This increase in utilization rates multiplied times actual enrollment of 11,000 created a variance of 55 additional admissions (11,000 × 0.005). We can then add this variance of 55 to the enrollment variance of 75 to produce a total variance of 130. This is the difference between budgeted admissions (750) and actual admissions (880). In a similar manner, the outpatient volume difference of 10,000 can be factored into 4,500 attributed to enrollment variance and 5,500 attributed to utilization variance. Multiplying these variations in volume by the budgeted costs of \$5,000 per case and \$82.50 per visit yield the variances calculated previously.

## Cost-Related Variances

The actual cost of treating an inpatient case was \$5,304 compared to a budgeted cost per case of \$5,000, a difference of \$304 per case. The outpatient difference between actual and budgeted cost per visit was \$9.50 (\$92.00 – \$82.50). These differences in costs contributed to the overall unfavorable variance, but, as before, there are two possible causes for this deviation in cost per unit:

1. Changes in the efficiency of production
2. Changes in the case mix of patients seen

## Efficiency Variance

Efficiency variances are a reflection of a change in the underlying cost of providing care, keeping case mix constant. The efficiency variance is the product of the difference between actual and budgeted costs for a constant case mix equal to one times the actual case mix of patients seen times actual volume of patients (TABLE 17-15).

In Table 17-11, we can see that the cost of an inpatient admission at a case mix of 1.0 increased from \$5,000 to \$5,200. Reasons for this increase could be related to the selection of hospitals by the health plan's subscribers. Assuming that negotiated rates are in existence, the subscribers may have selected hospital providers that have higher rates of payment. The data

**TABLE 17-14** Variance Definitions—Utilization

| Variance Formula | Calculation | Variance |
|---|---|---|
| Inpatient = $(APM^a - APM^b) \times E^a \times CPA^b \times ACMI^b$ | $(0.080 - 0.075) \times 11,000 \times \$5,000 \times 1.0$ | \$275,000 |
| Outpatient = $(VPM^a - VPM^b) \times E^a \times CPV^b \times VCMI^b$ | $(5.0 - 4.5) \times 11,000 \times \$75 \times 1.10$ | \$453,750 |
| Total utilization variance | | \$728,750 |

**TABLE 17-15** Variance Definitions—Efficiency

| Variance Formula | Calculation | Variance |
|---|---|---|
| Inpatient = (CPA$^a$ − CPA$^b$) × ACMI$^a$ × E$^a$ × APM$^a$ | (5,200 − $5,000) × 1.02 × 11,000 × 0.080 | $179,520 |
| Outpatient = (CPV$^a$ − CPV$^b$) × VCMI$^a$ × E$^a$ × VPM$^a$ | ($80 − $75) × 1.15 × 11,000 × 5.0 | $316,250 |
| Total efficiency variance | | $495,770 |

in Table 17-15 simply multiply that inpatient cost difference of $200 by the actual case-mix index of 1.02 to produce the actual change in cost due to efficiency of $204. The subscribers selected more expensive hospitals; this raised the cost of a standard admission by $200 but in addition the actual case mix also increased by 2%. That total increase in cost of $204 per admission multiplied times actual admissions of 880 produces the variance of $179,520.

## Case-Mix Variances

Case-mix variances reflect the change in cost per unit that result not from a change in efficiency, but from a change in case mix of patients seen. This variance may not be controllable by the providers and may be a reflection of the nature of the insured population. For example, recent enrollees in an Affordable Care Act exchange plan may be sicker than expected—requiring greater levels of service and having more complicated diseases. Case-mix variances are the product of the change in case mix times the expected cost per unit at a case-mix standard value of 1.0 times the actual volume (**TABLE 17-16**).

On the inpatient side we witnessed a 2% increase in case mix. This would have increased our cost per case by $100 (0.02 times $5,000). This difference in cost per case attributable to case mix is multiplied times actual cases of 880 to produce the variance of $88,000. On the outpatient side our case mix increased sizably—from 1.10, the budgeted value, to an actual case mix of 1.15. This 0.05 difference in case mix multiplied times the budgeted cost per visit of $75 produces a $3.75 cost increase per visit attributable to case-mix increases. This increase in cost per visit multiplied times actual visits of 55,000 produced a variance of $206,250.

It is now possible to summarize the variance analysis performed to date in a structure that may help management direct their attention to areas needing correction. This is done in **TABLE 17-17**.

Table 17-17 shows that the majority of the total variance can be attributed to enrollment variance and utilization variance. Of the two, enrollment variances accounted for approximately 32.9% of the total variation and is not likely to be a problem because increased enrollment most likely was offset by increased revenues. The utilization variances accounted for 32.2% of the total variation and could represent a serious problem that should be examined. Continuation of this trend could destroy the firm's profitability.

## ▶ SUMMARY

In general, within the framework for cost control, the following two approaches are possible: preventive and detection–correction (DC). The DC approach is usually based on some system of variance analysis.

**TABLE 17-16** Variance Definitions—Case Mix

| Variance Formula | Calculation | Variance |
|---|---|---|
| Inpatient = (ACMI$^a$ − ACMI$^b$) × CPA$^b$ × E$^a$ × APM$^a$ | (1.02 − 1.0) × $5,000 × 11,000 × 0.080 | $88,000 |
| Outpatient = (VCMI$^a$ − VCMI$^b$) × CPV$^b$ × E$^a$ × VPM$^a$ | (1.15 − 1.10) × $75 × 11,000 × 5.0 | $206,250 |
| Total case-mix variance | | $294,250 |

**TABLE 17-17** Individual Variance Analysis Summary

| Variance Cause | Inpatient Amount | Inpatient % | Outpatient Amount | Outpatient % | Amount | Total % |
|---|---|---|---|---|---|---|
| Enrollment | $375,000 | 40.9% | $371,250 | 27.6% | $746,250 | 32.9% |
| Utilization | 275,000 | 30.0% | 453,750 | 33.7% | 728,750 | 32.2% |
| Efficiency | 179,520 | 19.6% | 316,250 | 23.5% | 495,770 | 21.9% |
| Case mix | 88,000 | 9.6% | 206,250 | 15.3% | 294,250 | 13.0% |
| Total | $917,520 | 100.0% | $1,347,500 | 100.0% | $2,265,020 | 100.0% |

From a decision-theory perspective, the investigation of a variance is based on the cost of investigation, the probability that a correctable problem exists, the potential loss if the problem is not corrected, and the costs of problem correction. It may not always be possible to develop truly objective measures for these values, but sensitivity analysis may offer a useful aid in such situations.

## ASSIGNMENTS

1. Two general types of approaches to internal control are preventive approaches and detection approaches. Preventive approaches stress the elimination of problems, whereas detection approaches stress the early recognition and correction of problems. What sorts of things could you do if you used a preventive approach to reduce costs?
2. What is a coefficient of variation, and how can that information be used in budgeting?
3. Which would you investigate first—a budget variance that is 1.0 standard deviation away from the expected value or one that is 1.5 standard deviations away from the value? Why?
4. When is the use of a flexible budget likely to be most effective?
5. Standard cost accounting systems often separate variance into price and efficiency components. Why?
6. Ned Zechman is the dietary manager of a large convalescent center. He is disturbed by variances, all highly unfavorable, in his food budget for the past 3 months. Zechman has been reducing both the quantity and quality of delivered meals, but to date, there has been no reflection of this in his monthly budget variance report. A recent organizational change brought in Pat Schumaker, who is now responsible for all purchasing activity, including dietary. All purchased food costs are charged to dietary at the time of purchase. What do you think might explain Zechman's problem, and how would you determine the cause?
7. Assume that the budgeted cost for a department is $10,000 per week and the standard deviation is $500. The decision to investigate a variance requires a comparison of expected benefits with expected costs. Suppose an unfavorable variance of $1,000 is observed. The normal distribution indicates the probability of observing this variance is 0.0228 if the system is in control. Furthermore, assume that the benefits would be 50% of the variance and that investigation costs are $200. Should this variance be investigated? Assume that the variance is still $1,000, but it is favorable. Should it still be investigated?
8. Departmental costs may be out of control if (1) the variance is outside specified limits, or (2) the number of successive observations, above or below expected costs, is excessive. The binomial distribution can be used as a basis for determining what is or is not excessive. If we assume that the probability of being either above or below budgeted costs is 0.50, then the probability of $n$ successive observations of actual costs being greater than budgeted costs is $0.50^n$. What is the probability of observing six successive periods in which actual costs are greater than budgeted costs?
9. You are evaluating the performance of the radiology department manager. The service unit (SU) or output for this department is the number of procedures. A static budget was prepared at the beginning of the year. You are now examining that budget in relation to actual experience. The relevant data are included in **TABLE 17-18**.
   The department cost manager is pleased because he has a favorable $120,000 cost variance. Evaluate the effectiveness claims of the manager using the budgetary variance model described in this chapter.

**TABLE 17-18** Radiology Department Data

|  | Actual | Original Budget | Variance |  |
|---|---|---|---|---|
| Procedures | 100,000 | 120,000 | 20,000 | (unfavorable) |
| Variable costs | $1,200,000 | $1,320,000 | $120,000 | (favorable) |
| Fixed costs | 600,000 | 600,000 | – |  |
| Total costs | $1,800,000 | $1,920,000 | $120,000 | (favorable) |
| Average cost per unit | $18.00 | $16.00 |  |  |
| Variable cost per unit | $12.00 | $11.00 |  |  |
| Fixed cost per unit | $6.00 | $5.00 |  |  |

10. The data in **TABLE 17-19** were assembled for a laundry department during the period from 2016 to 2017. Break down the total change in cost, which is $7,422 ($86,378 less $78,956) into the variance categories described in this chapter: price, efficiency, intensity volume, and pure volume variances.

**TABLE 17-19** Laundry Department Data

|  | 2016 | 2017 |
|---|---|---|
| Weighted patient-days | 24,140 | 24,539 |
| Pounds of laundry | 333,225 | 328,624 |
| Pounds per day | 13.80385 | 13.39191 |
| Hours worked | 6,665 | 6,901 |
| Hours per pound | 0.020 | 0.021 |
| Average salary per hour | $10.50 | $11.00 |
| Total salary cost | $69,977 | $75,912 |
| Salary cost per pound | $0.210 | $0.231 |
| Supply units | 3,332 | 3,286 |
| Supply units per pound | 0.01 | 0.01 |
| Cost per supply unit | $2.69 | $3.18 |
| Total supply cost | $8,979 | $10,466 |
| Total cost | $78,956 | $86,378 |
| Cost per pound | $0.2369 | $0.2628 |

11. John Jones, CEO at Valley Hospital, is concerned by the rapid increase in cost per case during the last 5 years at his hospital. Five years ago, his average cost per case was $9,295; it is now $14,355. Using the data in **TABLE 17-20**, help Jones understand what factors have resulted in increased costs of $138,250 ($445,000 – $306,750) during the last 5 years.

12. You have just taken a position as a financial analyst with the American Health Plan, a partially integrated delivery system, contracting with major employers for healthcare services. The financial and utilization data in **TABLE 17-21** were presented to you regarding the previous completed year.

   You have been asked to make some sense of this data and factor the total variance of $1,156,000 ($10,406,000 – $9,250,000) into some subaccounts that suggest possible causes. Please review these data and calculate variances for inpatient and outpatient into the following areas:

   - Enrollment variance
   - Utilization variance
   - Efficiency variance (note that there is no case-mix intensity standard)

   Even in situations when one person does have responsibility for both components, the separation is useful because it provides information for focused management correction.

**TABLE 17-20** Valley Hospital DRG Costs

| | Total Cost | Present Volume | Average Cost |
|---|---|---|---|
| DRG A | $150,000 | 10 | $15,000 |
| DRG B | 200,000 | 20 | 10,000 |
| DRG C | 95,000 | 1 | 95,000 |
| | $445,000 | 31 | $14,355 |

| | Total Cost | Five Years Ago Volume | Average Cost |
|---|---|---|---|
| DRG A | $114,750 | 9 | $12,750 |
| DRG B | 192,000 | 24 | 8,000 |
| DRG C | 0 | 0 | 0 |
| | $306,750 | 33 | $9,295 |

**TABLE 17-21** American Health Plan Budget

| | Budget | Actual |
|---|---|---|
| Enrollees | 10,000 | 11,000 |
| Patient-days per 1,000 enrollees | 600 | 550 |

| | Budget | Actual |
|---|---|---|
| Patient-days | 6,000 | 6,050 |
| Visits per member | 5.0 | 5.5 |
| Visits | 50,000 | 60,500 |
| Cost per patient-day | $1,000 | $1,100 |
| Cost per visit | $65 | $62 |
| Inpatient costs | $6,000,000 | $6,655,000 |
| Outpatient costs | $3,250,000 | $3,751,000 |
| Total costs | $9,250,000 | $10,406,000 |
| Per-member per-year costs | $925 | $946 |

## SOLUTIONS AND ANSWERS

1. The following are some of the things you could do, using a preventive approach: improve employee training, increase inspection of material, improve equipment maintenance, and increase supervision.
2. The coefficient of variation is the ratio of the standard deviation to the mean. A large value implies great variability in the results. In a budgeting context, operations with large prior coefficients of variation typically require a more sophisticated budget model, such as a flexible budget, to account for deviations from average performance.
3. The budget variance that is 1.5 standard deviations from expected performance is more likely to be out of control and should be investigated first. However, adjustments for the relative differences in investigation costs and variance size should be considered.
4. A flexible budget is likely to be most effective when costs in a department are not fixed and are expected to vary with changes in output or other variables. A flexible budget is also more effective when variations in volume exist. If volume is constant across all budget periods, a fixed budget will be effective.
5. Standard cost accounting systems separate variances into price and efficiency components because, in many situations, one person does not have decision responsibility for both purchases and usage. Even in situations when one person does have responsibility for both components, the separation is useful because it provides information for focused management correction.
6. Prices paid for food may have increased significantly either because of recent changes in food prices or because of ineptness or fraud on the part of Schumaker. An audit of purchasing costs should be initiated, especially if other departments in the center have similar problems.
7. The following calculations should be made as a basis for deciding whether an investigation should be conducted:

$$\text{Expected benefits} - 0.5 \times \$1,000 \times (1 - 0.0228)^* = \$488.60$$

$$\text{Expected costs} = \$200$$

$$^*(1 - 0.0228) = \text{Probability that the variance is not a random occurrence}$$

Yes, the variance should be investigated, because the expected benefits are greater than the expected costs. Even if the variance is favorable, it should be investigated, because it may indicate that the budget is not accurate. A reduction of the budget may promote a future reduction in costs.

| **TABLE 17-22** Variances for Laundry Department | | | |
|---|---|---|---|
| Labor price | $3,451 | (unfavorable) | 46.5% |
| Supply price | $1,610 | (unfavorable) | 21.7% |
| Labor efficiency | $3,451 | (unfavorable) | 46.5% |
| Supply efficiency | $0 | | 0.0% |
| Pure volume | $1,305 | (unfavorable) | 17.6% |
| Intensity volume | –$2,395 | (favorable) | –32.3% |
| Total | $7,422 | | 100.0% |

Labor price = ($11.00 – 10.50) × 6,901 = $3,451 (unfavorable)
Supply price = ($3.18 – 2.69) × 3,286 = $1,610 (unfavorable)
Labor efficiency = (0.021 – 0.020) × 328,624 × $10.50 = $3,451 (unfavorable)
Supply efficiency = (0.01 – 0.01) × 328,624 × $2.69 = 0
Pure volume = (13.80385 × [24,539 – 24,140]) × $0.2369 = $1,305 (unfavorable)
Intensity volume = ([13.39191 – 13.80385] × 24,539) × $0.2369 = –$2395 (favorable)

8. The probability of observing six successive periods in which actual costs are greater than budgeted costs is $0.50^6 = 0.0156$.

9. In your evaluation, you can calculate spending and volume variances for the radiology department. The total variance would be calculated as:

Actual cost less assigned cost (actual costs less actual volume

times budgeted cost per unit)

or

$$\$1,800,000 - (100,000 \times \$16.00) = \$200,000 \text{ (unfavorable)}$$

The radiology department has an unfavorable variance of $200,000, as opposed to a favorable variance of $120,000. The $200,000 unfavorable variance can be broken into spending and volume variances:

Spending variance = Actual costs – Budgeted fixed costs – Budgeted variable

cost = $1,800,000 – $600,000 – ($11 × 100,000) = $100,000 (unfavorable)

Volume variance = (Budgeted volume – Actual volume) × Budgeted average fixed cost

= (120,000 – 100,000) × ($600,000 / 120,000) = $100,000 (unfavorable)

The department manager may not be responsible for the volume variance, but the unfavorable spending variance of $100,000 should be analyzed to see what caused it. More detail would permit further breakdowns by price and efficiency variances.

10. The causes of the change in cost and the resulting variances for the laundry department are presented in **TABLE 17-22**.

11. The primary cause for the increase in cost has been the initiation of a new DRG category that is expensive to produce. This case illustrates the importance of case mix and severity-adjusting cost data. **TABLE 17-23** breaks the variances into price and cost and volume variances.

**TABLE 17-23** Valley Hospital Variance Analysis

| | | Variance Analysis by DRG | | |
| | Cost | Volume | New | Total |
|---|---|---|---|---|
| DRG A | $22,500 | $12,750 | – | $35,250 |
| DRG B | 40,000 | (32,000) | – | 8,000 |
| DRG C | – | – | $95,000 | 95,000 |
| | $62,500 | $(19,250) | $95,000 | $138,250 |

Cost variance (DRG A) = ($15,000 – $12,750) × 10 = $22,500
Cost variance (DRG B) = ($10,000 – $8,000) × 20 = $40,000
Volume variance (DRG A) = (10 – 9) × $12,750 = $12,750
Volume variance (DRG B) = (20 – 24) × $8,000 = ($32,000)
New variance (DRG C) = $95,000 – 0 = $95,000

**TABLE 17-24** American Health Plan Variances

| | Inpatient | Outpatient | Total |
|---|---|---|---|
| Enrollment | $600,000 | $325,000 | $925,000 |
| Utilization | (550,000) | 357,500 | (192,500) |
| Efficiency | 605,000 | (181,500) | 423,500 |
| Total | $655,000 | $501,000 | $1,156,000 |

12. **TABLE 17-24** provides the variances in the required categories. The calculations for the variances are the following:
Enrollment:

$$Inpatient = 1,000 \times 0.600 \times \$1,000 = \$600,000 \text{ (unfavorable)}$$
$$Outpatient = 1,000 \times 5.0 \times \$65 = \$325,000 \text{ (unfavorable)}$$

Utilization:

$$Inpatient = (0.550 - 0.600) \times 11,000 \times \$1,000 = -\$550,000 \text{ (favorable)}$$
$$Outpatient = (5.5 - 5.0) \times 11,000 \times \$65 = \$357,500 \text{ (unfavorable)}$$

Efficiency:

$$Inpatient = (\$1,100 - \$1,000) \times 6,050 = \$605,000 \text{ (unfavorable)}$$
$$Outpatient = (\$62 - \$65) \times 60,500 = -\$181,500 \text{ (favorable)}$$

The data suggest that the vast majority of the variance was created by an increase in enrollment. Of the total $1,156,000 variance, $925,000 was the result of an increase in enrollment. This should not be a concern. There was, however, an increase in the price paid for inpatient care from $1,000 per day to $1,100 per day. It is not clear whether this is a result in the intensity of patients seen, or the use of more expensive hospitals. Inpatient utilization decreased significantly and created a favorable variance of $550,000. On the outpatient side, the situation was reversed. Outpatient utilization increased, resulting in an unfavorable variance of $357,500, whereas outpatient efficiency or prices paid actually declined, resulting in a favorable variance of $181,500.

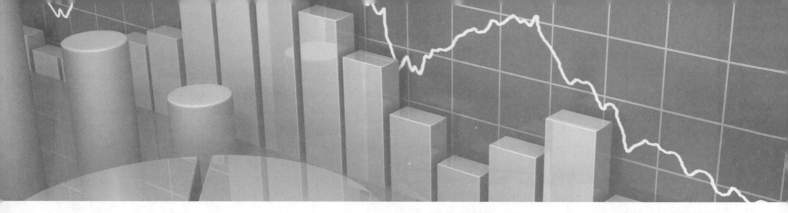

# CHAPTER 18

# Financial Mathematics

## LEARNING OBJECTIVES

After studying this chapter, you should be able to do the following:

1. Explain why a dollar today is worth more than a dollar in the future.
2. Define the terms *future value* and *present value*.
3. Explain the difference between an ordinary annuity and an annuity due.
4. Calculate the future value of an amount and annuity.

## REAL-WORLD SCENARIO

The critical aspect to understanding the value of any stock relates in part to the time value of money. The price of a stock is the sum of its anticipated future earnings or cash flow, adjusted by the time value of money and the uncertainty or risk of these future earnings. The "cost of capital" could be thought of as the investment hurdle or opportunity cost for similar risk investments. In other words, it is the minimum return an investor will accept to invest in a stock of similar risk.

Typically, this rate is greater than a return on U.S. Treasury securities. In February of 2016, rates for 10-year Treasury notes, which are guaranteed by the federal government, were around 2.4%. If an investor did not expect to achieve a return of at least 2.4% on a stock investment, then there would be no reason to take on the risk. However, over the past 70 years, most investors have received a premium of 6 to 7% above the bond rate to compensate for this risk. In other words, stocks have outpaced government bonds by 6 to 7%. Thus, the value of stock hinges on two factors: the cost of capital and the expected future earnings or cash flow streams, which depends on the time value of money.

In this chapter, we examine the concepts and methods of discounting sums of money received at various points in time through the use of **compound interest method** formulas and tables. This material is of special importance in the context of the next two chapters on capital budgeting (Chapter 19) and capital financing (Chapter 21). The present abbreviated discussion of financial mathematics is intended as a review for those who have had prior exposure; if this material is new to the reader, some background reading may be necessary.

The two major questions in the financial decision-making process of any business are the following: (1) Where shall we invest our funds? (2) How shall we finance our investment needs? Investment decisions involve expending funds today while expecting to realize returns in the future. Financing decisions involve the receipt of funds today in return for a promise to make payments in the future. The evaluation of the relative attractiveness of alternative investment and financing opportunities is a major task of management. Differences in the timing of either receipts or payments can have a significant impact on the ultimate decision to invest or finance in a certain way. A payment that is made or received in the first year has a greater value than an identical payment made or received in the tenth year. The concept underlying this point is often referred to as the **time value of money**. A time value for money is simply the assignment of a cost or interest rate for money.

Money or funds can be thought of as a commodity, like any other commodity that can be bought or sold. The price for the commodity called money is often stated as an interest rate, for example, 10% per year. An interest rate of 10% per year implies exchange rates between money at different periods. When the interest rate is 10%, a dollar received 1 year from today is worth only 0.9091 of a dollar received today, and a dollar received 10 years from today is worth only 0.3855 of a dollar today. Compound interest rate tables are merely values that provide relative weighting for money received or paid during different periods at specified prices or interest rates. With these relative weightings, money received or paid can be added or subtracted to produce some logical meaningful result. The major purpose of compound interest tables is to permit addition and subtraction of money paid or received during different periods. The resulting sums are usually expressed in dollars at one of the two following time points: (1) **present value** and (2) **future value**.

The compound interest tables we use in this chapter are categorized as either present value or future value tables. The present value tables provide the relative weights that should be used to restate money of future periods back to the present. Future value tables provide the relative weighting for restating money of one period to some designated future period.

## ▶ Single-Sum Problems

### Future Value: Single Sum

There are many situations in which a business would be interested in the future value of a single sum. For example, a nursing home may want to invest $100,000 today in a fund to be used in 2 years for replacement of a specific piece of equipment. It would like to know what sum of money would be available 2 years from now.

This type of problem is easily solved, using the values presented in **TABLE 18-1**. The first step in solving the problem is to set up a time graph. This involves

**TABLE 18-1** Future Value of $1 Received in *n* Periods

| Period | 2% | 4% | 6% | 8% | 10% | 12% | 14% |
|---|---|---|---|---|---|---|---|
| 1 | 1.0200 | 1.0400 | 1.0600 | 1.0800 | 1.1000 | 1.1200 | 1.1400 |
| 2 | 1.4040 | 1.0816 | 1.1236 | 1.1664 | 1.2100 | 1.2544 | 1.2996 |
| 3 | 1.0612 | 1.1249 | 1.1910 | 1.2597 | 1.3310 | 1.4049 | 1.4815 |
| 4 | 1.0824 | 1.1699 | 1.2625 | 1.3605 | 1.4614 | 1.5735 | 1.6890 |
| 5 | 1.1041 | 1.2167 | 1.3382 | 1.4693 | 1.6105 | 1.7623 | 1.9254 |

| 6 | 1.1262 | 1.2653 | 1.4185 | 1.5869 | 1.7716 | 1.9738 | 2.1950 |
| 7 | 1.1487 | 1.3159 | 1.5036 | 1.7138 | 1.9487 | 2.2107 | 2.5023 |
| 8 | 1.1717 | 1.3686 | 1.5938 | 1.8509 | 2.1436 | 2.4760 | 2.8526 |
| 9 | 1.1951 | 1.4233 | 1.6895 | 1.9990 | 2.3579 | 2.7731 | 3.2519 |
| 10 | 1.2190 | 1.4802 | 1.7908 | 2.1589 | 2.5937 | 3.1058 | 3.7072 |
| 11 | 1.2434 | 1.5395 | 1.8983 | 2.3316 | 2.8531 | 3.4785 | 4.2262 |
| 12 | 1.2682 | 1.6010 | 2.0122 | 2.5182 | 3.1384 | 3.8960 | 4.8179 |
| 13 | 1.2936 | 1.6651 | 2.1329 | 2.7196 | 3.4523 | 4.3635 | 5.4924 |
| 14 | 1.3195 | 1.7317 | 2.2609 | 2.9372 | 3.7975 | 4.8871 | 6.2613 |
| 15 | 1.3459 | 1.8009 | 2.3966 | 3.1722 | 4.1772 | 5.4736 | 7.1379 |
| 16 | 1.3728 | 1.8730 | 2.5404 | 3.4259 | 4.5950 | 6.1304 | 8.1372 |
| 17 | 1.4002 | 1.9479 | 2.6928 | 3.7000 | 5.0545 | 6.8660 | 9.2765 |
| 18 | 1.4282 | 2.0258 | 2.8543 | 3.9960 | 5.5599 | 7.6900 | 10.5752 |
| 19 | 1.4568 | 2.1068 | 3.0256 | 4.3157 | 6.1159 | 8.6128 | 12.0557 |
| 20 | 1.4859 | 2.1911 | 3.2071 | 4.6610 | 6.7275 | 9.6463 | 13.7435 |
| 30 | 1.8114 | 3.2434 | 5.7435 | 10.0627 | 17.4494 | 29.9599 | 50.9502 |
| 40 | 2.2080 | 4.8010 | 10.2857 | 21.7245 | 45.2593 | 93.0510 | 188.8835 |

the following four variables that make up any simple compound interest problem:

1. Number of periods during which the compounding occurs (*n*)
2. Present value of future sum (*p*)
3. Future value of present sum (*f*)
4. Interest rate per period (*i*)

If you know the values of any three of these variables, you can solve for the fourth. The *time line* is a simple device that helps you to conceptualize the problem and identify the known values to permit the problem to be solved. In the previous nursing home investment example, a 10% interest rate per period would be reflected in **FIGURE 18-1**.

The value 0 on this time graph represents the present time (today), whereas the values 1 and 2 represent year 1 and year 2. In the nursing home example, we know three of the four variables and can therefore

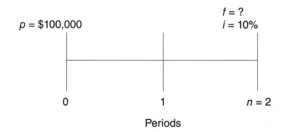

**FIGURE 18-1  Future Value of Present Sum**

solve the problem through substitution in the following formula:

$$f = p \times f(i, n)$$

The factor $f(i, n)$ is the future value of $1 invested today for $n$ periods at $i$ rate of interest per period. These values can be found in Table 18-1, using the previous generic formula. The following calculation then can be made to solve the problem:

$$f = \$100,00 \times f(10\%, 2) \text{ or}$$
$$f = \$100,000 \times 1.210 \text{ or}$$
$$f = \$121,000$$

In some situations, it may be the interest rate that we wish to determine. Assume that we can invest $8,576 today in a discounted note that will pay us $10,000 two years from today. **FIGURE 18-2** summarizes the problem.

The following calculation then can be made to solve the problem:

$$\$10,000 = \$8,576 \times f(i, 2) \text{ or}$$
$$f(i, 2) = 1.166$$

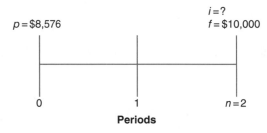

**FIGURE 18-2 Solving for the Interest Rate**

A check of the values in Table 18-1 indicates that the interest rate would be 8% ($f[8\%,2] = 1.166$). If the previous value had not exactly matched a figure in the table, some interpolation would have been required.

A microcomputer or a calculator with a financial mathematics function also could be used to solve the previous types of problems. It is still useful, however, to set up a time graph to conceptualize the problem before entering numbers into the calculator or computer.

## Present Value: Single Sum

In some situations, it is the present value of a future sum that is of interest. This type of problem is similar to those we examined regarding the future value of a single sum. In fact, the same table of values can be used, except that now we use division rather than multiplication.

The general equation used to solve present value, single-sum problems is the following:

$$p = f \times p(i, n)$$

The factor $p(i,n)$ represents the present value of $1 received in $n$ periods at an interest rate of $i$. Values for $p(i,n)$ can be found in **TABLE 18-2**.

Assume that your health maintenance organization (HMO) has a $100,000 debt service obligation

| **TABLE 18-2** Present Value of $1 Due in $n$ Periods | | | | | | | |
|---|---|---|---|---|---|---|---|
| **Period** | **2%** | **4%** | **6%** | **8%** | **10%** | **12%** | **14%** |
| 1 | 0.9804 | 0.9615 | 0.9434 | 0.9259 | 0.9091 | 0.8929 | 0.8772 |
| 2 | 0.9612 | 0.9246 | 0.8900 | 0.8573 | 0.8264 | 0.7972 | 0.7695 |
| 3 | 0.9423 | 0.8890 | 0.8396 | 0.7938 | 0.7513 | 0.7118 | 0.6750 |
| 4 | 0.9238 | 0.8548 | 0.7921 | 0.7350 | 0.6830 | 0.6355 | 0.5921 |
| 5 | 0.9057 | 0.8219 | 0.7473 | 0.6806 | 0.6209 | 0.5674 | 0.5194 |
| 6 | 0.8880 | 0.7903 | 0.7050 | 0.6302 | 0.5645 | 0.5066 | 0.4556 |
| 7 | 0.8706 | 0.7599 | 0.6651 | 0.5835 | 0.5132 | 0.4523 | 0.3996 |
| 8 | 0.8535 | 0.7307 | 0.6274 | 0.5403 | 0.4665 | 0.4039 | 0.3506 |
| 9 | 0.8368 | 0.7026 | 0.5919 | 0.5002 | 0.4241 | 0.3606 | 0.3075 |
| 10 | 0.8203 | 0.6756 | 0.5584 | 0.4632 | 0.3855 | 0.3220 | 0.2697 |

| | | | | | | | |
|---|---|---|---|---|---|---|---|
| 11 | 0.8043 | 0.6496 | 0.5268 | 0.4289 | 0.3505 | 0.2875 | 0.2366 |
| 12 | 0.7885 | 0.6246 | 0.4970 | 0.3971 | 0.3186 | 0.2567 | 0.2076 |
| 13 | 0.7730 | 0.6006 | 0.4688 | 0.3677 | 0.2897 | 0.2292 | 0.1821 |
| 14 | 0.7579 | 0.5775 | 0.4423 | 0.3405 | 0.2633 | 0.2046 | 0.1597 |
| 15 | 0.7430 | 0.5553 | 0.4173 | 0.3152 | 0.2394 | 0.1827 | 0.1401 |
| 16 | 0.7284 | 0.5339 | 0.3936 | 0.2919 | 0.2176 | 0.1631 | 0.1229 |
| 17 | 0.7142 | 0.5134 | 0.3714 | 0.2703 | 0.1978 | 0.1456 | 0.1078 |
| 18 | 0.7002 | 0.4936 | 0.3503 | 0.2502 | 0.1799 | 0.1300 | 0.0946 |
| 19 | 0.6864 | 0.4746 | 0.3305 | 0.2317 | 0.1635 | 0.1161 | 0.0829 |
| 20 | 0.6730 | 0.4564 | 0.3118 | 0.2145 | 0.1486 | 0.1037 | 0.0728 |
| 30 | 0.5521 | 0.3083 | 0.1741 | 0.0994 | 0.0573 | 0.0334 | 0.0196 |
| 40 | 0.4529 | 0.2083 | 0.0972 | 0.0460 | 0.0221 | 0.0107 | 0.0053 |

due in 2 years. You are interested in learning how much money must be set aside today to meet the obligation if the expected yield on the investment is 12%. The relevant time graph is depicted in **FIGURE 18-3**.

The calculation to solve the problem would be the following:

$$p = f \times p(i, n) \text{ or}$$
$$p = \$100,000 \times p(12\%, 2) \text{ or}$$
$$p = \$100,000 \times 0.7972 \text{ or}$$
$$p = \$79,720$$

It is important to note that the values of Table 18-1 and Table 18-2 are reciprocals of each other. That is

$$f(i, n) = 1 / p(i, n)$$

In effect, this means that only one of the two tables is necessary to solve either a present value or future value problem involving a single sum.

## ▶ Annuity Problems

### Future Value

In many business situations, there is more than one payment or receipt. In the case of multiple payments or receipts, when each payment or receipt is constant per time period, we have an **annuity** situation. **FIGURE 18-4** depicts a time graph for an annuity.

*Learning Objective 3*

Explain the difference between an ordinary annuity and an annuity due.

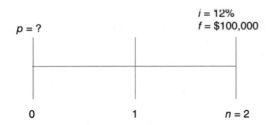

**FIGURE 18-3  Present Value of a Future Sum**

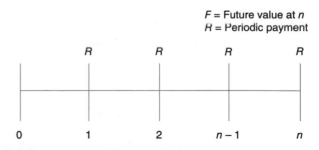

**FIGURE 18-4  Future Value of Annuity**

In the graph in Figure 18-4, $F$ represents the future value of the invested annuity deposits at the end of period $n$. (Note that $F$ is used to denote future value for annuities, while $f$ is used for single sums.) The values for $R$ represent the periodic deposits that are constant for each period. It should be emphasized that the deposits are made at the *end* of each period. Such a system of deposits is often described as an **ordinary annuity**. The values presented in **TABLES 18-3** and **18-4** assume an ordinary annuity situation in which deposits or receipts occur at the end of the period.

| **TABLE 18-3** Future Value of $1 Received Each Period for $n$ Periods | | | | | | | |
|---|---|---|---|---|---|---|---|
| **Period** | **2%** | **4%** | **6%** | **8%** | **10%** | **12%** | **14%** |
| 1 | 1.0000 | 1.0000 | 1.0000 | 1.0000 | 1.0000 | 1.0000 | 1.0000 |
| 2 | 2.0200 | 2.0400 | 2.0600 | 2.0800 | 2.1000 | 2.1200 | 2.1400 |
| 3 | 3.0604 | 3.1216 | 3.1836 | 3.2464 | 3.3100 | 3.3744 | 3.4396 |
| 4 | 4.1216 | 4.2465 | 4.3746 | 4.5061 | 4.6410 | 4.7793 | 4.9211 |
| 5 | 5.2040 | 5.4163 | 5.6371 | 5.8666 | 6.1051 | 6.3528 | 6.6101 |
| 6 | 6.3081 | 6.6330 | 6.9753 | 7.3359 | 7.7156 | 8.1152 | 8.5355 |
| 7 | 7.4343 | 7.8983 | 8.3938 | 8.9228 | 9.4872 | 10.0890 | 10.7305 |
| 8 | 8.5830 | 9.2142 | 9.8975 | 10.6366 | 11.4359 | 12.2997 | 13.2328 |
| 9 | 9.7546 | 10.5828 | 11.4913 | 12.4876 | 13.5795 | 14.7757 | 16.0853 |
| 10 | 10.9497 | 12.0061 | 13.1808 | 14.4866 | 15.9374 | 17.5487 | 19.3373 |
| 11 | 12.1687 | 13.4864 | 14.9716 | 16.6455 | 18.5312 | 20.6546 | 23.0445 |
| 12 | 13.4121 | 15.0258 | 16.8699 | 18.9771 | 21.3843 | 24.1331 | 27.2707 |
| 13 | 14.6803 | 16.6268 | 18.8821 | 21.4953 | 24.5227 | 28.0291 | 32.0887 |
| 14 | 15.9739 | 18.2919 | 21.0151 | 24.2149 | 27.9750 | 32.3926 | 37.5811 |
| 15 | 17.2934 | 20.0236 | 23.2760 | 27.1521 | 31.7725 | 37.2797 | 43.8424 |
| 16 | 18.6393 | 21.8245 | 25.6725 | 30.3243 | 35.9497 | 42.7533 | 50.9804 |
| 17 | 20.0121 | 23.6975 | 28.2129 | 33.7502 | 40.5447 | 48.8837 | 59.1176 |
| 18 | 21.4123 | 25.6454 | 30.9057 | 37.4502 | 45.5992 | 55.7497 | 68.3941 |
| 19 | 22.8406 | 27.6712 | 33.7600 | 41.4463 | 51.1591 | 63.4397 | 78.6992 |
| 20 | 24.2974 | 29.7781 | 36.7856 | 45.7620 | 57.2750 | 72.0524 | 91.0249 |
| 30 | 40.5681 | 56.0849 | 79.0582 | 113.2832 | 164.4940 | 241.3327 | 356.7868 |
| 40 | 60.4020 | 95.0255 | 154.7620 | 259.0565 | 442.5926 | 767.0914 | 1,342.0251 |

**TABLE 18-4**  Present Value of $1 Received Each Period for *n* Periods

| Period | 2% | 4% | 6% | 8% | 10% | 12% | 14% |
|--------|------|------|------|------|------|------|------|
| 1 | 0.9804 | 0.9615 | 0.9434 | 0.9259 | 0.9091 | 0.8929 | 0.8772 |
| 2 | 1.9416 | 1.8861 | 1.8334 | 1.7833 | 1.7355 | 1.6901 | 1.6467 |
| 3 | 2.8839 | 2.7751 | 2.6730 | 2.5771 | 2.4869 | 2.4018 | 2.3216 |
| 4 | 3.8077 | 3.6299 | 3.4651 | 3.3121 | 3.1699 | 3.0373 | 2.9137 |
| 5 | 4.7135 | 4.4518 | 4.2124 | 3.9927 | 3.7908 | 3.6048 | 3.4331 |
| 6 | 5.6014 | 5.2421 | 4.9173 | 4.6229 | 4.3553 | 4.1114 | 3.8887 |
| 7 | 6.4720 | 6.0021 | 5.5824 | 5.2064 | 4.8684 | 4.5638 | 4.2883 |
| 8 | 7.3255 | 6.7327 | 6.8017 | 5.7466 | 5.3349 | 4.9676 | 4.6389 |
| 9 | 8.1622 | 7.4353 | 7.3601 | 6.2469 | 5.7590 | 5.3282 | 4.9464 |
| 10 | 8.9826 | 8.1109 | 7.8869 | 6.7101 | 6.1446 | 5.6502 | 5.2161 |
| 11 | 9.7868 | 8.7605 | 8.3838 | 7.1390 | 6.4951 | 5.9377 | 5.4527 |
| 12 | 10.5753 | 9.3851 | 8.8527 | 7.5361 | 6.8137 | 6.1944 | 5.6603 |
| 13 | 11.3484 | 9.9856 | 9.2950 | 7.9038 | 7.1034 | 6.4235 | 5.8424 |
| 14 | 12.1062 | 10.5631 | 9.7122 | 8.2442 | 7.3667 | 6.6282 | 6.0021 |
| 15 | 12.8493 | 11.1184 | 9.7122 | 8.5595 | 7.6061 | 6.8109 | 6.1422 |
| 16 | 13.5777 | 11.6523 | 10.1059 | 8.8514 | 7.8237 | 6.9740 | 6.2651 |
| 17 | 14.2919 | 12.1657 | 10.4773 | 9.1216 | 8.0216 | 7.1196 | 6.3729 |
| 18 | 14.9920 | 12.6593 | 10.8276 | 9.3719 | 8.2014 | 7.2497 | 6.4674 |
| 19 | 15.6785 | 13.1339 | 11.1581 | 9.6036 | 8.3649 | 7.3658 | 6.5504 |
| 20 | 16.3514 | 13.5903 | 11.4699 | 9.8181 | 8.5136 | 7.4694 | 6.6231 |
| 30 | 22.3965 | 17.2920 | 13.7648 | 11.2578 | 9.4269 | 8.0552 | 7.0027 |
| 40 | 27.3555 | 19.7928 | 15.0463 | 11.9246 | 9.7791 | 8.2438 | 7.1050 |

### *Learning Objective 4*

Calculate the future value of an amount and annuity.

The basic equation for a future value annuity is

$$F = R \times F(i, n)$$

The factor $F(i, n)$ represents the future value of $1 invested each period for $n$ periods at $i$ rate of interest. Values for $F(i, n)$ can be found in Table 18-3. Again, if three of the four variables ($F$, $R$, $i$, and $n$) in the previous equation are known, the equation can be solved to determine the fourth. Thus, if we know $F$, $i$, and $n$, we can solve for $R$.

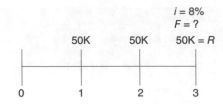

**FIGURE 18-5** **Determining the Future Value of an Annuity**

Assume that a hospital wants to know what the value of $50,000 worth of annual deposits in a trust fund for professional malpractice insurance will be in 3 years if the fund earns 8% per year. The time graph for this problem is depicted in **FIGURE 18-5**.

The calculation to solve the problem would be as follows:

$$F = R \times F(i, n) \text{ or}$$
$$F = \$50,000 \times F(8\%, 3) \text{ or}$$
$$F = \$50,000 \times 3.2464 \text{ or}$$
$$F = \$162,320$$

The values in Table 18-3 also could be determined through simple addition of the values for a single sum in Table 18-1. This can be seen easily by further examining our hospital example. **TABLE 18-5** summarizes the relevant data.

Notice that the future value total in Table 18-5 is identical to that in the earlier annuity formula. Also

note that the summation of the individual **future value factors (FVF)** yields the value of the annuity factor (3.2464). In general, a future value annuity factor can be expressed as follows:

$$F(i, n) = f(i, 1) + f(i, 2) + \cdots + f(i, n-1) + 1.0$$

In many situations, a financial mathematics problem may be part annuity and part single sum. In such cases, the use of a time graph will help you spot this duality and solve the problem correctly. Assume that a hospital has a sinking fund payment requirement for the last 10 years of a bond's life. At the end of that period, there must be $45 million available to retire the debt. The hospital has created a $5 million fund today, 20 years before debt retirement, to offset part of the future sinking fund requirement. If the investment yield is expected to be 10% per year, what annual deposit must be made to the sinking fund? **FIGURE 18-6** summarizes the problem.

The first step is to determine the future value of the $5 million deposit, which is

$$f = \$5,000,000 \times f(10\%, 20) \text{ or}$$
$$f = \$5,000,000 \times 6.7275 \text{ or}$$
$$f = \$33,637,500$$

This means that the amount of money that must be generated by the 10 sinking fund deposits must

| | | | Year Invested | | |
|---|---|---|---|---|---|
| **Year** | **Future Value Factor (8%)** | **Future Value** | **1** | **2** | **3** |
| 1 | 1.1664 | $58,320 | $50,000 | | |
| 2 | 1.0800 | 54,000 | | $50,000 | |
| 3 | 1.0000 | 50,000 | | | $50,000 |
| Total | 3.2464 | $162,320 | | | |

**TABLE 18-5**  Using Sum of Simple Future Value Factors to Calculate Annuity Value

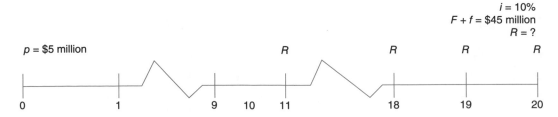

**FIGURE 18-6** **Determining the Annual Sinking Fund Deposit**

equal $11,362,500 ($45,000,000 − $33,637,500). The following calculation provides the solution:

$$F - f = R \times F(i, n) \text{ or}$$

$$\$11,362,500 = R \times F(10\%, 10) \text{ or}$$

$$\$11,362,500 = R \times 15.9374 \text{ or}$$

$$R = \$712,946$$

## Present Value

While determining the present value of an annuity, the procedure is analogous to that used to determine the **future value of an annuity**, except that our attention is now on present value rather than future value. **FIGURE 18-7** represents the typical present value annuity problem.

As noted earlier, this is an ordinary annuity situation because the payments are at the end of the period. The basic equation used to solve a **present value of an annuity** problem is the following:

$$P = R \times P(i, n)$$

The factor $P(i, n)$ represents the present value of $1 received at the end of each period for $n$ periods when $i$ is the rate of interest. Values for $P(i, n)$ are found in Table 18-4. (Note that $P$ is used to denote an annuity problem, while $p$ is used to denote a single-sum problem.)

Assume that a hospital is considering buying an older hospital and consolidating its operations in another nearby facility. An actuary has estimated that pension payments of $100,000 per year for the next 4 years will be required to satisfy the obligation to vested employees. The hospital wants to know what the present value of this obligation is so that it can be subtracted from the negotiated purchase price. The obligation's discount rate is assumed to be 12%. The time graph for this problem is depicted in **FIGURE 18-8**. The calculation to solve the problem is as follows:

$$P = \$100,000 \times P(12\%, 4) \text{ or}$$

$$P = \$100,000 \times 3.0373$$

$$P = \$303,730$$

Present value annuity problems can be thought of as a series of individual single-sum problems. The present value annuity factor $P(i, n)$ is the sum of the individual single-sum values of Table 18-2. The data in **TABLE 18-6** summarize this calculation in our hospital example.

The small differences between the annuity values and the single-sum values in Table 18-6 are due to rounding errors.

The present value annuity factor $[P(i, n)]$ can be expressed as follows:

$$P(i, n) = p(i, 1) + p(i, 2) + \cdots + p(i, n)$$

In many business situations, ordinary annuity problems do not arise. The classic exception to the ordinary annuity situation is a lease with front-end payments. Assume that a clinic wants to lease a computer for the next 5 years with quarterly payments of $1,000 due at the *beginning* of each quarter. If the clinic's discount rate is 16% per annum, what is the present value of the lease liability? The relevant time graph is presented in **FIGURE 18-9**.

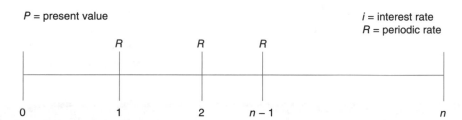

FIGURE 18-7 **Typical Present Value Annuity**

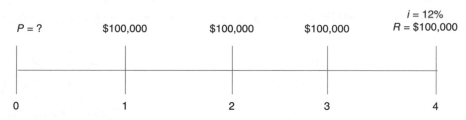

FIGURE 18-8 **Present Value of the Pension Obligation**

**TABLE 18-6** Using Sum of Simple Present Value Factors to Calculate Annuity Value

| Year | Present Value Factor (12%) | Present Value | Year of Payment | | | |
|------|---------------------------|---------------|-----------|-----------|-----------|-----------|
| | | | 1 | 2 | 3 | 4 |
| 1 | 0.8929 | $89,290 | $100,000 | | | |
| 2 | 0.7972 | $79,720 | | $100,000 | | |
| 3 | 0.7118 | $71,180 | | | $100,000 | |
| 4 | 0.6355 | $63,550 | | | | $100,000 |
| Total | 3.0374 | $303,740 | | | | |

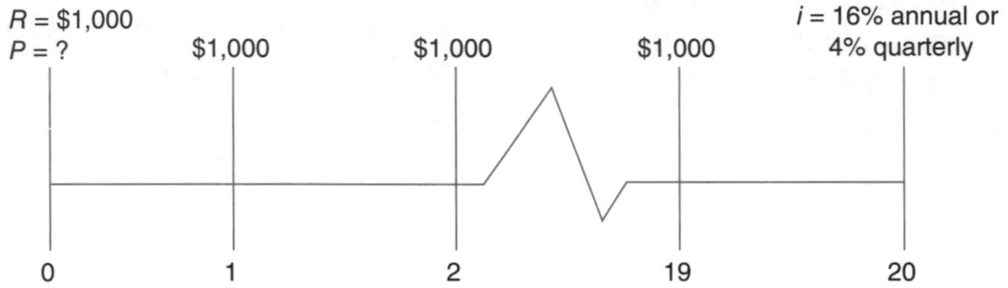

**FIGURE 18-9** **Present Value of a Lease Liability**

The graph in Figure 18-9 indicates that the clinic has a 19-period ordinary annuity, with each period lasting 3 months. The effective interest rate for each quarter is 4% (16% divided by 4). The present value of the first payment is $1,000 because it occurs at the beginning of the first quarter. The following calculation provides the solution to the problem:

$$P = \$1,000 + \$1,000 \times P(4\%, 19) \text{ or}$$
$$P = \$1,000 + \$1,000 \times 13.1339 \text{ or}$$
$$P = \$14,134$$

## ▶ SUMMARY

In the area of financial mathematics, compound interest rate tables provide us with values with which we can weight money flows that are received or paid during different periods. The relative weighting assigned to each period's money flow is a function of the price of money or the interest rate. The relative weightings permit us to add or subtract money flows from different periods and produce a meaningful measure. The value of money is usually expressed in terms of present value or value at some future specified date.

## ASSIGNMENTS

1. Steven Hudson has agreed to settle a debt of $100,000 by paying $14,903 at the end of each year for 10 years. What effective rate of interest is Hudson paying under this agreement?
2. Findling Hospital is planning a major expansion project. The construction cost of the project is to be paid from the proceeds of serial notes. The notes are of equal amounts and include a provision for interest at an annual rate of 8% payable semiannually over the next 10 years. It is expected that receipts from the hospital will provide for the repayment of principal and interest on the notes. Allan Klein, controller of the hospital, has estimated that the cash flow available for repayment of principal and interest will be $450,000 per year. The construction project is expected to cost $3,420,000. Can the hospital meet the peak debt service with existing cash flows?
3. Jerry Scott has just accepted a position with a state agency that has a retirement pension plan calling for joint contributions by the employee and the employer. Scott is now 10 years from retirement age of 65 and expects

to contribute $4,000 per year to the plan, which would make him eligible for payments of $10,000 per year for the remainder of his life, starting in 10 years. Because this retirement plan is optional, Scott is considering the alternative of investing annually an amount equal to his $4,000 per year contribution. If Scott assumes that his investments would earn 8% annually, and that his life expectancy is 80 years, should he invest in his own plan or should he make contributions to his employer's fund?

4. Meany Hospital wishes to provide for the retirement of an obligation of $10,000,000 that becomes due July 1, 2026. The hospital plans to deposit $500,000 in a special fund each July 1 for 8 years, starting July 1, 2018. In addition, the hospital wishes to deposit on July 1, 2018, an amount that, with accumulated interest at 10% compounded annually, will bring the total value of the fund to the required $10,000,000 at July 1, 2026. What dollar amount should the hospital deposit?

5. Jim Hubert, an investment banker with The Ohio Company, is arranging a financing package with Bill Andrews, president of Lebish Hospital. The financing package calls for $20 million in bonds to be repaid in 20 years. A decision must be made regarding the amount that must be deposited on an annual basis in a sinking fund. It is estimated that the sinking fund will earn interest at the rate of 8% compounded annually. What dollar amount must be set aside annually at year-end in the sinking fund to meet the $20 million payment in the twentieth year?

6. General Hospital is evaluating a zero-interest capital financing alternative. General would borrow $100,000,000 and receive $62,100,000 in cash. The $100,000,000 note would carry no interest payment but would be due at the end of the fifth year. The lender would require an annual year-end sinking fund payment over the next 5 years to meet the maturity value of $100,000,000. If the fund is scheduled to earn interest at the rate of 6% annually, what amount must be deposited annually?

7. ABC Hospital is embarking on a major renovation program. The total cost of construction will be $50,000,000. Payments will be $10,000,000 at the end of year 1, $30,000,000 at the end of year 2, and $10,000,000 at the end of year 3. ABC wants to set aside sufficient funds today to meet the expected construction draws. If the fund can be expected to earn 8% per annum, what amount should be set aside?

8. If you issue $100,000 of 10% bonds with interest payable semiannually over the next 5 years, what is the market value of the bonds if the required market rate of interest is 12% annually? Assume that no payment of principal is made until maturity.

9. You have agreed to buy an adjacent medical office building with quarterly payments of $100,000 for the next 5 years. Payments are due at the end of each quarter. If the cost of money to you is 16% per annum, would you pay $1,200,000 in cash today to the present owners?

10. You plan to invest $1 million per year for the next 3 years at year-end to meet future professional liability payments. If the fund earns interest at a rate of 10% per annum, how large will the balance be in 5 years? Assume that no payments for claims are made until then.

## SOLUTIONS AND ANSWERS

1. The graph in **FIGURE 18-10** and the following calculations show the effective rate of interest Hudson is paying.

$$P = R \times P(i,n)$$

$$\$100,000 = \$14,903 \times P(i,10)$$

$$P(i,10) = 6.710$$

$$I = 8\%$$

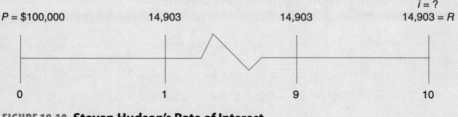

**FIGURE 18-10  Steven Hudson's Rate of Interest**

2. In this hospital expansion project, it is necessary to recognize that debt service will be at the maximum or peak in the first year. This is the pattern that results with a serial note. Thus:

$$\text{Debt principal payment} = \$3,420,000/20 = \$181,000 \text{ every 6 months}$$

$$\text{Interest in first 6 months} = 0.04 \times \$3,420,000 = \$136,800$$

$$\text{Interest in second 6 months} = 0.04 \times (\$3,420,000 - \$171,000) = \$129,960$$

$$\text{Total first-year debt service} = \$171,000 + \$136,800 + \$171,000 + \$129,960 = \$608,760$$

Thus, Findling Hospital's project cannot be financed with the existing cash flow of $450,000.

3. The graph in **FIGURE 18-11** and the following calculations are relevant to Scott's retirement fund decision.

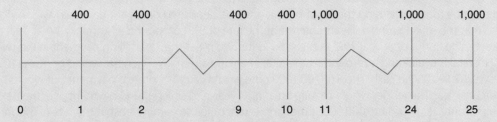

**FIGURE 18-11 Jerry Scott's Annual Investments**

We first need to determine the expected value of the state's pension payments at Scott's retirement in year 10. Calculation of the value of the state agency's payments at year 10 is as follows:

$$P = \$10,000 \times P(8\%, 15)$$

$$P = \$10,000 \times 8.559$$

$$P = \$85,590$$

We next determine the expected value of Scott's deposits, assuming that he can realize an 8% yield at the end of year 10. Calculation of the value of Scott's deposits at year 10 is as follows:

$$F = \$4,000 \times F(8\%, 10)$$

$$F = \$4,000 \times 14.4866$$

$$F = \$57,950$$

Thus, Scott is better off with the state agency's retirement plan. His deposits of $400 would not provide a fund large enough to give him $1,000 per year for 15 years.

4. The relevant calculations for Meany Hospital are as follows and depicted in **FIGURE 18-12**.

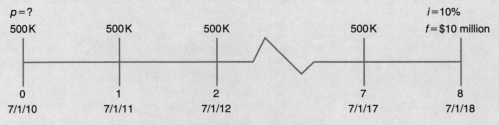

**FIGURE 18-12 Meany Hospital Required Fund Deposit**

Calculation of the value of annual deposits at July 1, 2026 is as follows:

$$\text{Future value of deposits} = \$500,000 \times f(10\%, 8) + [\$500,000 \times F(10\%, 7)] \times f(10\%, 1)$$

$$F = \$500,000 \times 2.1436 + (\$500,000 \times 9.4872) \times 1.10$$

$$F = \$1,071,800 + \$5,217,960 = \$6,289,760$$

Calculation of the required deposit at July 1, 2018 is as follows:

Required amount at July 1, 2026 must equal $10,000,000 − $6,289,760, or $3,710,240

$$p = \$3,710,240 \times p(10\%, 8) = \text{Required deposit at July 1, 2018}$$

$$p = \$3,710,240 \times 0.467$$

$$p = \$1,732,682 = \text{Deposit required at July 1, 2018}$$

5. **FIGURE 18-13** and the following calculations show the dollar amount that must be set aside annually in the sinking fund to meet the $20 million repayment in the twentieth year.

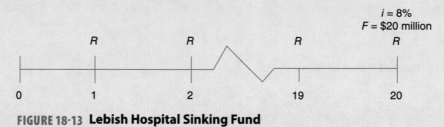

**FIGURE 18-13** **Lebish Hospital Sinking Fund**

$$F = R \times F(i, n)$$

$$\$20,000,000 = R \times F(8\%, 20)$$

$$\$20,000,000 = R \times 45.7620$$

$$R = \$437,044$$

6. **FIGURE 18-14** and the following calculations show the amount that General Hospital will have to deposit in the sinking fund each year.

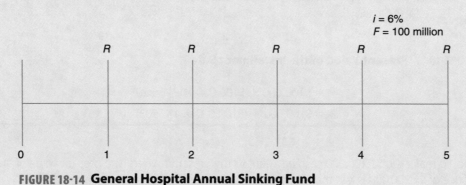

**FIGURE 18-14** **General Hospital Annual Sinking Fund**

$$F = R \times F(i, n)$$

$$\$100,000,000 = R \times F(6\%, 5)$$

$$\$100,000,000 = R \times 5.6371$$

$$R = \$17,739,618$$

7. **FIGURE 18-15** and the following calculations show the amount that ABC Hospital must set aside to meet expected construction draws.

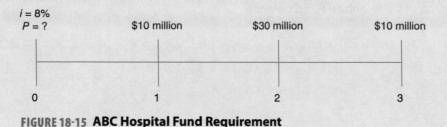

**FIGURE 18-15** **ABC Hospital Fund Requirement**

Present value = $10,000,000 × $p$(8%, 1) + $30,000,000 × $p$(8%, 2) + $10,000,000 × $p$(8%, 3)

Present value = $10,000,000 × 0.926 + $30,000,000 × 0.857 + $10,000,000 × 0.794

Present value = $42,910,000

8. The market value of the bonds may be calculated as follows (**FIGURE 18-16**):

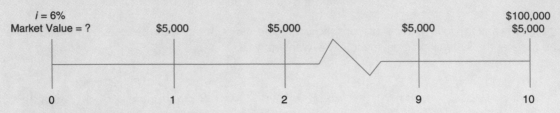

**FIGURE 18-16** **Market Value of Bonds**

Market value = $5,000 × $P$(6%, 10) + $100,000 × $p$(6%, 10)

Market value = $5,000 × 7.360 + $100,000 × 0.558

Market value = $92,600

9. To determine whether you should pay $1,200,00 in cash today to the present owners, **FIGURE 18-17** and the following calculations are relevant.

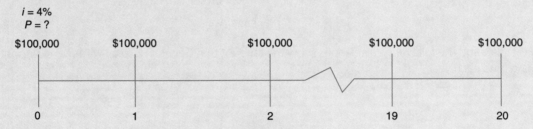

**FIGURE 18-17** **Present Value of the Installment Sale**

$P$ = $100,000 + $100,000 × $P$(4%, 20)

$P$ = $100,000 + ($100,000 × 13.5903)

$P$ = $1,359,030

Yes, you should make the $1,200,000 cash payment to the present owners. The present value of an outright purchase price of $1,200,000 is less than the present value of the installment sale arrangement.

10. **FIGURE 18-18** and the following calculations show the amount of the fund balance in 5 years.

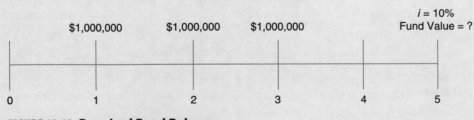

**FIGURE 18-18** **Required Fund Balance**

Fund value = $1,000,000 × $F$(10%, 3) × $f$(10%, 2)

Fund value = $1,000,000 × 3.310 × 1.210

Fund value = $4,005,100

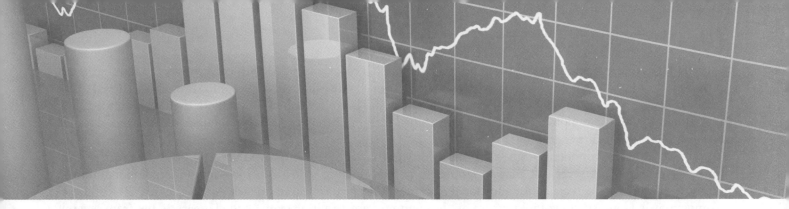

# CHAPTER 19

# Capital Project Analysis

## LEARNING OBJECTIVES

After studying this chapter, you should be able to do the following:

1. Explain who is involved in the capital investment decision process.
2. Describe the kinds of decisions that are made in capital investment decision analysis.
3. Explain the four stages of the capital decision-making process.
4. List some of the kinds of information that is needed to evaluate a capital investment project.
5. Calculate a project's net present value, profitability index, and equivalent annual cost.
6. Explain the concept of a discount rate and what the weighted average cost of capital is.

## REAL-WORLD SCENARIO

The phone rang in the office of Jack Smith, an executive at Specialized Medical Devices, Inc. (SMD), a firm that manufactures specialized digital mammography devices. On the line was Dr. Sipparo, Chief of Radiology at Academic Medical Center (AMC). Dr. Sipparo explained that she needed Smith's help in understanding an analysis prepared by the staff of Dr. Alexander, AMC's Chief Executive Officer, of the pending purchase of new imaging equipment for the evaluation of patients presenting for breast cancer screening. AMC is evaluating two types of imaging equipment—standard screen-film mammography equipment and a machine offered by SMD that allows for full-field digital mammography with tomosynthesis. Dr. Sipparo explained the situation as follows:

Based on his staff's cost analysis, Dr. Alexander believes the hospital should purchase the conventional mammography equipment rather than the digital mammography machine. The physicians in the radiology department are very upset by this. They want the hospital to purchase the tomosynthesis scanner because it incorporates the latest imaging technology. In addition, Dr. Sipparo is not convinced by Dr. Alexander's staff's analysis that the conventional equipment is really the better choice even from a purely financial perspective.

The capital budget committee meets next week, and Dr. Sipparo needs Smith's help. Dr. Sipparo has asked Smith to evaluate the analysis prepared by Dr. Alexander's staff and to recommend changes to his analysis if he believed they were warranted.

Digital mammography, which eliminates the film and lab costs associated with conventional mammography, provides the ability to combine multiple images taken from slightly different angles into three-dimensional (3D) images. Tomosynthesis is a relatively new technology that has been developed for use with digital mammography that allows for multiple high-resolution cross-sectional images of the breast to be obtained at the same dose as conventional screen-film mammography.

Tomosynthesis proponents argue that this 3D image may allow for improved detection of breast cancer and for fewer false-positive screening mammograms. In current practice, 7 to 15% of women undergoing mammography screening may be recalled for additional mammography or ultrasound images. Approximately 50% of these women may have a suspicious-looking area on the mammogram, resulting from normal breast tissues from several areas of the breast that are superimposed to look like a lesion or other abnormality. Tomosynthesis, which allows cross-sectional viewing of the breast, may allow the radiologist to differentiate between superimposed tissue and actual lesions, thereby allowing for a reduction in the recall rate. Reducing the recall rate is an important goal because of the anxiety associated with being asked to return for additional views. It is also possible that tomosynthesis may increase the positive biopsy rate. Tomosynthesis might also allow the complete patient workup in one visit for many women, a significant goal given the noncompliance with recommended follow-up after abnormal screening studies.

Dr. Alexander remains skeptical, however. He is concerned that full-field digital mammography with tomosynthesis will increase the hospital's initial fixed costs of screening, while many of the reduced costs will accrue to the patient and to the payer, for which the hospital is not remunerated or tangibly rewarded. He also is concerned about the increased time it will take for radiologists to learn how to use this new technology.

Dr. Alexander's staff had analyzed the two alternatives using an equivalent annual cost (EAC) method. Because the alternatives have different useful lives, EAC appeared to be the best way to determine which type of equipment would be more cost effective for the hospital. Essentially, EAC is the amount of an annuity that has the same life and present value as the investment option being considered. Thus, Dr. Alexander based the cost comparison on the initial outlay costs of both types of imaging equipment and on the annual maintenance, personnel-related, and other costs associated with the two equipment types. Dr. Alexander wants to purchase the conventional mammography equipment because it results in lower cost for AMC.

Dr. Sipparo, however, remains convinced that full-field digital mammography with tomosynthesis is the right decision. She believes the technology is superior, offers better care, and, ultimately, will reduce many of the long-term costs associated with breast cancer screening and diagnosis. Without a strong financial background, she is unsure how to convince Dr. Alexander of this, which is why she contacted Smith. She wants his help to prepare an alternative analysis using the latest financial decision-making tools.

---

*Capital project analysis* occurs during the programming phase of the management control process. (See Figure 16-3 in Chapter 16.) Whereas zero-base budgeting or zero-base review can be considered as the programming phase of management control concerned with old or existing programs, capital project analysis is the phase primarily concerned with new programs. Here, it is broadly defined to include the selection of investment projects.

Capital project analysis is an ongoing activity, but it is not usually summarized annually in the budget. The capital budget is the yearly estimate of resources that will be expended for new programs during the coming year. Capital budgeting may be considered as less comprehensive and shorter term than capital project analysis.

> ### Learning Objective 1
>
> Explain who is involved in the capital investment decision process.

## ▶ Participants in the Analytical Process

The capital decision-making process in the healthcare industry is complex for several reasons. First, a healthcare firm, whether nonprofit or investor owned, is likely to have more complex and less quantifiable objectives than firms in other industries. Provision of care to the indigent and community access to services as well as meeting quality standards are often critical objectives for healthcare firms in addition to profits. Second, the number of individuals involved in the process, either directly or indirectly, is likely to be greater in the healthcare industry than in most other industries. **FIGURE 19-1** illustrates the relationships of various parties involved in the capital decision-making process of a healthcare facility.

## External Participants

### Financing Sources

The option of obtaining funds externally for many new programs is an important variable in the capital decision-making process. A variety of individual organizations are involved in the credit-determination process, including investment bankers, bond-rating agencies, bankers, and feasibility consultants. Many of these entities and their roles are discussed in Chapter 21. At this juncture, it is important to recognize that, collectively, these entities may influence the amount of money that can be borrowed and the terms of the borrowing, and this can affect the nature and size of capital projects undertaken by a given healthcare facility.

## Rate-Setting and Rate-Control Agencies

Some states control or limit the rates that hospitals and other healthcare firms can charge for services. The influence exerted by rate-setting or rate-control organizations on capital decision making is indirect but still extremely important. Control of rates can limit both short-term and long-term profitability. This control can reduce a healthcare firm's ability to repay indebtedness and thus limit its access to the capital markets. More directly, rate-setting organizations can limit the amount of money available for financing capital projects by reducing the amount of profits that may be retained. One of the major effects of rate control is to significantly reduce the level of capital expenditures by healthcare firms.

## Third-Party Payers

Like rate-setting and rate-control agencies, third-party payers can indirectly influence the capital decision-making process. Through their reimbursement provisions, third-party payers can affect both capital expenditure levels and sources of financing. For example, many people believe that third-party cost reimbursement provides a strong incentive for

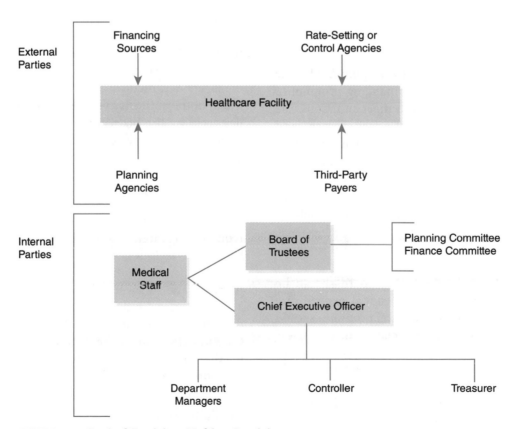

**FIGURE 19-1** **Capital Decision-Making Participants**

increased capital spending: in most situations, such cost reimbursement provides for the reimbursement of depreciation and interest expense, which then may be used to repay financial requirements associated with any indebtedness. As a result, the risk associated with hospital-indebted indebtedness is reduced. In the past, third-party cost reimbursement favorably affected the availability of credit. Currently, cost reimbursement is almost nonexistent except for Critical Access Hospitals that are paid on a cost basis by Medicare.

## Planning Agencies

In many states, state approval of capital expenditures is still required. Planning agencies review certificate-of-need (CON) applications and their recommendations are then passed on to the state authority responsible for final approval or disapproval. An unfavorable decision by the state may be appealed in court. The Federal Trade Commission and the U.S. Justice Department have pressed states to abandon these laws, decrying them as bad for competition. Many states have also engaged in debates over the matter. But none of these efforts—whether through courts, politics, or federal agencies—have led to much change. Thirty-five states and the District of Columbia still have CON programs as of 2016.

## Internal Participants

### Board of Trustees

Ultimately, the board of trustees is responsible for the capital expenditure and capital financing program of the healthcare firm. However, in most situations, the board delegates this authority to management and special board committees. The board's major function should be to clearly establish defined goals and objectives. The statement of goals and objectives is a prerequisite to the programming phase of management control, which includes capital expenditure analysis. Without a clear statement of goals and objectives, capital expenditure programs cannot be adequately defined and analyzed.

Another role of the governing board should be to approve a preliminary 5-year capital expenditure program. This capital expenditure program should link back to the strategic financial plan. (This was discussed in Chapter 13.) The list of capital expenditures should be generated by management and should reflect not just a "wish list" of capital expenditures that would be desirable to make, but should represent management's best guess concerning what future capital expenditures will be essential to meet and maintain the organization's mission.

## Planning Committee

Many healthcare facility boards of trustees have established planning committees whose primary function is to define, analyze, and propose programs to help the organization attain its goals and objectives. These committees are specialized groups within the board of trustees that are directly involved in capital expenditure analysis.

## Finance Committee

Some boards of trustees also have established finance committees that have authority in several key financial functional areas, including budgeting and capital financing. In the latter two areas, a finance committee may be involved with translating programs, perhaps identified by the planning committee, into financing requirements. These requirements may be operational or capital. The finance committee's major responsibility is to ensure adequate financing to meet program requirements. Many of the finance committee's budgetary functions are delegated to the controller; many of its capital financing functions are delegated to the treasurer.

## Chief Executive Officer

The chief executive officer (CEO) is responsible on a day-to-day basis for implementing approved capital expenditure programs and developing related financing plans. The CEO must develop an organizational system that responds to the requests of department managers and medical staff for capital expenditures. Much of the authority vested in the CEO's position is delegated by the board of trustees. Additionally, the administration may seek board approval for its own programs.

## Department Managers

Department managers make most of the internal requests for capital expenditure approval. In many healthcare facilities, formal systems for approving capital expenditures have been developed to receive, process, and answer departmental requests. The allocation of a limited capital budget to competing departmental areas is a difficult task for management. Careful definition of the criteria for capital decision making can help make this problem less political and more objective.

## Medical Staff

Medical staff demands for capital expenditures are a problem unique to the healthcare industry. Medical staff members, in most situations, are not employees of the healthcare firm but rather use it to treat their private patients. Because of their ability to change a firm's utilization dramatically and thus affect financial solvency, executives listen to, and frequently honor, the wishes of medical staff members. Healthcare firms thus encounter strong pressure from individuals who have little financial interest in the organization and whose financial interest may, in fact, be contrary to that of the healthcare firm.

## Controller

The controller facilitates approval of capital expenditures. The controller is usually responsible for developing capital expenditure request forms and for assisting department managers with preparing their capital expenditure proposals. The controller usually serves as an analyst, assisting the administrator with allocating the budget to competing departmental areas. In many small healthcare firms, the controller's function may be merged with that of the treasurer.

## Treasurer

The treasurer is responsible for obtaining funds for both short- and long-term programs. The treasurer may work with the finance committee to negotiate for funds necessary to implement approved programs.

### Learning Objective 2

Describe the kinds of decisions that are made in capital investment decision analysis.

## ▶ Classification of Capital Expenditures

A **capital expenditure** is a commitment of resources that is expected to provide benefits during a reasonably long period, at least 2 or more years. Any system of management control must take into account the various types of capital expenditures. Different types of capital expenditures create different problems; they may require specific individuals to evaluate them or special methods of evaluation.

The more important classifications of capital expenditures are as follows:

- Period during which the investment occurs
- Types of resources invested
- Dollar amounts of capital expenditures
- Types of benefits received

## Period of Investment

Determining the amount of resources committed to a capital project depends heavily on the definition of the period. For example, how would you determine the capital expenditures needed by a project that had a low initial investment cost but will have a significant investment cost in future years? Should just the initial capital expenditure be considered, or should total expenditures over the life of the project be considered? If the latter is the answer, is it appropriate just to add the total expenditures together, or should expenditures made in later years be weighted to reflect their lower present value? If so, at what discount rate? These are not simple questions to answer, but they are important when evaluating capital projects.

A classic example of this type of problem in the healthcare industry is the initiation of programs that have been funded by grants. In many such situations, there appears to be little or no investment of capital, because the amounts are funded almost totally through the grant. The programs thus appear to be highly desirable. However, if there is a formal or informal commitment to continue the programs for a longer period, capital expenditures and additional operating funds for later periods may be required. In such cases, it is imperative that the grant-funded projects be classified separately and their long-run capital cost requirements be identified. The healthcare facility may very well not have a sufficient capital base to finance a program's continuation. Thus, granting agencies should assess the healthcare facility's financial capability to continue funded programs after the grant period expires.

## Types of Resources Invested

When discussing capital expenditures, many people are apt to limit their attention to the expenditure or resources invested in **capital assets**, that is, tangible fixed assets. This narrow focus has several shortcomings, however, and may result in ineffective capital expenditure decisions.

First, focusing on tangible fixed assets implies ownership; yet, many healthcare facilities **lease** a significant percentage of their fixed assets, especially in the major movable equipment area. If a lease is not construed to be a capital expenditure, it may escape the normal review and approval system. Lease payments should be considered as a capital expenditure. Furthermore, the contractual provisions of the lease should be considered when determining the total expenditure amount. Weight should be given to future payments or to the alternative purchase price of the asset.

Second, the capital costs of a capital expenditure are only one part of total cost; indeed, in the labor-intensive healthcare industry, capital costs may be just the "tip of the iceberg." All of the operating costs associated with beginning and continuing a capital project should be considered. Programs with low capital investment costs may not be considered as favorable when their operating costs are taken into account.

**Lifecycle costing** is a method for estimating the cost of a capital project that reflects total costs, both operating and capital, over the project's estimated useful life. The lifecycle cost of all contemplated programs should be considered; failure to do this can cause errors in the capital decision-making process, especially in the selection of alternative programs. Consider, for example, two alternative renal dialysis projects; both may have the same capacity, but one may have a significantly greater investment cost because it uses equipment requiring less monitoring and lower operating costs. Failure to consider the operating cost differences between these two projects may bias the decision in favor of the project with lower capital expenditures and result in higher expenses in the long run.

## Amounts of Expenditures

Different systems of control and evaluation are required for different-sized projects. It would not be economical to spend $500 in administrative time evaluating the purchase of a $100 calculator. Nor would it be wise to spend only $500 to evaluate a $25 million building program. Obviously, control over capital expenditures should be conditioned by the total amount involved; and, if appropriate, the amount should be based on the total lifecycle cost.

Control of capital expenditures in most organizations, including healthcare firms, typically follows one of three patterns:

1. Approval required for all capital expenditures
2. Approval required for all capital expenditures above a preestablished limit
3. No approval required for individual capital expenditure projects below a total budgeted amount

Retaining final approval of all capital expenditures allows management to exert maximum control over the resource-spending area. However, the cost of management time to develop and review expenditure proposals is high. In most organizations of any size, management review of all capital expenditure requests is not productive. However, some review is needed, so a limit must be established. For example, a given responsibility center or department need not submit any justification for

individual capital expenditure projects requiring less than $2,000 in investment costs. In such cases, there is usually some formal or informal limitation on the total dollar amount of the capital budget that will be available for small-dollar capital expenditures. This prevents responsibility-center managers from making excessive investments in capital expenditures that have no formalized reviewing system.

Another form of management control over capital expenditures is an absolute dollar limit; that is, any responsibility center manager may spend up to an authorized capital budget amount on any items. The real negotiation involves determining the size of the capital budget that will be available for individual departments. However, this system, although least costly in terms of review time, does not ensure that the capital expenditures that are made are necessarily in the best interests of the organization.

## Types of Benefits

Depending on the types of benefits envisioned for a capital expenditure, different systems of management control and evaluation may be necessary. For example, investment in a medical office building results in different benefits than investment in an alcoholic rehabilitation unit. Such differences make it inappropriate to rely exclusively on any one method of evaluating projects. It is important to note that traditional methods of evaluating capital budgeting may not be appropriate in the healthcare industry. Traditional methods evaluate only the financial aspects of a capital expenditure. However, projects in the healthcare industry may produce benefits that are much more important than a reduction in cost or an increase in profit.

The following are major categories of investment in which benefits may be differentially evaluated:

- Operational continuance
- Financial
- Other

The first category of investment produces benefits that permit continued operations of the facility along present lines. Here, the governing board or management must usually answer the following two questions: (1) Are continued operations in the present form desirable? (In most cases, the answer is yes.) and (2) Which alternative investment project can achieve continued operations in the most desirable way (for example, with lowest cost, patient safety, and so on)? A classic example of this type of investment is based on a licensure requirement for installation of a sprinkler system in a nursing home. Failure to make the investment may result in discontinuance of operations.

The second category of investment provides benefits that are largely financial, in terms of either reduced costs or increased profits to the organization. Many people may believe that these two are identical, that is, that reduced costs imply increased profits. However, as we will determine, this may not be true if cost reimbursement for either operating or capital costs is present (as they would be for Critical Access Hospitals). The important point to remember is that if the major benefits are financial, traditional capital budgeting methods may be more appropriate.

The third category of investments is a catch-all category. Investments here would range from projects that activate major new medical areas (such as outpatient or mental health services) to projects that improve employee working conditions (such as employee gymnasiums). In this category, benefits may be more difficult to quantify and evaluate. Traditional capital budgeting methods thus may be appropriate only in the selection of least costly ways to provide designated services.

# ▶ The Capital Project Decision-Making Process

Making decisions that will form the basis on which capital projects will be undertaken is not an easy task. In many respects, this may represent the most difficult and important management decision area. The allocation of limited resources to specific project areas will directly affect the organization's efficiency and effectiveness and, ultimately, its continued viability.

### Learning Objective 3

Explain the four stages of the capital decision-making process.

For our purposes, we can divide the capital decision-making process into four interrelated activities or stages:

1. Generation of project information
2. Evaluation of projects
3. Decisions about which projects to fund
4. Project implementation and reporting

### Learning Objective 4

List some of the kinds of information that is needed to evaluate a capital investment project.

## Generation of Project Information

In this stage of the decision-making process, information is gathered that can be analyzed and evaluated later. This is an extremely important stage because inadequate or inaccurate information can lead to poor decision making. Specifically, there are six major categories of information that should be included in most capital expenditure proposals:

1. Available alternatives
2. Available resources
3. Cost data
4. Benefit data
5. Prior performance
6. Risk projection

## Available Alternatives

A major deficiency related to many capital expenditure decisions is the failure to consider possible alternatives. Too many times, capital expenditures are presented on a "take it or leave it" basis; yet there usually are alternatives. For example, different manufacturers might be selected; different methods of financing could be used; or different boundaries in the scope of the project could be defined.

## Available Resources

Capital expenditure decisions are not made in a vacuum. In most situations, there are constraints on the amount of available funding. This is the rationale behind capital expenditure decision making: scarce resources must be allocated among a virtually unlimited number of investment opportunities. There is little question that top-level management needs information concerning the availability of funding.

However, there is some question about its importance at the departmental level. On one hand, a budgetary constraint may temper requests for capital expenditures. On the other hand, it may encourage a department manager to submit only those projects that are in the department's best interests. These may, in fact, conflict with the broader goals and objectives of the organization as a whole.

## Cost Data

It goes without saying that cost information is an important variable in the decision-making process. In all cases, the lifecycle costs of a project should be presented. Limiting cost information to capital costs can be counterproductive.

## Benefit Data

We can divide benefit data into the following two categories: quantitative and nonquantitative. Some believe that much of the benefit data in the healthcare industry is nonquantitative. To a large extent, quantitative data are viewed as being synonymous with financial data. And because financial criteria are sometimes viewed as less important in the not-for-profit healthcare industry, the assumption is that quantitative data are also less important. This is not true. Quantitative data can and should be used. Effective management control is predicated on the use of numbers that relate to the organization's stated goals and objectives. It may not be easy to develop quantitative estimates of benefits, but it is not impossible. For example, assume that a hospital in an urban area opens a clinic in a medically underserved area. One of the stated goals for the clinic is the reduction of unnecessary use of the hospital's emergency room for nonurgent care. A realistic and quantifiable benefit of this project should be a numerical reduction in the use of the hospital's emergency room for nonurgent care by individuals from the clinic area. However, no quantitative assessments are either projected or reported; the only quantitative statistics used are those of a financial nature. The management control process in this situation is less valuable than it should have been.

## Prior Performance

Information on prior operating results of projects proposed by responsibility center managers can be useful. A comparison of prior actual results with forecast results can give a decision maker some idea of the manager's reliability in forecasting. In too many cases, project planners are likely to overstate a project's benefits if the project interests them. Review of prior performance can help a manager evaluate the accuracy of the projections.

It is generally acknowledged that most people requesting capital expenditure approval for their projects will overstate benefits (revenues) and understate costs. This type of behavior is not necessarily intentional, but may reflect sincere faith and interest in the project. Individuals reviewing proposals must recognize this inherent bias and also recognize that not all people make the same magnitude of errors in forecasts.

## Risk Projection

As the saying goes, nothing is certain in this world except death and taxes—especially when evaluating capital expenditure projects. It is important to ask "what if" questions. For example, how would costs and benefits change if volume changed? Volume of service is a key variable in most capital expenditure forecasts, and its effects should be understood. In some situations, requiring projections for the highest, lowest, and most likely projections of volume can help answer these questions. The same types of calculations can be made for other key factors, such as prices of key inputs and technological changes. This is an important area to understand, because some capital expenditure projects are inherently more risky than others. Specifically, programs with extremely high proportions of fixed or sunk costs are much more sensitive to changes in volume than those with low percentages of fixed or sunk costs.

## Evaluation of Projects

Although financial criteria are clearly not the only factors that should be evaluated while making capital expenditure decisions, there are few, if any, capital expenditure decisions that can omit financial considerations. Our focus is on the following two prime financial criteria: solvency and cost.

## Solvency

A project that cannot show a positive rate of return in the long run should be questioned. If implemented, such a program will need to be subsidized by some other existing program area. For example, should a hospital subsidize an outpatient clinic? If so, to what extent? This is the kind of policy and financial question the governing board of the organization needs to determine. The fairness of some patients subsidizing other patients is one of the basic qualitative issues in capital project analysis. Operation of an insolvent program eventually can threaten the solvency of the entire organization. Thus, organizations that plan to subsidize insolvent programs must be in good financial condition, and assessment of financial condition can be done only after the organization's financial statements are examined.

## Cost

Cost is the second important financial concern. An organization needs to select the projects that contribute most to the attainment of its objectives, given resource constraints. This type of analysis is often called cost-benefit analysis. Benefits differ from project to project. While evaluating alternative programs, decision makers must weigh the benefits according to their own preferences and then compare them with cost.

There is a second dimension to the cost criterion. All projects that are eventually selected should cost the least to provide the service. This type of evaluation is sometimes called cost-effectiveness analysis. Least cost should be defined as the present value of both operating and capital costs (methods for determining this are discussed later in the chapter).

## Decisions About Which Projects to Fund

At this juncture of the capital expenditure decision-making process, it is time to make the decisions. The decision makers possess lists of possible projects that may be funded. Each project should represent the lowest cost of providing the desired service or output. In addition, various benefit data on each project should be described. These data should be consistent with the criteria that the decision makers used in their capital expenditure decision making.

To illustrate this process, assume that the members of the governing board are deciding on how many, if any, of three proposed programs they will fund in the coming year. The three programs are a burn care unit, a hemodialysis unit, and a commercial laboratory. Assume further that the members have decided that there are only four criteria of importance to them:

1. Solvency
2. Incremental management time required
3. Public image
4. Medical staff approval

Because none of the three projects clearly dominates, it is not clear which, if any, should be funded. Thus, the decision makers must weight the criteria according to their own preferences and determine the overall ranking of the three projects. For example, one manager might weight solvency and management time highly, relative to public image and the medical staff, and thus select the commercial laboratory project. Another manager might weight medical staff and public image more heavily and thus select the hemodialysis or burn care unit project.

In this example, the three projects can be ranked in terms of their relative standing on each of the four criteria in **TABLE 19-1**, with 1 being best and 3 being worst.

## Project Implementation and Reporting

Most capital expenditure control systems are concerned primarily, if not exclusively, with analysis and evaluation prior to selection. However, a real concern should be focused on whether the projected benefits are actually being realized as forecast. Without this feedback on the actual results of prior investments, the capital expenditure control system's feedback loop is not complete.

The following are some of the specific advantages of establishing a capital expenditure review program:

- Capital expenditure review could highlight differences between planned versus actual performance that may permit corrective action. If actual performance is never evaluated, corrective action may not be taken. This could mean that the projected benefits might never be realized.
- Use of a review process may result in more accurate estimates. If people realize that they will be held responsible for their estimates, they may be more careful with their projections. This will ensure greater accuracy in forecast results.
- Forecasts by individuals with a continuous record of biased forecasts can be adjusted to reflect that bias. This should result in a better forecast of actual results.

## ▶ Justification of Capital Expenditures

In most healthcare organizations, there is a formal process for approval of a capital expenditure. Usually, a department or responsibility center manager initiates the process by completing a capital expenditure approval form. Both the approval form and the

**TABLE 19-1** Capital Project Ranking

| Criterion | Project | | |
|---|---|---|---|
| | Hemodialysis Unit | Burn Care Unit | Commercial Laboratory |
| Solvency | 2 | 3 | 1 |
| Management time | 2 | 3 | 1 |
| Public image | 2 | 1 | 3 |
| Medical staff | 1 | 2 | 3 |

approval process may vary across healthcare organizations, depending on the nature of the management control process in each case.

The approval provides a detailed summary of the following key aspects involved in capital expenditure approval:

- Amount and type of expenditure
- Attainment of key decision criteria
- Detailed financial analysis

In most firms, small capital expenditures are usually not subjected to detailed analysis and do not require justification. For example, capital expenditures of less than $2,000 may not be not reviewed under the formal capital expenditure process. This does not mean that a department has an unlimited capital expenditures budget if it spends less than $2,000 per item; the department is most likely subject to some overall level for small capital expenditures. For example, a department such as physical therapy might have an $8,000 limit on small capital expenditure items. No justification for capital expenditure items less than $2,000 would be required if the aggregate limit of $8,000 is not violated.

Replacement items are specially recognized. For example, a replacement expenditure less than $20,000 my not be subject to review. The rationale for this higher limit relates to the operational continuance of capital expenditures. Replacement expenditures are often viewed as essential to the continuation of existing operations. They are, therefore, not as closely evaluated as are expenditures for new pieces of equipment.

In any decision-making process, it is important to carefully define the criteria that will be used in the selection process. At a minimum, these criteria usually include:

1. Need (management goals, hospital goals)
2. Economic feasibility
3. Acceptability (physicians, employees, community)

An important point to recognize is that project selection usually involves the consideration of criteria other than financial criteria. Failure to collect data on the attainment of those additional criteria for specific projects often will lead to greater subjectivity in the process. Without relevant data, individuals may make inferences that are not legitimate.

A key aspect of the capital expenditure approval process is the financial or economic feasibility of the project. In most capital expenditure forms, there is some summary statistic that measures the project's overall financial performance. In general, such measures are usually categorized as either (1) discounted cash-flow methods (DCF) or (2) nondiscounted cash-flow methods. In the present discussion, we will not be concerned with nondiscounted cash-flow methods because they are usually regarded as less sophisticated than DCF methods.

*Learning Objective 5*

Calculate a project's net present value, profitability index, and equivalent annual cost.

# ▶ Discounted Cash-Flow Methods

In this section, we examine three DCF methods that are relatively easy to understand and use:

1. Net present value
2. Profitability index
3. Equivalent annual cost

Before examining these three methods, a word of caution is in order: In our view, the calculation of specific DCF measures is an important, but not a critical, phase of capital expenditure review. We strongly believe that the most important phase in the capital expenditure review process is the generation of quality project information. Specifically, the set of alternatives being considered must include the best ones; it does a firm little good to select the best 5 projects from a list of 10 inferior ones. As Peter Drucker, noted management expert, said, "It's more important to do the right things than to do things right." Beyond that, the validity of the forecasted data is critical; small changes in projected volumes, rates, or costs can have profound effects on cash flow. Determination of possible changes in both of these parameters is much more important than discussions about the appropriate discount rate or cost of capital where much of the current corporate finance literature exists.

Each of the previous three DCF methods is based on a time-value concept of money. Each is useful in evaluating a specific type of capital expenditure or capital financing alternative. Specifically, their areas of application are:

| Method of Evaluation | Area of Application |
|---|---|
| Net present value | Capital financing alternative |
| Profitability index | Capital expenditures with financial benefits |
| Equivalent annual cost | Capital expenditures with nonfinancial benefits |

## Net Present Value

A **net present value (NPV)** analysis is a useful way to analyze alternative methods of capital financing. In most situations, the objective in such a situation is clear: the commodity being dealt with is money, and it is management's goal to minimize the cost of financing operations. (We consider shortly how this goal may conflict with solvency when the effects of cost reimbursement are considered.)

The NPV equals discounted cash inflows less discounted cash outflows. When calculating the NPV, only **incremental cash flows** (i.e., the additional cash inflows and outflows that accrue as a result of taking on the capital project) should be considered. Nonincremental costs, such as sunk costs, should not be included in the cash flows. In addition, financing costs, such as interest expense, should not be included as a cash outflow as these costs are represented by the **discount rate**. When using NPV analysis to compare two alternative financing packages, the one with the highest NPV should be selected.

For example, assume that an asset can be financed with a 4-year annual $1,000 lease payment or can be purchased outright for $2,800. Assume further that the discount rate is 10%, which may reflect either the borrowing cost or the investment rate, depending on which alternative is relevant. (We will discuss the issue of an appropriate discount rate shortly.) The present value cost of the lease is $3,169. This amount is greater than the present value cost of the purchase, $2,800. With no consideration given to cost reimbursement, the purchase alternative is the lowest cost alternative method of financing.

In this era of prospective payment and capitation, the effects of cost reimbursement are declining for many providers, with the exception of designated critical access hospitals under the Medicare program. However, the effects of *cost reimbursement* should be considered, if applicable. Reimbursement of costs would mean that the facility would be entitled to reimbursement for depreciation if the asset was purchased, or the facility would be entitled to the rent payment if the asset were leased. (Some third-party cost payers limit reimbursement on leases to depreciation and interest if the lease is treated as an installment purchase.) Assuming that straight-line depreciation is used and that 20% of capital expenses are reimbursed by third-party cost payers, the present value of the reimbursed cash inflow would be as presented in **TABLE 19-2**. (Use the discount factors from Table 18-4.)

If the asset were purchased, the organization would pay $2,800 immediately. For each of the next 4 years, it would be reimbursed for the noncash expense item of depreciation in the amount of $700 per year ($2,800 ÷ 4). However, because only 20% of the patients are capital cost payers (i.e., patients who are covered by third-party payers who reimburse the facility for capital costs), only $140 per year would be received (0.20 × $700). If the asset were leased, the organization would be permitted reimbursement of the lease payment in the amount of $1,000 per year. However, because only 20% of the patients are capital cost payers, only $200 (0.20 × $1,000) would be paid.

The NPV of the previous two financing methods for considering cost reimbursement would be as presented in **TABLE 19-3**.

**TABLE 19-2** Present Value of Reimbursement

| | | Annual Reimbursement | | Discount Factor (10%) | | % of Cost Reimbursement | | |
|---|---|---|---|---|---|---|---|---|
| Present value of reimbursed depreciation | = | $2,800/4 | × | 3.170 | × | 20 | = | $444 |
| Present value of reimbursed lease payments | = | $1,000 | × | 3.170 | × | 20 | = | $634 |

**TABLE 19-3** Net Present Value of Financing Alternatives

| | | Present Value of Reimbursement (Cash Inflows) | | Present Value of Payments (Cash Outflows) | | NPV |
|---|---|---|---|---|---|---|
| NPV of purchase | = | $444 | – | $2,800 | = | –$2,356 |
| NPV of lease | = | $634 | – | $3,170 | = | –$2,536 |

In this example, it is clear that the best method of financing is outright purchase. By purchasing the asset, annual expenses will be $700 in depreciation, compared with $1,000 per year with the leasing plan. In addition, purchasing is also a plan that results in a lower NPV. Relative ratings regarding NPV could change quickly, however, given higher percentages of capital cost reimbursement. To see the impact of cost reimbursement on NPV, now assume that 80% of capital costs will be reimbursed. When this change is reflected in the calculations in Table 19-2, the lease NPV (–$634) is better (i.e., less negative) than the purchase NPV (–$1,025).

## Profitability Index

The **profitability index** method of capital project evaluation is of primary importance in cases when the benefits of the projects are mostly financial, for example, a capital project that saves costs or expands revenue with a primary purpose of increased profits. In these situations, there is usually a constraint on the availability of funding. Thus, those projects with the highest rate of return per dollar of capital investment are the best candidates for selection. The profitability index attempts to compare rates of return. The numerator is the NPV of the project, and the denominator is the investment cost.

$$\text{Profitability index} = \frac{\text{NPV}}{\text{Investment cost}}$$

To illustrate the use of this measure, let us assume that a hospital is considering an investment in a laundry service shared with a group of neighboring hospitals. The initial investment cost is $100,000 for the purchase of new equipment and delivery trucks. Savings in operating costs are estimated to be $20,000 per year for the entire 10-year life of the project. If the discount rate is assumed to be 10%, the following calculations could be made, ignoring the effect of cost reimbursement and using the discount factors. (See Table 18-4.)

$$\text{Present value of operating savings} = \$20,000 \times 6.145$$
$$= \$122,900$$

$$\text{NPV} = \$122,900 - \$100,000 = \$22,900$$

$$\text{Profitability index} = \frac{\$22,900}{\$100,000} = 0.229$$

Values for profitability indices that are greater than zero imply that the project is earning at a rate greater than the discount rate. Given no funding constraints, all projects with profitability indices greater than zero should be funded. However, in most situations, funding constraints do exist, and only a portion of those projects with profitability indices greater than zero can be accepted.

The previous calculations give no consideration to the effects of cost reimbursement. If we assume that 40% of the facility's capital expenses are reimbursed and 40% of its operating expenses are reimbursed, then the following additional calculations must be made:

$$\text{Present value of reimbursed depreciation}$$
$$= (\$100,000/10) \times 6.145 \times 0.40 = \$24,580$$
$$\text{Present value of lost reimbursement from operating}$$
$$\text{savings} = \$20,000 \times 6.145 \times 0.40 = \$49,160$$
$$\text{NPV} = \$22,900 + \$24,580 - \$49,160 = -\$1,680$$
$$\text{Profitability index} = -\$1,680/\$100,000 = -0.0168$$

The previous calculations require some clarification. We are adjusting the initially calculated NPV of $22,900 to reflect the effects of cost reimbursement. Depreciation is the first item to be considered. Because 40% of the facility's patients are associated with capital cost reimbursement formulas, it can expect to receive 50% of the annual depreciation charge of $10,000 ($100,000/10) or $4,000 per year as a reimbursement cash flow. The present value of this stream, $24,580, is added to the initial net present value of $22,900.

The second item to be considered is the operating savings. If the investment is undertaken, the facility can anticipate a yearly savings of $20,000 for the next 10 years. However, that savings will reduce its reimbursable costs by $20,000 annually, which means that 40% of that amount, or $10,000, will be lost annually in reimbursement. The present value of that loss for the 10 years is $49,160, which is subtracted from the initial NPV. The effect of cost reimbursement reduces increased costs associated with new programs, but it also reduces the cost savings associated with new programs.

The preceding example illustrates an important financial concept. (This concept is discussed further in Chapter 3.) When cost reimbursement exists, as it does for critical access hospitals under Medicare, there is less incentive to invest in projects that reduce costs. In the previous example, the laundry facility's profitability index decreased from 0.229 to –0.168 when the effects of capital and operating cost reimbursement were considered.

## Equivalent Annual Cost

Equivalent annual cost is of primary value when selecting those capital projects for which alternatives exist. Usually, these are capital expenditure projects that are classified as operational continuance or other.

The profitability index measure discussed previously is used for projects in which the benefits are primarily financial in nature.

**Equivalent annual cost** is the expected average cost, considering both capital and operating cost, over the life of the project. It is calculated by dividing the sum of the present value of operating costs over the life of the project and the present value of the investment cost by the discount factor for an annualized stream of equal payments (as derived from Table 18-4):

$$\text{Equivalent annual cost} =$$
$$\frac{\text{Present value of operating cost} + \text{Present value of investment cost}}{\text{Present value of annuity}}$$

To illustrate use of this measure, assume that an extended care facility must invest in a sprinkler system to maintain its license. After investigation, two alternatives are identified. One sprinkler system would require a $5,000 investment and an annual maintenance cost of $500 during each year of its estimated 10-year life. An alternative sprinkler system can be purchased for $10,000 and would require only $200 in maintenance cost each year of its estimated 20-year life. Ignoring cost reimbursement and assuming a discount factor of 10%, the following calculations can be made:

Equivalent annual cost of a $5,000 sprinkler system:

$$\text{Present value of operating costs} = \$500 \times 6.145 = \$3,073$$
$$\text{Present value of investment} = \$5,000$$
$$\text{Equivalent annual cost} = \frac{\$3,073 + \$5,000}{6.145} = \$1,314$$

Equivalent annual cost of a $10,000 sprinkler system:

$$\text{Present value of operating costs} = \$200 \times 8.514 = \$1,703$$
$$\text{Present value of investment} = \$10,000$$
$$\text{Equivalent annual cost} = \frac{\$1,703 + \$10,000}{8.514} = \$1,375$$

From this analysis, it can be determined that the $5,000 sprinkler system would produce the lowest equivalent annual cost, $1,314 per year, compared with the $1,375 equivalent annual cost of the $10,000 system.

Two points should be made regarding this analysis. First, the equivalent annual cost method permits comparison of two alternative projects with different lives. In this case, a project with a 10-year life was compared with a project with a 20-year life. It is assumed that the technology will not change and that in 10 years the relevant alternatives still will be the two systems being analyzed. However, in situations of estimated rapid technological changes, some subjective weight should be given to projects of shorter duration. In the previous example, this is not a problem, because the project with the shorter life also has the lowest equivalent annual cost.

Second, equivalent annual cost is not identical to the reported or accounting cost. The annual reported accounting cost for the two alternatives would be the annual depreciation expenses plus the maintenance cost. Thus,

Accounting expense per year ($5,000 sprinkler system)
$$= \frac{\$5,000}{10} + \$500 = \$1,000$$

Accounting expense per year ($10,000 sprinkler system)
$$= \frac{\$10,000}{20} + \$200 = \$700$$

Reliance on such information that does not incorporate the time-value concept of money can produce misleading results, as it does in the previous example. The second alternative is not the lowest cost alternative when the cost of capital is included. In this case, the savings of $5,000 in investment cost between the two systems can be used either to generate additional investment income or to reduce outstanding indebtedness. It is assumed that the appropriate discount rate for each of these two alternatives would be 10%.

Once again, the effects of cost reimbursement should be considered. In our example, we assume that 50% of the extended care facility's costs will be reimbursed. The following adjustments result:

Equivalent annual cost of a $5,000 sprinkler system:

Present value of reimbursed operating costs
$$= \$500 \times 6.145 \times 0.50 = \$1,536.25$$
Present value of reimbursed depreciation
$$= \frac{\$5,000}{10} \times 6.145 \times 0.50 = \$1,536.25$$

Equivalent annual cost of $10,000 sprinkler system (reflecting cost reimbursement):

Present value of reimbursed operating costs
$$= \$200 \times 8.514 \times 0.50 - \$851.40$$
Present value of reimbursed depreciation
$$= \frac{\$10,000}{2} \times 8.514 \times 0.50 = \$2,128.50$$

Equivalent annual cost (reflecting cost reimbursement)
$$= \$1,375 - \frac{(\$851.40 + \$2,128.50)}{8.514} = \$1,025$$

Again, some clarification of the calculations may be useful. To reflect the effect of cost reimbursement, the reimbursement of reported expenses for the two alternative sprinkler systems must be considered. The reported expense items for both sprinkler systems are depreciation and maintenance costs, which are referred to as operating costs. Depreciation for the $5,000 sprinkler system will be $500 per year ($5,000/10), and 50% of this amount ($250) will be paid for reimbursement each year. The present value of the reimbursed depreciation ($250 × 6.145) is $1,536.25. Using the same procedure, the present value of reimbursed depreciation for the $10,000 sprinkler system is $2,128.50 ($250 × 8.514). In a similar fashion, payment for reimbursement of the maintenance costs for the two sprinkler systems also will be made. For the $5,000 system, the annual $500 maintenance cost will yield $250 in new reimbursement (0.50 × $500) per year. The present value of this reimbursement inflow is $1,536.25. Using the same calculations for the $10,000 sprinkler system yields a present value of $851.40. The present values of both reimbursed depreciation and maintenance costs are then annualized and subtracted from the initially calculated equivalent annual cost to derive new equivalent annual costs that reflect cost reimbursement effects.

In this case, cost reimbursement did not change the decision. The lower-cost sprinkler system, after consideration of the effects of reimbursement, is still the best alternative.

---

### Learning Objective 6

Explain the concept of a discount rate and what the weighted average cost of capital is.

---

▶ ## Selection of the Discount Rate

In the three DCF methods just discussed, to specify the discount rate we arbitrarily selected a number for each of our examples. In an actual case, however, the issue of how to select the appropriate discount rate requires careful attention.

Before discussing methods of determining the appropriate discount rate, it may be useful to evaluate the role of the discount rate in project selection. A natural question at this point is, would an alternative discount rate affect the list of capital projects selected? For example, if we used a discount rate of 10% and later learned that 12% should have been used, would our list of approved projects change? The answer is maybe. In some cases, alternative values for

the discount rate would alter the relative ranking and therefore the desirability of particular projects.

Again, we believe that the definition of the discount rate is an important issue, but not a critical one—especially for healthcare organizations. This is true for several reasons. First, in the case of healthcare organizations, the financial criterion is not likely to be the only criterion. Other areas, such as need, quality of care, and teaching, also may be important. Second, a change in the relative ranking of projects is much more likely to result from an accurate forecast of cash flows than it is from an alternative discount rate. Efforts to improve forecasting would appear to be much more important than esoteric discussions about the relevancy of cost-of-capital alternatives.

In this context, we can examine three primary methods for defining a discount rate or the cost of capital for use in a DCF analysis:

1. Cost of specific financing source
2. Yield achievable on other investments
3. Weighted cost of capital

The *cost of a specific financing source* is sometimes used as the discount rate. Usually, the identified financing source is debt. For example, if a firm can borrow money at 8% in the bond market, that rate would become its cost of capital or discount rate.

Another alternative is to use the *yield rate* possible on other investments. In many cases, this rate might be equal to the investment yield possible in the firm's security portfolio. For example, if the firm currently earned 10% on its security investments, then 10% would be its discount rate. This method, based on an opportunity cost concept, is relatively easy to understand.

The last alternative is to use the **weighted average cost of capital (WACC)**. This is the most widely discussed and used method of defining the discount rate. The WACC is calculated as follows:

$$\text{Weighted average cost of capital} = [\text{Debt}/(\text{Debt} + \text{Equity}) \times \text{Cost of debt}] + [\text{Equity}/(\text{Equity} + \text{Debt}) \times \text{Cost of equity}]$$

The advantage of this method is that it clearly represents the cost of capital to the firm. A major problem with its use, however, is the definition of the cost of equity capital. This is an especially difficult problem for not-for-profit firms. How do you define the cost of equity capital? Detailed exploration of this issue and other aspects of discount rate selection are beyond the scope of the present discussion. Valuation methods are discussed in Chapter 20. Readers who are interested in examining these topics in greater depth are referred to any good introductory finance textbook.

## ▶ Valuation

It is becoming an almost everyday occurrence to read about one healthcare entity buying or acquiring another related healthcare business. Hospitals buy other hospitals, nursing homes, physician practices, durable medical equipment firms, and other types of businesses. Nursing homes buy other nursing homes, home health firms, and other businesses. Although there are many tasks that need to be accomplished in any business acquisition, one of the most difficult and most important is valuation. Exactly what is the value of the business being acquired?

Valuation is really a subset of capital expenditure analysis. The business being acquired can be thought of as a capital expenditure that needs to be evaluated just as any other capital expenditure made in the organization. Nonfinancial criteria should be considered, and the contribution that the acquired business will make toward the acquiring firm's mission must be addressed.

## ▶ SUMMARY

The capital decision-making process in the healthcare industry is complex, involving many independent decision makers. In this chapter, we examined the process and focused on methods for evaluating capital projects. Although capital expenditure decisions in the healthcare industry are not usually decided exclusively on the basis of financial criteria, most healthcare decision makers regard financial factors as important elements in the process. In that context, the three DCF methods we examined can serve as useful tools in capital project analysis for healthcare facilities.

## ASSIGNMENTS

1. A healthcare firm's investment of $1,000 in a piece of equipment will reduce labor costs by $400 per year for the next 5 years. Thirty percent of all patients seen by the firm have a third-party payer arrangement that pays for capital costs on a retrospective basis. Thirty percent of all patients also reimburse for actual operating costs. What is the annual cash flow of the investment? Assume a 5-year life and straight-line depreciation.

2. A hospital has just experienced a breakdown of one of its boilers. The boiler must be replaced quickly if the hospital is to continue operations. Should this investment be subjected to any analysis?

3. Few firms ever track the actual results achieved from a specific capital investment against projected results. What are the likely effects of such a management policy?

4. Santa Cruz Community Hospital is considering investing $90,000 in new laundry equipment to replace its present equipment, which is completely depreciated and outmoded. An alternative to this investment is a long-term contract with a local firm to perform the hospital's laundry service. It is expected that the hospital would save $20,000 per year in operating costs if the laundry service was performed internally. Both the expected life and the depreciable life of the projected equipment are 6 years. Salvage value of the present equipment is expected to be zero. Assuming that Santa Cruz Community Hospital can borrow or invest money at 8%, calculate the payback, the NPV, and the profitability index. Ignore any reimbursement effects.

5. Frances Gebauer, president of Lucas Valley Hospital System, is investigating the purchase of 36 computer game systems for rental purposes. The sets have an expected life of 2 years and cost $500 apiece. The possible rental income flows are presented in **TABLE 19-4**. If funds cost Lucas Valley 10%, calculate the expected NPV of this project.

6. Mr. Dobbs, administrator at Innovative Hospital, is considering opening a new health screening department in the hospital. However, he is concerned about the financial consequences of this action, because his board has indicated that because the current financial position of the hospital is not good, the project must pay for itself. Dobbs is thus especially interested in the establishment of a rate for the service and wishes to consult with you for your expert financial advice. He has prepared the cost and utilization data found in **TABLE 19-5** for your review. Dobbs is aware of the rapid pace of technologic change and anticipates that the current equipment, costing $350,000, will need to be replaced at the end of year 5 for $500,000. He is not concerned about price inflation for his other operating costs because he believes that the increased costs can be recovered by increased charges. However, he is concerned about establishing a current charge for the new service that will generate a fund of sufficient size to meet the year 5 replacement cost. Dobbs believes that any invested funds will earn interest at a rate of 8% compounded annually. Assume that all payments and receipts are made at year-end. What rate would you recommend charging for the new health screening service? Assume this rate to be effective for the entire 5-year period.

**TABLE 19-4**  Rental Revenues from Computer Game Systems

| Year 1 | | Year 2 | |
|---|---|---|---|
| **Rental Income** | **Conditional Probability** | **Rental Income** | **Conditional Probability** |
| $12,000 | 0.40 | $4,000 | 0.40 |
| | | 7,000 | 0.60 |
| | | 6,000 | 0.30 |
| $15,000 | 0.60 | 8,000 | 0.70 |

**TABLE 19-5**  Projected Costs of Health Screening Unit

| Year | Variable Cost | Fixed Costs* | Patients Screened |
|---|---|---|---|
| 1 | $96,000 | $120,000 | 2,400 |
| 2 | 144,000 | 135,000 | 3,600 |
| 3 | 192,000 | 150,000 | 4,800 |
| 4 | 192,000 | 150,000 | 4,800 |
| 5 | 192,000 | 150,000 | 4,800 |

*Includes annual depreciation of $70,000.

7. Scioto Valley Convalescent Center is considering buying a $25,000 computer to improve its medical record and accounting functions. It is estimated that, with the computer, operating costs will be reduced by $7,000 per year. The computer has an estimated 5-year life with an estimated $5,000 salvage value. What is this investment's profitability index if the discount rate is 8%? Ignore reimbursement considerations.

8. In problem 7, assume that costs are reimbursed 30%. Further assume that Scioto Valley is a tax-paying entity with a marginal tax rate of 40%. What is the profitability index for this project now?

## SOLUTIONS AND ANSWERS

1. The cash flow of the equipment investment by the healthcare firm will be equal to the annual reimbursed depreciation plus the reduced operating costs net of the cost reimbursement effect and may be calculated as follows:

Cash flow = Annual depreciation $\times$ Proportion of capital cost payers

+ (Annual operating savings $\times$ [1 − Proportion of operating cost payers])

= $200 $\times$ 0.30 + ($400 $\times$ [1 − 0.30])

= $60 + $280 = $340

2. The investment in a new boiler would benefit the hospital in the area of operational continuance. Failure to make the needed investment would mean discontinued service. In this case, less analysis is needed, but care still should be exercised when identifying alternatives. The lowest-cost alternative to meet the need should be selected.

3. If it does not compare actual with projected results, management may lose some of the benefits that were originally expected to be realized with its investment. If the control loop is not closed, management will not know, and therefore cannot correct for, deviations from forecasted results. It is also possible that some department managers will overstate benefits for their favorite capital projects and that such actions will not be perceived as having any adverse consequences, because no comparison of forecast with actual results was made.

4. The calculations in **TABLE 19-6** show the payback, the NPV, and the profitability index for the laundry service investment.

## TABLE 19-6  Laundry Alternative Analysis

Payback = Investment cost/Annual cash flow = $90,000/$20,000 = 4.5 years

Net present value = Present value of cash inflows – Investment cost

= $20,000 × P(8%, 6) – $90,000

= $20,000 × 4.623 – $90,000 = $2,460

Profitability index = Net present value/Investment cost = $2,460/$90,000 = 0.0273

5. The NPV of Lucas Valley's computer game system purchase project is shown in the data in **TABLE 19-7**.
6. The first step in determining the rate that Dobbs should charge for the new health screening service is to calculate the present value of the cash flow requirements that need to be covered by the charge for the service (**TABLE 19-8**). The second step is to define the rate that will generate the required present value as calculated in Table 19-8. If we define $r$ as the required rate per screening, the following calculation can be made:

$$\$1,255,929 = (2,400 \times r \times p[8\%,1]) + (3,600 \times r \times p[8\%,2])$$
$$+ (4,800 \times r \times p[8\%,3]) + (4,800 \times r \times p[8\%,4])$$
$$+ (4,800 \times r \times p[8\%,5])$$
$$\$1,255,929 = (2,400r[0.926]) + (3,600r[0.857]) + (4,800r[0.794])$$
$$+ (4,800r[0.735]) + (4,800r[0.681])$$
$$\$1,255,929 = 15,915.6r$$
$$r = \frac{\$1,255,929}{15,915.6}$$
$$r = \$78.91$$

7. The profitability index for the computer investment by Scioto Valley Convalescent Center is calculated as follows:

$$\text{Present value of cash in flows} = (\$7,000 \times p[8\%,5]) + (\$5,000 \times p[8\%,5])$$
$$= (\$7,000 \times 3.993) + (\$5,000 \times 0.681)$$
$$= \$31,356$$
$$\text{Profitability index} = \frac{\$31,356 - \$25,000}{\$25,000} - 0.254$$

8. The calculation of the profitability index for the computer investment in these new circumstances is computed here. The impact of cost reimbursement and income taxation has made this cost saving opportunity less beneficial.

Calculation of present value of cash inflows:

Operating savings

$$\$7,000 \times (1 - 0.30) \times (1 - 0.40) \times 3.993 = \$11,739$$

**TABLE 19-7** Expected NPV of Computer Game System Purchase

| Item | Amount | Year | Probability | Expected Value | Present Value Factor | Expected Present Value |
|---|---|---|---|---|---|---|
| Rental income | $12,000 | 1 | 0.40 | $4,800 | 0.9090 | $4,363.20 |
| Rental income | 15,000 | 1 | 0.60 | 9,000 | 0.9090 | 8,181.00 |
| Rental income | 4,000 | 2 | 0.16 (0.4×0.4) | 640 | 0.8260 | 528.64 |
| Rental income | 7,000 | 2 | 0.24 (0.4× 0.6) | 1,680 | 0.8260 | 1,387.68 |
| Rental income | 6,000 | 2 | 0.18 (0.6× 0.3) | 1,080 | 0.8260 | 892.08 |
| Rental income | 8,000 | 2 | 0.42 (0.6× 0.7) | 3,360 | 0.8260 | 2,775.36 |
| TV cost | (18,000) | 0 | 1.00 | (18,000) | 1.0000 | (18,000.00) |
| Expected NPV | | | | | | $127.96 |

**TABLE 19-8** Present Value of Cash Operating Expenses

| Item | Amount | Year | Present Value Factor (8%) | Present Value |
|---|---|---|---|---|
| Costs less depreciation | $146,000 | 1 | 0.926 | $135,196 |
| Costs less depreciation | 209,000 | 2 | 0.857 | 179,113 |
| Costs less depreciation | 272,000 | 3 | 0.794 | 215,968 |
| Costs less depreciation | 272,000 | 4 | 0.735 | 199,920 |
| Costs less depreciation | 272,000 | 5 | 0.681 | 185,232 |
| Replacement | 500,000 | 5 | 0.681 | 340,500 |
| | | | | $1,255,929 |

Reimbursed depreciation

$$\$4,000 \times 0.30 \times (1 - 0.40) \times 3.993 = 2,875$$

Depreciation tax shelter effect

$$\$4,000 \times 0.40 \times 3.993 = 6,389$$

Salvage value

$$\$5,000 \times 0.681 = 3,405$$

Total present value $24,408

$$\text{Profitability index} = \frac{(\$24,408 - \$25,000)}{\$25,000} = -0.0237$$

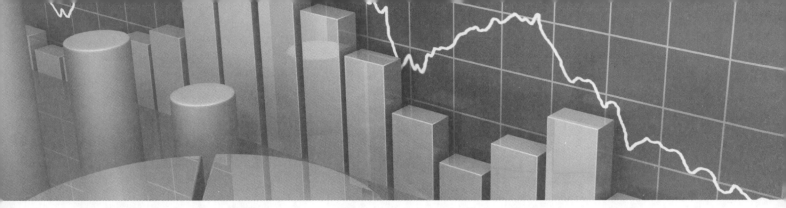

# CHAPTER 20

# Consolidations and Mergers

## REAL-WORLD SCENARIO

Jace Olin, CEO of Linworth Medical Center, has been approached by a major investor-owned hospital chain about a possible acquisition of one of their local hospitals. Jace knows that other hospitals in town have received similar overtures because the chain has made known their intent to sell this hospital within a year. The acquisition hospital, Orca Memorial, had been part of another investor-owned chain until 6 months ago when it was acquired by the present system in a stock swap arrangement. Orca Memorial does not meet the present system's criteria for ownership. It is the only investor-owned hospital in town, and it has experienced several years of declining profitability. Jace is very interested in acquiring this hospital because his major competitors have all been engaged in merger mania during the last 3 years. Jace's hospital is the only remaining nonaligned hospital in town. Jace's declining market share has hurt him at the negotiating table with major health plans. Although Jace is very interested in buying Orca Memorial, he is concerned about the possible price that he may have to pay to acquire the hospital. Jace's board is very conservative and does not want to expose the hospital to a burdensome level of debt or to erode their sizable cash reserve position. This situation has been made more complex by the current lack of profitability at Orca Memorial. Joel Thomas, the board chairperson at Linworth Medical Center, has told Jace on numerous occasions that he will examine the numbers very closely and will not approve any acquisition above a fair market value.

Jace's dilemma is just what is a "fair market value" given the historic lack of earnings. Jace believes that his management team could turn Orca Memorial around in 2 years and restore it to profitability, but Thomas is very skeptical about rose-colored projections of future profitability. Jace is examining the financial summary presented in **TABLE 20-1** for Orca Memorial, hoping to find a way to convince his board to move forward.

Opener image: © A1Stock/Shutterstock

**TABLE 20-1** Financial Summary for Orca Memorial

| Key indicator | Value |
| --- | --- |
| Hospital beds | 125 |
| Total operating revenue | $57,042,000 |
| Total expenses | $57,629,000 |
| Net income before tax | −$587,000 |
| Interest expense | 0 |
| Depreciation expense | $3,100,000 |
| Book value | $25,800,000 |

Strong evidence indicates that a $14 million bid would buy Orca Memorial. Olin believes that Orca is a "steal" at $14 million because the assets alone are valued at $25.8 million with no outstanding long-term debt. Olin has also learned that investor-owned chains are being valued at 1 to 1.4 times sales, which makes Orca Memorial worth $57 to $80 million. Earnings before interest, taxes, depreciation, and amortization multiples for investor-owned hospitals are averaging 6 to 7, which would create a valuation of $15.1 to $17.6 million. The more Olin examines the data, the more he becomes convinced that a bid of $14 million for Orca Memorial makes good economic sense. He is still concerned, however, about his ability to convince Thomas and the other board members that they should move forward with a bid.

It is becoming an almost everyday occurrence to read about one healthcare entity buying or acquiring another related healthcare business. Hospitals buy other hospitals, nursing homes, physician practices, durable medical equipment firms, and other types of businesses. Nursing homes buy other nursing homes, home healthcare firms, and other businesses. The way these firms combine is through acquisition, merger, or consolidation. The objective of this chapter is to define what is meant by consolidations, mergers, and acquisitions and to understand why they happen. The impact of these deals on shareholders (in the case of investor-owned firms) of both the acquiring and acquired companies is investigated, and the reasons some mergers succeed while others fail are examined. Finally, to determine the value of a firm, several valuation frameworks are provided.

### Learning Objective 1

Understand the terminology used in the field of consolidations, mergers, and acquisitions.

## ▶ Defining the Terms

Mergers and acquisitions (M&As) have long played an important role in the growth of firms. Growth is generally viewed as vital to the well-being of a firm. There are three basic ways to acquire another company:

1. Merger or consolidation
2. Acquisition of the stock of the target company
3. Acquisition of the target company's assets but not its corporate shell

In a **consolidation** two or more corporations combine into a brand new corporation. A **merger** is the combination of two or more companies, with one continuing as a legal entity while all others cease to exist; the former company's assets and liabilities become part of the continuing company. In both a merger and a consolidation, the surviving corporation has direct ownership of the assets and liabilities of the target company (or companies).

An **acquisition of stock** differs from a merger in two important respects. First, the target company remains in existence as a separate legal entity. Second, because the legal person (i.e., the target corporation) is still in existence, the acquiring company owns stock of the target, not the target's individual assets such as inventory, equipment, or land. In many respects this type of transaction is very similar to purchasing publicly traded stock in the open market, except the acquirer of the stock buys a majority of the outstanding shares.

An **acquisition of assets** is not exactly like either a merger or an acquisition of stock, but it is more similar to the former. Like a merger, the acquiring company ends up directly owning the target's assets. However, it may or may not directly have responsibility for liabilities. That depends on the terms of the bargain between the parties. Moreover, sale of assets does not directly affect the legal entity, the target corporation. The target corporation can either continue to exist or be liquidated. Thus, if assets, but not liabilities, are acquired and if the target's corporate shell remains as the holder of the funds given for target's assets, a merger and an acquisition of assets are similar but also meaningfully different. On the other hand, if all the assets and all the liabilities are acquired and if the target's corporate shell is liquidated and consideration from the acquiring company is distributed to the target's shareholders, a merger and an acquisition of assets are functionally identical.

There are several different types of mergers. **Horizontal mergers** involve two firms operating in the same kind of business. **Vertical mergers** involve different stages of production and operations, and **conglomerate mergers** involve firms engaged in unrelated business activity. Acquisition means that company X buys company Y and acquires control. An example of a horizontal acquisition is the purchase of Frye Regional Medical Center by Duke LifePoint Healthcare in 2015. An example of vertical integration is when a medical center purchases a skilled nursing facility when it previously did not offer such services.

When discussing M&As, a number of other terms are often used. **Leveraged buyouts** involve the purchase of the entire public stock interest of a firm, or division of a firm, financed primarily with debt. If the transaction is by management, it is referred to as a **management buyout**. If the shares are owned exclusively by the acquiring party (e.g., management) rather than by third-party investors, the transaction is called **going private**, and there is no market for trading its shares. **Joint ventures** involve the joining together of two or more firms in a project or even in a new company founded jointly by the two companies. In these cases equity participation and control are decided by mutual agreement in advance of the joint venture.

**Sell-offs** are considered the opposite of M&As. The two major types of sell-offs are spin-offs and divestitures. In a **spin-off**, a separate new legal entity is formed with its shares distributed to existing shareholders of the parent company in the same proportions as in the parent company. In contrast, **divestitures** involve the sale of a portion of the firm to an outside party with cash or equivalent consideration received by the divesting firm.

## ▶ M&A Activity

As with many industries, the healthcare industry long has reflected the belief that "bigger is better." Healthcare systems have existed for decades and continue to expand. **TABLE 20-2** shows that this trend has continued throughout the 2000s The number of acute care hospitals declined, whereas revenue increasingly was concentrated in the larger hospital segments.

In other healthcare sectors, M&A activity has differed significantly (**FIGURE 20-1**). Long-term care has continued to lead all healthcare sectors for M&A activity. The sector labeled "other" includes a variety of healthcare companies and services, such as urgent-care clinics, ambulatory surgery centers, and pharmacy benefit management. In sum across all sectors, however, consolidations have increased. Presumably, many of these mergers and acquisitions are creating

**TABLE 20-2** Number of Acute Care Hospitals by Annual Revenue, 2007–2014

| Annual Revenue | Number of Hospitals | |
|---|---|---|
| | 2007 | 2014 |
| < $25 million | 573 | 339 |
| $25–$75 million | 978 | 751 |
| $75–$150 million | 823 | 715 |
| $150–$300 million | 696 | 746 |
| $300–$500 million | 314 | 410 |
| > $500 million | 248 | 390 |
| | 3,652 | 3,476 |

Courtesy of Cleverley and Associates. (2016). State of the Hospital Industry. 2016 Edition, Worthington, OH, Cleverley & Associates.

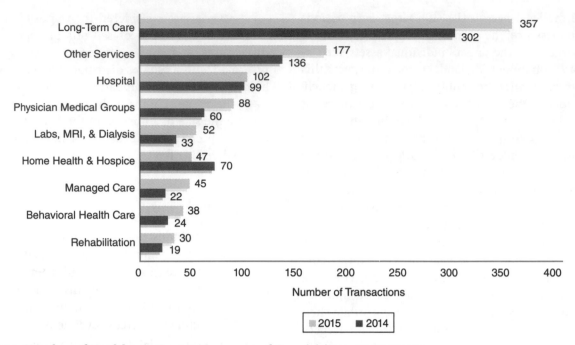

**FIGURE 20-1** **Number of Healthcare Sector Mergers and Acquisitions, 2014–2015**
Reproduced from The Health Care M&A Information Source. www.HealthcareMandA.com. March 2016.

larger integrated provider networks that are able to deliver more coordinated care in "bundled" or "episodic" care as a result of the Patient Protection and Affordable Care Act (ACA).

Some specific information regarding hospital industry M&A activity is presented in **TABLE 20-3**. The data show that 11 organizations announced two or more hospital acquisitions in 2015, which contrasts

| **TABLE 20-3** Companies Announcing Two or More Hospital Acquisitions in 2015 | | | |
|---|---|---|---|
| **Company** | **Number of Deals** | **Number of Hospitals** | **Number of Beds** |
| Prime Healthcare Services | 4 | 4 | 610 |
| LifePoint Health | 3 | 3 | 459 |
| University Hospitals Health System | 3 | 3 | 376 |
| Nobilis Health Corp. | 3 | 3 | 62 |
| Medical Properties Trust, Inc. | 2 | 9 | 1,330 |
| Prospect Medical Holdings, Inc. | 2 | 3 | 650 |
| Trinity Health System | 2 | 2 | 601 |
| UPMC | 2 | 2 | 571 |
| Community Health Systems, Inc. | 2 | 7 | 495 |
| BJC HealthCare | 2 | 2 | 443 |
| Carter Validus Mission Critical REIT II | 2 | 2 | 49 |

Reproduced from The Health Care M&A Information Source. www.HealthcareMandA.com. March 2016.

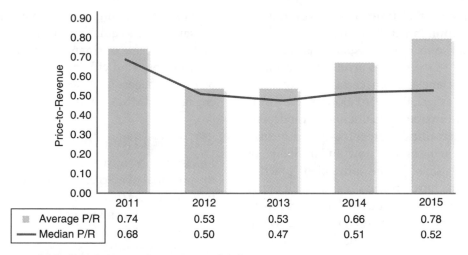

**FIGURE 20-2 Average and Median Price-to-Revenue Multiples, 2011–2015**

Reproduced from The Health Care M&A Information Source. www.HealthcareMandA.com. March 2016.

with 7 organizations in 2014. In addition, **FIGURE 20-2** shows the price-to-revenue values over 5 years averaging approximately 0.7; however, there was a significant drop between 2012 and 2014.

Accurate price to EBITDA (earnings before interest, taxes, depreciation, and amortization) multiples have been more challenging to calculate in the hospital market because the financial data reports tend to lag the announcements of deals. Revenue values, though, tend to fluctuate less than cash flow. Finally, some examples of the largest M&A hospital deals in 2015 are shown in **TABLE 20-4**.

Though partially offset by the Balanced Budget Relief Act, the Balanced Budget Act of 1997 put reimbursement pressure on many healthcare sectors, leading to deteriorating financial condition and less financial and operating flexibility. In 2008 and 2009 the stock prices of many publicly owned companies

**TABLE 20-4** Large Hospital Transactions, 2015

| Acquirer | Target | Price | Hospitals | Beds |
|---|---|---|---|---|
| Mediclinic International Ltd. | Al Noor Hospitals Group Plc | $2,300,000,00 | N/A | N/A |
| Ventas, Inc. | Ardent Health Services | $1,750,000,000 | 10 | 2,045 |
| Medical Properties Trust, Inc. | Capella Healthcare, Inc. | $900,000,000 | 7 | 1,169 |
| WellStar Health System | 5 Tenet hospitals | $661,000,000 | 5 | 1,004 |
| LCMC Health | West Jefferson Medical Center | $540,000,000 | 1 | 405 |
| Equity Group Investments, LLC | Ardent Health hospital operations | $475,000,000 | N/A | N/A |
| UnitedHealth Group Inc. | Hospital Samaritano | $350,000,000 | 1 | N/A |
| LifeBridge Health | Carroll Hospital Center | $250,000,000 | 1 | 193 |
| BlueMountain Capital Management, LLC | Daughters of Charity Health System | $250,000,000 | 5 | 1,563 |
| Tenet Healthcare Corporation | Aspen Healthcare Ltd. | $215,000,000 | 9 | N/A |

Reproduced from The Health Care M&A Information Source. www.HealthcareMandA.com. March 2016.

in the industry traded at all-time lows; however, stock prices began to rebound in 2009 to 2010.

In recent years some of the hospital mergers were severed by consent of the parties involved. The ability to realize cost efficiencies from certain mergers has been questionable, especially in situations where medical professionals are anxious to maintain their independence to determine medical protocols and treatments.

In certain markets there is now an "undoing" of previous consolidations. Some physician practice management groups have broken up as a result of the failure of management companies to deliver on promised business efficiencies. In the managed-care sector, health maintenance organizations have been accused of hampering the ability of physicians to deliver medical care, and a consumer and medical backlash against health maintenance organization business practices has been unleashed. At the same time, relatively new managed-care models, such as Accountable Care Organizations, have similar constructs. Many hospital consolidations have failed to realize the hoped-for efficiencies of management and operations, although, the negotiating position of these larger organizations has been enhanced on the revenue side.

However, despite the potential challenges of successfully integrating systems and cultures, significant health plan mergers still are occurring; the primary objective is market share capture. Providers continue to consolidate in order to increase negotiating leverage with payers, and payers continue to consolidate to create more power with providers. There may be limitations, however, as we have seen when the U.S. government sued to block the Anthem-Cigna and Aetna-Humana mergers to keep the "big five" insurers from becoming the "big three." Only time will tell how much consolidation will occur.

---

> ### *Learning Objective 2*
>
> Explain some of the possible reasons why consolidations, mergers, and acquisitions occur.

---

## ▶ Overview of Theories of M&A Activity

Numerous theories have been proposed to explain M&A activity and, more specifically, the reasons why M&As occur. Some of the reasons firms give for wanting to acquire or merge with another firm are to increase market share, to expand the firm's geographical reach, to expand quickly into new products or services, to gain immediate financial results (such as tax savings or to quickly grow revenue or earnings), or to gain strategic or financial synergistic effects. These theories focus on efficiency, synergy, and motivation of the managers and factors that influence them in engaging in M&A activity.

### Efficiency Theories

*Efficiency theories* are the most optimistic views about the potential of mergers for social benefits. By merging two companies there is a possibility of lower unit costs, stronger purchasing power, or gaining of management efficiencies. Economies of scale are an example of an efficiency that might be gained through a merger. The differential efficiency theory argues that there are differences in the effectiveness of management between companies. In theory, if the management of firm A is more efficient than the management of firm B, after firm A acquires firm B, the efficiency of firm B is brought up to the level of efficiency of firm A. Efficiency represents the real gain in merging businesses.

Efficiency theories also include the possibility of achieving some form of synergy. If synergy occurs, the value of the combined firm exceeds the value of the individual firms brought together by the mergers. This theory makes the assumption that economies of scale do exist in the industry and that before the merger, the firms were operating at a level of activity that fell short of achieving the potential for economies of scale. One potential problem in merging firms with existing organizations is the question of how to combine and coordinate the good parts of the organizations and eliminate what is not required.

### Information Theories

*Information theories* refer to the revaluation of the ownership shares of firms due to new information that is generated during the merger negotiations, the tender offer process, or the joint venture planning. This is explained in two ways. The first is the "kick in the pants" explanation where management is stimulated to implement a higher-valued operating strategy. The second is the "sitting on a gold mine" hypothesis where negotiations or tendering activity may involve the dissemination of new information or lead the market to judge that the bidders have superior information. The market may then revalue previously "undervalued" shares.

### Agency Problems

An *agency problem* arises when managers, or agents acting on behalf of the principals (all shareholders), own no shares or only a fraction of the shares of the firm. This partial ownership may cause managers to work less vigorously than otherwise and/or consume more perquisites (known as "perks"; examples are lavish trips, expense accounts, club memberships, etc.) because most owners bear most of the cost.

Two different types of theories emerge from the agency problem. Some believe that the threat of a takeover may mitigate the agency problem by substituting for the need of individual shareholders to monitor the managers. If the managers have a stake in the business, they will do what is best for the company, thus doing what is best for all shareholders. However, others argue that mergers may be a manifestation of the agency problem because managers are motivated to increase the size of their firms further and, consequently, adopt lower investment **hurdle rates**.

## Market Power

Another reason given for mergers is that they increase a firm's market share. In a horizontal merger, if a company acquires one of its competitors, then it will have a greater share of the market. Increased **market power** (resulting from increased market share) should permit the firm to achieve pricing leverage in its market. This means that the firm can either negotiate higher rates with managed-care firms or simply establish higher posted prices for its services. The government is very interested in merger cases where a potential for abuse of market power exists, and most mergers where this possibility exists are carefully reviewed for antitrust issues.

## Tax Considerations

*Tax considerations* are also involved in mergers. One example is where a firm is sold with accumulated tax losses. In some instances a firm with tax losses can shelter the positive earnings of another firm with which it is joined. Consequently, the acquiring firm gains value for its shareholders by paying less tax than it would have without the acquisition.

## ▶ Factors Affecting M&A Activity

To successfully complete a M&A transaction, a number of factors must come together: corporate will (the company's goals and strategy), funding, relative values of the two companies, and a conducive economic environment. Because these and other factors must be "in sync," there tend to be cycles in M&A activity.

Factors affecting M&A activity can be categorized as external and internal. *External factors* include monetary policy, general economic activity, political issues, and regulatory policy (competition policy, foreign investment policy). Monetary policy affects M&A activity because, generally speaking, when interest rates are high, stocks are out of favor (valuations are low) and well-funded companies can buy other companies at a good price. Low valuation multiples for stocks can also hamper M&As because the acquiring companies' currency, its own stock, may be depressed. The *internal factors* that can influence M&A activity, such as management capabilities and type of product, vary from company to company and from industry to industry. When one combines the internal and external factors, the result is an M&A cycle. The predominant influence at any one peak or trough may differ. However, typically a peak is a time when corporations have access to funds, valuations are low, interest rates are low, and bank financing is available.

## ▶ Why Do Mergers Succeed or Fail?

Any company contemplating an acquisition must familiarize itself with the simple facts that external growth is extremely competitive, and the probability of increasing its shareholders' wealth via M&A is low. In the case of mergers, the average return (around the time of the announcement) to shareholders of the acquired company is 20%, whereas the average return to the acquiring company is 0%. In the case where a tender offer for takeover has occurred (i.e., a company makes a public offer to the shareholders of a target company), the acquired company's shareholders receive an average return of 30%, whereas the shareholders of the acquiring company receive 4%.

Clearly, the acquired company's shareholders can expect significant returns, whereas the acquiring company's shareholders do not see the gains they might expect. Some research tends to paint a bleak picture with respect to the success of M&As. In an analysis conducted by McKinsey & Company consultants of 116 acquisition programs undertaken between 1972 and 1983, 61% were failures, 23% were successes, and 16% were unknown. (An acquisition was deemed successful if it earned its cost of equity capital or better on funds invested in the acquisition program. In other words, income after taxes as a percentage of equity invested in the acquisition had to exceed the acquirer's opportunity cost of equity.) If the successes and failures are probed further by looking at the rates by type of acquisition, a company acquiring another company in a related business has a greater chance of success than one acquiring a company in an unrelated business.

With statistics suggesting high failure rates of M&As, the question remains: Why do they fail? A number of reasons can be cited for the failure of acquisitions. Poor management and unfortunate circumstances (bad luck) are two such reasons. However, the most likely reason is that acquirers pay too much.

Companies overpay for a variety of reasons. One reason is that acquirers are overoptimistic in their assumptions. *Assumptions*, such as rapid growth continuing indefinitely, a market rebounding from a cyclical slump, or a company "turning around," can sometimes lead acquirers to overpay. A second possible reason is an *overestimation* of the synergies that the merged company will experience. One of the most difficult aspects of any merger is the integration of the two firms afterward. Suppose Company X is known for having a strong marketing department. Company Y takes over Company X and assumes in its valuation that it will be able to take advantage of this marketing strength. However, with the merger, key people from Company X exit the merged company, leaving the firm with a weaker marketing department than the acquiring company had hoped. The third possible reason for overpaying is simply that the acquiring company *overbids*.

In the heat of the deal, the acquirer may find it all too easy to bid up the price beyond the limits of reasonable valuations. A fourth possible reason is poor post acquisition *integration*. Integration can be difficult, and during this time relationships with customers, employees, and suppliers can easily be disrupted, and this disruption may cause damage to the value of the business.

*Learning Objective 3*

Understand common methods for valuation of a potential target firm.

# ▶ Valuations

Although many tasks need to be accomplished in any business acquisition, one of the most difficult and most important is valuation. Exactly what is the value of the business being acquired? In this section, frameworks are provided for numerous valuation methods. **FIGURE 20-3** provides an overview of the major valuation methods. These basic valuation methods can be used in any valuation circumstance, not only with respect to M&A activity. (The final section presents a model that highlights distinctions between the "standard" discounted cash flow valuation model and valuation in an M&A context.)

Valuation is really a subset of capital expenditure analysis. The business being acquired can be thought of as a capital expenditure that needs to be evaluated just as any other capital expenditure made in the organization. Nonfinancial criteria should be considered, and the contribution that the acquired business will make toward the acquiring firm's mission must be addressed.

Valuation of a business is not a scientific process that results in one objective measure of value. Different measures of value result for the following three reasons:

1. Different methods of valuation are used.
2. Different expectations regarding future performance of the acquired business are assumed.
3. Different values may be assigned by different prospective buyers.

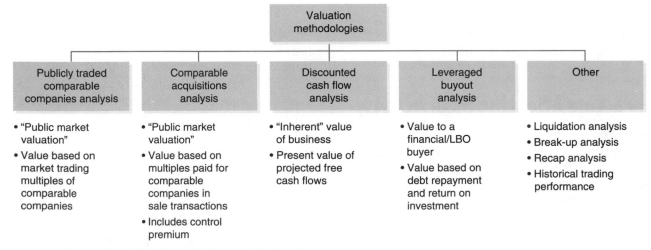

**FIGURE 20-3 Overview of Business Valuation Methods**

Before discussing the valuation methods in detail, descriptions of some general terms of valuation are helpful. The equity value of an investor-owned firm represents value attributable to the "owners" of the business (i.e., residual value after paying debt). The **market value** of a company's equity equals the product of the number of shares outstanding and the current stock price. The value of debt is typically assumed to be its market value (if observable). An organization's **enterprise value** (also termed *firm value* or *total value*) represents the value of all capital invested in the business, as follows:

Enterprise value = Market value of equity + Net debt

where

Net debt = Short-term debt + Long-term debt
(including current portion) +
Minority interest + Preferred stock +
Capitalized leases − (Cash +
Cash equivalents)

## Alternative Valuation Methods

In general, four major methods of valuation are often cited in practice:

1. Income/cash flow (discounted cash flow [DCF])
2. Asset based
3. Comparable sales
4. Breakup value

In the paragraphs to follow we explore these different valuation methods.

## Method One: Income/Cash-Flow Valuation

The most common methods of valuing healthcare firms are usually based on some projections of income or cash flow. The three most common methods are

1. Direct capitalization
2. Price earnings multiple
3. DCF

**Direct Capitalization Approach** In direct capitalization, a projected value for cash flow is determined. That number is then divided by some discount rate. The discount rate ideally represents the acquiring firm's cost of capital, but it is often adjusted up or down to reflect the risk of the business being acquired. For example, if a **durable medical equipment (DME)** firm was thought to have cash flow of $100,000 per year for the foreseeable future and the purchasing

firm's cost of capital was 12%, the value of the DME firm would be the following:

$$\text{Value of DME firm} = \frac{\$100,000}{0.12} = \$833,333$$

To reflect greater risk in the business, the discount rate could be increased to 20%. This increase would effectively reduce the value to $500,000. A preferable way to reflect risk, rather than adjusting the discount rate, is to conduct a sensitivity analysis on the forecast of cash flows. It is highly desirable to forecast at least the following three scenarios: most likely, pessimistic, and optimistic.

**Price Earnings Approach** A price earnings approach is similar to direct capitalization, except that it uses earnings rather than cash flow to discount, and multiplication rather than division is used. The key formula in this approach is as follows:

$$P_0 = \text{"Multiple"} \times EPS_1$$

where $P_0$ is the price of the share in year 0 and $EPS_1$ is the projected earnings per share in year 1.

In this valuation approach the multiple is the projected price to earnings (P/E) ratio. A P/E ratio for a company can be determined by looking for a similar company within the industry. A similar company is one that has similar operational characteristics (e.g., industry, product, markets, customers) and financial characteristics (size, leverage, margins, growth, etc.) as your target company. Remember the following guidelines when comparing companies: higher growth for a company results in a higher P/E ratio, and higher risk results in a lower P/E ratio. When comparing companies, if one company has higher financial leverage (all else equal), it will have a lower P/E ratio because financial leverage is related to increased risk. Similarly, a typical company in a high-growth industry will tend to have a higher P/E ratio (all else equal) than a typical company in a low-growth industry. **TABLE 20-5** presents price earnings multiples for selected firms in several major sectors of the healthcare industry.

Two major points should be made with respect to the data presented here. First, P/E multiples for future earnings are usually lower than for historical earnings. This is a direct result of **discounting**, because future earnings have lower value than current earnings and are also less certain. Second, differences in P/E multiples exist largely because of different expectations for future growth. In Table 20-5 Merck, a pharmaceutical company, has the highest trailing P/E multiple of any

**TABLE 20-5** Valuation Multiples—September 26, 2016

| | P/E Ratio Trailing 12 Months | Forward P/E Ratio (1 year) |
|---|---|---|
| Anthem (ANTM) | 14.46 | 11.61 |
| LifePoint Health, Inc. (LPNT) | 19.64 | 16.75 |
| Kindred Healthcare (KND) | 13.45 | 11.51 |
| Merck (MRK) | 34.15 | 16.83 |
| Dow Industrial | 19.62 | 17.69 |
| S&P 500 | 24.81 | 18.43 |

**TABLE 20-6** Tenet Healthcare Corporation Valuation (in Millions, except EBITDA multiple)

| | Fiscal Year Ending 12/31/15 |
|---|---|
| Net income | $76 |
| + Interest | 912 |
| + Income taxes | 68 |
| + Depreciation and amortization | 797 |
| EBITDA × | $1,853 |
| EBITDA multiple | 9.5 |
| Value | $17,604 |
| – Debt (Long-term + CMLTD) | $14,510 |
| Equity value | $3,094 |
| Tenet stock value (9/26/16) | $3,108 |

firm listed, which would suggest the market believes there is greater earnings growth for Merck than for other firms.

Assume that the previously mentioned DME firm had earnings (not cash flow) of $125,000. If the purchasing firm applied a P/E ratio of 8 to the earnings, the value would be the following:

Value of DME firm = 8.0 × $125,000 = $1,000,000

A variation of the price earnings multiple is EBITDA. The higher the EBITDA multiple, the greater the value assigned to the firm. It is important to note that using an EBITDA multiple provides an estimate of the total value of the business. To value the equity portion, the outstanding debt must be subtracted. **TABLE 20-6** illustrates this concept for Tenet, a national, investor-owned hospital company, under the assumption that its EBITDA multiple is 9.5.

**Discounted Cash Flow (DCF) Approach** DCF methods are most commonly used in healthcare firm valuations. The typical approach estimates cash flows for each of the next 5 years. These cash flows are then discounted to reflect the present value of the firm. The last remaining requirement is to estimate what the value of the acquired firm will be at the end of year 5, or whenever annual cash flows are no longer estimated. Generically, the value of a firm would be stated as follows:

Value = Present value of estimated future cash flows + Present value of terminal value

*Steps in the DCF Approach* In the DCF approach the value of a business is the future expected cash flow discounted at a rate that reflects the riskiness of the projected cash flows. This model is used to evaluate capital spending projects as well as entire businesses, which are effectively just collections of individual projects.

**Step 1. Calculate Cost of Capital.** The first step in a DCF analysis is to determine the cost of capital. The cost of capital is the minimum acceptable rate of return on new investments based on the rate investors can expect to earn by investing in alternative, identically risky securities. Using the acquiring company's target capital structure, the weighted average cost of capital is calculated. The weighted average cost of capital is generally a weighted average of the company's cost of debt (on an after-tax basis) and cost of equity. The acquiring company uses its own cost of capital only when it can be safely assumed that the acquisition will not affect the risk profile of the acquirer. If the acquisition will affect the acquirer's risk, then the discount rate must be adjusted.

**Step 2. Determine Free Cash Flows.** Cash flow is usually defined more broadly than net income plus depreciation for valuation purposes. Often, the term **free cash flow** is used. Free cash flow is typically used in the DCF calculation. "Free" refers to those cash flows that are available to stakeholders (e.g., equity and debt holders) after consideration for taxes, capital expenditures, and working capital needs. Cash flow should be considered as the cash flow contribution that the target is expected to make to the acquiring company. The following formula is used to calculate free cash flows:

$$\text{EBIT} \times (1 - t) + \text{Noncash expenses} -$$
$$\text{Capital expenditures} - \text{Incremental working capital}$$

where EBIT is earnings before interest and taxes and $t$ is the marginal tax rate of the firm. Noncash expenses include items such as depreciation and amortization. These are added back because they do not affect the company's cash position. Capital expenditures are purchases of fixed assets that are not reflected in the company's income statements but rather are accounted for through depreciation and amortization over the life of the asset. However, capital expenditures do represent cash outlays and are subtracted from EBIT. Incremental working capital is the amount of additional cash that will be tied up in items such as accounts receivable and cash required for the operations of the merged firm. Increased working capital is often estimated as a percentage of the increase in sales. It is subtracted from EBIT because it does not represent a "free" cash flow to the firm.

Most analysts think of depreciation plus net income as cash flow. Interest is added back in the previous concept of free cash flow to recognize that the business may be financed in a manner different from the way it is presently financed, and that financing is incorporated in the cost of capital. If a business was purchased and the existing debt of that business was assumed by the purchaser, then interest should not be subtracted because the interest expense would be a cash expense assumed by the buyer. In addition, any principal payments on debt would also be subtracted to derive free cash flow when the acquired firm's debt is being assumed. Capital expenditures are subtracted to recognize that businesses need to renovate and replace their physical assets if they are to stay in business, and this, in fact, represents a reduction of available cash flow. In the same manner, expenditures for working capital also represent a drain on available funds, or free cash flow. A buildup in accounts receivable means that not all of the firm's net income is available.

The free cash flows should be determined for a particular projected time frame. This time frame should extend to a time after which it is believed the company will experience constant growth. Five to 10 years is often used somewhat arbitrarily, but the exact time frame used should be tailored to the particular valuation scenario.

**Step 3. Calculate Present Value of Cash Flows.** Calculate the present value of the cash flows based on the determined cost of capital. This is a simple matter of discounting the amounts back to year zero. Generally, only one cost of capital is used throughout the entire forecast period, although it is possible that this value may change over the forecast period. Another assumption made in these calculations is that all cash flows occur at the end of the period.

**Step 4. Add Present Value of Terminal Value.** At this point, we have not accounted for the cash flows generated by the entity beyond the forecast period. To account for this, the present value of the **terminal value** is added to the present value of cash flows. The terminal value is the present value of the resulting cash flow perpetuity beginning 1 year after the forecast period.

The most common method calculates the discounted cash flow, assuming constant growth of cash flows. To do this calculation, the cash flow in the year following the forecast period is calculated. Assuming the terminal value of cash flow projections is year $T$, the terminal value (as of year $T$) is

$$\frac{CF_T \times (1 + g)}{K - g}$$

where $CF_T$ is the cash flow in year $T$, $g$ is the constant growth rate assumed for the firm beyond year $T$, and $K$ is the cost of capital.

Applying the direct capitalization method to cash flows is not the only way to construct a residual value. In some cases an estimate of the resale value of the firm might be used. Other methods might also be used in certain situations. The following point, however, is important: The residual value may be uncertain, and, as a result, some alternative scenarios should be tested. One value should never be accepted. Alternative valuations under different assumptions should be sought.

**Step 5. Subtract Debt and Other Obligations Assumed.** When valuing equity in a firm, it must be recognized that the shareholders, as owners of the firm, have an obligation to pay any debt holders. Consequently, repayment of these obligations (the market value of the debt and any other similar obligations) must be subtracted from the present value of the cash flows of the firm.

### Learning Objective 4

Apply analytical methods and tools to value potential acquisitions.

*Valuation Example* Suppose an analyst has been asked to assess the value of Meredith Dean Hospital. The analyst first determines the cost of capital for the hospital. The beta for Meredith Dean Hospital is 1.38. Assume that long-term risk-free interest rates are at 5.85%. Using the capital asset pricing model (CAPM) and assuming a market risk premium of 6%, the cost of equity ($K_e$) is calculated as follows:

$$K_e = K_f + \beta_{\text{Dean}} (R_m + R_f)$$
$$K_e = 5.85\% + 1.38 (6\%)$$
$$K_e = 14.13\%$$

The hospital can acquire debt at a rate of 8.50% and has a tax rate of 45%. Therefore, the cost of debt ($K_d$) is calculated as follows:

$$K_d = \text{Debt} \times (1 - t)$$
$$K_d = 8.50\%(1 - 0.45)$$
$$K_d = 4.68\%$$

Assume the hospital's balance sheet for the present year indicates a capital structure of 35% debt and 65% equity. Assuming this is also the target capital structure, the result is a weighted average cost of capital ($K$) calculated as follows:

$$K = (35\% \times 4.68) + (65\% \times 14.13)$$
$$K = 1.64\% + 9.18\%$$
$$K = 10.82\%$$

The next step for the analyst is to review the financial statements provided. From these financial statements the expected cash flows are projected. The EBIT can be estimated from past income statements.

Over the past 3 years (years 0, –1, and –2) Meredith Dean Hospital has experienced an annual increase in its EBIT of over 10%. The analyst assumes, based on industry data, that a growth level of 10% is sustainable for the next 2 years but beyond this period believes that a growth level of 2% is more reasonable. The analyst believes that with the growth this hospital will be experiencing over the next 10 years, new medical equipment will have to be installed in 3 years worth approximately $2 million with a depreciation rate of 30%. No other major capital expenditures are anticipated. However, it will be necessary for Meredith Dean Hospital to maintain its capital base. To do this, the analyst assumes that in all years other than year 3 the company will spend an equal amount on capital expenditures and depreciation. Working capital in the past 3 years has increased proportionately with increases in revenues. Therefore, the projected free cash flows for the next 5 years are as presented in **TABLE 20-7**.

Based on the calculated cost of capital of 10.82%, the projected cash flows are discounted back to the present year, year 0. The result is a present value of $8,103,065. The terminal value can now be calculated. The analyst believes that annual growth of 2% is sustainable for Meredith Dean Hospital beyond year 5. Therefore, the cash flow in year 6 is calculated by increasing the cash flow in year 5 by 2%. The resulting cash flow is $2,704,320 (1.02 × $2,651,294), which is the numerator in the following formula:

$$\text{Terminal value: } \frac{CF_T \times (1 + g)}{K - g}$$

| TABLE 20-7 Cash Flow Projections | | | | | |
|---|---|---|---|---|---|
| | **Year 1** | **Year 2** | **Year 3** | **Year 4** | **Year 5** |
| EBIT | 4,675,000 | 5,142,500 | 5,245,350 | 5,350,257 | 5,457,262 |
| EBIT ($1 - t$) | 2,571,250 | 2,828,275 | 2,884,942 | 2,942,641 | 3,001,494 |
| – Noncash expenses | 750,000 | 750,000 | 750,000 | 1,350,000 | 1,350,000 |
| – Capital expenditures | 750,000 | 750,000 | 2,000,000 | 1,350,000 | 1,350,000 |
| – Incremental working capital | 300,000 | 330,000 | 336,600 | 343,332 | 350,200 |
| Total FCF | 2,271,250 | 2,498,275 | 1,298,342 | 2,599,309 | 2,651,294 |
| Present value (at 10.82%) | 2,049,495 | 2,034,248 | 953,970 | 1,723,397 | 1,586,234 |

The result is a terminal value of $30,661,223 ($2,704,320/0.0882). The present value of this terminal value is $18,344,196 ($30,661,223 discounted at 10.82% for 5 years). The sum of the present value of the year 1 through year 5 cash flows and the present value of the terminal value is $26,691,539. The company's long-term debt is then subtracted, which according to Meredith Dean Hospital's balance sheet is $7,000,000. The analyst therefore has come up with a value for Meredith Dean Hospital of $19,691,539. These calculations are only the beginning of the analyst's work. The next step is to do some sensitivity analysis to test the assumptions made. Is the 10.82% discount rate appropriate? Is an ongoing growth rate of 2% reasonable in the hospital industry? After completing this analysis, the analyst will be left with a range of values based on different assumptions.

*Cost of Equity in Not-for-Profit and Private Firms* When valuing not-for-profit or private companies, it is difficult to estimate the cost of equity. There is no equity information to use for calculating the firm's beta. A common solution is to take an average beta of comparable publicly traded companies. Be careful, however, to "unlever" the betas of the public companies (using their respective debt-to-equity ratios) to arrive at their asset betas. Then, average the asset betas of the public companies and "relever" for the company being evaluated using its debt-to-equity ratio.

## Method Two: Asset-Based Valuation

Asset-based approaches to valuation rely on the availability of objective measures for the assets being acquired. Usually, three alternative asset-based valuation approaches are identified. One approach is simply to take the tangible **book value** of the acquired firm's assets. Although this method is objective, there is great doubt regarding the relevance of the resulting value. For example, consider a computed tomograph that was acquired 2 years ago at a cost of $700,000 that now has a book value of $500,000, which reflects 2 years of depreciation. The $500,000 value is most likely not a good measure of this asset's value to an acquiring firm.

A second asset-based method is to use the replacement cost of the assets. For example, assume that the computed tomograph in the previous example now has a current replacement cost of $1,400,000. Recognizing 2 years' worth of depreciation produces an adjusted replacement cost of $1,000,000.

| Current replacement cost | $1,400,000 |
| – Allowance for depreciation | 400,000 |
| Estimated replacement cost | $1,000,000 |

This estimate of value is useful for a firm that anticipated using the computed tomograph in the future. Replacement cost is often associated with "a going concern" basis of operation. A going concern basis simply means the business is expected to continue and will not be terminated. The acquired firm will continue to operate basically as it currently does, and therefore the existing capital assets will be needed.

The third asset-based approach assumes that the assets are not really needed and will be sold. For example, the computed tomograph referenced previously will be sold in a secondhand market for $600,000. This value is often associated with liquidation.

## Method Three: Comparable Sales Valuation

Comparable sales methods are widely used in real estate valuation. Real estate appraisers look at properties similar to the one being valued that have sold in that location during a recent time interval. This method of valuation is not often used for healthcare businesses because there are not enough comparable sales to make the valuation meaningful. Common rules of thumb based on sales around the country are sometimes used. Although these comparable sales values are useful, they usually are only a benchmark against which a calculated value is determined from an appraisal based on income or cash flow.

## Method Four: Breakup Value Valuation

Another way to value a company is by assessing its breakup value. In this method, the book value of the assets of the target company is added to the value of any hidden assets, such as real estate, brand names, and copyrights. The market value is then assessed for each piece if it were to be sold separately. There are a number of reasons the pieces sold separately might be worth more than the whole. These include hidden assets, improved earnings through cost savings, unused debt capacity or tax implications, or the division has not been carefully researched or followed. This approach attempts to determine what others would pay to gain control of each piece.

### Goodwill

It is also important to understand the term **goodwill**. Goodwill is defined as the price or value paid for a business less the fair market value of the **tangible assets** acquired. For example, assume that a hospital paid $4,000,000 for a 100-bed nursing home. All tangible assets of the nursing home would be appraised at fair market value. A piece of land may have a recorded cost of $100,000 on the nursing home's books, but its current market value might be $800,000. The fair market value of the land is $800,000. Alternatively, some equipment items might be reduced below their historical cost because they are no longer of value.

Goodwill is an intangible asset that, until recently, was amortized over future years. The next section describes a recent change in the accounting for goodwill. For example, assume that the fair market value of the acquired assets in the nursing home was $3,000,000. The amount of goodwill is $1,000,000 ($4,000,000 – $3,000,000) and would have been written off as a cost of operation in the future. Goodwill plus fair market value equals the price paid for the business.

## Accounting for Business Combinations

Until 2001 two methods were used to account for mergers: purchase accounting and pooling of interests. Under purchase accounting, target assets are reported at fair market value. Anything paid above this amount is considered goodwill. In July 2001, however, the Financial Accounting Standards Board issued Statement 141, Business Combinations, and Statement 142, Goodwill and Other Intangible Assets. Statement 141 requires that the purchase method of accounting be used for all business combinations initiated after June 30, 2001, effectively prohibiting the use of the pooling-of-interests method.

Pooling of interests allowed companies to ignore goodwill, instead combining all assets without recording the premium paid above fair market value of tangible assets. Management of acquiring companies often favored this method because of its simplicity and because of the avoidance of recording goodwill. Many accountants criticized the method, however, arguing

that it allowed corporations to make overpriced acquisitions without having to suffer the consequences in their earnings.

Statement 142 changes the accounting for goodwill from an amortization method to an impairment-only approach, meaning that the amortization of goodwill, including goodwill recorded from past business combinations, will cease upon adoption of that statement, which for companies operating with calendar year-ends will be January 1, 2002. Until this statement, accounting rules required companies to amortize goodwill assets over periods of up to 40 years.

## ▶ SUMMARY

The healthcare business environment is characterized by change, including the level of technology, reimbursement methods, and labor availability. The general trend in health care has been toward consolidation. Most healthcare managers today will be involved in some capacity with some type of consolidation, merger, or acquisition of another entity. Thus, they should understand why and how these acquisitions occur. Although purely financial considerations might not dominate the decision criteria, the financial implications of any possible deal must be considered. In that context, the valuation methods we examined can serve as useful tools in capital project analysis for healthcare facilities. Just as importantly, understanding how value will be added through the deal is critical to the success of the new, combined entity. Finally, remember that every type of consolidation involves change for the employees and customers or patients of all the affected firms. Thus, just as financial planning is important, so too is planning for the effects on the people involved. Managers must therefore be prepared to deal with numerous post-deal issues that invariably arise.

## ASSIGNMENTS

1. Two hospitals are considering merging their laundry departments and constructing a new facility to take care of their future laundry requirements. Relevant cost data are presented in **TABLE 20-8**.

   The new laundry facility will cost approximately $40,000 to construct and will be located between the two hospitals in a leased building. Average life of the equipment is assumed to be 8 years, which generates a $5,000 yearly depreciation charge. Lease payment is fixed at $3,000 per year for the next 8 years. Financing for the project will be generated from available funds in each institution: $12,000 from Hospital A and $28,000 from Hospital B. Expenses will be shared using the same ratios (30% and 70%, respectively). Both hospitals use a discount factor of 10% on their cost-reduction investment projects. Given this information, do you believe the merger is beneficial to both hospitals? What other information would you like to have to help you evaluate this investment project?

**TABLE 20-8** Laundry Merger Data

| | Hospital A | Hospital B | Merged C |
|---|---|---|---|
| Variable cost/pound | 0.030 | 0.032 | 0.024 |
| Pounds of laundry | 300,000 | 700,000 | 1,000,000 |
| Fixed costs/year | | | |
| Depreciation (lease) | $1,000 | $5,000 | $8,000 |
| Maintenance | 1,400 | 2,500 | 3,000 |
| Administrative salaries | 8,000 | 16,000 | 20,000 |
| Transportation | 0 | 0 | 3,000 |
| Total fixed cost | $10,400 | $23,500 | $34,000 |

2. In the preceding laundry merger problem, assume that Hospital B expects to replace its present equipment with new equipment in 2 years at a cost of $64,000. The equipment would have an 8-year life. Ignoring cost-reimbursement considerations, does the merger make economic sense for Hospital B under these conditions?

3. You have been asked to provide an estimate of the value for a nursing home that your client is interested in buying. Financial data and projections are presented in **TABLE 20-9**.

**TABLE 20-9** Projected Nursing Home Cash Flows

| | Year 1 | Year 2 | Year 3 | Year 4 | Year 5 |
|---|---|---|---|---|---|
| Net income | $2,000 | $2,200 | $2,400 | $2,700 | $3,000 |
| – Depreciation | 1,400 | 1,500 | 1,700 | 2,000 | 2,200 |
| – Working capital | 500 | 600 | 700 | 800 | 1,000 |
| – Capital expenditures | 4,000 | 4,000 | 5,000 | 300 | 300 |
| Free cash flow | ($1,100) | ($900) | ($1,600) | $3,600 | $3,900 |

Use an assumed discount rate of 10% to value the firm and assume that the fifth-year cash flow will carry into the future. After you have completed your valuation, what additional information or steps would you suggest to the client?

4. Assume that as of January 2, 20X2, Mountview Healthcare sold at $48.75 per share with 175,215,000 outstanding shares. This creates a market value of Mountview Healthcare shares of $8,541,731,000 ($48.75 × 175,215,000). Calculate the multiple of EBITDA that Mountview Healthcare is trading, assuming the values in **TABLE 20-10**.

| TABLE 20-10 Mountview Healthcare Valuation Data | |
|---|---|
| Net income | $285,964,000 |
| Interest | 771,000 |
| Income taxes | 170,205,000 |
| Depreciation and amortization | 94,458,000 |
| EBITDA | $551,398,000 |
| Debt | $38,970,000 |

## SOLUTIONS AND ANSWERS

1. The relevant data and calculations in the laundry service merger between Hospital A and Hospital B are presented in **TABLE 20-11**. Thus, given present data, the merger would be beneficial to Hospital A but not to Hospital B. A key piece of additional data that is needed is the replacement cost of the existing equipment. If Hospital B needed to acquire new equipment in the near future, the merger also might be favorable to it. The effects of cost reimbursement also should be considered.

| TABLE 20-11 Discounted Cash Flow Analysis of Laundry Merger | Hospital A | Hospital B |
|---|---|---|
| Cash outflow: unmerged | | |
| Variable costs | $9,000 | $22,400 |
| Maintenance | 1,400 | 2,500 |
| Salaries | 8,000 | 16,000 |
| Total | $18,400 | $40,900 |
| Cash outflow: merged | | |
| Variable costs | 7,200 | 16,800 |
| Lease | 900 | 2,100 |
| Maintenance | 900 | 2,100 |

| | | |
|---|---|---|
| Salaries | 6,000 | 14,000 |
| Transportation | 900 | 2,100 |
| | $15,900 | $37,100 |
| Net savings | $2,500 | $3,800 |

Hospital A: Present value of savings = $2,500 × P(10%, 8) = $2,500 × 5.335 = $13,337.50
Profitability index = $1,337.50/$12,000.00 = 0.111
Hospital B: Present value of savings = $3,800 × P(10%, 8) = $3,800 × 5.335 = $20,273
Profitability index = −7,727/28,000 = −0.276

2. The laundry merger project in these new circumstances requires use of the equivalent annual cost method. The alternative of a merger (**FIGURE 20-4**) has an 8-year life, whereas the alternative not including a merger (**FIGURE 20-5**) has a 10-year cycle.

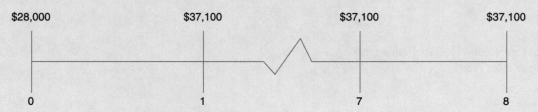

**FIGURE 20-4  Cost of Merger—Hospital B**

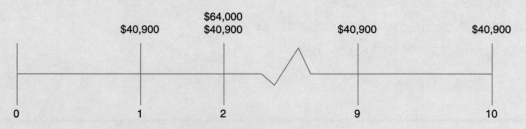

**FIGURE 20-5  Costs Unmerged—Hospital B**

Hospital B merged equivalent annual cost:

$$\text{Equivalent annual cost} = \frac{[\$37,100 \times P(10\%, 8)] + \$28,000}{P(10\%, 8)}$$

$$\text{Equivalent annual cost} = \frac{[\$37,100 \times 5.335] + \$28,000}{5.335}$$

$$= \$42,348$$

Hospital B unmerged equivalent annual cost:

$$\text{Equivalent annual cost} = \frac{[\$40,900 \times P(10\%, 10)] + [\$64,000 \times p(10\%, 2)]}{P(10\%, 10)}$$

$$\text{Equivalent annual cost} = \frac{[\$40,900 \times 6.145] + [\$64,000 \times .826]}{6.145}$$

$$= \$49,503$$

The alternative of a merger is now more desirable for Hospital B because it has a lower equivalent annual cost compared with the alternative that does not include a merger.

3. Using the data in Table 20-9 (along with the present value factors from Table 18-2) the estimate of value in **TABLE 20-12** results.

| **TABLE 20-12** Nursing Home Valuation | | | |
| --- | --- | --- | --- |
| **Present Value of Cash Flows** | **Amount** | **Present Value Factor** | **Present Value** |
| Year 1 | ($1,100) | 0.909 | ($1,000) |
| Year 2 | (900) | 0.826 | 743 |
| Year 3 | (1,600) | 0.751 | (1,202) |
| Year 4 | 3,600 | 0.683 | 2,459 |
| Year 5 | 3,900 | 0.621 | 2,422 |
| Present value of residual value cash flows after year 5 | $39,000 | 0.621 | $24,220 |
| Total value | | | $26,156 |

4. (EBITDA × Multiple) − Debt = Market value

($551,398,000 × Multiple) − $38,970,000 = $8,541,731,000

EBITDA Multiple: $8,580,701/$551,398,000 = 15.56

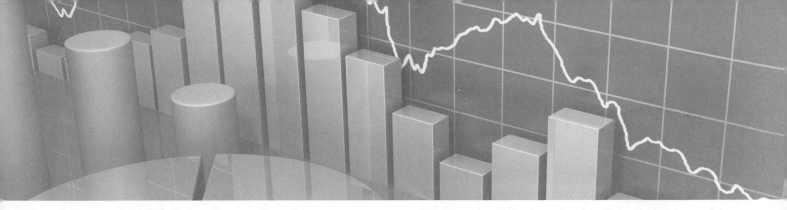

# CHAPTER 21

# Capital Formation

## REAL-WORLD SCENARIO

Michelle Marshall, CFO at Wrangler Medical Center, has been reviewing the center's most recent audited financial statements delivered that morning by the auditors. For the past year Wrangler Medical Center has been in violation of its debt service coverage ratio in the trust indenture related to its 2015 revenue bond financing. The required debt service coverage ratio in the trust indenture is 1.05, and Wrangler Medical Center's last fiscal year debt service coverage ratio was 1.01.

Marshall has known of the debt service coverage violation for some time, and in fact, she alerted the bond trustee to this issue 6 months ago. The bond trustee had two options available. First, they could have called the entire $80 million issue immediately, which would have forced Wrangler Medical Center into bankruptcy. Second, they could appoint an outside consultant to work with the hospital to correct the current debt service coverage deficiency. Fortunately, the trustee chose to appoint an outside consulting firm 3 months ago to work with Marshall and others on the hospital staff to correct the current cash-flow deficiency.

Marshall's concern was the auditor's treatment of the current noncompliance with its debt service coverage provision. The auditor could have qualified its opinion and reclassified the entire $80 million of long-term bonded debt to a current liability. Alternatively, the auditor could choose a footnote disclosure in the financial statements. Marshall was relieved to find that the auditor had chosen the latter alternative. The footnote in the most recent audited financial statement states that Wrangler Medical Center is in violation of their debt service coverage covenant, and that an outside consulting firm has been selected. The auditor then stated: "Accordingly, the 2015 revenue bonds have been classified as noncurrent liabilities in the accompanying balance sheet."

Marshall realizes that significant changes must be made to return the hospital to solvency, but she is confident that major strides can be made in the upcoming year to push their debt service coverage ratio above 1.05 and remove the operating constraints imposed by the bond trustee.

---

In this chapter we examine the concepts and principles of capital formation in the healthcare industry. Few areas are more important to the financial well-being of a healthcare firm. A firm that cannot obtain the amounts of capital specified in its strategic financial plan cannot achieve its long-term objectives. Indeed, if the firm finds it difficult to acquire any amount of capital at a reasonable cost, its future survival may be questionable. Successful firms have the capability to provide capital financing when needed and at a cost that is reasonable.

Two key questions are relevant to our discussion of capital formation in the healthcare industry. First, how much capital is needed? Ideally, the firm should have defined its capital needs in its strategic financial plan. Capital needs should include working capital

requirements and replacement reserves, as well as the funding needs for buildings and equipment.

Second, what sources of capital financing are available? Tax-exempt financing has been the largest source of capital for the hospital industry for the last 30 years, however, this source is available primarily to nonprofit facilities.

**TABLE 21-1** presents a summary of investment and financing patterns in the hospital industry for the years 2012 and 2014. Note the increase in equity financing during the period as long-term liability growth (2.6%) was exceeded by equity growth (22.5%).

In general, we can classify the sources of financing into the following two categories: equity and debt. Historically, the hospital industry has financed approximately 50% of total assets with equity and 50% with

**TABLE 21-1** Average Acute Care Hospitals' Consolidated Balance Sheet (in Thousands), 2012 and 2014

|  | 2012 | 2014 | % Change |
|---|---|---|---|
| Cash | $25,228 | $28,253 | 12.0% |
| Accounts receivable | $33,394 | $41,099 | 23.1% |
| Inventory | $3,280 | $3,702 | 12.9% |
| Other current assets | $14,064 | $18,736 | 33.2% |
| Total current assets | **$75,967** | **$91,790** | **20.8%** |
| Net property, plant, and equipment | $102,992 | $112,209 | 8.9% |
| Investments | $43,067 | $52,417 | 21.7% |
| Other assets | $27,503 | $31,648 | 15.1% |
| Total assets | **$249,527** | **$288,064** | **15.4%** |
| Current liabilities | $36,981 | $42,601 | 15.2% |
| Long-term liabilities | $74,953 | $76,886 | 2.6% |
| Equity | $137,594 | $168,577 | 22.5% |
| Total liabilities and equity | **$249,527** | **$288,064** | **15.4%** |

Courtesy of Cleverley & Associates

debt. The relative reduction in debt financing levels recently is a result of improving financial conditions in the industry. In addition, hospitals have increasingly relied on equity financing since the 2008–2009 market meltdown, when access to capital deteriorated. Even after access improved, hospitals have remained more cautious about issuing and maintaining the levels of debt that were present before the Great Recession.

In different sectors of the healthcare industry, however, financing patterns may vary somewhat. For example, many long-term care facilities have much higher proportions of debt. Debt financing in such facilities may run as high as 90%.

---

### Learning Objective 1

Explain the differences between debt and equity financing and the sources of each.

---

## ▶ Equity Financing

In general, a firm can generate new equity capital in one of three ways: profit retention, contributions, and sale of equity interests. We already have stressed the importance of earning adequate levels of profit. Hence, our discussion at this point is focused primarily on contributions and sales of new equity. A contribution may be given to a firm for a variety of reasons. Normally, in tax-exempt healthcare firms a contribution is given with no expectation of a future return. The donor may derive some immediate or deferred tax benefit, but there is no expectation of a financial return to be paid by the healthcare entity. In contrast, contributions are given to a taxable healthcare entity with the expectation of a future financial return. The contribution may be in the form of a stock purchase

or a limited partnership unit. It is important to note that this form of contribution also may be available to tax-exempt entities through a corporate restructuring arrangement. We discuss this point in more detail shortly.

*Philanthropy* is definitely not dead in our nation. In 2015 approximately 2.1% of our nation's gross domestic product, or $373.3 billion, was in the form of philanthropic gifts. **TABLE 21-2** and **TABLE 21-3** provide data showing the sources and the distribution of giving, respectively, for the years 1995, 2005, and 2015. These data present an encouraging picture. Total giving increased during the 20-year period from 1995 to 2015 on an inflation-adjusted basis by 95%. Individuals were clearly the largest source of giving, representing about 71% of total giving.

To be successful a major philanthropic program should have the following key elements:

- **Case statement**: This document should carefully and persuasively define why you need money.
- **Designated development officer**: This individual may not be a full-time employee, but duties and expectations should be precisely defined. Incentives for development officers should be related to expectations for giving.
- **Trustee and medical staff involvement**: People give to people, not to organizations.
- **Prospect lists**: You should know who in the community is a prime prospect for giving.
- **Programs for giving**: This is critical. You should have a variety of methods and means to encourage giving. For example, you may have a number of deferred giving plans, such as unitrusts, annuity trusts, or pooled-income funds. Your development officer should be familiar with these methods.
- **Goals**: You need to define realistic targets for long-range planning.

**TABLE 21-2** Sources of Giving (dollars in billions)

| | 1995 (inflation adj.) | % | 2005 (inflation adj.) | % | 2015 | % |
|---|---|---|---|---|---|---|
| Individuals | $147.4 | 77% | $268.0 | 76% | $264.6 | 71% |
| Bequests | 16.2 | 8% | 29.1 | 8% | 31.8 | 9% |
| Foundations | 16.4 | 9% | 39.3 | 11% | 58.5 | 16% |
| Corporations | 11.4 | 6% | 18.5 | 5% | 18.5 | 5% |
| Total | $191.5 | 100% | $354.9 | 100% | $373.3 | 100% |

Giving USA 2016: The Annual Report on Philanthropy for the Year 2015. Researched and written by Indiana University Lilly Family School of Philanthropy.

**TABLE 21-3** Distribution of Giving (dollars in billions)

| | 1995 | | 2005 | | 2015 | |
|---|---|---|---|---|---|---|
| | Giving (inflation adj.) | % | Giving (inflation adj.) | % | Giving | % |
| Religion | $90.3 | 47% | $110.3 | 31% | $119.3 | 32% |
| Education | 25.6 | 13% | 42.5 | 12% | 57.5 | 15% |
| Human services | 16.6 | 9% | 36.8 | 10% | 45.2 | 12% |
| Health | 27.9 | 15% | 24.7 | 7% | 29.8 | 8% |
| Arts and culture | 8.2 | 4% | 15.1 | 4% | 17.1 | 5% |
| Other | 22.9 | 12% | 125.6 | 35% | 104.4 | 28% |
| Total | $191.5 | 100% | $354.9 | 100% | $373.3 | 100% |

Giving USA 2016: The Annual Report on Philanthropy for the Year 2015. Researched and written by Indiana University Lilly Family School of Philanthropy. Sponsored by Giving USA Foundation, a public service initiative of The Giving Institute.

There are many ways to encourage people to give to charitable, tax-exempt healthcare firms. Many large firms employ full-time development staff. These individuals can do much to increase charitable giving.

One of the most promising areas of philanthropic giving is in deferred gift arrangements. In a deferred giving plan, a taxpayer donor may get an immediate tax benefit in return for a gift to be given to the tax-exempt firm later. An example of this is a **charitable gift annuity** or deferred gift annuity. A charitable gift annuity provides a way for a donor to make a contribution to a charity while ensuring a future income stream now or at some point in the future (in the "deferred" form). These arrangements represent a contract between the donor and the charity, in which the charity agrees to pay a fixed sum of money to the donor (or an individual the donor specifies) over a period of time in exchange for the current transfer of cash or other property. The person who receives payments is called the "annuitant" or "beneficiary." Typically, the annuitant is also the donor, but that is not always true. The maximum number of annuitants is two, and payments can be made to them jointly or successively. The payments are guaranteed by the charity's assets and are set at a fixed amount that will not change over time, regardless of market performance. For this reason the annuity rate is typically lower than that of an insurance or other investment vehicle. The benefits for the donor are three, (1) tax benefits for the initial contribution; (2) annuity payments, securing a fixed/future payment stream for living expenses; and (3) being able to support a charity of interest. The charity benefits from the initial gift can be used for operating, capital, or endowment projects; however, strong financial management is required to ensure proper use of the funds and care in meeting the obligations to donors. This form of giving is increasing as our society ages and more people create structured retirement and giving plans. While healthcare providers can use these and other forms of giving to help fund projects of interest, donors increasingly are using similar structures to arrange for financing of long-term care.

Both taxable and tax-exempt healthcare providers have shown great interest in the *issuance of equity* to investors. For taxable healthcare firms this interest is not new; for most such firms the issuance of equity has been a major source of financing over the years. Most taxable healthcare firms began with a small amount of venture capital. They were able to use that original funding to develop a successful track record of operations. Based on that record of success, an initial **public offering** of stock was made. The resulting funds were then used to expand operations, part of which was fueled by leveraging funds acquired during the initial public offering.

The technique of expanding operations quickly through the issuance of equity and then leveraging that equity through the issuance of debt has been used extensively in the taxable sector. **TABLE 21-4** illustrates the growth potential of a taxable entity.

These data indicate that a taxable entity could raise approximately 14 times the amount of total capital than

**TABLE 21-4** Capital Growth in Alternative Organizations

| Organizational Type | Historical Net Income | Equity Issue (Stock) | Debt Addition | Possible Total Capital |
|---|---|---|---|---|
| Tax-exempt | $1.00 | $0.0 | $2.0 | $3.0 |
| Taxable | $0.07 | $14.0 | $28.0 | $42.7 |

a tax-exempt entity. Let us examine these data and their related assumptions more closely to clearly understand the underlying process behind capital formation. It is assumed that some business unit or firm has generated $1 million in before-tax income. If the firm was a taxable entity, it is required to pay approximately 30% of this income as tax. However, the taxable firm could issue stock, limited partnership units, or some other type of equity security. Furthermore, it is assumed that a price-to-earnings multiple of 20 is in effect. This means that the taxable firm could raise $14 million in equity based on its net income of $700,000. Both the tax-exempt and the taxable firms could issue debt based on their equity positions. We have assumed that a leverage ratio of 2 to 1 exists; that is, the firms could borrow $2 for every $1 of equity. The taxable firm could issue $28 million in debt, whereas the tax-exempt firm would be limited to $2 million in debt. Total capital, both debt and equity, is $3 million for the tax-exempt firm and $42.7 million for the taxable firm.

In the preceding example some assumptions might be changed, but the relative growth potential would remain the same. In this situation, is there any way that a tax-exempt firm can take advantage of this growth potential? The answer is yes: a tax-exempt firm could change its status to taxable. This is not an easy thing to do, but it is not impossible. Several large health maintenance organizations (HMOs) started out as tax-exempt firms but changed their ownership status to maximize their growth potential.

An easier, alternative method is to restructure the firm. **FIGURE 21-1** presents a generic structure used by many tax-exempt healthcare firms to create an equity capital formation alternative. This structure involves the creation of taxable entities that can issue equity securities directly to investors. In the parent holding company

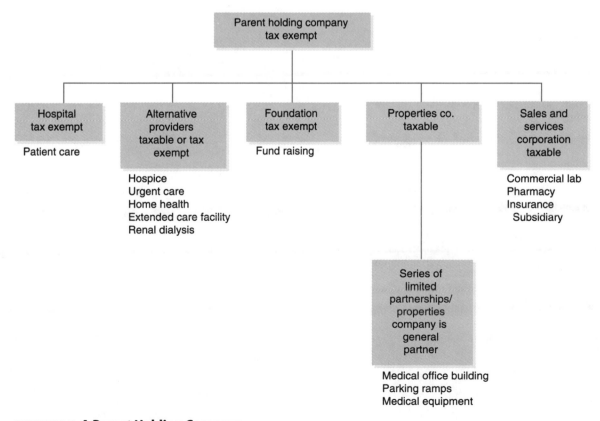

**FIGURE 21-1  A Parent Holding Company**

model in Figure 21-1, there are several taxable entities that could issue equity to investors and help generate capital for the entire consolidated structure.

An actual case example may help to illustrate the potential for capital formation created by restructuring a tax-exempt healthcare firm. ABC Hospital needed to replace its computed tomography (CT) scanner with a new one. The estimated cost of the new scanner was $1,160,000. The hospital did not wish to use any of its debt capacity for this project. The solution was to create a limited partnership and joint venture with its physicians. A new entity was created, called ABC Scanner, which was a limited partnership. The ABC Properties Company, which was a **subsidiary** of the hospital's parent holding company, was the general partner. A bank loan of $1,180,000 was obtained; the loan was guaranteed by the limited partners (30 limited partners) and the general partner. The source and use-of-funds statement for the new structure is presented in **TABLE 21-5**.

Table 21-5 documents the capability of the new structure to enhance ABC Hospital's capital position with little funding commitment from the hospital. The general partner, a member of the restructured healthcare entity, has contributed only $50,000 of cash and guaranteed $295,000 in loans. For this relatively modest level of commitment, total funding of $1,380,000 was made available. However, although the level of required capital was reduced, the expected future returns from the investment are also reduced because of the presence of physician limited partners.

*Learning Objective 2*

Explain the factors that influence the desirability of alternative sources of financing.

## ▶ Long-Term Debt Financing

An examination of the specific sources of long-term debt financing in the healthcare industry can be a complex and confusing process. Part of the problem stems from the use of jargon by those involved. Unless one is familiar with this jargon, meaningful communication

| **TABLE 21-5** Source and Use of Funds for CT Scanner | | |
|---|---|---|
| Sources of bank loan | | $1,180,000 |
| Guaranteed by | | |
| General partner | $295,000 | |
| Limited partners (@$29,500) | 885,000 | |
| General partner's cash contribution | | 50,000 |
| Limited partner's cash contribution (@ $5,000) | | 150,000 |
| Total sources | | $1,380,000 |
| Uses of funds | | |
| Purchase and installation of computed topography scanner | | $1,160,000 |
| Leasehold (suite) improvements | | 95,000 |
| Loan placement fee | | 35,400 |
| Legal and other organizational expenses | | 15,000 |
| Reserve for working capital | | 74,600 |
| Total uses | | $1,380,000 |

with financing professionals may be difficult. Before describing the alternatives for long-term debt financing in the healthcare industry, we should note five key characteristics of financing that greatly affect the relative desirability of alternative sources of financing. As we describe these characteristics, we introduce new terminology to facilitate later discussion. The five key characteristics are as follows:

1. Cost
2. Control
3. Risk
4. Availability
5. Adequacy

## Cost

Interest rates are the most important characteristic that affects the cost of alternative debt financing. The fixed return of a long-term debt instrument is often called the **coupon rate**. For example, a 7.0% revenue bond indicates that the issuer will pay the investor $70 annually for every $1,000 of principal. Sometimes the term **basis point** is used to describe differences in coupon rates. A basis point is 1/100 of 1%. For example, the difference between a coupon rate of 7.00% and 6.50% is 50 basis points.

Although interest is the primary measure of financing cost, it is not the only aspect of cost that should be considered. **Issuance costs** can be sizable in some types of financing. Issuance costs are simply those expenditures that are essential to consummate the financing. There is a great difference in the amount of issuance costs for publicly placed and privately placed issues. A privately placed issue is not sold to the general market but rather is purchased directly by only a few major buyers. In a publicly placed issue, a number of costs must be incurred to legally sell the securities to the general public. Printing costs are associated with producing the official statements that are sent to prospective clients. There are costs for attorneys and accountants who must certify various aspects of the issue, such as its financial feasibility and its tax-exempt status. Finally, there is the underwriter's spread that is charged by the investment banking firm that arranges the sale of the securities. The underwriter's spread represents the difference between the face value of the bonds and the price the underwriter or investment banker pays to purchase the bonds. When aggregated, issuance costs can sometimes amount to as much as 7% of the total issue. This means that an issuer must borrow $100 to get $93.

Another large cost of financing is **reserve requirements**. Some types of financing require the creation of fund balances in escrow accounts under the custody of the bond trustee. The bond trustee is designated by the issuer to represent the interests of the bondholders. The obligations of the trustee are defined in the Trust Indenture Act of 1939, which is administered by the Securities and Exchange Commission. There are two primary categories of reserve requirements. The first is the **debt service reserve**. This fund represents a cushion for the investors if the issuer gets into some type of fiscal crisis. It is usually set equal to 1 year's worth of principal and interest payments. The second category of reserve requirement is the **depreciation reserve**. This fund is sometimes set up to equal the cumulative difference between debt principal repayment and depreciation expense on the depreciable assets financed with debt. Usually, the amount of depreciation expense is greatest during the immediate years after a major construction program has been completed, when debt principal may be at its lowest level. Because depreciation may represent the primary source of debt principal payment, there is a need to accumulate these funds to ensure their availability in later years, when the amount of debt principal payment exceeds depreciation. **FIGURE 21-2** presents a graphic display of this relationship.

## Control

Ideally, when issuing debt financing, the issuer would like to have little or no interference in management by the investors. It is usually not possible to avoid such interference, however. The investors often specify some conditions or restrictions that they would like included in the bond contract. Such conditions or restrictions are often known as **covenants**. These are explained in great detail in the **indenture**, which is the written contract between the investors and the issuing company.

One category of restrictive covenants concerns specific financial performance indicators. For example, most indentures define values for the firm's debt service coverage ratio and its current ratio. If actual values for these indicators are below the defined values, the bond trustee may take certain actions. The trustee may assume a position on the board of trustees, replace current management, or require the entire outstanding principal to be paid immediately.

Another category of covenants concerns future financing. A section in the indenture referred to as **additional parity financing** defines the conditions that must be satisfied before the firm can issue any additional debt. The most important condition is usually prior and projected debt service coverage.

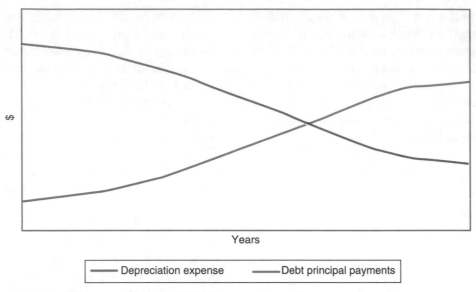

**FIGURE 21-2** **Depreciation Reserve Requirement: Relationship Between Depreciation Expense and Debt Principal Payments**

There is a trend developing in the issuance of tax-exempt bonds to replace the projected debt service coverage provision with a stated level of debt to equity. For example, the initial bond placement may specify that new financing can be issued if long-term debt does not equal a multiple of 1.5 times present equity or net assets. This would permit large healthcare systems more flexibility when issuing future debt and is more closely akin to provisions that exist in the corporate taxable debt markets.

## Risk

From the issuer's perspective, flexibility of repayment terms is highly desirable. An issuer with flexible repayment terms can alter payments to meet the issuer's current cash flow. The investor, however, wants some guarantee that the principal will be repaid in accordance with some preestablished plan.

One of the most important indenture elements is the **prepayment provision**. This provision specifies the point in time at which the debt can be retired and the penalty imposed for an early retirement. For example, the indenture may prohibit the issuer from prepaying the debt for the first 10 years of issue life. Thereafter, the debt may be repaid, but only if there is a call premium. The *call premium* is some percentage of the par or face value of the bonds. Thus, a call premium of 5% would mean that a $50 premium is paid for each $1,000 of bonds. The issuer would like to have the option of retiring outstanding debt at any point with no call premium. However, investors usually do not permit this for debt with a fixed interest rate.

Another aspect of risk relates to the debt principal amortization pattern. Most debt retirement plans can be categorized as **level-debt service** or *level-debt principal*. In a level-debt service plan the amount of interest and principal repaid each year remains fairly constant. This type of repayment is usually associated with home mortgages. In the early years the amount of interest is much greater than the debt principal. Over time, this pattern changes and the amount of principal repaid each year begins to exceed the interest payment. **FIGURE 21-3** presents a graphic view of a level-debt service plan.

Level-debt principal means that equal amount of debt principal is repaid each year. In this pattern of debt retirement, the total debt service payment decreases over time. **FIGURE 21-4** shows this relationship.

Many financing plans resemble a level-debt service plan. This pattern of debt amortization extends the debt retirement life and may benefit the issuer. The benefit is predicated on three factors:

1. The ability of the issuer to earn a return greater than the interest rate on the debt
2. The presence of reimbursement for capital costs
3. The availability of tax-exempt financing

To illustrate the desirability of principal repayment delay, we examine a simple case. Let us assume that we have two alternative financing plans. One plan permits us to borrow $10 million for 5 years with no payment of principal until the fifth year. We are required to pay 10% per year as our interest payment for each of the 5 years. The second financing plan permits us to borrow the same $10 million for

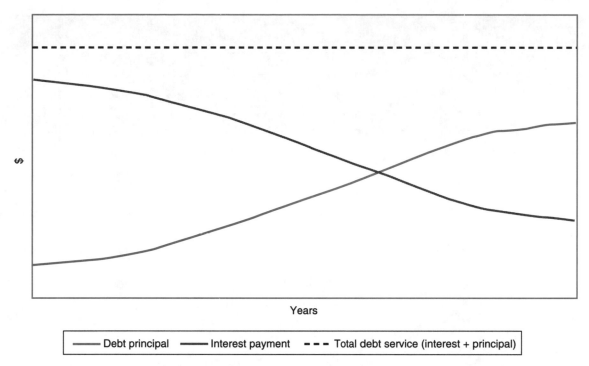

**FIGURE 21-3** **Level-Debt Service: Relationship Between Interest Payment and Debt Principal**

5 years; however, there is an annual payment of principal equal to $2 million per year. The interest rate on this financing plan is 8% per year, which is below the interest rate in the first plan. Let us further assume that 80% of our interest expense will be repaid by our third-party payers, who still pay us for the actual costs of capital incurred because this is a critical access designated hospital. Finally, let us assume that any differences in cash flow between the two plans could be invested at 10%.

**TABLE 21-6** provides a comparison of the net present values for these two financing plans. The values indicate that the higher-interest balloon payment plan is the lower cost source of financing. This is a direct result of the large percentage (80%) of capital cost payment. An 80% capital cost payment means

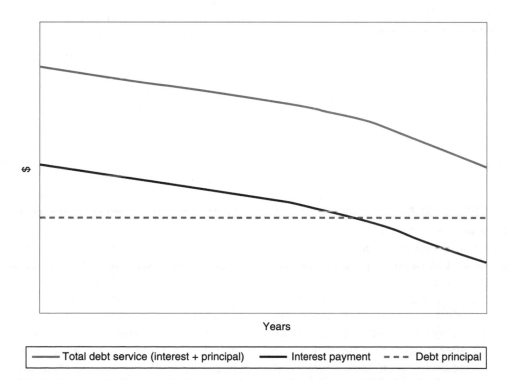

**FIGURE 21-4** **Level-Debt Service: Relationship Between Interest Payment and Total Debt Principal**

**TABLE 21-6** Cost of Alternative Debt Amortization Plans

| Item | Amount Before Reimbursement Effect | Amount After Reimbursement Effect | Years | Present Value Factor (10%) | Present Value |
|---|---|---|---|---|---|
| **Equal Principal Payment: 8%** | | | | | |
| Principal | $2,000,000 | $2,000,000 | | 3.791 | $7,582,000 |
| Interest | 800,000 | 160,000 | | 0.909 | 145,440 |
| Interest | 640,000 | 128,000 | | 0.826 | 105,728 |
| Interest | 480,000 | 96,000 | | 0.751 | 72,096 |
| Interest | 320,000 | 64,000 | | 0.683 | 43,712 |
| Interest | 160,000 | 32,000 | | 0.621 | 19,872 |
| Net present value cost | | | | | $7,968,848 |
| **Balloon Principal: 10%** | | | | | |
| Interest | $1,000,000 | $200,000 | 1–5 | 3.791 | 758,200 |
| Principal | 10,000,000 | 10,000,000 | 5 | 0.621 | 6,210,000 |
| Net present value | | | | | $6,968,200 |

that the effective interest rate is (1 – 0.80) times the interest rate. This means the effective interest rate for the balloon repayment plan is 2% and the corresponding value for the equal principal plan is 1.6%. The difference in interest rates has decreased from 2% to 0.4 of 1%. An investment yield of 10% means that we can make money from delaying principal payment. In short, our cost is less than our return. It is only natural to want to retain money as long as possible.

## Availability

Once a healthcare firm decides it needs debt financing, it usually wants to obtain the funds as quickly as possible. A delay can result in severe consequences and may postpone the start of a construction program. This might increase the cost of the total program because of normal inflation in construction costs. A delay also could result in an unexpected increase in interest rates. Although privately placed issues usually can be arranged more quickly than publicly placed issues, there is usually a higher interest rate associated with privately placed issues. However, the difference in interest rates may more than offset the costs of delay.

## Adequacy

A key requirement of any proposed plan of financing is that it covers all associated costs. One of the key areas of adequacy is that of refinancing costs. In many situations a new construction program that requires financing may not be possible unless existing financing can be retired or refinanced. Not all types of financing permit the issuer to include the costs of refinancing in the amount borrowed.

Funding during construction is another important area of financing. Some types of financing do not permit the issuer to borrow during the construction period. A loan is issued only after the construction has been completed and the new assets are available for operations. In this situation the issuer must arrange for a separate source of funding to finance the construction. Permanent financing must then be arranged upon completion of the construction program.

Interest incurred during construction can be sizable. For example, a $50 million construction program might incur $5 to $10 million in interest during the construction period. It is thus important to have a source of financing that permits the issuer to borrow to cover interest costs.

Finally, the percentage of financing available varies across financing plans. Some plans permit up to 100% of the cost, whereas others may limit the amount to 70 or 80%. Depending on the availability of other funds, these limitations may pose real problems in some situations.

# ▶ Alternative Debt Financing Sources

## Sources

Presently, the following four major alternative sources of long-term debt are available to healthcare facilities:

1. Tax-exempt revenue bonds
2. Federal Housing Administration (FHA)-insured mortgages
3. Public taxable bonds
4. Conventional mortgage financing

**TABLE 21-7** compares these four sources of financing regarding the factors that affect capital financing desirability.

## Tax-Exempt Revenue Bonds

Tax-exempt revenue bonds permit the interest earned on them to be exempt from federal income taxation. The primary security for such loans is usually a pledge of the revenues of the facility seeking the loan, plus a first mortgage on the facility's assets. If the tax revenue of a government entity is also pledged, the bonds are referred to as **general obligation bonds**. Because of the income tax exemption, interest rates on a tax-exempt bond are usually 1.5 to 2% lower than other sources of financing.

Most tax-exempt revenue bonds are issued by a state or local authority. The healthcare facility then

**TABLE 21-7** Comparative Analysis: Long-Term Debt Alternatives for Hospitals

| Program Characteristics | Conventional Mortgage | Taxable Bonds | Tax-Exempt Bonds | FHA 242 Mortgage Insurance Program* |
|---|---|---|---|---|
| Security | First mortgage given to lender; pledge of gross revenues (substantially all hospital assets pledged); generally requires an appraisal | First mortgage given to trustee bank for benefit of bondholder; pledge of gross revenue (substantially all assets pledged) | First mortgage or negative pledge if A rated or higher, given to trustee bank for benefit of bondholders; pledge of gross revenue (substantially all assets pledged) | First mortgage given to FHA-approved mortgage for benefits of HUD; pledge of gross revenue (substantially all assets pledged) |
| Timing for alternative | 2–6 months | 4–6 months | 3–6 months | 9–12 months |
| Percentage financing available | Usually 60–80% of eligible assets available to be pledged (as determined by appraisal) | Up to 100%, limited by available cash flow and available assets in some cases | Up to 100%, subject to available cash flow | 90% of value; up to 100% of cost |
| Construction financing | Normally required | Optional | Not required | Generally not required |
| Financing costs | Covers all costs of assets, excluding some movable equipment | Covers all cost | Maximum of 2% issuance cost covered by bond proceeds | Tax-exempt financing can include up to 2% of par amount; taxable has no reimbursement limitations |

*(continues)*

**TABLE 21-7** Comparative Analysis: Long-Term Debt Alternatives for Hospitals *(continued)*

| Program Characteristics | Conventional Mortgage | Taxable Bonds | Tax-Exempt Bonds | FHA 242 Mortgage Insurance Program* |
|---|---|---|---|---|
| Term of financing | 5–15 fixed balloon 20–25 amortization | 10–20 years (occasionally with balloon payment based on longer amortization) | 30–40 years depending on useful life of assets | 25 years fully amortizing starting after completion of construction, plus construction period |
| Front-end fees | 1–2% commitment fee subject to amount financed; other fees $5–$25,000 | 1–2% underwriting (private placement) or 2–4% underwriting (public offering); other expenses approximately 1/2 of 1% plus feasibility study | Generally no front-end fees | 0.80% filing fee, 0.5% insurance (FHA) fee, plus a maximum of 2.0% financing and 1.5% placement fees |
| Continuing annual fee | 1/8 of 1% servicing if multiple lenders | Trustee fees (nominal) | Trustee fees (nominal) | 0.5% FHA insurance fee; 0.25% GNMA fee |
| Prepayment provisions | Make whole provision with lender | Make whole provision or borrower pays higher rate for 10 year optional call feature | Normally no prepayment for 10 years | Normally 10 year no call |
| Required reserves | Usually none; depreciation reserve optional | None | Debt service reserve equal to 1 year's principal and interest (P&I); depreciation reserve equal to deficiency amount | A "Mortgage Reserve Fund" is required, to equal 1 year's debt service after 5 years and 2 years' debt service after 10 years—other reserves depending on taxable/tax-exempt structure may be required |
| Restriction on leasing | Yes; subject to cash-flow levels by covenant | None | None | None |
| Additional parity financing | Yes; normally subject to lender approval | Yes; subject to approval of underwriter or to provisions of financing agreement; normally required coverage of 110–150% | Yes; subject to meeting coverage requirement of 110–120% on both historical and pro forma basis | Generally, none allowed because the FHA mortgage requires a first lien; a very "soft" second mortgage is allowed; FHA has the Section 241 program to finance renovations secured by second mortgage liens |
| Payment reporting | Monthly lender(s) only | Quarterly reporting to bond trustee and other related parties | Quarterly reporting to bond trustee and other related parties | Monthly debt service payments to HUD-approved lender; annual financial statement reporting requirement |

*Debt can be issued taxable or tax-exempt

enters into a lease arrangement with the authority. Title to the assets remains with the authority until the indebtedness is repaid.

Congress has issued legislation that has begun to limit both the total amount of tax-exempt revenue bonds that can be issued and the purpose for which the financing can be used. For example, a hospital can no longer issue tax-exempt revenue bonds to finance the construction of a medical office building.

## FHA-Insured Mortgages

FHA-insured mortgages are sponsored by the Federal Housing Administration, but initial processing begins in the Department of Health and Human Services. Through the FHA program, the government provides mortgage insurance for both proprietary and nonproprietary hospitals. This guarantee reduces the risk of a loan to investors and thus lowers the interest rate that a hospital must pay. However, obtaining the appropriate approvals often can be a time-consuming process.

## Public Taxable Bonds

Public taxable bonds are issued in much the same way as tax-exempt revenue bonds, except that there is no issuing authority and no interest income tax exemption. An investment banking firm usually underwrites the loan and markets the issue to individual investors. Interest rates are thus higher on this type of financing than they are on a tax-exempt issue.

## Conventional Mortgage Financing

Conventional mortgage financing is usually privately placed with a bank, pension fund, savings and loan institution, life insurance company, or real estate investment trust. This source of financing can be arranged quickly but, compared with other alternatives, does not provide as large a percentage of the total financing requirements for large projects. Thus, greater amounts of equity must be contributed.

## Parties Involved

**FIGURE 21-5** is a schematic representation of the parties involved and their relationships when issuing a public tax-exempt revenue bond. This schematic also could be used to illustrate the process of issuing a public taxable bond. The only change would be the deletion of the issuing authority and addition of a line showing the direct issuance of the bonds by the healthcare facility.

The specific parties involved in financing a bond include the following:

- Issuing authority
- Investment banker
- Healthcare facility
- Market
- Trustee bank
- Feasibility consultant
- Legal counsel
- Bond-rating agency

## Issuing Authority

The issuing authority is involved only in tax-exempt financing. In most cases the issuing authority is some state or local governmental authority, which may be specially created for the sole purpose of issuing revenue bonds. The issuing authority serves as a conduit between the healthcare facility and the investment banker. In a public taxable issue or in a situation in which tax-exempt revenue bonds are issued directly by the healthcare facility, the role of the issuing authority may be eliminated.

---

### *Learning Objective 3*

Explain what an investment banker does.

---

## Investment Banker

In public or private issues **investment bankers** have a dual role. First, they serve as advisors to the healthcare facility that is issuing the bonds. In many circumstances they are the focal point for coordinating the services of the feasibility consultant, the legal counsel, and the **bond-rating agencies**. Their advice can be extremely important for obtaining timely funding under favorable conditions. Second, investment bankers serve as brokers between the market and the issuer of the bond. If investment bankers **underwrite** the issue, it means that they technically buy the entire issue and are at risk for the sale of the bonds to individual investors. If investment bankers place the issue on a *best-efforts* basis, they do not purchase the issue, and any unsold bonds become the property of the issuer.

## Healthcare Facility

The healthcare facility is the ultimate beneficiary of the bond issue. The healthcare facility is also responsible for repayment of the loan principal. The healthcare

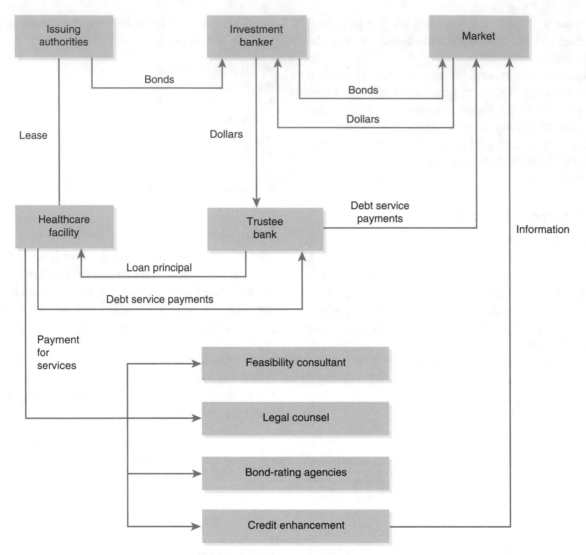

**FIGURE 21-5  Parties Involved in a Public Tax-Exempt Revenue Bond Issue**

facility's financial condition and its ability to repay the indebtedness are thus the central concerns of the investor. To provide evidence of its financial condition and the risk of the investment to the market, the healthcare facility usually employs independent consultants who assess various aspects of the facility. Such consultants include the feasibility consultant, the legal counsel, and the bond-rating agencies.

## Market

For any given bond issue the market may consist of a large number of individual investors or it may consist of a small number of large institutional investors. In any case the market purchases the bonds of the issuer with the expectation of some stated rate of return. The market also wants assurances that the bonds will be repaid on a timely basis and that there is not an unreasonable amount of risk.

## Trustee Bank

A trustee bank serves as the market's agent once the bonds are sold. Typically, the trustee bank is a commercial bank—in some cases the same bank at which the healthcare facility has its accounts. The trustee bank may receive the proceeds from the sale of the bond issue and deliver the monies directly to the hospital or to the contractor, as required. The trustee bank also receives the debt service payments from the healthcare facility and distributes these to the market or investors. It may retire outstanding bonds according to a prearranged schedule of retirement and hold additional reserve requirements deposited by the healthcare facility. Finally, the trustee bank ensures that the healthcare facility is adhering to the provisions of the bond contract or indenture, such as those concerning adequate debt service coverage and working capital positions.

## Feasibility Consultant

The feasibility consultant is usually an independent, certified public accountant who may or may not be the healthcare facility's outside auditor. The feasibility consultant's primary function is to assess the financial feasibility of the project and the ability of the healthcare facility to meet the associated indebtedness. Financial projections are usually made for a 5-year period. These projections provide a basis for the investor and the bond-rating agency to assess the risk of default.

## Legal Counsel

Legal counsel is needed for several reasons. First, in a tax-exempt revenue bond issue, the market is concerned with the legality of the tax exemption. If the interest payments are determined not to be tax-exempt by the Internal Revenue Service, the investors will suffer a significant loss. Second, legal opinion is necessary to ensure that the security pledged by the healthcare facility, whether it is revenue or assets, is legal and enforceable.

---

### *Learning Objective 4*

List the major bond-rating agencies and explain their role in the debt market.

---

## Bond-Rating Agencies

Moody's, Standard & Poor's, and Fitch are the three primary bond-rating agencies, although other smaller agencies exist. By some estimates, Moody's and Standard & Poor's hold roughly 80% of the global market share. The primary function of a bond-rating agency is to assess the relative risk associated with a given bond issue. The agencies have developed detailed coding systems to assess risk (**TABLE 21-8**). The resulting bond rating has important implications. First, there is a definite correlation between the interest rate that an **issuer** must pay and the bond rating associated with the issue. Generally speaking, the higher the bond rating, the lower the interest rate. Thus, a bond rated AAA by Standard & Poor's is likely to have a much lower rate of interest than one rated BBB. Second, issues rated below BBB by Standard & Poor's or Baa by Moody's are not classified as **investment grade**. Many institutional investors are prohibited from investing in bonds that carry a rating lower than investment grade. Thus, the market for such issues is likely to be small.

**TABLE 21-8** Bond Ratings

| Classification | Moody's | Standard & Poor's |
|---|---|---|
| Investment grade | Aaa | AAA |
| | Aa | AA |
| | A | A |
| | Baa | BBB |
| Not investment grade | Ba | BB |
| | B | B |
| | Caa | CCC |
| | Ca | CC |
| | C | C |

Moody's assigns subcategory ratings of 1, 2, and 3. A Baa rating would be at the higher end of the rating and the modifier 3 would be at the lower end. Standard and Poor's uses plus and minus modifiers for their rating categories.

## Credit Enhancement

*Credit enhancement* is a term that has come into use in the healthcare financing field only recently. A credit enhancement device is simply a mechanism by which the risk of default can be shifted from the issuer to a third party. Thus, the FHA-insured mortgage program provides a form of credit enhancement.

The **municipal bond insurance** industry collapsed in 2008–2009 as a result of the mortgage loan securitization debacle. Before September 2008 there were seven AAA-rated bond insurers that were active in both the new issue and secondary traded bond markets. Investors purchasing insured tax-exempt bonds often disregarded the underlying credit strength (or weakness) of the hospital being insured and relied almost exclusively on the bond insurer's guarantee of repayment. After the mortgage-backed market meltdown in late 2008 and 2009, the bond-rating agencies lowered ratings on all seven insurers. For certain cases the ratings were lowered to below investment grade. This debacle in the bond insurance industry had a devastating impact on hospitals. Where bond insurers were used for fixed-rate issuances, the investors who purchased those bonds took a huge market valuation decline. Where hospitals issued variable-rate debt supported by bond insurance, it required the hospital to refinance into other fixed-rate structures. This failure of bond insurers to maintain their AAA ratings and credibility in the market cost U.S. not-for-profit hospitals hundreds of millions of dollars.

The other form of credit enhancement is an *irrevocable letter of credit* from a highly rated U.S. or foreign bank. The letter of credit market, like bond insurers, also underwent massive bond-rating declines making the letters of credit issue, in many cases, worthless and thus drawing up the interest rates needed to "market" the bonds. Credit enhancement now represents a very small percentage of all new hospital issues. Before 2008, credit enhancement accounted for over 60% of all new issuances. At the time of publication, that figure stands at less than 10%. Beyond the difficulty in the bond insurance market, the primary reason credit enhancement is not being utilized is due to the current low cost of borrowing across risk levels. In a higher interest rate environment, there is a greater differential on the cost of borrowing for a higher-risk provider. Because the relative costs of borrowing are lower, the provider paying a premium for credit enhancement is not justified.

## ▶ More Recent Developments

The following four more recent modifications in the traditional sources of long-term debt should be noted at this juncture:

1. Variable-rate financing
2. Pooled or shared financing
3. Zero-coupon and original issue discount bonds
4. Interest rate swaps

### Variable-Rate Financing

Before the 2008–2009 market meltdown in the healthcare sector, as well as in other industries, there had been a shift to the use of *variable-rate financing*. In variable-rate financing the outstanding debt principal is fixed, but the interest rate on the principal is variable. This contrasts with the traditional situation in which the interest rate is fixed for the life of the bonds.

Variable-rate financing requires that the interest rate be adjusted periodically—in some cases, weekly—to a current market index.

A feature that is often associated with variable-rate financing is the use of a **tender option** or *put*. A tender option or put permits investors to redeem their bonds at some predetermined interval—perhaps daily—at

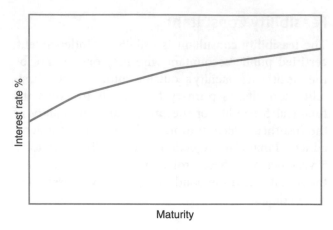

**FIGURE 21-6** **The Yield Curve**

the face value. In reality, this type of financing is short term, not long term. As a result the interest rate may be significantly below a comparable long-term rate at the initiation of the financing. Many firms—not just healthcare firms—have opted to use variable-rate financing to achieve a lower cost of financing. Sometimes this strategy is referred to as "moving down the yield curve." **FIGURE 21-6** shows a typical upward-sloping yield curve.

### Pooled Financing

In the healthcare sector there has been increasing interest in developing financing packages that encompass more than one entity. The major rationale for this interest lies in the relationship between size and cost of debt; larger organizations are better able to obtain debt capital and to realize lower costs of financing.

In general, there are three ways in which pooled or shared arrangements have been created in the healthcare sector. The first is through the use of **master indenture financing** by healthcare systems. In such cases master indenture financing means that the debt is guaranteed by all members who are a part of the master indenture. For example, a system of 10 hospitals could finance through a master indenture arrangement in which all 10 hospitals, or some subset of the 10 hospitals, would be involved in the financing. The subset of hospitals involved in the financing is referred to as the "obligated group."

A second alternative is the use of **pooled equipment financing programs**. These programs are often sponsored by the state hospital association or a regional association. Individual hospitals are involved in the financing and can obtain funds from the pool. The interest rate is usually much lower because the risk is spread across several hospitals.

The third alternative is an arrangement similar to the previous, except that the sponsor is different. Here, the pooled approach is used either for equipment needs or, in some cases, for major building programs. The issuer and sponsor of the pool is not the state or regional association, however, but some voluntary association of healthcare entities. The Voluntary Hospitals of America has created pooled financing for their members, and other associations are developing similar financing programs for their members.

## Zero-Coupon and Original Issue Discount Bonds

Bonds that do not pay interest during the life of the security are referred to as **zero-coupon bonds**. This does not mean that there is no interest paid to the investor; however, it means that the interest is paid in one lump sum at maturity, as opposed to incrementally throughout the life of the bond. In zero-coupon situations the purchaser buys the bond at a deep discount from the **face value** (the amount the bond will be worth when it "matures" in the future). When a zero-coupon bond matures, the investor will receive one lump sum equal to the initial investment plus the imputed interest. A simple example is a person who purchases a bond with a face value of $50 for $30. When the bond matures, let's assume after 10 years, the investor would receive $50, having earned $20 in "delayed" interest.

The maturity dates on zero-coupon bonds are usually long term—many do not mature for 10, 15, or more years. These long-term maturity dates allow an investor to plan for a long-range goal, such as paying for a child's college education. Larger purchasers, such as pension funds, may find these investments beneficial for helping to meet beneficiary payments in the future. With the deep discount, an investor can put up a smaller amount of money that can grow over many years. Beyond healthcare zero-coupon issues,

investors can also purchase these bonds from a variety of sources, including the U.S. Treasury, corporations, and state and local government entities.

The major advantage for the issuer is the delay of interest payments. This can conserve needed cash flow and may match the cash needs of the issuer. There is also the possibility that the after-reimbursement cost of the debt will be below the investment yield. It is important to note that in most zero-coupon situations, there is a periodic payment to a **sinking fund**. The sinking fund is an account under the control of the bond trustee, and the proceeds of the fund are used to retire the bonds at maturity.

The mechanics of a zero-coupon situation may be illustrated in the following case example. Assume that General Hospital issues $100,000,000 in zero-coupon, 5-year bonds. General Hospital would receive $62,100,000 from the market if the current **market rate of interest** is 10%. Although no interest is paid, each year an amount is recorded for interest expense. This amount is an amortization of the difference between the face value of the bonds ($100,000,000) and the actual cash received ($62,100,000). Thus, during the 5-year period, $37,900,000 will be recognized as interest expense. General Hospital also is required to make semiannual payments of $7,586,793 to a sinking fund. This fund is assumed to earn interest at 12% annually or 6% semiannually. Assume also that equal amounts of the total discount will be recognized as interest expense each year. This would amount to $7,580,000 ($37,900,000/5). The calculation in **TABLE 21-9** shows the net present value cost of this financing, assuming that 50% of capital costs are reimbursed and that the appropriate discount rate for the hospital is its investment yield of 12%.

The net present value cost of General Hospital's financing is $46,174,086, which is significantly less than the $62,100,000 that the hospital will receive. The sinking fund is not recognized as a capital

**TABLE 21-9** Net Present Value of Zero-Coupon Financing

| Item | Amount Before Reimbursement | Amount After Reimbursement | Years (Periods) | Present Value Factor (12%) | Present Value |
|---|---|---|---|---|---|
| Sinking fund | $7,586,793 | $7,586,793 | 1–10* | 7.8869 | $59,836,278 |
| Interest expense (amortization) | (7,580,000) | (3,790,000) | 1–5 | 3.6048 | (13,662,192) |
| Net present value cost | | | | | $46,174,086 |

*Ten semiannual payments; the present value factor Is for 10 periods at 6%.

expense item, which explains why the before and after reimbursement amounts are the same. The annual amortization of the discount, which is recognized by third-party payers as a reimbursable capital item, reduces the cost of the financing significantly. In some cases this pattern of amortization may not be permitted by the payers. Instead, the payer may require a type of amortization called *effective yield*. This type of amortization requires that the same total amount of interest expense be recorded over the 5 years ($37,900,000), but the amounts in the earlier years would be less. This would reduce the present value of the benefit somewhat.

## Interest Rate Swaps

Many hospitals and other healthcare providers have used interest rate swaps to lock in fixed rates after originally issuing **variable-rate debt**. Interest rate swaps may enable firms to deal with the volatility in the financial markets and obtain lower-cost financing that better meets their needs. To understand an interest rate swap, three questions must be answered:

1. What is an interest rate swap?
2. Why are interest rate swaps beneficial? For every winner, won't there be a loser?
3. How can a swap arrangement be analyzed?

An interest rate swap is merely an exchange of interest rate payments between two firms, with a bank usually acting as a broker. For example, a firm that has issued **fixed-rate debt** may wish to make floating-rate payments. If a firm that makes floating-rate payments can be found that would like to substitute this type of payment with fixed-rate payments, a swap may be arranged. It is also possible to swap two different types of floating-rate debt. In a swap, only the coupon payments are exchanged, not the principal.

The basic nature of the swap is easy to understand. The aspect that is often puzzling is how both parties benefit from the swap. Many people believe the only party that truly benefits is the broker.

The rationale for swaps is purely and simply a function of a supposed market imperfection. This means that one borrower has a better relative position in one maturity market than another. This difference is often ascribed to differential information and institutional restrictions that lead to differences in transaction costs. Because of these imperfections, the opportunity for financial arbitrage occurs.

To understand this concept more fully, let us assume that Hospital A and Hospital B encounter the interest rates in **TABLE 21-10**. In this example, Hospital A has a better relative position in both markets, fixed and floating. The differential, however, is much larger in the fixed-rate market (95 basis points) than in the floating-rate market (15 basis points). The net differential is 80 (95 − 15). This difference implies a swap opportunity is present and the total advantage is 80 basis points. It is this 80–basis point differential that will be split among Hospital A, Hospital B, and the broker.

Assume now that both hospitals issue $50 million of debt. Hospital A issues fixed-rate debt and Hospital B issues floating-rate debt. A broker could put these two hospitals together, and the set of payments in **TABLE 21-11** might result. The data in Table 21-11 show that all parties have realized some financial advantage as a result of the swap.

Hospital A has reduced its floating rate to variable minus 10 basis points from variable plus 25 basis points. This is a savings of 35 basis points from its initial position. Hospital B also has gained. It now has fixed-rate debt at 7.80%, which is 30 basis points under its projected rate of 8.10%. Of course, the broker has kept 15 basis points for the time and effort required to bring the parties together.

This is the way in which a swap is supposed to work. Everyone has benefited. It is not always true, however, that every party will benefit, and each swap opportunity must be carefully analyzed to ensure that benefits will be realized. You can see information regarding an interest rate swap arrangement in the sample audit (Appendix 9-A).

| **TABLE 21-10** Interest Rates for Two Hospitals | | | |
|---|---|---|---|
| **Type of Debt** | **Hospital A** | **Hospital B** | **Rate Differential** |
| Fixed | 7.15% | 8.10% | 95 bps |
| Floating | Variable + 25 bps* | Variable + 40 bps | 15 bps |

*bps = basis point (1/100 of 1%).

**TABLE 21-11** Interest Rate Swap Payments

| Payments | Hospital A | Hospital B | Broker |
|---|---|---|---|
| To bondholders | 715 bps | Variable 40 bps | 0 |
| To broker | Variable +15 bps | 750 bps | Variable +765 bps |
| From broker to A | 740 bps | 0 | 740 bps |
| From broker to B | 0 | Variable +10 bps | Variable +10 bps |
| Net payment | Variable −10 bps | 780 bps | 15 bps |
| Advantage | 35 bps | 30 bps | 15 bps |

# ▶ Early Retirement of Debt

In many cases an issuer would like to retire an existing debt issue before its maturity. There are a variety of reasons for wanting to do this. One important reason is that it permits the issuer to take advantage of a reduction in interest rates. An issue may have been marketed several years ago when interest rates were 10% and rates may now have decreased to 7%. If the present lower interest rate could be substituted for the original rate, a major improvement in net income could result.

The following are other reasons for wishing to retire an existing indebtedness:

- To avoid onerous covenants in the existing indenture
- To take advantage of changes in bond ratings
- To take advantage of changes in policy regarding tax-exempt financing

Whatever the reason, most healthcare issues do not remain outstanding for their full life cycles; most are retired early.

There are two common ways of retiring an issue early: refinancing and refunding. In a **refinancing** situation the issuer buys back the outstanding bonds from the investors. This can be accomplished in either of two ways. First, the issuer may have the option of an early call. If the outstanding bonds are callable, the issuer would notify the present bondholders that the bonds are being called and should be tendered for payment. The principal or face value would then be paid, along with any call premium plus accrued interest. Second, the issuer buys back the bonds in open-market transactions or sends a letter to existing bondholders, offering to buy the bonds at some stated dollar amount.

Early retirement of existing bonds also can be accomplished through **refunding**. In a refunding situation the outstanding bonds are not acquired by the issuer, and the present bondholders continue to maintain their investment. Although the refunding does not actually retire the bonds, the bonds are not shown on the issuer's financial statements, and the covenants present in the indenture are now voided. The process of voiding existing indenture covenants and removing the bonds from the issuer's financial statements is called **defeasance**. In effect, defeasance in a refunding situation involves the deposit of a sum of money with the bond trustee, which is then used to buy specially designated securities of the federal government. With these securities there is a guarantee that all future interest and principal payments can be met from the proceeds controlled by the bond trustee.

The following is a simple example to illustrate the refunding process: On January 1, 2017, $1 million of 15%, level-debt service bonds are issued. The bonds have a 5-year life. The earliest call date is January 1, 2019. No call premium is involved. On January 1, 2018, interest rates have decreased to 7%, and management advance-refunds the January 1, 2017, issue. In this example the original issue would have the debt service schedule included in **TABLE 21-12**.

To retire or advance-refund the issue on January 1, 2018, management must place on deposit with a trustee a sum of money that guarantees payment of

**TABLE 21-12** Debt Service Schedule of January 2017 Issue

| Date | Interest | Principal | Total Debt Service | Ending Debt Principal |
|------|----------|-----------|--------------------|-----------------------|
| Jan. 1, 2018 | $150,000 | $148,320 | $298,320 | $851,680 |
| Jan. 1, 2019 | 127,750 | 170,570 | 298,320 | 681,110 |
| Jan. 1, 2020 | 102,170 | 196,150 | 298,320 | 484,960 |
| Jan. 1, 2021 | 72,740 | 225,580 | 298,320 | 259,380 |
| Jan. 1, 2022 | 38,940 | 259,380 | 298,320 | 0 |

the following amounts on January 1, 2019 (the earliest call date):

| | |
|---|---|
| Interest due Jan. 1, 2019 | $127,750 |
| Debt principal due Jan. 1, 2019 | 170,570 |
| Ending debt principal on Jan. 1, 2019 | 681,110 |
| | $979,430 |

If management borrows all the funds necessary to meet the $979,430 payment on January 1, 2019, how much must it borrow on January 1, 2018? Ignoring placement fees and other debt issuance costs, the hospital would borrow $915,360. Why $915,360? It is assumed that the hospital will be able to invest the proceeds at 7%, the effective interest rate on January 1, 2018 (1.07 times $915,360 = $979,430). In tax-exempt issues, an arbitrage restriction limits investment yields for all practical purposes to the interest rate of the refunding issue.

Are there any real savings in debt service costs? Yes; the new issue schedule in **TABLE 21-13** shows annual savings of $28,080 ($298,320 – $270,240) for the next 4 years.

Thus far, the refinancing looks good. However, there is an accounting loss that must be recorded. At the end of the first year (January 1, 2018), the value for the old debt, $851,680, will be removed from the balance sheet. But the defeased debt will be replaced by $915,360 of new debt, and this will reduce income in that year by $63,680 ($915,360 – $851,680). This will be treated as an extraordinary loss during the period in which refunding takes place.

A real-world case may make the magnitude of these numbers more apparent. A hospital recently refunded $65 million of 2-year-old debt with $79 million of new debt at a lower effective interest rate. Estimated savings in debt service over the life of the issue were $22 million, but there was an accounting loss of approximately $13 million during the initial year. More important, this loss reduced the hospital's ratio of equity to assets from 26 to 16%. This is a sizable reduction that could have some impact on future credit availability. Many lenders establish target equity-to-debt ratios beyond which they will not lend funds at reasonable interest rates.

In sum, refunding to take advantage of reduced interest rates usually makes a lot of economic sense. But the presence of an accounting loss should be considered, especially when considering its potential impact on future credit availability.

**TABLE 21-13** Debt Service Schedule of January 2018 Issue

| Date | Interest | Principal | Total Debt Service | Ending Debt | Savings in Debt Service |
|------|----------|-----------|--------------------|-------------|-------------------------|
| Jan. 1, 2019 | $64,080 | $206,160 | $270,240 | $709,200 | $28,080 |
| Jan. 1, 2020 | 49,640 | 220,600 | 270,240 | 488,600 | 28,080 |
| Jan. 1, 2021 | 34,200 | 236,040 | 270,240 | 252,560 | 28,080 |
| Jan. 1, 2022 | 17,680 | 252,560 | 270,240 | 0 | 28,080 |

# ▶ SUMMARY

The major sources of capital financing available to healthcare firms may be categorized as equity and debt. Equity has become an important source of capital, even for traditional tax-exempt healthcare firms. Corporate restructuring can greatly facilitate the process of accessing equity capital. However, long-term debt probably will continue to represent the major source of capital for most healthcare firms. Evaluation of alternative sources of long-term debt requires more than a simple comparison of interest rates. The impact of other factors also should be carefully reviewed to determine the overall attractiveness of alternative financing packages.

## ASSIGNMENTS

1. Explain the term *defeasance*. What does it mean?
2. Assuming a normal or typical yield curve (that is, upward sloping), discuss the advantages and disadvantages of borrowing money for a major construction program with 3-year term financing.
3. When is a master trust indenture used, and what is its value?
4. Under what circumstances might your firm be interested in issuing zero-coupon bonds?
5. In an advance refunding of debt, accounting gains or losses usually occur. Under what conditions could there be an accounting gain?
6. United Hospital has received a leasing proposal from Leasing, Inc. for a cardiac catheterization unit. The terms are as follows:

   - Five-year lease
   - Annual payments of $200,000 payable 1 year in advance
   - Payment of property tax estimated to be $23,000 annually
   - Renewal at end of year 5 at fair market value

   Alternatively, United Hospital can buy the catheterization unit for $725,000. United Hospital must debt-finance this equipment. It anticipates a bank loan with an initial down payment of $125,000 and a 3-year term loan at 16% with equal principal payments. The residual value of the equipment at year 5 is estimated to be $225,000. The lease is treated as an operating lease. Depreciation is calculated on a straight-line basis. Assuming a discount rate of 14%, what financing option should United Hospital select? Assume that there is no reimbursement of capital costs.

7. Nutty Hospital wishes to advance-refund its existing 15% long-term debt. The present $30,000,000 is not callable until 5 years from today. The payout on the issue over the next 5 years is as presented in **TABLE 21-14**.

| **TABLE 21-14** Nutty Hospital Debt Service Schedule | | | |
|---|---|---|---|
| | **Interest** | **Principal** | **Total** |
| End of year 1 | $4,500,000 | $1,000,000 | $5,500,000 |
| End of year 2 | 4,350,000 | 1,000,000 | 5,350,000 |
| End of year 3 | 4,200,000 | 1,000,000 | 5,200,000 |
| End of year 4 | 4,050,000 | 1,000,000 | 5,050,000 |
| End of year 5 | 3,900,000 | 1,000,000 | 4,900,000 |

At the end of the fifth year the debt ($25,000,000 outstanding balance at that time) may be called with a 10% penalty. If present interest rates are 10% and the investment rate on the funds to be received from the new issue cannot exceed 10%, what amount must Nutty Hospital borrow today? Assume that underwriting fees and other issuance costs will be 5% of the issue and that all debt service on the old issue must be met from the proceeds of the refunding issue and related investment income.

8. You have the option of leasing an asset for $100,000 per year, with payments to be made at the end of each year of use. This lease cannot be canceled. Alternatively, you may buy the asset for $248,700. For reimbursement purposes, the lease must be capitalized. If the asset is purchased, it will be debt-financed with $210,000 of 3-year serial notes (that is, $70,000 of principal will be repaid each year). The effective interest rate on this loan will be 8%. Assume that the asset has an allowable useful life of 3 years with no estimated salvage value.

   - Determine the amount of expense that would be reported during each of the 3 years under the two financing plans.
   - Assuming that 80% of all reported capital expenses are reimbursed and that the discount rate is 6%, determine the present value of the asset in these two methods of financing.

9. Happy Valley is considering moving from its present location into a new 200-bed facility. The estimated construction cost for the new facility is $40 million. The hospital has no internal funds and is considering a 20-year mortgage with interest scheduled to be 8%. The issue will be repaid over 20 years with equal annual principal payments of $2 million. Interest expense would decline each year by $160,000.

   The cost of the plant and fixed equipment would be 80% of the total cost or $32 million, and the movable equipment would be $8 million. The movable equipment would need to be replaced in 10 years, and it is estimated that the replacement cost would be $17,271,200 (inflation is assumed to be 8% per year). The plant and fixed equipment would need to be replaced in 30 years at a cost of $322,006,400 (inflation again assumed to be 8% per year). All costs reflect only the investment required to provide inpatient services. A separate analysis will be done for outpatient services.

   Happy Valley anticipates that its operation will generate about 9,700 discharges per year. The hospital anticipates that its operating costs, excluding capital costs, will be $4,000 per discharge, or $38,800,000 in the first full year of operation.

   The payer mix at Happy Valley is expected to be 60% Medicare and Medicaid on the inpatient side. These payers will pay approximately $4,400 per discharge. This payment reflects both operating and capital cost payments. Approximately 10% of Happy Valley's operating and capital costs is paid by payers who reimburse the hospital on a cost-related basis for both capital and operating costs. The remaining 30% of Happy Valley's business will be charge-based, but it is expected that discounts to commercial insurers and bad-debt and charity write-offs will average 30%.

   Assuming that Happy Valley wishes to break even on a cash-flow basis during the first year of operation, what charge per discharge must be set? If the hospital wanted to include an element in its rate structure to reflect replacement cost of the building and movable equipment, what additional amount would that be? Assume that 50% of the movable equipment cost would be debt-financed and 80% of the building and fixed equipment would be debt-financed. Also assume that the hospital can earn 10% on any invested money, so use 10% as your discount rate.

10. Mayberry Hospital is considering a joint venture relationship with your physicians to acquire a full-body computed tomography (CT) scanner. Projected revenues and expenses for the scanner are presented in **TABLE 21-15**.

**TABLE 21-15** Computed Tomography (CT) Scanner Financial Forecast

|  | Year 1 | Year 2 | Year 3 | Year 4 | Year 5 |
|---|---|---|---|---|---|
| Revenues | $521,000 | $531,000 | $542,000 | $533,000 | $564,000 |
| Less bad debts and discounts | 52,100 | 53,100 | 54,200 | 53,300 | 56,400 |
| Net revenues | 468,900 | 477,900 | 487,800 | 479,700 | 507,600 |
| Expenses |  |  |  |  |  |
| Wages and employee benefits | 60,000 | 63,000 | 66,150 | 69,459 | 72,930 |
| Maintenance | 55,000 | 57,750 | 60,638 | 63,669 | 66,853 |

| | | | | | |
|---|---|---|---|---|---|
| Supplies | 20,000 | 21,000 | 22,050 | 23,153 | 24,310 |
| Rent | 18,000 | 18,900 | 19,845 | 20,837 | 21,879 |
| Administrative | 10,000 | 10,500 | 11,025 | 11,576 | 12,155 |
| Utilities | 5,000 | 5,250 | 5,513 | 5,788 | 6,078 |
| Insurance | 5,000 | 5,250 | 5,513 | 5,788 | 6,078 |
| Taxes | 10,000 | 10,000 | 10,000 | 10,000 | 10,000 |
| Depreciation | 94,050 | 137,940 | 131,670 | 131,670 | 131,670 |
| Other expense | 40,620 | 33,384 | 25,271 | 16,176 | 5,977 |
| Total expenses | 317,670 | 362,974 | 357,675 | 358,116 | 357,930 |
| Net income before tax or interest | $151,230 | $114,926 | $130,125 | $121,585 | $149,670 |

The scanner is expected to cost $627,000 and have a useful life of 5 years. Two possible financing plans have been proposed. The first plan would be a limited partnership arrangement. There would be 34 shares: 33 would be sold to investors for $19,000 each (total funds generated would be $627,000) and 1 share would be retained by the hospital for its development effort. In the second financing plan, a $380,000 level-debt service plan with a 5-year maturity and interest at 10% would be arranged. The remainder of the funding would be generated through the sale of 33 limited partnership shares at $7,485 per share ($247,000). Again, the final share would be issued to the hospital for its development efforts. Assuming that a 30% marginal tax rate exists, project cash flow per partnership unit under each financing alternative for each of the 5 years.

## SOLUTIONS AND ANSWERS

1. *Defeasance* means that upon final payment of all interest and principal, the rights of the bond trustee cease to exist; that is, they are defeased. The security covenants in an indenture also may be satisfied through the creation of a trust (escrow) in which sufficient monies are held to guarantee payment at some future date. Defeasance means that the issue defeased is no longer an obligation of the issuer and can be removed from the issuer's books.
2. The typical upward-sloping yield curve implies that a 3-year interest rate probably will be much lower than a 20- to 25-year rate. Therefore, cost will be lower with a 3-year construction loan. At the end of the third year, however, permanent financing must be sought; also, there is no guarantee that interest rates will not have increased during the period or that financing will be available at the end of the third year.
3. A master trust indenture usually pledges the assets and revenues of several firms in a combined financing package. It is often used by healthcare systems to gain better access to capital and lower interest rates.
4. Zero-coupon bonds are especially desirable if the issuer's effective interest rate on the bonds is well below the yield or discount rate of the issuer. In a zero-coupon bond issue, the postponement of interest payment maximizes the possibility for additional arbitrage, that is, for investing at a yield greater than the cost of funds.
5. Accounting gains usually take place when the advance-refunding issue has a higher rate of interest than the refunded issue. Accounting losses often occur when the reverse is true, or the refunding interest rate is less than the initial borrowing rate.
6. United Hospital's financing options for the cardiac catheterization unit are detailed in **TABLE 21-16**. From the data in Table 21-16, it can be seen that purchase of the catheterization unit would produce a lower net present value cost, compared with a lease.

**TABLE 21-16** · Lease/Purchase Analysis

| Item | Amount Before Reimbursement | Amount After Reimbursement | Years | Present Value Factor (14%) | Present Value |
|---|---|---|---|---|---|
| Lease | | | | | |
|   Rent | $200,000 | $200,000 | 0 | 1.000 | $200,000 |
|   Rent | 200,000 | 200,000 | 1–4 | 2.914 | 582,800 |
|   Property tax* | 23,000 | 23,000 | 1–5 | 3.433 | 78,959 |
|   Net present value cost of lease | | | | | $861,759 |
| Purchase | | | | | |
|   Down payment | $125,000 | $125,000 | 0 | 1.000 | $125,000 |
|   Principal | 200,000 | 200,000 | 1–3 | 2.322 | 464,400 |
|   Interest | 96,000 | 96,000 | 1 | 0.877 | 84,192 |
|   Interest | 64,000 | 64,000 | 2 | 0.769 | 49,216 |
|   Interest | 32,000 | 32,000 | 3 | 0.675 | 21,600 |
|   Salvage | (225,000) | (225,000) | 5 | 0.519 | (116,775) |
|   Net present value of purchase | | | | | $627,633 |

*Property tax would be passed on to the lessee or hospital. There is no property tax on the purchase because the hospital is a tax-exempt firm

7. Nutty Hospital's present borrowing needs are detailed in **TABLE 21-17**.

**TABLE 21-17** Nutty Hospital Refunding Requirements

| Item | Amount Required | Years | Present Value Factor (10%) | Present Value |
|---|---|---|---|---|
| Debt service year 1 | $5,500,000 | 1 | 0.909 | $4,999,500 |
| Debt service year 2 | 5,350,000 | 2 | 0.826 | 4,419,100 |
| Debt service year 3 | 5,200,000 | 3 | 0.751 | 3,905,200 |
| Debt service year 4 | 5,050,000 | 4 | 0.683 | 3,449,150 |
| Debt service year 5 | 4,900,000 | 5 | 0.621 | 3,042,900 |

| Principal at year 5 | 25,000,000 | 5 | 0.621 | 15,525,500 |
| Call premium | 2,500,000 | 5 | 0.621 | 1,552,500 |
| Net present value | | | | $36,893,850 |

Amount borrowed = $36,893,850/0.95 = $38,835,631

8. The data in **TABLE 21-18** and **TABLE 21-19** show the comparative expense and present values for leasing versus debt-financing the asset during the 3-year period.

**TABLE 21-18**　Leasing Versus Purchase Analysis

| | Year 1 | Year 2 | Year 3 |
|---|---|---|---|
| **Leasing Expenses** | | | |
| Lease payment per year (3 y @ 10%) | $100,000 | $100,000 | $100,000 |
| Interest @ 10% | $24,870 | $17,357 | $9,073 |
| Principal payment | $75,130 | $82,643 | $90,927 |
| Ending principal | $173,570 | $90,927 | $0 |
| Depreciation expense | $82,900 | $82,900 | $82,900 |
| Total expenses (Int + Dep) | **$107,770** | **$100,257** | **$91,973** |
| **Debt Financing Expenses** | | | |
| Interest @ 8% | $16,800 | $11,200 | $5,600 |
| Principal payment | $70,000 | $70,000 | $70,000 |
| Ending principal | $140,000 | $70,000 | $0 |
| Depreciation expense | $82,900 | $82,900 | $82,900 |
| Total expenses (Int + Dep) | **$99,700** | **$94,100** | **$88,500** |
| **Expense Difference** | | | |
| Leasing less debt | $8,070 | $6,157 | $3,473 |

9. **TABLE 21-20** reflects the required charge that Happy Valley must set to break even on a cash-flow basis and the additional charge required to cover the funded depreciation requirement necessary for eventual replacement.

**TABLE 21-19** Leasing Versus Debt Finance: Present Value Analysis

| Item | Amount Before Reimbursement | Amount After Reimbursement (80%) | Years | Present Value Factor | Present Value |
|---|---|---|---|---|---|
| Lease financing | | | | | |
| Depreciation | −$82,900 | −$66,320 | 1–3 | 2.673 | −$177,273 |
| Interest | $24,870 | $4,974 | 1 | 0.943 | $4,690 |
| Interest | $17,357 | $3,471 | 2 | 0.890 | $3,090 |
| Interest | $9,073 | $1,815 | 3 | 0.840 | $1,524 |
| Principal | $75,130 | $75,130 | 1 | 0.943 | $70,848 |
| Principal | $82,643 | $82,643 | 2 | 0.890 | $73,552 |
| Principal | $90,927 | $90,927 | 3 | 0.840 | $76,379 |
| Net present value cost of lease | | | | | **$52,809** |
| Debt financing | | | | | |
| Depreciation | −$82,900 | −$66,320 | 1–3 | 2.673 | −$177,273 |
| Down payment | $38,700 | $38,700 | Present | 1.000 | $38,700 |
| Principal payment | $70,000 | $70,000 | 1–3 | 2.673 | $187,110 |
| Interest | $16,800 | $3,360 | 1 | 0.943 | $3,168 |
| Interest | $11,200 | $2,240 | 2 | 0.890 | $1,994 |
| Interest | $5,600 | $1,120 | 3 | 0.840 | $941 |
| | | | | | **$54,640** |

**TABLE 21-20** Happy Valley Required Rate Structure

| Cash expenditures | |
|---|---|
| Principal amount | $2,000,000 |
| Interest payment | $3,200,000 |
| Operating costs | $38,800,000 |
| Total cash costs | $44,000,000 |

| | |
|---|---|
| Reimbursement | |
| Medicare and Medicaid ($4,400 × 0.6 × 9,700) | $25,608,000 |
| Reimbursed interest (0.10 × $3,200,000) | $320,000 |
| Reimbursed operating costs (0.10 × $38,800,000) | $3,880,000 |
| Reimbursed equip. depreciation (0.10 × $800,000) | $80,000 |
| Reimbursed build. depreciation (0.10 × $1,066,667) | $106,667 |
| Total payments | $29,994,667 |
| Required charge to cover cash expenditures | |
| Remaining cash costs to be covered | $14,005,333 |
| Number of charge paying discharges (0.3 × 9,700) | 2,910 |
| Required charge without discount | $4,812.83 |
| Required charge with discount (30%) | $6,875.47 |
| Additional requirements for replacement | |
| Equipment (0.5 × $17,271,200/F(10%,10 years)) | $541,838 |
| Plant (0.2 × $322,006,400/F(10%,30 years)) | $391,506 |
| Total annual deposit | $933,344 |
| Number of charge paying discharges | 2,910 |
| Required charge without discount | $320.74 |
| Required charge with discount | $458.20 |

10. The data in **TABLE 21-21** show the projected cash flow per partnership unit under the two financing alternatives.

**TABLE 21-21** Computed Tomography (CT) Scanner Cash Flow per Share

| | Years | | | | |
|---|---|---|---|---|---|
| | 1 | 2 | 3 | 4 | 5 |
| Alternative 1: no debt | | | | | |
| Income before tax and interest | $151,230 | $114,926 | $130,125 | $121,585 | $149,670 |
| Less income tax | 45,369 | 34,478 | 39,038 | 36,476 | 44,901 |

*(continues)*

**TABLE 21-21** Computed Tomography (CT) Scanner Cash Flow per Share    *(continued)*

| | Years | | | | |
|---|---|---|---|---|---|
| | **1** | **2** | **3** | **4** | **5** |
| Income after tax | $105,861 | $80,448 | $91,088 | $85,110 | $104,769 |
| Add depreciation | 94,050 | 137,940 | 131,670 | 131,670 | 131,670 |
| Cash flow | 199,911 | 218,388 | 222,758 | 216,780 | 236,439 |
| Cash flow per share (34 shares) | 5,880 | 6,423 | 6,552 | 6,376 | 6,954 |
| Percentage return (cash flow/$19,000) | 30.9% | 33.8% | 34.5% | 33.6% | 36.6% |
| Alternative 2: debt financing | | | | | |
| Income before tax and interest | $151,230 | $114,926 | $130,125 | $121,585 | $149,670 |
| Less interest | 38,000 | 31,776 | 24,929 | 17,398 | 9,111 |
| Taxable income | 113,230 | 83,150 | 105,196 | 104,187 | 140,559 |
| Less income tax | 33,969 | 24,945 | 31,559 | 31,256 | 42,168 |
| Income after tax | 79,261 | 58,205 | 73,637 | 72,931 | 98,391 |
| Add depreciation | 94,050 | 137,940 | 131,670 | 131,670 | 131,670 |
| Less principal | 62,243 | 68,467 | 75,314 | 82,845 | 91,132 |
| Cash flow | $111,068 | $127,678 | $129,994 | $121,756 | $138,930 |
| Cash flow per share (34 shares) | $3,267 | $3,755 | $3,823 | $3,581 | $4,086 |
| Percentage return (cash flow/$7,485) | 43.6% | 50.2% | 51.1% | 47.8% | 54.6% |
| Debt service for $380,000 loan | | | | | |
| Total debt service (5 yr @ 10%) | $100,243 | $100,243 | $100,243 | $100,243 | $100,243 |
| Interest @ 10% | $38,000 | $31,776 | $24,929 | $17,398 | $9,111 |
| Principal payment | $62,243 | $68,467 | $75,314 | $82,845 | $91,132 |
| Ending principal | $317,757 | $249,290 | $173,977 | $91,132 | $0 |

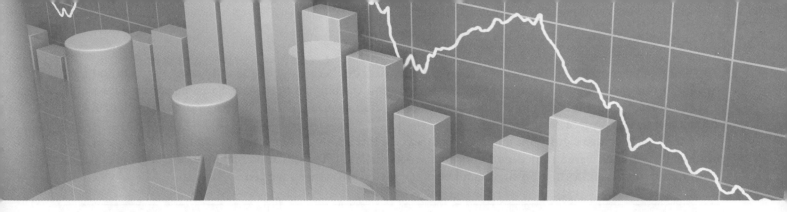

# CHAPTER 22

# Working Capital and Cash Management

## REAL-WORLD SCENARIO

Dr. Noah Johnson, chair of the ear, nose, and throat (ENT) department in a hospital, tracked his department's revenues one month, and as the end of the month approached he decided that the revenues for the current month already were above budget. Therefore, he decided to hedge his bets for the following month by delaying some of the end-of-month revenues until the following month. This was not difficult to accomplish. The charges simply were not submitted for a few days. The few days were followed by a weekend, and before charges were actually posted to the account 7 days had passed without posting any charges.

The loss of revenues became evident in accounting. An inquiry into the situation found no problems with the charging system but rather that the delay was intentional. Soon, everyone was angry. The ENT department had not followed the hospital's charging policy. Accounting was angry because the delay distorted the monthly revenues.

Accrual accounting matches the revenue and expenses in the month they actually occur. The chair of the ENT department had bypassed the process and moved charges into the wrong month. This distorted reporting of the results of operations for the period. Also, this information is used for forward planning. Therefore, the cyclical nature of revenues may be distorted going forward.

Finally, billing was upset. They collect charges 4 days after discharge, and on the fifth day they create and send the bill. In this case they had some charges not posted until the bill had been sent. Some minor charges would never be billed, because it costs more to bill them than the cash received. Other charges would be rebilled, but the additional cost was unnecessary.

In the end, the most significant financial result was the lost reimbursement on some of the late charges. Organizationally, relations were strained, and information was distorted. This situation highlights the principle that the collection of financial information should not be manipulated but rather analyzed.

---

Few topics in finance are more important than cash and investment management. Cash is the lifeblood of a business operation. A firm that controls its access to cash and the generation of cash usually will survive and thrive. A firm that ignores or manages its cash position poorly may fail. Experience has shown that more firms fail because of a lack of ready cash than for any other reason—even firms with sound profitability. It is important, therefore, to recognize and appreciate that profit and cash management are not the same thing.

It would seem logical to expect that great volumes of literature would be devoted to such an important topic as cash and investment management. Unfortunately, this is not the case. Although a major portion of a financial manager's time is devoted to working capital problems, relatively little space is devoted to them in most financial management textbooks. A typical text often contains only several chapters that deal with working capital management and perhaps a single chapter that discusses cash management.

**Cash management** is probably more important in the healthcare industry than in many other industries, but it is often less understood. Healthcare financial executives frequently advance through the accounting route. Finance texts provide little coverage on cash management, and accounting texts provide almost no coverage. Traditionally, many healthcare financial executives think of cash management in terms of receivables control. They often believe that better cash management will result if accounts receivable can be reduced or the collection cycle shortened. Although accounts receivable management in healthcare organizations is clearly important, limiting attention to this one area is myopic. Good cash management should focus not only on the acceleration of receivables but also on the complete cash conversion cycle. Reduction of the cash conversion cycle, along with the related investment of surplus funds, should be a critical objective of financial managers.

Many hospitals and healthcare firms often are willing to allow their banks to handle most of their cash-management decisions. Although this strategy is acceptable in some situations, it may produce a result that is less than optimal. Risks are sometimes unnecessarily increased or yields on investments are sacrificed. Real or perceived conflicts of interest also exist if the bank is represented on the healthcare firm's governing board.

### Learning Objective 1

Explain why cash management is especially crucial in most sectors of the health industry.

Why is cash and investment management important to healthcare executives? Compared with firms of similar size in other industries, hospitals have large sums of investment-eligible funds. Hospitals and other healthcare firms are also more likely to have greater investment management needs than other industries for several reasons:

- Many healthcare firms are voluntary, not-for-profit firms and must set aside funds for replacement of plants and equipment. Investor-owned firms can rely on the issuance of new stockholders' equity to finance some of their replacement needs.
- Healthcare firms are increasingly beginning to self-insure all or a portion of their professional liability risk. This requires sizable investment pools to be available to meet estimated actuarial needs.
- Many healthcare firms receive gifts and endowments. Although these sums may not be large for individual firms, they can provide additional sources of investment.
- Many healthcare firms also have sizable funding requirements for defined-benefit pension plans and debt service requirements associated with the issuance of bonds. These funds are usually held by a trustee.

With greater investments, one should expect to find greater levels of investment income. The level of reported investment income taken from 2014 Medicare cost reports was $7.8 billion, compared to total reported net income of $48.1 billion. Investment income comprised 16% of total net income.

# ► Cash and Investment Management Structure

Effective cash management is often related to the *cash conversion cycle*, as depicted in **FIGURE 22-1**. In its simplest form, the cash conversion cycle represents the time it takes a firm to go from an outlay of cash to purchase the needed factors of production, such as labor and supplies, to the actual collection of cash for the produced product or service, such as a completed treatment for a given patient. Usually, the objectives in cash management are to minimize the collection period and to maximize the payment period. Trade-offs often exist; for example, accelerating collection of receivables may result in lost sales, and delaying payments to vendors could result in increased prices.

## *Learning Objective 2*

Explain what working capital is and why it is needed.

The primary tool used in cash planning is the **cash budget**. (Cash budgeting is discussed more fully in Chapter 23.) Cash balances are affected by changes in working capital over time. **Working capital** may be defined as the difference between current assets and current liabilities. The following items are usually included in these two categories:

- Current assets
  - Cash and investments
  - Accounts receivable
  - Inventories
  - Other current assets

- Current liabilities
  - Accounts payable
  - Accrued salaries and wages
  - Accrued expenses
  - Notes payable
  - Current position of long-term debt

## *Learning Objective 3*

Describe the activities covered in the cash budget that affect working capital.

The cash budget focuses on four major activities that affect working capital:

1. Purchasing of resources
2. Production/sale of service
3. Billing
4. Collection

These activities represent intervals in the cash conversion cycle. The **purchasing** of resources relates to the acquisition of supplies and labor, such as the level of inventory necessary to maintain realistic production schedules and the staff required to ensure adequate provision of services. *Production and sale* are virtually the same in the healthcare industry; there is no inventory of products or services. However, there is a delay between the production of service and final delivery. A patient may be in the hospital for 10 to 15 days or in a skilled nursing facility for 2 months, which could be regarded as the final point of sale. *Billing* represents the interval between the release or discharge of a patient and the generation of a bill. **Collection** represents the interval between the generation of a bill and the actual collection of the cash from the patient or the patient's third-party payer.

Estimating these four intervals is critical to cash budgeting and therefore to cash planning. For example, the average collection period dramatically influences the need for cash assets. During periods when sales are expected to increase, a long collection period requires the hospital to finance a larger amount of working capital in the form of increased receivables. The hospital must pay for its factors of production (that is, supplies and labor) at the beginning of the cycle and wait to receive payment from its customers at the end of the cycle.

The previous example also illustrates why a focus on a static measure of liquidity, such as a current ratio, sometimes can be deceiving. A rapid buildup in sales results in a large increase in accounts receivable, which increases the current ratio. Liquidity position, however, might not be improved in this case. The speed

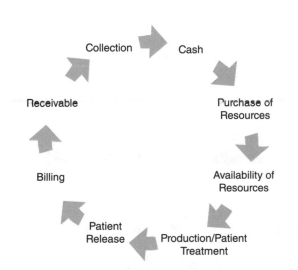

**FIGURE 22-1 Cash Conversion Cycle**

with which these receivables can be turned into cash is also an extremely important measure of liquidity.

The major purpose of a cash budget, an example of which is shown in **TABLE 22-1**, is to prepare an accurate estimate of future cash flows. With this estimate the firm can arrange for **short-term financing** from a bank through a line of credit if it projects a period of cash deficiency, or it can invest surplus funds. Because yields are usually higher on longer-term investments, an investment for a 6-month term is likely to result in greater income than an investment broken down into two 3-month cycles. The cash budget, then, is the key document in terms of providing information regarding **short-term investment** and short-term financing decisions. A key factor in these projections is the desired level of cash balances the firm would like to maintain. Firms that set low cash requirement levels are assuming more risks. The entire cash-management process can be broken down into five sequential steps:

1. Understand and manage the cash conversion cycle. In most situations the objective is to minimize the required investment in working capital, when working capital is defined as current assets less current liabilities.
2. Develop a sound cash budget that accurately projects cash inflows and cash outflows during the planning horizon.
3. Establish the firm's minimum required cash balance. This level should be set in a manner consistent with the firm's overall risk assumption posture.
4. Establish working capital loans during those periods when the cash budget indicates that short-term financing will be needed.
5. Invest cash surpluses in a way that will maximize the expected yield to the firm, subject to a prudent assumption of risk.

**TABLE 22-1** Sample Cash Budget

| | First Quarter | | | Second Quarter | Third Quarter | Fourth Quarter |
|---|---|---|---|---|---|---|
| | **January** | **February** | **March** | | | |
| Recipients from operations | $300,000 | $310,000 | $320,000 | $1,000,000 | $1,100,000 | $1,100,000 |
| Less disbursements from operations | 280,000 | 280,000 | 300,000 | 940,000 | 1,000,000 | 1,000,000 |
| Cash available from operations | $20,000 | $30,000 | $20,000 | $60,000 | $100,000 | $100,000 |
| Other receipts | | | | | | |
| Increase in mortgage payable | | | | 500,000 | | |
| Sale of fixed assets | | 20,000 | | | | |
| Unrestricted income, endowed | | | 40,000 | 40,000 | 40,000 | 40,000 |
| Total other receipts | 0 | $20,000 | $40,000 | $540,000 | $40,000 | $40,000 |
| Other disbursements | | | | | | |
| Mortgage payments | | | 150,000 | | 150,000 | |
| Fixed-asset purchase | | | | 480,000 | | |

| | | | | | | |
|---|---|---|---|---|---|---|
| Funded depreciation | | | 30,000 | 130,000 | 30,000 | 30,000 |
| Total other disbursements | 0 | 0 | 180,000 | 610,000 | 180,000 | 30,000 |
| Net cash gain (loss) | $20,000 | $50,000 | ($120,000) | ($10,000) | ($40,000) | $110,000 |
| Beginning cash balance | 100,000 | 120,000 | 170,000 | 50,000 | 40,000 | 0 |
| Ending cash | $120,000 | $170,000 | $50,000 | $40,000 | $0 | $110,000 |
| Desired level of cash | 100,000 | 100,000 | 100,000 | 100,000 | 100,000 | 100,000 |
| Cash above minimum needs (financing needs) | $20,000 | $70,000 | ($50,000) | ($60,000) | ($100,000) | $10,000 |

## ▶ Management of Working Capital

The management of working capital items is related to short-term bank financing and investment of cash surpluses, discussed further later in the chapter. The balance sheet for ABC Medical Center in **TABLE 22-2** presents a useful way to examine the relevant items of working capital management.

As examples, the following two categories are discussed: receivables and accounts payable, and accrued salaries and wages.

### Learning Objective 4

Describe the tools an organization manager can use to manage receivables.

**TABLE 22-2** ABC Medical Center, Consolidated Balance Sheets, June 30, 20X9 and 20X8

| | Assets | |
|---|---|---|
| | 20X9 | 20X8 |
| Current assets | | |
| Cash | $1,216,980 | $362,422 |
| Investments | 4,042,407 | 4,597,806 |
| Patient accounts receivable (20X9, $7,356,120; 20X8, $6,253,629), less allowance for uncollectibles | 5,892,339 | 5,143,471 |
| Other receivables | | |
| Medicare | 2,672,612 | 2,113,655 |
| Miscellaneous | 213,726 | 164,631 |

*(continues)*

**TABLE 22-2** ABC Medical Center, Consolidated Balance Sheets, June 30, 20X9 and 20X8 *(continued)*

| | Assets | |
|---|---|---|
| | **20X9** | **20X8** |
| Inventories | 1,302,598 | 1,174,295 |
| Prepaid expenses | 1,021,972 | 249,455 |
| Current portion of deferred receivables from Medicare | 454,404 | 502,904 |
| Assets held by trustee | 180,000 | 247,181 |
| Total current assets | $16,997,038 | $14,555,820 |
| Other assets | | |
| Investments | $10,642,621 | $10,983,125 |
| Accounts receivables, affiliated companies | 4,510,105 | 2,036,436 |
| Notes receivable, affiliated company | 700,000 | 700,000 |
| Assets held by trustee | | |
| Temporary cash account | 0 | 0 |
| Construction fund | 2,717,846 | 59,643 |
| Sinking fund | 6,751,942 | 4,018,948 |
| Interest receivable | 118,142 | 6,112,530 |
| Self-insurance funds | 10,942,749 | 94,231 |
| Unamortized debt issuance expenses | 934,535 | 7,875,602 |
| Investment in ABC Insurance, Ltd. | 209,655 | 954,078 |
| Deferred receivables for Medicare | 2,620,162 | 0 |
| Prepaid pension cost | 840,449 | 3,074,567 |
| Unamortized past service cost | 1,784,160 | 0 |
| Total other assets | $42,772,366 | $35,909,160 |
| Property, plant, and equipment | | |
| Land | $1,654,394 | $1,649,912 |
| Buildings | 36,505,277 | 34,504,398 |
| Improvements to land and leaseholds | 1,272,205 | 1,263,959 |

| | 20X9 | 20X8 |
|---|---|---|
| Fixed equipment | 8,812,615 | 8,713,615 |
| Movable equipment | 20,290,037 | 15,461,276 |
| Capitalized leases | 2,998,295 | 3,293,693 |
| Total property, plant, and equipment | $71,532,823 | $64,886,853 |
| Less allowance for depreciation | 27,763,195 | 22,037,503 |
| | 43,769,628 | 42,849,350 |
| Construction and other work in progress | $4,396,463 | $3,869,866 |
| Total property, plant, and equipment | $48,166,091 | $46,719,216 |
| Total assets | $107,935,495 | $97,184,196 |

| | **Liabilities and Net Assets** | |
|---|---|---|
| | **20X9** | **20X8** |
| Current liabilities | | |
| Accounts payable trade | $2,297,672 | $2,531,257 |
| Accrued salaries and wages | 1,366,777 | 1,035,496 |
| Accrued liability for compensated balances | 1,232,586 | 1,119,800 |
| Accrued Medicare liability | 317,302 | 1,881,895 |
| Accrued indigent care assessment | 1,170,001 | 1,061,742 |
| Other accrued liabilities | 611,230 | 444,916 |
| Current portion of long-term debt | 1,528,910 | 1,442,420 |
| Total current liabilities | $8,524,478 | $9,517,526 |
| Other liabilities | | |
| Accounts payable, affiliated companies | 1,993,815 | 0 |
| Self-insurance liabilities | 8,904,000 | 7,048,000 |
| Total other liabilities | 10,897,815 | 7,048,000 |
| Long-term, less current maturities | | |
| Bonds payable | $45,745,652 | $46,063,575 |
| Notes payable | 3,902,113 | 1,888,504 |

*(continues)*

| **TABLE 22-2** ABC Medical Center, Consolidated Balance Sheets, June 30, 20X9 and 20X8 *(continued)* | | |
|---|---|---|
| | **Liabilities and Net Assets** | |
| | **20X9** | **20X8** |
| Capital leases payable | 127,535 | 595,407 |
| | $49,775,300 | $48,547,486 |
| Net assets | $38,737,952 | $32,071,204 |
| Total liabilities and net assets | $107,935,545 | $97,184,216 |

## Receivables

Industry experience suggests that receivables constitute the most critical, but not exclusive, area of importance in cash management. In general, accounts receivable usually represent about 40 to 50% of a hospital's total investment in current assets. ABC Medical Center has $8,778,677 ($5,892,339 + $2,672,612 + $213,726) of receivables, or 51.6% of its total current assets, in 20X9. This value is below the range cited previously, largely because ABC Medical Center has a relatively low value for days in accounts receivable (50.3 days). This situation, of course, is favorable and is an objective of most financial managers. In general, the following three objectives are usually associated with accounts receivable management:

1. Minimize lost charges
2. Minimize write-offs for uncollectable accounts
3. Minimize the accounts receivable collection cycle

All three objectives are important, but our attention is directed at the third—minimizing the collection cycle. **FIGURE 22-2** provides a schematic that predicts intervals involved in the entire accounts receivable cycle. The following intervals usually exist in the hospital inpatient accounts receivable collection cycle:

- Admission to discharge
- Discharge to bill completion
- Bill completion to receipt by payer
- Receipt by payer to mailing of payment
- Mailing of payment to receipt by hospital
- Receipt by hospital to deposit in bank

Figure 22-2 also provides the estimated time that could be involved in each interval, but these numbers vary widely among hospitals and payer categories within hospitals. They are intended only to show the relative importance of each interval in the overall accounts receivable collection cycle. The total number of days represented in Figure 22-2 is 55, which is reasonably close to the national average of 54 days during 2014.

## Admission to Discharge (5 Days)

Shortening this interval is not the critical objective from an accounts receivable perspective. This does not imply, however, that a reduction in length of stay is not an objective, because clearly it is. With fixed prices per case, reduced length of stay is particularly desirable from an overall cost management viewpoint.

In terms of managing the accounts receivable cycle, the real solution appears to be what occurs during this interval to expedite later collection. The following specific suggestions are provided:

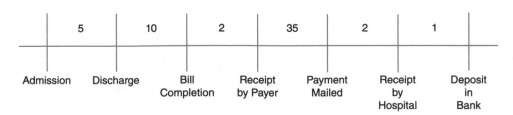

**FIGURE 22-2 Accounts Receivable Collection Cycle in Days**

- Determine whether interim billings are possible for patients with a long length of stay. Some third-party payers permit interim billings if the length of stay exceeds a specified interval. Often, this is 21 days. Although there may be relatively few patients in this category, it is important to recognize the absolute value of accounts receivable represented by these patients can be large.
- Use advance deposits for nonemergent admissions. If insurance coverage can be verified, estimates of the total deductible and copayment amounts can be made. This is becoming especially important as the number of "high deductible" health plans increases as employers attempt to shift more of the payment risk to their employees. The deductible and copayment portion can be requested from the patient before or during admission. In situations when this is not possible, a financing plan should be developed jointly between the hospital and the patient. Many patients appreciate being told beforehand what their insurance will pay and what their individual liability is likely to be.
- Obtain required insurance and eligibility information before admission for nonemergent patients. For emergency admissions, obtain the same data during the hospital stay. This permits the preparation of a bill during or shortly after discharge.
- For patients with health saving account coverage, arrange for the deductible payment portion during patient registration.

## Discharge to Bill Completion (10 Days)

Ideally, this interval should be reduced as much as possible. Although this may be an objective, clearly some cost-to-benefit trade-offs need to be evaluated. For example, speeding up the processing of bills is desirable only if the cost involved does not exceed the benefits of more rapid bill preparation. An acceleration of the billing process can also create a reduction in final payments if the acceleration results in some late charges not being posted to the final bill. Inaccurate coding could also result from an acceleration of billing that could cause later delays in payment or inaccurate payment amounts. Basic suggestions are as follows:

- Implement more timely billing and remove bottlenecks. Usually, bills are not prepared during discharge so that late charges can be posted. If certain ancillary departments constantly experience delays, corrective steps should be taken to improve posting. A holding period longer than 2 to 3 days is probably not reasonable.
- Develop educational programs for physicians to show the effects of delays in completing medical charts. Often, an incomplete medical chart is the reason for delay in billing. Physicians must be informed of the effect these delays have on the hospital. Some hospitals have suspended admitting privileges of physicians who constantly are delinquent. Although this strategy may not be useful in many hospitals, it is worth considering in some situations.

## Bill Completion to Receipt by Payer (2 Days)

The estimated 2-day length of this interval may be overstated where electronic claim submission is used.

Several steps may be useful in shortening this interval, including the following:

- Consider electronic invoicing for large payers when this alternative is available. This decreases mail time to zero.
- Try to settle all outpatient accounts at the point of discharge or departure. Each outpatient should be presented with a bill at the point of departure, and payment should be requested at that time.
- Submit a bill for any deductible and copayment amounts for hospital inpatients at the point of discharge. Settlement should take place at this point if the patient has been advised previously of the total amount due.

## Receipt by Payer to Mailing of Payment (35 Days)

This interval varies greatly by type of payer. Some self-pay patients may have outstanding accounts for more than a year. Insurance companies may take an inordinate amount of time to settle bills because of disputes over coverage or reasonableness. The following steps should be considered:

- Selling some accounts receivable. Until recently, hospitals could not legally sell Medicare accounts, but this is no longer true. More and more hospitals are considering selling accounts receivable because the rates of interest charged for these loans are relatively low. On a taxable basis, the interest rate will be slightly below prime for these asset-backed transactions.
- Using discounts for prompt payment. Many businesses have long provided discounts as financial incentives for early payment. This strategy may be used for self-pay portions of hospital bills and also for insurance payers. Sufficiently large discounts also can greatly reduce collection costs and write-offs. How large an inducement should be offered?

This decision, of course, is firm specific, but a 5% reduction for payment during discharge does not seem excessive.

- Creating a system to respond quickly to third-party requests for additional data. Third-party payers often delay payment until requested information has been received and reviewed. At a minimum, a log should be maintained that shows dates of requests and responses.

- Claiming all bad debts on the Medicare deductible and copayment portion of hospital bills. Medicare is liable for payment of a percentage of bad debts experienced on their patients. It is important, however, to document reasonable collection efforts on the part of the hospital before Medicare liability for payment can be ensured.

- Making frequent follow-up telephone calls to detect problems or concerns with bills. In many situations self-pay hospital bills are not paid because there is disagreement over the amount of the bill. This type of dispute can be avoided by having a nonthreatening hospital employee promptly contact the patient and inquire about the patient's health and the amount of the bill. Sometimes this may be better handled by an independent party. When this approach has been used, reductions in bad debt write-offs have been large.

## Payment Mailed to Receipt by Hospital (2 Days)

Mail time is the cause for this 2-day interval. These delays cannot be prevented for most small, personal accounts. In the case of a government or large insurance payer, a courier service can be used. Checks are picked up as they become available. For large, out-of-town payers, a special courier arrangement can be used or direct deposits to an area bank can be initiated. Relatively large sums of money must be involved for these strategies to be cost effective. In addition, direct **wire transfer** of funds between payer and the healthcare provider's bank is also an alternative that makes great sense if available. Many major commercial payers and public programs such as Medicare and Medicaid arrange for wire transfer of payments.

## Receipt by Hospital to Deposit in Bank (1 or More Days)

Perhaps the only effective way this interval can be shortened is through the use of a lock-box arrangement in which payments go directly to a post office box that is cleared at least once a day by bank employees. Bank employees deposit all payments, usually

photocopy the checks, and send the copies—along with any enclosures—to the hospital for proper crediting. There is usually a cost for this service. The hospital must determine whether improvement in the cash flow, plus potential reduction in clerical costs, are worth the fee charged.

## Accounts Payable and Accrued Salaries and Wages

Accounts payable and accrued salaries and wages represent spontaneous sources of financing. This means these amounts are not usually negotiated but vary directly with the level of operations. Table 22-2 shows that ABC Medical Center had $2,297,672 in accounts payable trade and $1,366,777 in accrued salaries and wages in 20X9. In addition, $1,993,815 of accounts payable from affiliated companies also existed. These amounts are not small and represent a sizable proportion of ABC's total financing.

Managing accounts payable and accrued salaries is similar to the management of accounts receivable, except in a reverse direction. Instead of acceleration, most financial managers would like to slow payment to these accounts. A number of approaches, as discussed in the literature, attempt to do this. Several relevant approaches for a free-standing healthcare provider are as follows:

- Delay payment of an account payable until the actual due date. Often, many healthcare providers process invoices upon receipt and initiate payment even when the invoices are not due for several weeks or months. For example, many invoices for subscriptions to journals are sent out 3 to 5 months before their due dates. There is no reason to pay these invoices until they are actually due.

- Stretch accounts payable. This technique has been described frequently in the literature and is familiar to most individuals. Stretching accounts payable simply means delaying payment until some point after the due date. Although this technique is often used, the ethics of the method are clearly debatable. In addition, delays may cause a hospital's credit rating to deteriorate. Vendors eventually will be unwilling to grant credit, or they may alter payment terms.

- Change the frequency of payroll. Although not a popular decision with employees, lengthening the payroll period can provide a significant amount of additional financing that is virtually free. For example, ABC Medical Center has an estimated weekly payroll of approximately $1,150,000. If

ABC changes its payroll period from a weekly to a biweekly basis, it can create an additional source of financing equal to 1 week's payroll, or $1,150,000. Investing that money at 4% provides $46,000 in annual investment income. Fewer payroll periods may also reduce bookkeeping costs.

- Use banks in distant cities to pay vendors and employees. This method may delay check clearing and create a day or two of "float." Float is defined as the difference between the bank balance and the checkbook balance. It also may be a questionable practice, depending on applicable state laws. With the advent of direct deposit for most employees, float is no longer a possibility.

- Schedule deposits to checking accounts to match expected disbursements on a daily basis. A daily cash report can be prepared for each account, using information obtained daily by calling the bank or accessing the account electronically. The report can reconcile data on beginning cash balances and disbursements expected to be made that day. Separate accounts for payroll are often maintained to recognize the predictability of check clearing. For example, payroll checks issued on a Friday may have a highly predictable pattern of check clearing. Knowledge of this distribution enables the treasurer to minimize the amount of funds needed in the account on any given day to meet actual disbursements and thus maximize the amount of invested funds.

---

*Learning Objective 5*

List the external resources available to an organization for its short-term financing needs.

---

## ▶ Short-Term Bank Financing

Many healthcare firms may experience a short-term need for funds during their operating cycles. The need for funds may have resulted from a predictable seasonality in the receipt and disbursement of cash or it may represent an unexpected business event, such as a strike. Commercial banks are the predominant sources of short-term loans, but other sources are also available. Several common arrangements used by healthcare firms to arrange for short-term loans are discussed here.

### Single-Payment Loan

The single-payment loan is the simplest credit arrangement and is usually given for a specific purpose, such as the purchase of inventory. The note can be on either a discount or an add-on basis. In the discount arrangement, the interest is computed and deducted from the face value of the note. The actual proceeds of the loan, then, would be in an amount less than the face of the note. In an add-on note, the interest is added to the final payment of the loan. In this arrangement the borrower receives the full value of the loan when the loan is originated.

### Line of Credit

A **line of credit** is an agreement that permits a firm to borrow up to a specified limit during a defined loan period. For example, a commercial bank may grant a $2 million line of credit to a hospital during a specific year. In that year the hospital could borrow up to $2 million from the bank with presumably little or no additional paperwork required. Lines of credit are either committed or uncommitted. In an uncommitted line, there is no formal or binding agreement on the part of the bank to loan money. If conditions change, the bank could decide not to loan any funds at all. In a committed line of credit, there is a written agreement that conveys the terms and conditions of the line of credit. The bank is legally required to lend money under the line as long as the borrower has met the terms and conditions. To cover the costs and risks incurred by the commercial bank in a committed line of credit, the bank charges a **commitment fee**. The fee is usually based on either the total credit line or the unused portion of the line.

### Revolving Credit Agreements

A revolving credit is similar to a line of credit except that it is usually for a period longer than 1 year. Revolving credit agreements may be in effect for 2 to 3 years. Most revolving credit agreements are renegotiated before maturity. If the renegotiation occurs more than 1 year before maturity, a revolving credit agreement loan may be stated as a long-term debt and never appear as a current liability on a firm's balance sheet. Terms of revolving credit agreements are similar to those of lines of credit. Interest rates are usually variable and based on the prime rate or other money-market rates.

### Term Loans

**Term loans** are made for a specific period, usually ranging between 2 and 7 years. The loans usually require periodic installment payments of the principal. This type of loan is frequently used to finance a tangible asset that produces income in future periods, such as a computed tomography (CT) scanner. The asset acquired with the loan proceeds may be pledged as collateral for the loan.

## Letters of Credit

Some hospitals use letters of credit as a method of bond insurance. A letter of credit is simply a letter from a bank stating that a loan will be made if certain conditions are met. In hospital bond financing, a letter of credit from a bank guarantees payment of the loan if the hospital defaults.

---

### Learning Objective 6

List and explain the criteria that should be used when investing an organization's cash in the short term.

---

## ▶ Investment of Cash Surpluses

The term *surplus* is confusing, even among financial executives. For the purpose of this discussion, **cash surplus** is defined as money exceeding a minimum balance that the firm prefers to maintain to meet immediate operating expenses and minor contingencies, plus any **compensating balance** required at its banks.

The balance sheet for ABC Medical Center shown in Table 22-2 lists a cash balance of $1,216,980 plus $4,042,407 in short-term investments as of June 30, 20X9. These funds are most often referred to as surplus cash when discussing short-term investment strategy. It is important to note that ABC Medical Center has significant investments in other areas. Most hospitals follow this procedure. For example, ABC Medical Center, as of June 30, 20X9, has $10,642,621 in an investments account under the "other assets" section of the balance sheet. These funds probably are designated for the eventual replacement of the hospital plant. In addition, sizable balances of funds are maintained with a trustee. For example, there is $2,717,846 in the construction fund account, $6,751,942 in the sinking fund account, $118,142 in the interest receivable account, and $10,942,749 in the self-insurance fund account. Most hospitals and healthcare firms maintain similar fund balances. It is critical for management to make investments to meet the objectives of each specific fund and maximize the potential yield to the firm.

Often, a portion of a firm's investment funds is restricted to money-market investments. The term money market refers to the market for short-term securities, including U.S. Treasury bills, **negotiable certificates of deposit**, bankers' acceptances, **commercial paper**, and repurchase agreements.

Maturities for money-market investments can range from 1 day to 1 year. Funds invested in money-market securities usually serve two roles. They represent (1) a **liquidity** reserve that can be used if the firm experiences a need for these funds and (2) a temporary investment of surplus funds that can result in the earning of a return.

If the funds are invested for periods longer than 1 year (for example, the investment of a replacement reserve fund), higher yields often result. These longer-term maturity investments may not be referred to as money-market securities.

When evaluating alternative investment strategies, five basic criteria are usually reviewed:

1. Price stability
2. Safety of principal
3. Marketability
4. Maturity
5. Yield

## Price Stability

The importance of price stability, especially for money-market investments, cannot be overemphasized. If a firm has a sudden need for cash, most major money-market investments can be sold without any serious capital losses. Generally, U.S. **Treasury bills** are the most credit-worthy money-market investments, followed closely by other U.S. Treasury obligations and federal agency issues. Investment in securities with long-term maturities is subject to risk if interest rates increase. This explains why money-market investments are usually restricted to maturities of less than 1 year.

## Safety of Principal

Financial managers expect that the principal of their investment is generally not at risk. Treasury and federal agency obligations have little risk of principal loss through default. Bank securities (such as negotiable certificates of deposit and bankers' acceptances) and corporate obligations (such as commercial paper) are different matters. There may be a loss of principal through default, and care should be exercised when choosing these instruments. Information on banks is available in *Polk's World Bank Directory* and *Moody's Bank and Finance Manual*. There is no reason why a firm should not review the creditworthiness of its banks as carefully as banks review the financial position of loan applicants. It should be noted, however, that erosion of principal can occur through increases in money-market interest rates, and these increases subsequently have an impact on fixed-rate securities.

## Marketability

Marketability varies among money-market instruments. The term refers to the ability to sell a security quickly and with little price concession before maturity. In general, an active secondary trading market must exist to ensure the presence of marketability. Most major money-market instruments do have active **secondary markets**, especially obligations of the U.S. Treasury. Some commercial paper, especially that of industrial firms, may be difficult to redeem before maturity.

## Maturity

There is a clear relationship between the yield of a security and its maturity that can be summarized in a yield curve. **TABLE 22-3** shows a set of values for U.S. Treasury securities on June 13, 2016.

Some firms use a strategy of investment described as "riding the yield curve." This strategy relies on the existence of an upward-sloping yield curve. Investments are made in longer-term securities that are sold before maturity.

## Yield

Yield is a measure of the investment's return and is an important consideration. Yield is usually affected by maturity, expected default risk of principal, marketability, and price stability. In addition, taxability is often an issue. A tax-exempt healthcare firm has no incentive to invest in securities that are exempt from federal income taxes.

## ▶ SUMMARY

Working capital management involves decisions that have an impact on operating cash flows of the firm.

Ideally, the objective of most working capital management systems is to accelerate the collection of cash from customers and to slow down the payment to suppliers and employees. Investment management is important in many healthcare firms because of the relative size of their investment portfolios. Hospitals, for example, generate about 30% of their total net income from nonoperating sources, largely investment income. With so much at stake, healthcare firms need to improve performance in the cash and investment management area.

**TABLE 22-3**  Yield to Maturity for U.S. Treasuries, June 13, 2016

| Maturity | Yield (%) |
|---|---|
| 30 day | 0.18 |
| 90 day | 0.26 |
| 180 day | 0.42 |
| 1 year | 0.57 |
| 2 years | 0.73 |
| 3 years | 0.87 |
| 5 years | 1.17 |
| 7 years | 1.44 |
| 10 years | 1.64 |
| 20 years | 2.02 |
| 30 years | 2.44 |

## ASSIGNMENTS

1. Data from Table 22-2 indicate that $8,778,677 of accounts receivable was present at the end of 20X9. If this value represented 50 days of average net patient revenue and the hospital believed this value could be reduced to 40 days, what dollar amount of new cash flow would be generated? If these funds were invested at 8.5%, how much additional investment income would result per year?

2. Alpha Home Health, Inc. has received an invoice for medical supplies for $5,000 with terms of a 2% discount if paid within 10 days. The invoice is due on the 30th day. What is the annual effective cost of interest on this invoice?

3. Pauly Hospital has been thinking about changing its payroll period from biweekly to monthly. Pauly currently has 600 employees with an annual payroll of $18,000,000. If Pauly could earn 9.5% on invested funds, what amount of new investment income could be generated on an annual basis? If the cost of writing a payroll check is $1.50, what additional amount could be saved on an annual basis from switching to a monthly payroll period?

4. Your firm has negotiated a $1,000,000 line of credit with your local bank. The terms of the line of credit call for an interest rate of 2% above prime on any borrowing plus 0.5% on any unused balance. If the line is not used during the year, what cost will your firm incur?

5. ABC Medical Center (Table 22-2) expects its revenues to increase by 10% next year. If the firm can increase its current liabilities by 12% through payment extensions and limit its increase in current assets, excluding cash and investments, to 8%, what additional cash will be required to finance working capital?

## SOLUTIONS AND ANSWERS

1. The amount of new cash flow is $1,755,735:

$$[(\$8,778,677) / 50] \times [50 - 40]$$

The amount of additional investment income per year is $149,238 (0.085 × $1,755,735).

2. The 2% discount would be realized for making payment 20 days before required. The annual interest cost is approximately 36%:

$$2\% \times [360\,\text{days} / 20\,\text{days}] = 36\%$$

3. There are two ways to estimate the annual savings. The easiest method is to multiply the difference in average wages payable by 9.5%:

$$\left[\frac{(18,000,000 \div 12)}{2} - \frac{(18,000,000 \div 26)}{2}\right] \times 0.095 = \$38,365$$

Alternatively, the difference in average payable amount per day can be calculated and multiplied times the average daily interest rate (0.095/360), shown in **TABLE 22-4**.
Assuming that the pattern presented in Table 22-4 holds, the annual return would be $39,353 (12 × $3,279.42). The savings from reduced checks would be $12,600 = [600 (26 − 12) × $1.50].

4. The firm must pay 0.5% on the entire $1,000,000, or $5,000 (0.005 × $1,000,000).

5. The schedule presented in **TABLE 22-5** shows the increase in net working capital.

**TABLE 22-4** Investment Payable Income from Longer Payroll Cycle

| Day | Average Payable Balance* | | Incremental Amount Invested | Investment Income |
| --- | --- | --- | --- | --- |
| | **Monthly** | **Biweekly** | | |
| 1 | $49,315 | $49,315 | $— | $— |
| 2 | 98,630 | 98,630 | — | — |
| 3 | 147,945 | 147,945 | — | — |
| 4 | 197,260 | 197,260 | — | — |
| 5 | 246,575 | 246,575 | — | — |
| 6 | 295,890 | 295,890 | — | — |

| | | | | |
|---|---|---|---|---|
| 7 | 345,205 | 345,205 | — | — |
| 8 | 394,521 | 394,521 | — | — |
| 9 | 443,836 | 443,836 | — | — |
| 10 | 493,151 | 493,151 | — | — |
| 11 | 542,466 | 542,466 | — | — |
| 12 | 591,781 | 591,781 | — | — |
| 13 | 641,096 | 641,096 | — | — |
| 14 | 690,411 | 690,411 | — | — |
| 15 | 739,726 | 49,315 | 690,411 | 182.19 |
| 16 | 789,041 | 98,630 | 690,411 | 182.19 |
| 17 | 838,356 | 147,945 | 690,411 | 182.19 |
| 18 | 887,671 | 197,260 | 690,411 | 182.19 |
| 19 | 936,986 | 246,575 | 690,411 | 182.19 |
| 20 | 986,301 | 295,890 | 690,411 | 182.19 |
| 21 | 1,035,616 | 345,205 | 690,411 | 182.19 |
| 22 | 1,084,932 | 394,521 | 690,411 | 182.19 |
| 23 | 1,232,877 | 443,836 | 690,411 | 182.19 |
| 24 | 1,183,562 | 493,151 | 690,411 | 182.19 |
| 25 | 1,232,877 | 542,466 | 690,411 | 182.19 |
| 26 | 1,282,192 | 591,781 | 690,411 | 182.19 |
| 27 | 1,331,507 | 641,096 | 690,411 | 182.19 |
| 28 | 1,380,822 | 690,411 | 690,411 | 182.19 |
| 29 | 1,430,137 | 49,315 | 1,380,822 | 364.38 |
| 30 | 1,479,452 | 98,630 | 1,380,822 | 364.38 |
| Monthly total | | | | $3,279.42 |

*Average Payable Balance = $18,000,000/365 Days

**TABLE 22-5** Net Increase in Working Capital

| | |
|---|---|
| Present current assets | $16,997,038 |
| – Cash | 1,216,980 |
| – Investments | 4,042,407 |
| Noncash current assets | $11,737,651 |
| 8% increase | 0.08 |
| Increase in noncash current assets | $939,012 |
| Present current liabilities | $8,524,478 |
| × 12% increase | 0.12 |
| Increase in current liabilities | $1,022,937 |
| Net increase in working capital | ($83,925) |

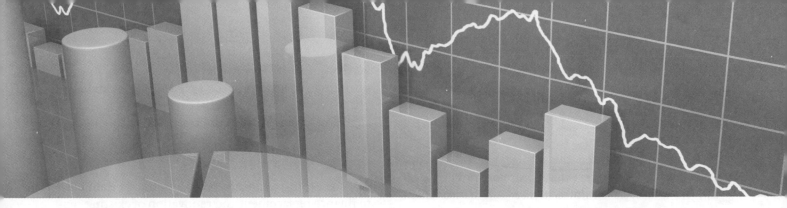

# CHAPTER 23
# Developing the Cash Budget

## LEARNING OBJECTIVES

After studying this chapter, you should be able to do the following:

1. Explain the importance of a cash budget.
2. Explain why an organization needs to carry cash balances.
3. List and describe where cash is generated by an organization and where an organization uses its cash.
4. Understand how to prepare a cash budget.

## REAL-WORLD SCENARIO

Ainsley Campbell, CEO of Mikaela Grace Medical Center (MGMC), the largest hospital in their market area, was being briefed by her CFO, Joshua Douglas, regarding their current liquidity crisis. Douglas informed Campbell that their cash balances had been eroded by about $25 million in the last 6 months. The primary cause for this erosion has been the medical center's removal from the network of the largest commercial payer in their region. The loss of that contract meant that all beneficiaries of the plan were now considered out of network if they received care at the MGMC. A large number of their physicians, especially their cardiovascular surgeons, have begun to do procedures at their primary competitor in the market. Major elective procedures are being shifted to their competitor, and revenues are down almost 5% from budget in the first 6 months.

Campbell questioned Douglas regarding their financial ability to withstand another 6 months of reduced volume if a new contract cannot be negotiated. Douglas said their large existing reserves of capital funds will protect them from any default on existing obligations, but they will be forced to use their present line of credit from the local bank. Douglas wanted to give special credit to Riley Ilene, the controller, who had anticipated the current crisis when developing the hospital's cash budget last year. Her forecast was almost perfect, and as a result MGMC had negotiated a new expanded line of credit with the bank. Campbell instructed Douglas to try to finalize negotiations with the health plan as quickly as possible to avoid a permanent reduction in their service lines, especially cardiology, which was the hospital's most profitable line.

Explain the importance of a cash budget.

Previously, we stressed the importance of developing a sound cash budget that accurately projects cash inflows and cash outflows in the cash-management process. Cash budgets embody the key source of information that permits management to determine the firm's short-term needs for cash. When a cash budget is modified to include the effects of alternative outcomes, financial executives can better assess the issue of liquidity risk and make decisions that will reduce the probability of a liquidity crisis. One of the following three courses of action can be taken:

1. Increase the level of cash and investment reserves.
2. Restructure the maturity of existing debt.
3. Arrange a line of credit with a bank.

Explain why an organization needs to carry cash balances.

# ▶ Determining Required Cash and Investment Reserves

Businesses maintain cash and investments for four primary purposes:

1. Short-term working capital needs
2. Capital investment needs
3. Contingencies
4. Supplement operating earnings

## Short-Term Working Capital Needs

The area of need most easily projected is usually short-term working capital transactions. In 2016 the average not-for-profit U.S. hospital held between 20 and 30 days of short-term cash and investments to meet short-term working capital needs. This represents less than 1 month of cash transactions, and standards do not vary much across different industry sectors. It is safe to assume that most healthcare firms should carry approximately 20 days of expected cash transactions at any point in time to meet normal short-term working capital needs for cash. However, it is not safe to say that a not-for-profit healthcare firm would need only 20 days of cash. Twenty days of cash meets current operating short-term needs such as payroll and supplies. It would not cover the larger long-term needs for capital replacement and contingencies.

## Capital Investment Needs

Not-for-profit healthcare providers must retain cash to finance replacement and renovation of existing capital assets as well as for investment in new product and service line areas. Their position is very different from that of taxable firms, whose access to capital for both replacement and new capital assets can and should be directed back to equity investors. Shareholders decide whether they wish to supply more capital to the firm based on their expected return. Not-for-profit entities in general and not-for-profit healthcare firms in particular must routinely set aside funds for replacement. Unlike investor-owned healthcare firms, there is no access to the equity capital markets. The amount of money that a nonprofit healthcare firm should reserve for capital assets depends on two factors:

1. Percentage of debt financing to be used
2. Projected future levels of capital expenditures

Healthcare firms that choose or are forced to limit their debt financing of capital assets must clearly set aside larger sums of money for capital replacement and expansion. The absence of debt in a firm's capital structure should permit a greater accumulation of capital reserves because there is no interest being paid to decrease earnings and lower cash reinvestment potential. The absence of debt in a healthcare firm's capital structure also reduces the financial risk and lowers the probability of failure.

It is the board's responsibility to establish appropriate levels of debt financing. Boards usually make trade-offs between the risk associated with debt financing and the firm's needs for capital to meet mission-related goals. Access to debt capital is usually related to both historical and projected financial performance. Not-for-profit healthcare firms that maintain high levels of cash and reserves usually have greater access to debt financing with lower interest rates.

Projecting future levels of capital expenditures over a long period of time is very difficult. Capital expenditure decisions result from both routine replacement factors as well as strategic considerations regarding the future direction of the firm. Most healthcare firms also experience years when capital expenditures are especially large due to major replacement needs. In general, however, most firms spend more on new capital expenditures than they depreciate in any given year.

One method commonly used to estimate future capital expenditures is based on present levels of allowances for depreciation. If all of a firm's existing assets were to be replaced, if no inflation in replacement cost occurred, and if no new capital assets other than replacement items were purchased, the present allowance-for-depreciation balance would be an accurate estimate of future capital expenditures. A simple example may help to illustrate this concept. If a digital mammography unit were acquired today for $500,000 and had a 5-year estimated life, it would be depreciated at a rate of $100,000 per year. At the end of the first year, the allowance for depreciation would be $100,000 and would increase each year by $100,000. Not-for-profit hospitals without access to equity capital often adopt a program called *funding depreciation*. If this practice were adopted, the hospital would place $100,000 in a fund each year. At the end of the 5-year useful life, it would have $500,000 available for replacement, assuming no pricing increase. However, new capital assets not presently in the firm's capital asset pool are purchased, and replacement capital assets do typically increase in price.

Although it is true that some capital assets are not replaced, in most situations projected capital expenditures exceed present allowance-for-depreciation balances. To adjust this forecast of capital expenditures, an inflation factor is usually applied in the following way. The present allowance-for-depreciation balance is increased at some projected inflation rate compounded at the average age of the firm's present capital assets. The formula can be stated as follows:

Estimated capital expenditures = [Allowance for depreciation] $\times$ [1 + Inflation rate]$^{\text{average age of plant}}$

As a general rule, most voluntary healthcare firms should try to have the following amount of cash available for replacement needs:

(100% − Desired debt policy %) $\times$ Estimated capital expenditures

## Contingencies

Many firms try to sequester some funding to meet **contingencies**, or unexpected demands for cash flow. The amount they reserve reflects their tolerance for risk as well as their estimates of unexpected cash demands on the firm. Values for underfunded pension or professional liability claims should be considered contingency funds. Payment of these liabilities requires funding at some future date. This investment is over and above short-term working capital needs.

## Supplement Operating Earnings

A number of not-for-profit healthcare firms in the United States have established "**operating endowments**." The purpose of these funds is to provide a dependable flow of investment earnings that can be used to supplement expected weaknesses in operating earnings. Although this practice is not widespread, it is worthy of consideration if a significant deterioration in operating earnings is expected or if current operating margins have been weak, with no expectation of future improvement.

## Case Example: Defining Required Cash Balances

**TABLE 23-1** identifies the sources of cash and investments available at our case example firm, Saint Alexis Health System, as of December 31, 20X9. Cash and investments are limited to those balances not restricted by a third party.

Based on calendar year 20X9 data, Saint Alexis Health System should carry $114,860,000 to maintain a 20-day cash-on-hand position. The estimated days of cash expenses are defined by taking 20X9 total operating expenses ($2,186,536,000) and subtracting depreciation ($90,339,000) to derive annual cash expenses ($2,096,197,000). This value is then divided by 365 to yield daily cash expenses ($5,743,005). Multiplying that number by 20 (which is short-term working capital need) produces the $114,860,000 requirement.

A desirable cash and investment position for capital asset needs can be estimated using the methodology described earlier. To estimate projected future capital asset expenditures based on the December 31, 20X9, allowance-for-depreciation balance of $1,203,185,000, we assumed a range of possible inflation factors ranging from 4 to 8%.

Inflation factors were compounded at the present average age of plant at Saint Alexis Health System (13.3 years). Finally, we assumed that the percentage of debt financing to be used would be 40%, 50%, 60%,

**TABLE 23-1** Saint Alexis Health System Cash and Investment Position (in Thousands)

| | |
|---|---|
| Current asset cash and short-term investments | $201,013 |
| Assets limited as to use, board designation | 540,211 |
| Total | $741,224 |

| TABLE 23-2 Required Capital Fund (in Thousands) | | | |
|---|---|---|---|
| | **Inflation Rate** | | |
| **Debt** | **4%** | **6%** | **8%** |
| 40% | $1,216,266 | $1,566,937 | $2,009,184 |
| 50% | 1,013,552 | 1,305,781 | 1,674,320 |
| 60% | 810,841 | 1,044,625 | 1,339,456 |
| 70% | 608,131 | 783,469 | 1,004,592 |

or 70%. For example, the replacement cost of the plant and equipment, assuming a 6% inflation rate would be $2,611,562,000 ($1,203,185,000 × 1.06$^{13.3}$). If it was determined that a 40% debt and 60% equity financing mix was to be used, the required level of funding would be $1,566,937,000 (0.60 × $2,611,562,000). **TABLE 23-2** presents the required cash and investment position under these scenarios.

## Contingency Needs

There is no really good methodology for establishing a desired contingency reserve. To a large extent the desired balance is a reflection of the firm's propensity to tolerate risk. Specifically, we identified two areas where funds must be set aside. First, Saint Alexis Health System reported a negative funded status for its defined benefit retirement plan of $111,552,000 in 20X9. This is a sizable deficit and has been increasing. The comparable 20X8 value was $87,381,000. Second, Saint Alexis Health System reported $90,194,000 of accrued liability for medical malpractice in 20X9 that was not currently funded. This value is also increasing dramatically; the comparable 20X8 value was $63,496,000. Although it is unclear at what future point actual funds will be used, the deficits are very large and indicate that funding for these liabilities must be established.

No supplement to operating earnings was established because prior operating earnings are assumed to be adequate. **TABLE 23-3** summarizes the determination of required cash balances at Saint Alexis Health System.

*Learning Objective 3*

List and describe where cash is generated by an organization and where an organization uses its cash.

| TABLE 23-3 Required Cash and Investment Position (in Thousands) | | |
|---|---|---|
| **Investment Need** | **Desired Balance** | **Days Cash** |
| Working capital | $114,860 | 20 |
| Capital asset | 783,469 | 136 |
| Contingency | 201,746 | 35 |
| Supplement operating earnings | 0 | 0 |
| Total required | $1,100,075 | 191 |
| Present available funds | 741,224 | 129 |
| *Surplus (deficit)* | *($358,851)* | *(62)* |

## ▶ Sources and Uses of Cash

In its most basic form, a cash budget is a statement that projects how the firm's cash balance position changes between two points in time. Changes to cash position are categorized as either sources of cash flow (sometimes called "receipts") or uses of cash flow (sometimes called "disbursements"). The following are some sources of cash:

- Collection of accounts receivable
- Cash sales
- Investment income
- Sale of assets
- Financings
- Capital contributions

The following are some uses of cash:

- Payments to employees
- Payments to suppliers
- Payments to lenders for interest and principal
- Purchase of fixed assets
- Investments

It is important to note that the definition of income and the definition of cash flows are not the same. This means that the amount reported for revenues in any given period most likely will not equal the actual amount of cash realized. The only exception is a case in which all revenues were produced by cash sales. In most healthcare settings, there is a lag between the recording of revenue and the collection of the resulting account receivable. In the same manner, expenses reported for wages and salaries and supplies may not actually equal the amount of cash expended within the period. As the period expands, for example, from a month to a year, the differences between revenues and expenses and receipts and disbursements begin to narrow. If one expanded the period from 1 year to 20 years, the difference between cash flows and income would be minimal. Unfortunately, most financial managers are interested in cash flows over much shorter periods. Many firms have cash budgets defined on at least a monthly basis, and some have biweekly or weekly cash budgets.

When cash flows are extremely volatile but can be reasonably forecasted, cash budgets for shorter terms are desirable. If cash flows are reasonably stable, a cash budget defined on a quarterly basis may be appropriate. Although most firms develop cash budgets on a monthly basis, it is common for these budgets to be revised periodically because original budget assumptions often prove to be inaccurate.

The primary factor affecting the validity of the cash budget is the accuracy of the forecasts for individual cash-flow categories. The greater the degree of possible variation between actual and forecasted cash flow, the higher the liquidity need of the firm. Firms that cannot predict cash flow with much certainty should increase their cash balances or negotiate lines of credit to escape the possibility of severe cash insolvency problems.

---

### *Learning Objective 4*

Understand how to prepare a cash budget.

---

## ▶ Preparing the Cash Budget

The most important area in cash budgeting is the revenue forecast. The revenue for healthcare providers is a function of two factors: volumes by product line and expected prices by payer category.

Most firms use a variety of methods to estimate volumes of services during the cash budget period. As shown in **FIGURE 23-1**, the revenue budget is critically related to the statistics budget. (See Chapter 15 for further discussion.) In general, two major categories of methods are used to develop estimates of volumes: subjective forecasts and statistical forecasts.

In reality, most forecasts probably combine elements of both subjective and statistical methods. **Subjective forecasts** are often referred to as "seat of the pants" methods and other less flattering names. Subjective forecasts do, however, have a place in the estimation of product line volumes. The critical factors in the reliability of a subjective forecast are the

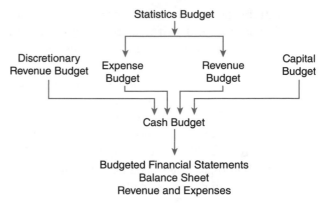

**FIGURE 23-1 Integration of the Budgetary Process**

wisdom and understanding of the forecaster. In cases when future volumes are likely to deviate from historical patterns, subjective forecasts may be the most reliable method of forecasting. Surveying medical staff members regarding their expected utilization during the next year is a form of subjective forecasting, but one that may be extremely reliable.

**Statistical forecasts** run the gamut from major econometric studies to simple time series techniques. Whatever the method, an underlying assumption surrounds a statistical forecast that states that the future can be predicted based on some mathematical model extrapolated from the past. If the relationships or models on which the forecasts are based have changed, future forecasts can be misleading.

In some cases predicting prices for the firm's products and services may be almost as difficult as projecting volumes. Healthcare firms are price takers in most situations. This means they rely on someone else to establish prices for their services. Medicare and Medicaid are two organizations that set prices and exert tremendous influence on a major portion of the total revenue budget. One would believe these payers would establish prices far enough in advance so that forecasting prices would be a simple matter. Unfortunately, interim prices sometimes stay interim for longer than expected, and promised increases never materialize. Although the differences between expected and actual prices may be relatively small, the volume of the Medicare and Medicaid book of business is so large that small changes in prices have a major impact on net cash flows. Most healthcare providers operate with relatively small margins—somewhere between 1 and 5%. When Medicare and Medicaid account for 50% or more of a firm's total business, a small forecast error of 1 or 2% in the final prices to be paid by Medicare and Medicaid can have a disastrous impact on final operating margins.

Also, healthcare firms increasingly are being asked to discount more and more of their business to other major groups such as health maintenance organizations, preferred provider organizations, commercial insurers, and self-insured employers. This makes projecting actual realized net prices more and more difficult.

Projecting revenues does not equate to projecting cash flows. Collections will lag the actual booking of revenues for some period. One common way to develop forecasts of patient receipts is through the use of "**decay curves.**" These curves relate future collections to past billings. **FIGURE 23-2** depicts a decay curve with the following pattern of collections:

1. The first 15% of any month's revenue is collected in the first month.
2. The next 30% of any month's revenue is collected in the second month.
3. The next 25% of any month's revenue is collected in the third month.
4. The next 20% of any month's revenue is collected in the fourth month.
5. The next 5% of any month's revenue is collected in the fifth month.
6. The remaining 5% of any month's revenue is written off and not collected.

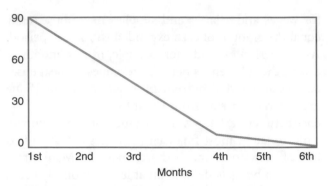

**FIGURE 23-2 Decay Curve Analysis: Percentage Uncollected by Month After Billing**

**TABLE 23-4** presents a cash receipts summary for the first 6 months of the year.

The collection pattern reflected in the decay curve of Figure 23-2 can be seen in Table 23-4. For example, of the $2,000,000 of January revenue, 15% ($300,000) is collected in January, 30% ($600,000) is collected in February, 25% ($500,000) is collected in March, 20% ($400,000) is collected in April, 5% ($100,000) is collected in May, and the remaining 5% ($100,000) is written off and not collected. The revenues in the following months reflect

| **TABLE 23-4** Cash Receipts Summary (in Thousands) | | | | | | | |
|---|---|---|---|---|---|---|---|
| | | **January** | **February** | **March** | **April** | **May** | **June** |
| Beginning accounts receivable revenue | $3,600 | $1,600 | $1,000 | $500 | $100 | | |
| January sales | 2,000 | 300 | 600 | 500 | 400 | 100 | 0 |
| February sales | 2,100 | 0 | 315 | 630 | 525 | 420 | 105 |
| March sales | 2,000 | 0 | 0 | 300 | 600 | 500 | 400 |
| April sales | 1,900 | 0 | 0 | 0 | 285 | 570 | 475 |
| May sales | 1,800 | 0 | 0 | 0 | 0 | 270 | 540 |
| June sales | 1,800 | 0 | 0 | 0 | 0 | 0 | 270 |
| Subtotal | | 1,900 | 1,915 | 1,930 | 1,910 | 1,860 | 1,790 |
| Other cash receipts Investment income | | 20 | 20 | 50 | 20 | 20 | 50 |
| Sale of assets | | 0 | 0 | 25 | 0 | 0 | 0 |
| Subtotal | | $20 | $20 | $75 | $20 | $20 | $50 |
| Estimated cash receipts | | $1,920 | $1,935 | $2,005 | $1,930 | $1,880 | $1,840 |

the same collection pattern. Although cash receipts and revenues are most often correlated, it is not always true that the months producing the highest revenue will be the months with the highest cash collection. For many health-care firms, the highest cash collection month is often 1 to 2 months after the highest revenue month.

Changes in collection patterns of major third-party payers can have a significant effect on cash flows and should be reflected immediately in revised cash budgets. For example, if Medicaid decides to delay the payment of patient bills by 60 days to conserve cash, the cash budget must be revised to reflect this new payment pattern. Increasing values for deductibles and copayments under many healthcare insurance plans also may delay collection patterns and increase eventual write-offs because the self-pay portion of the total healthcare bill may not be paid by the patient.

Additional cash receipts may come from sources other than revenue collection. Investment income and sale of assets are identified as the only other sources in Table 23-4, but other sources may exist. Contributions, sale of stock, and the issuance of new debt are also possibilities.

After forecasting cash receipts, a schedule of expected cash disbursements is necessary before the cash budget is complete. The two largest categories in most healthcare firms are labor and supplies. Labor costs or payroll most often represent about 60% or more of a healthcare firm's total expenses. The **expense budget** identifies expected labor or payroll expenses by month, but payroll expenses do not translate into cash disbursements. Most healthcare firms meet the majority of their payroll obligations on a biweekly basis, which necessitates some accruals. For example, labor expense in January might be $1,200,000, but actual payroll might be $1,731,000 because there were three biweekly payroll periods. (There are 26 biweekly payroll periods in a year. Every month has at least two payroll periods, but 2 months have three.) Conversely, in other months during which only two biweekly pay periods were present, actual payroll disbursements might be less than labor expense.

Payroll expense also must be adjusted for with-holding and other deductions. For example, the January payroll of $1,731,000 might be broken down as presented in **TABLE 23-5**. In Table 23-5 the figure for net payroll—$1,190,000—does not include additional payroll taxes, such as workers' compensation, unemployment, and the employer's share of social security. Other fringe benefits such as pension and health insurance also are not included. The employee deductions such as income tax and social security involve a cash outlay, but the payment goes to the federal government.

| **TABLE 23-5** Payroll Disbursements | |
|---|---|
| Total payroll | $1,731,000 |
| Less employee deductions | |
| Income taxes | 330,000 |
| Social Security | 126,000 |
| Other deductions | 85,000 |
| Net payroll disbursed to employees | $1,190,000 |

As with payroll, the expense budget includes a value for supplies expense, but that value will not equal the actual disbursement for supplies. **TABLE 23-6** presents a schedule of expected cash disbursements.

The only remaining task is to combine the cash receipts summary and the cash disbursements summary to create the cash budget. Before doing so, a desired level of cash balances must be defined. For this example, it is assumed that a short-term cash balance of $1,350,000 is required to meet the firm's short-term working capital needs. If the firm cannot maintain this balance, it must make a decision whether it will transfer funds from its replacement reserves or whether it will borrow short-term through a line-of-credit arrangement. **TABLE 23-7** combines the cash receipt and cash disbursement summaries to produce the cash budget.

The cash budget shows the firm will experience negative cash flows in some months. However, in this initial 6-month forecast, no month will show a balance less than the required cash balance of $1,350,000. If the forecast proves to be accurate, the firm will not need to arrange any short-term financing or transfer any replacement reserves. In fact, it could transfer some of the short-term cash balances that are more than the required minimal balance of $1,350,000 to replacement reserves. The firm could transfer all $50,000 in cash flow that occurs in January to replacement reserves, but only $160,000 of the $300,000 net cash flow in February could be transferred because the March cash flow will be a negative $140,000.

By examining the pattern of expected cash flows, the treasurer of the firm can better decide the duration and maturity of possible investments. Usually, longer-term securities yield higher returns. Therefore, if the funds are not expected to be needed for 6 months, the firm would be better off to invest in a 6-month treasury bill than a 30-day treasury bill.

**TABLE 23-6**  Cash Disbursements Summary (in Thousands)

|  | January | February | March | April | May | June |
|---|---|---|---|---|---|---|
| Salary and wages | $1,190 | $900 | $980 | $880 | $850 | $840 |
| Payroll deductions | $541 | $400 | $446 | $400 | $386 | $382 |
| Fringe benefits | 155 | 130 | 135 | 125 | 115 | 110 |
| Purchases | 315 | 385 | 405 | 390 | 385 | 385 |
| Other disbursements | 185 | 205 | 225 | 190 | 210 | 250 |
| Capital expenditures | 25 | 15 | 100 | 350 | 45 | 60 |
| Debt service | 0 | 0 | 300 | 0 | 0 | 300 |
| Estimated disbursement | $2,411 | $2,035 | $2,591 | $2,335 | $1,991 | $2,327 |

**TABLE 23-7**  Cash Budget Summary (in Thousands)

|  | January | February | March | April | May | June |
|---|---|---|---|---|---|---|
| Beginning cash balance | $1,350 | $1,400 | $1,700 | $1,560 | $1,555 | $1,830 |
| Add receipts | 2,461 | 2,335 | 2,451 | 2,330 | 2,266 | 2,222 |
| Less disbursements | 2,411 | 2,035 | 2,591 | 2,335 | 1,991 | 2,327 |
| Cash flow | 50 | 300 | (140) | (5) | 275 | (105) |
| Ending cash balance | $1,400 | $1,700 | $1,560 | $1,555 | $1,830 | $1,725 |

# ▶ SUMMARY

Cash budgets are critical pieces of information that financial executives in all healthcare firms need to prepare and monitor closely. The forecast of cash flows should help management determine whether additional financing will be needed, in what amounts, and for what duration. The information also permits the short-term investment of surplus funds so that yields on those investments might be improved.

Cash budgets are forecasts, and there is no guarantee that the results forecast will be achieved. It is important for management to test the sensitivity of the forecasts regarding alternative scenarios, such as slowdowns in collections or declines in revenues.

## ASSIGNMENTS

1. Morgan Village is a voluntary, nonprofit, continuing care retirement center. Presently, it has $1,200,000 set aside for replacement and renovation. Its current accumulated depreciation is $1,800,000, and the average age of the plant is 10 years. If it can be assumed that capital assets for Morgan Village are inflating at 6% per year, what balance would Morgan Village need to have set aside today to meet their replacement needs if they will not be using any debt financing?

2. Huntley Hospital must maintain $3.3 million in a debt service reserve fund maintained by the bond trustee. The board members would like to count this balance when determining the amount of cash that they should carry for meeting normal transaction needs. Is this reasonable?
3. Dean Nursing Home has a payer mix of approximately 60% Medicaid and 40% private pay. The state Medicaid program recently has experienced major funding problems, and the frequency of payment for Medicaid beneficiaries is unclear for the next year. How might this information affect Dean's cash management?
4. Prepare a cash budget for Aztec Home Health Agency for the months of May, June, and July. The firm wishes to maintain a $200,000 minimum cash balance during the period, and it presently has a $220,000 balance as of April 30. Revenues are presented in **TABLE 23-8**.

The firm collects 30% of its revenue in the month billing occurred, 30% in the next month, and 25% in the following month. The firm fails to collect 15% of its revenue because of either bad debt or contractual allowances. Expense budget relationships are presented here:

Payroll = $50,000 per month plus 0.50 × revenues
Supplies = 0.10 × revenues
Rent = $50,000 per month
Debt service = $150,000 in July
Capital expenditures = $75,000 in June

Eighty percent of payroll expense is paid in the month this expense was incurred, and 20% is paid in the following month. Supplies expense is paid in the following month. All other items are paid in the month reported. Determine during which months Aztec can invest surplus funds and during which months it might need to borrow.

**TABLE 23-8** Revenues for Aztec Home Health Agency

| | |
|---|---|
| January | 500,000 |
| February | 500,000 |
| March | 600,000 |
| April | 600,000 |
| May | 700,000 |
| June | 800,000 |
| July | 1,000,000 |
| August | 1,000,000 |

## SOLUTIONS AND ANSWERS

1. The total amount of required replacement reserves should be

   $1,800,000 × (1.06)^{10}$, or $3,223,400

2. No. The debt service reserve fund is not under the control of Huntley Hospital management and could not be used to meet normal transactional needs for cash such as payroll and purchases.
3. Because cash flows are likely to be more volatile next year, Dean should consider enhancing its liquidity position. This might be accomplished by increasing the amount of short-term cash reserves or negotiating a line of credit.
4. Surplus funds will be available during May and June, but a loan will need to be obtained during July, as the cash budget in **TABLE 23-9** shows.

**TABLE 23-9** Cash Budget for Aztec Home Health Agency

|  | May | June | July |
|---|---|---|---|
| Receipts |  |  |  |
| March revenue | $150,000 | $0 | $0 |
| April revenue | 180,000 | 150,000 | 0 |
| May revenue | 210,000 | 210,000 | 175,000 |
| June revenue | 0 | 240,000 | 240,000 |
| July revenue | 0 | 0 | 300,000 |
| Total receipts | $540,000 | $600,000 | $715,000 |
| Disbursements |  |  |  |
| Payroll |  |  |  |
| April | $70,000 | $0 | $0 |
| May | 320,000 | 80,000 | 0 |
| June | 0 | 360,000 | 90,000 |
| July | 0 | 0 | 440,000 |
| Total payroll disbursed | $390,000 | $440,000 | $530,000 |
| Supplies | 60,000 | 70,000 | 80,000 |
| Rent | 50,000 | 50,000 | 50,000 |
| Debt service | 0 | 0 | 150,000 |
| Capital expenditures | 0 | 75,000 | 0 |
| Total disbursements | $500,000 | $635,000 | $810,000 |
| Net cash flow | $40,000 | ($35,000) | ($95,000) |
| Beginning balance | $220,000 | $260,000 | $225,000 |
| Ending cash | 260,000 | 225,000 | 130,000 |
| Less required minimum | 200,000 | 200,000 | 200,000 |
| Net investment (borrowing) | $60,000 | $25,000 | ($70,000) |

# Glossary

**501(c)(3)** Provision of the Internal Revenue Code that relates to charitable purpose. Provides that not-for-profit hospitals qualify for tax exemption.

# A

**Accounting** The process and principles for preparing and disseminating financial information. The third phase of the management control process.

**Accounting entity** The organization for which financial information is recorded and reported.

**Accounting period** The elapsed time between financial statements. Common accounting periods include a month, a quarter, and a year.

**Accounts** Term used to refer to the individual assets and liabilities.

**Accounts payable** Amounts the organization is obligated to pay others, including suppliers and creditors.

**Accounts receivable** Amounts due to the organization from patients, third parties, and others.

**Accrual (basis of) accounting** The system of accounting that recognizes revenues when earned and expenses when resources are used. *See also* Cash-basis accounting.

**Accrued liabilities** Expenses that have been incurred but not yet paid.

**Accumulated depreciation** The cumulative amount of depreciation recognized on an asset since its purchase. An asset's book value is equal to its purchase price less the amount of accumulated depreciation.

**Acid test ratio** [(cash + marketable securities)/current liabilities] A liquidity ratio that measures how much cash and marketable securities are available to pay off all current liabilities.

**Acquisition (or historical) cost** Alternative method of asset valuation. Assessing in this method means the value of the asset is not changed over time to reflect changing market values.

**Acquisition of assets** An acquisition in which the acquiring company ends up directly owning the target's assets and may or may not directly have responsibility for liabilities. The target corporation can either continue to exist or be liquidated.

**Acquisition of stock** An acquisition in which the target company remains in existence as a separate legal entity while the acquiring company owns stock of target, but does not own target's individual assets such as inventory, equipment, or land.

**Activity-based costing (ABC)** A method to determine the costs of a service, product, or customer by tracing the resources consumed. ABC focuses on (1) controlling and calculating costs, (2) tracing as opposed to allocating costs, and (3) the importance of indirect costs. *See also* Step-down method.

**Activity ratios** Ratios that measure how efficiently an organization is using its assets to produce revenues.

**Actual level of volume** A level of activity that is critical in cost variance analysis, because if management has established a set of expectations concerning how costs should behave, given changes in volume from budgeted levels, an adjustment to budgeted cost can be made for a change in volume.

**Additional parity financing** A section in the indenture that defines the conditions that must be satisfied before the firm can issue any additional debt.

**Administrative cost centers** Organizational units responsible for their own costs that provide administrative support to other organizational units or the organization as a whole.

**Admitting diagnosis** The initial diagnosis made upon admission to a hospital.

**Adverse risk selection** Term used to describe the inclusion of patients who will become high resource users in a health plan.

**Age of plant ratio** (accumulated depreciation/depreciation expense) This ratio indicates the average number of years an organization has owned its plant and equipment.

**Allocation base** A statistic used to allocate costs from a cost center based on a cause-and-effect relationship. For example, a common allocation base to allocate the costs of maintaining medical records is number of visits. *See also* Cost driver.

**Allowance for depreciation** The accumulated depreciation taken on the asset to the date of the financial statement.

**Allowance for uncollectibles** A balance sheet account that estimates the total amount of patient accounts receivable that will not be collected. Also called allowance for bad debts and allowance for doubtful accounts.

**Ambulatory payment classifications (APCs)** Groups of outpatient services paid on a prospective basis to hospitals by CMS.

**Amortization of a loan** The gradual process of paying off debt through a long series of equal periodic payments. Each payment covers a portion of the principal plus current interest. The periodic payments are equal over the lifetime of the loan, but the proportion going toward principal gradually increases.

**Analysis and reporting** The last phase in management control, which reports and explains deviations from budgets.

**Ancillary service usage** The types of services that a patient requires while in a facility; one of the factors that determine service intensity.

**Annuity** A series of equal cash flows made or received at regular time intervals. "Ordinary annuities" describe annuities where the cash flows occur at the end of each period, whereas "annuities due" the cash flows occur at the beginning of each period.

**Appropriations** Monies provided by governmental agencies to organizations.

**Asset mix** The percentage of each asset relative to total assets.

**Assets** The resources owned by the organization. It is one of the three major categories on the balance sheet.

**Assets that have limited use** Funds, excluding those restricted by donors, that have been set aside for specific purposes and are not available for general use. The balance sheet presentation of assets limited as to use must differentiate between current and noncurrent assets limited as to use and separate internally designated amounts from externally designated amounts either on the balance sheet or in the notes to the financial statements.

**Assignment over time** Determines the total value or cost of a resource that is used to produce a final product.

**Audited financial statements** The collective term used for financial statements once they are prepared and reviewed by an external, independent accounting firm.

**Authority** The entity (usually governmental) that formally issues tax-exempt revenue bonds on behalf of the beneficiary. It is not responsible for payment of the bonds and plays no active role once the bonds are issued.

**Average charge per Medicare discharge CMI Adj.** Defines the average price for a Medicare discharge with a case-mix weight of 1.0.

**Average charge per Medicare visit RW Adj.** Uses the weights assigned by Medicare to pay for outpatient procedures to case-mix adjust individual claims. A concept similar to the average charge per Medicare discharge case-mix adjusted measure.

**Average payment period** {current liabilities/[(total expenses – depreciation expense)/365]} This ratio measures how long, on average, it takes an organization to pay its bills.

**Average relative weight per outpatient visit (service mix index)** The total APC paid weight in an outpatient visit.

**Avoidable fixed cost** A fixed cost that is avoided or eliminated if a particular service is no longer offered.

# B

**Bad debt (doubtful account)** An amount owed to the organization that will not be paid. Charity care is not considered a bad debt because nothing is owed to the organization for services provided.

**Bad-debt provisions** Recognition of the amount of charges that will not be collected from patients from whom payment was expected. *See also* Allowance for uncollectibles.

**Balance sheet** One of the four major financial statements of a healthcare organization. It presents a summary of the organization's assets, liabilities, and net assets as of a certain date.

**Balanced scorecards** Neatly formatted reports that provide information on the organization's performance in a limited number of areas. The reports help focus attention to key performance indicators (also referred to as key metrics or measures) that are typically defined by senior leadership.

**Basic accounting equation** (assets = liabilities + owners' equity) In nonprofit, business-oriented healthcare organizations, the analogous equation is assets = liabilities + net assets.

**Basis point** A method to describe the change in a bond's interest rate where a 1% change equals 100 basis points. One basis point is one-hundredth of 1% in the yield of an investment.

**Beginning inventory** The amount of inventory on hand at the beginning of an accounting period. *See also* Ending inventory.

**Benchmarking data** Comparative reference points used to help determine how a business is doing with respect to similar firms in any given industry, or how it is doing relative to its primary competitors.

**Benefit period (spell of illness), Medicare** The unit of time for measuring use of Part A benefits. The period begins upon the beneficiary's admission to a hospital or other facility and ends after 60 consecutive days during which the individual was not an inpatient of any hospital, skilled nursing facility, or rehabilitative facility. Although there are limits to covered benefits per benefit period, there is no limit to the number of benefit periods a beneficiary can have. The beneficiary must pay the Part A deductible for each new period.

**Bond rating** An assignment or grading of the likelihood that an organization will not default on a bond.

**Bond-rating (or credit-rating) agency** Agencies that assess the credit worthiness of an organization. The three major agencies are Moody's, Standard & Poor's, and Fitch.

**Bonds** A form of long-term financing whereby the issuer receives cash and in return issues a note. The issuer agrees to make principal and/or interest payments on specific dates to the holders of the note.

**Book value** The cost of a capital asset minus accumulated depreciation.

**Break-even analysis** An approach to analyzing the relationship among revenues, costs, and volume. It is also called cost-volume-profit or CVP analysis.

**Break-even point** The point at which total revenues equal total costs. It is described by the equation: (price × volume) = fixed costs + (variable cost per unit × volume).

**Budget** The central document of the planning/control cycle that identifies revenues and resources that will be needed by an organization to achieve its goals and objectives. It is a quantitative expression of a plan of action stated in monetary terms and typically covers a period of 1 year.

**Budget variance** The difference between what was planned (budgeted) and what was achieved (actual).

**Budgetary committee** A committee composed of several department managers, headed by the controller that is often used to aid in budget development and approval.

**Budgeted or expected volume** Critical in cost variance analysis. It is on this expected volume level that management establishes its commitments for resources and therefore incurs cost. An unjustified faith in volume forecasts can lock management into a sizable fixed-cost position, especially regarding labor costs.

**Bundled services** Services provided to a patient in an encounter of care aggregated into one payment unit.

**Bundling** The pricing mechanism that combines services that are charged for separately into a single package with a single price.

# C

**Callable bonds** Bonds that may be redeemed by the issuer before they mature.

**Cannibalization** A situation that occurs when a new service decreases the revenues or cash flows from existing services.

**Capital** The sources of funds to finance the noncurrent assets of the organization. It is also considered the debt and equity of the organization.

**Capital appreciation** The increase in the value of an investment from the time it is purchased until the time it is sold.

**Capital assets** Assets that have a useful life greater than 1 year, such as plant, property, and equipment. Plant and equipment are depreciated over time; land (property) is not.

**Capital budget** The budget used to forecast, and in some cases justify, the expenditures (and in some cases the sources of financing) for capital expenditures.

**Capital costs (or capital expenditures)** Costs associated with the investment in equipment and facilities. Capital expenditure items are expected to provide benefits during a reasonably long period, at least 2 or more years.

**Capital investment decisions** Decisions regarding the acquisition of capital assets. This decision should be separate from the decision on how to finance capital assets.

**Capital lease** A lease in which the lessor aims to lease an asset for virtually all its economic life. In return, the lessee is committed to lease payments for the entire lease period. Also called a financial lease.

**Capital structure decisions** Decisions regarding the relative amount of debt and equity used to finance the organization's noncurrent assets.

**Capital structure ratios** Ratios that measure how the organization's assets are financed and/or whether the organization can take on new debt.

**Capitation** A payment system in which providers receive a specific amount in advance to care for specific healthcare needs of a defined population over a specific period. Providers are usually paid on a per-member-per-month (PMPM) basis, and they assume the risk of caring for the covered population for the PMPM amount. The payments are derived from premiums paid by enrollees, and typically, administrative fees for claims payment, case management, profit, and other costs are taken out of the premium before any payment is made to providers.

**Case management** The coordination of services provided to a patient by a specific entity. It is often provided by a primary physician or by clinical experts who have the responsibility to approve, monitor, and/or evaluate the care given to a patient.

**Case mix** The mix of patients served by a provider classified by one or more salient characteristics (age, sex, diagnosis, acuity, etc.).

**Case rates** A fixed reimbursement amount depending on the type of case (hip replacement, normal newborn delivery, cardiac catheterization, etc.).

**Cash and cash equivalents** The balance sheet category that includes actual money on hand as well as money equivalents, such as savings and checking accounts. It excludes money restricted for something other than current operations.

**Cash-basis accounting** The system of accounting that recognizes revenues when cash is received and expenses when cash is paid out. *See also* Accrual basis of accounting.

**Cash budget** The budget that projects the organization's cash inflows and outflows. The bottom line is the amount of cash available at the end of the period.

**Cash flows from financing activities** Cash inflows and outflows resulting from activities such as obtaining grants or endowments or from borrowing or paying back long-term debt.

**Cash flows from investing activities** Cash inflows and outflows resulting from activities such as purchasing and selling investments or investing in itself by purchasing or selling noncurrent assets. It also includes transfers to and from the parent corporation.

**Cash flows from operating activities** The changes in cash resulting from the normal operating activities of the organization.

**Cash management** Processes and techniques focused on the acceleration of receivables and the cash conversion cycle. Reduction of the cash conversion cycle, along with the related investment of surplus funds, should be a critical objective of financial managers.

**Cash surplus** Money exceeding a minimum balance that the firm prefers to maintain to meet immediate operating expenses and minor contingencies, plus any compensating balance required by creditors.

**CC/MCC capture rate** Comorbidity or complication (CC) and major complication and comorbidity (MCC) rates based on the MS-DRG system ranks how hospitals are performing based on the national average. It is a standard comparison that hospitals can use in order to determine whether they are properly coding the severity of a patient's illness.

**Certificate of need (CON)** The process by which a provider justifies the necessity for capital expenditures to obtain approval from an independent agency, such as the government. If approved, a CON is issued.

**Certified public accountant (CPA)** An accountant who has passed certain examinations and met all other statutory and licensing requirements of a U.S. state to be certified.

**Charge-based system** A system in which providers set the rates for services. Reimbursement is based on the charge rather than being predetermined by the payer.

**Charge capture** Accumulation of actual paper documents or charge slips used to identify services performed, which are then posted to a patient's account in a batch-processing mode by data processing or the business office. Alternatively, an order entry system may involve direct entry of charges to the patient's account through a computer terminal.

**Charge code** A unique code reflected in the order entry system or the charge slips and also represented on the firm's charge master (also known as CDM). There one code for each service procedure, supply item, or drug in the CDM.

**Charge description master (CDM)** A list of all items for which a firm has established specific prices.

**Charge explosion** A system used to better organize charge entry for selective services. One code is used, which then explodes into the list of supply codes used for that surgery.

**Charitable gift annuity** A type of gift transaction where an individual transfers assets to a charity in exchange for a tax benefit and a lifetime annuity.

**Charity allowance** The difference between established gross charge service rates and the amounts actually charged to indigent patients.

**Charity care** Free care provided to those who cannot pay for service. Also called indigent care. Each organization must have rules to differentiate it from bad debt. Some healthcare institutions may receive appropriations from the government to help offset the costs.

**Claim** A request by a provider for payment for services provided to a beneficiary.

**Coefficient of variation** The ratio of the standard deviation divided by the mean. Large values for this ratio in a budgeting context imply large control limit corridors.

**Coinsurance (Medicare)** That portion of covered hospital and medical expenses, after subtraction of any deductible, for which the beneficiary is responsible. Under Part A, there is no coinsurance for the first 60 days of inpatient hospital care; from the 61st through the 90th day of inpatient care, the daily coinsurance amount is equal to one-fourth of the inpatient hospital deductible. For each of the 60 lifetime reserve days used, the daily coinsurance amount is equal to one-half of the inpatient hospital deductible. There is no coinsurance for the first 20 days of skilled nursing facility (SNF) care; from the 21st through the 100th day of SNF care, the daily coinsurance amount is equal to one-eighth of the inpatient hospital deductible. Under Part B, after the annual deductible has been met the beneficiary must generally pay 20% of the approved amount (plus any charges above the approved amount).

**Collateral** A borrower's assets on which a lender has legal claim if a borrower defaults on a loan.

**Collection** The interval between the generation of a bill and the actual collection of the cash from the patient or the patient's third-party payer.

**Commercial paper (CP or C.P.)** A negotiable promissory note (essentially an IOU) issued at a discount by large corporations.

**Commitment fee** A percentage of the unused portion of a credit line charged to the potential borrower. The annual fee is a function of the credit risk of the borrower and the reason for the line of credit.

**Common stock** Stock that entitles its holders to ownership rights in the corporation and to dividends only after the rights of preferred stockholders have been satisfied.

**Community benefit** Related to nonprofit hospitals. Term used to describe the scope of services and support that a hospital provides in return for its tax-exempt status. Services include charity care and setting lower prices, or offering services that, from a financial perspective, might not be viable for for-profit firms.

**Community Value Index® (CVI)** An index created to provide a measure of the value a hospital provides to its community. It is composed of 10 measures that assess a hospital's performance in 4 areas. It suggests that a hospital provides value to the community when it is financially viable, is appropriately reinvesting back into the facility, is maintaining a low-cost structure, has reasonable charges, and is providing high-quality care to patients.

**Compensating balance** The amount required to be maintained on deposit with the bank for such things as maintaining a credit line and fee-free checking.

**Compounding** (1) Calculating interest using the compound interest method. (2) Adjusting for the time value of money forward in time to a future value. *See also* Compound interest method *and* Discounting.

**Compound interest method** The method of determining the future value of money in which interest is calculated on the cumulative principal and interest earned up to that point. *See also* Simple interest method.

**Concurrent review** Monitoring the continued medical necessity of hospital treatment and assessing discharge needs to determine the appropriateness of payment.

**Conglomerate mergers** Mergers that involve firms engaged in unrelated business activity.

**Consolidation** Two or more corporations combine into a brand new corporation.

**Constant dollars** Alternative unit of measurement in financial reporting. This measurement reports the effects of all financial transactions in terms of constant purchasing power. The unit that is usually used is the purchasing power of the dollar at the end of the reporting period or the average during the fiscal year. The measurement is made by multiplying the unadjusted, or nominal, dollars by a price index to convert to a measure of constant purchasing power.

**Contingencies** Uncontrollable changes in the environment that may affect the financial condition of the organization (changes in the payment system, labor shortages, and catastrophic events).

**Continuing care retirement communities (CCRCs)** Providers with a continuum of care that runs the gamut from independent living, to assisted living, to skilled care.

**Contra asset** An asset that, when increased, decreases the value of a related asset. Two primary examples are accumulated depreciation, which is the contra asset to properties and equipment, and the allowance for doubtful accounts, which is the contra asset to accounts receivable.

**Contractual allowances** The difference between rates billed to a third-party payer, such as Medicare, and the amount that actually will be paid by that third-party payer.

**Contribution margin** The amount remaining after subtracting variable costs from revenues. When the organization is not at capacity, it is the "profit" the organization makes on providing each new unit that is available to cover all other costs. It may be determined on a total or per unit basis.

**Control chart** A chart that always has a central line for the average, an upper line for the control limit, and a lower line for the lower control limit.

**Controllable costs** Costs that can be influenced by a designated responsibility center or departmental manager within a defined control period.

**Construction in progress** This is a long-term asset account that accumulates the cost of a project that has not yet been placed into service.

**Coordination of benefits** The process of assigning payment responsibility when multiple insurers exist.

**Copayments** The part of a healthcare bill for which the patient is responsible. These payments are used to prevent overutilization of services.

**Cost** The resources used to produce a good or service.

**Cost allocation** The process of assigning pooled indirect costs to specific cost objects using an allocation base that represents a major function of a business.

**Cost-based systems** A payment system that uses provider cost, as opposed to charges, as the starting point to determine the amount of payment.

**Cost basis** The process by which a value is assigned to each and every resource transaction occurring between the entity being accounted for and another entity.

**Cost centers** Organizational units responsible for providing services and controlling their costs. There are two major types: clinical and administrative.

**Cost driver** An activity or event that causes activities to occur and thus resources to be used and costs to be incurred.

**Cost object** Anything for which a cost is found (a test, a visit, a patient day).

**Cost of capital** The rate of return required to undertake a project. *See also* Discount rate *and* Hurdle rate *and* Weighted average cost of capital (WACC).

**Cost-payment basis** The underlying method for payment will be the provider's cost.

**Cost shifting** The increasing payment from payers to cover losses from governmental and charity patients.

**Cost structure** The relative proportion of each type of cost present in a firm.

**Cost variance analysis** A type of analysis whose successful use requires a sound system of standard setting, or budgeting, and a related system of cost accounting. It has great potential importance to the healthcare industry.

**Coupon** A certificate attached to a bond representing the amount of interest to be paid to the holder.

**Coupon rate** The stated interest rate on a bond, as promised by the issuer.

**Courtesy allowance** The difference between established rates for services and rates billed to special patients, such as employees, physicians, and clergy.

**Covenant** Legal provisions in a bond that must be followed by the issuer. Also called a loan covenant.

**Creditor** An entity that is owed money for lending funds or supplying goods or services on credit.

**Current assets** Assets that will be used or consumed within 1 year. Some organizations use a period of less than 1 year.

**Current liabilities** An organization's financial obligations that are to be paid within 1 year.

**Current portion (or maturities) of long-term debt** The amount of principal that will be repaid on the indebtedness within the coming year. It does not equal the total amount of the payments that will be made during that year.

**Current procedural terminology (CPT) codes** Codes for reporting medical services and procedures performed by physicians. *See also* Healthcare Common Procedure Coding System (HCPCS).

**Current ratio (current assets to current liabilities)** A liquidity ratio that measures the proportion of all current assets to all current liabilities to determine how easily current debt can be paid off. It is one of the most commonly used ratios.

**Current (or replacement) value** Alternative method of asset valuation. This method of valuation revalues the assets in each reporting period. The assets are stated at their current value rather than their acquisition cost. This method recognizes gains or losses from holding assets before sale or retirement.

**Current value–general price level adjusted (CV-GPL)** Alternative method of financial reporting. Often referred to as *current cost accounting*.

# D

**Dashboards** Subset of balanced scorecards. Neatly formatted reports that provide information on the organization's performance in a limited number of areas. The reports help focus attention to key performance indicators (also referred to as key metrics or measures) that are typically defined by senior leadership.

**Days cash on hand** {[cash marketable securities]/ [(operating expenses – depreciation)/365]} A ratio that indicates the number of days' worth of expenses an organization can cover with its most liquid assets (cash and marketable securities).

**Days in accounts receivable** [net accounts receivable/ (net patient revenues/365)] This ratio indicates how quickly a hospital is converting its receivables into cash. It provides an estimate of how many days' revenues are yet to be collected.

**Debenture** An unsecured bond, one that is not backed by any specific lien on the property.

**Debt financing** Borrowing money from others at a cost in the form of interest. It is an alternative to equity financing. *See also* Equity financing.

**Debt policy** The percentage of the firm's investment that the board permits to be financed with debt.

**Debt service coverage** [(excess of revenues over expenses + interest expense + depreciation expense)/(interest expense + principal payments)] A ratio that measures an organization's ability to pay back a loan.

**Debt service reserve** This fund represents a cushion for the investors if the issuer gets into some type of fiscal crisis.

**Decay curves** Curves that relate future collections to past billings that are a common way to develop forecasts of patient receipts.

**Deductible** A set amount the patient is responsible for paying before third-party coverage begins. These are used to prevent overutilization of services.

**Deduction percentage** It is one of several measures for contract negotiation assessment. Specifically, it shows the amount of contractual allowances deducted from gross charges. A lower percentage is clearly more desirable because additional net revenue results with the lower value.

**Defeasance** The process of voiding existing indenture covenants and removing the bonds from the issuer's financial statements.

**Deferred revenues** Monies received that have not yet been earned. One of the most common types of deferred revenues is the receipt of capitation on the basis of per member per month.

**Depreciation** An estimate/measure of how much a tangible asset (such as plant or equipment) has been "used up" during an accounting period. It is an expense that does not require any cash outflow under the accrual basis of accounting. *See also* Accumulated depreciation.

**Depreciation reserve** This fund is sometimes set up to equal the cumulative difference between debt principal repayment and depreciation expense on the depreciable assets financed with debt.

**Diagnosis-related groups (DRGs)** A patient classification system that categorizes patients into groups that are clinically coherent and homogeneous with respect to resource use. The prospective payment system uses approximately 550 DRGs as the basis for payment to hospitals.

**Direct costs** Costs that are traced to a cost object. *See also* Indirect costs *and* Cost object.

**Discount** (1) A reduction in the charge for services. (2) When the market rate is higher than the coupon rate, a bond is said to be selling at a discount from its par value. *See also* Premium.

**Discount rate** (1) The returns that must be generated on a project to compensate the organization for its risk. (2) The returns the organization is forgoing by investing its money in one project as opposed to an alternative of similar risk. *See also* Cost of capital *and* Hurdle rate *and* Weighted average cost of capital (WACC).

**Discounted cash flows** Cash flows that have been adjusted (discounted) to their present value to account for the cost of capital (over time) and the time value of money.

**Discounting** The process of adjusting for the time value of money backward in time to present value. *See also* Compounding.

**Discounts from billed charges** A negotiated reduction from list price granted to a health plan or uninsured patient.

**Disproportionate share hospital** A hospital that serves a relatively large volume of low-income patients.

**Disproportionate share payment** A separate Medicare payment that is provided to a hospital that treats a large percentage of Medicaid and Medicaid-eligible patients.

**Divestitures** The sale of a portion of the firm to an outside party with cash or equivalent consideration received by the divesting firm.

**Dividends** The portion of profit an organization distributes to investors. By law, only investor-owned healthcare organizations can distribute dividends outside the organization.

**Donation** Funds provided by a private entity or individual without the requirement of repayment. Donations can be either restricted or unrestricted. Also called philanthropy.

**Double-distribution** Method of cost allocation that is a refinement of the step-down method. Instead of closing the individual department after allocating its costs, it is kept open and receives the costs of other indirect departments. After one complete allocation sequence, the former departments are then closed, using the normal step-down method.

**Doubtful account allowance** The difference between rates billed and amounts expected to be recovered.

**DRGs** *See* Diagnosis-related groups.

**Dual entitlement (dual eligible)** Indicates that an individual is entitled for both Medicare and Medicaid coverage.

**Duality principle** A principle that states that the value of assets must always equal the combined value of liabilities and residual interest (also called net assets). This basic accounting equation may be stated as follows: assets = liabilities + net assets

**Due to third-party payers** Money that is due to an intermediary payer (Medicare, Blue Cross, etc.) from the organization that is, as yet, unpaid.

**Durable medical equipment (DME)** Under Medicare, this includes certain medical supplies and items such as hospital beds and wheelchairs used in a patient's home.

**Dynamic coding** When codes are left off the charge master and entered later by health information management personnel. Also referred to as soft coding.

# E

**Economic obligations** Responsibilities to transfer economic resources or provide services to other entities in the future, usually in return for economic resources received from other entities in the past through the purchase of assets, the receipt of services, or the acceptance of loans.

**Economic resources** Scarce means, limited in supply but essential to economic activity. They include supplies, buildings, equipment, money, claims to receive money, and ownership interests in other enterprises.

**Effectiveness** The relationship of the firm's outputs to its stated goals and objectives.

**Efficiency** (1) Measuring inputs against outputs. (2) The cost of service per unit rendered.

**Efficiency variances** The difference between actual quantity ($I^a$) and budgeted quantity ($I^b$) multiplied by budgeted price ($P^b$).

**Electronic billing** A process whereby bills are sent electronically to third parties through electronic data interfacing.

**Employee benefits** Indirect and non-cash compensation paid to an employee that includes such items as social security, unemployment, workers compensation, vacation, pension, and health insurance.

**Encounter of care** All services and products provided to the patient during a specific treatment at a healthcare firm.

**Ending inventory** The amount of inventory on hand at the end of an accounting period. *See also* Beginning inventory.

**Endowment funds** Funds contributed to be held intact for generating income. The income may or may not be restricted for specific purposes.

**Enterprise value** The value of all capital invested in the business, represented as follows: market value of equity + net debt. Also termed firm value or total value.

**Equivalent annual cost** The expected average cost, considering both capital and operating cost, over the life of the project. Calculated by dividing the sum of the present value of operating costs over the life of the project and the present value of the investment cost by the discount factor for an annualized stream of equal payments

**Equity financing** The purchase of assets with contributed and internally generated funds. *See also* Debt financing.

**Equity growth** The rate at which a firm's equity position is increasing. It is a critical measure of long-term financial success and a direct indicator of the firm's asset growth potential.

**Estimated third-party payer settlements** Amounts due to (or from) third-party payers for advances or overpayments (or underpayments) from third parties.

**Excess of revenues over expenses** Operating income plus other income. This is analogous to net income before taxes in for-profit entities.

**Expenditure** An actual outlay of cash that may or may not be recognized as an accounting expense at the time of payment.

**Expense** A measure of the resources used to generate revenue and/or provide a service. Often used synonymously with costs. *See also* Cost.

**Expense budget** The budget used to forecast operating expenses.

**Expense cost variance** [(actual cost per unit – budgeted cost per unit) × actual volume] The difference between the variable expenses that would have been expected at the actual volume and those actually incurred.

**Expense volume variance** [(actual volume – budgeted volume) × budgeted cost per unit] The portion of total variance that is due to actual volume being either higher or lower than budgeted volume. It is the difference between the expenses forecast in the original budget and what would have been expected at the actual volume.

**Extraordinary item** An extremely unusual and infrequent occurrence.

# F

**Face value** The amount the bond will be worth when it "matures" in the future.

**Factoring** The selling of accounts receivable at a discount, usually to a bank, to obtain cash.

**Favorable variance** (1) When actual revenues are higher than budgeted revenues. (2) When actual expenses are lower than budgeted expenses. *See also* Unfavorable variance.

**Feasibility study** A study that looks at factors affecting an issue's ability to generate the necessary cash flows to meet principal and interest requirements.

**Federal Housing Administration (FHA) program loans** Mortgage insurance provided by the Federal Housing Administration that guarantees the principal and interest on a loan for a healthcare provider.

**Fee-for-service arrangement (FFS)** Arrangements in which providers receive payment for "necessary" services as the services are provided.

**Fee-schedule basis** The actual payment is predetermined and is unrelated to either the provider's cost or the provider's actual prices.

**Financial accounting** The branch of accounting that provides general-purpose financial statements or reports to aid many decision-making groups, internal and external to the organization, in making a variety of decisions.

**Financial counseling** Staff at the healthcare firm can advise the patient regarding eligibility for discounts through the firm's charity care policy or governmental programs such as Medicaid. Staff can help the patient complete the necessary documents required for coverage.

**Financial Strength Index** An index that attempts to measure the four areas of financial position that collectively determine a firm's financial strength: profits, liquidity, debt structure, and age of physical facilities.

**Financing activities** A section of the statement of cash flows used to report activities such as borrowing and paying back loans.

**Financing mix** How an organization chooses to finance its working capital needs.

**Fiscal intermediary (FI)** A Medicare contractor that processes and pays Medicare institutional claims.

**Fixed assets** Literally, nonmovable assets. Generally used to refer to buildings and equipment.

**Fixed asset turnover ratio** [total revenues/net plant and equipment] A ratio that measures the number of dollars generated for each dollar invested in an organization's plant and equipment.

**Fixed budget period** Covers some defined time from a given budget date, usually 1 year.

**Fixed costs** Costs that stay the same in total over the relevant range as volume increases but that change inversely on a per unit basis.

**Fixed income securities** Securities that pay a fixed amount of interest periodically, usually semiannually, over the lifetime of the bond.

**Fixed-(interest) rate debt** A security with an interest rate that does not change during the lifetime of the bond.

**Fixed labor budget** The section of the expense budget that forecasts salary and benefits that do not change with volume.

**Fixed supplies budget** The section of the expense budget that forecasts the cost of those supplies that will not vary as a direct result of changes in the amount of services provided (such as administrative office supplies).

**Flexible budget** A budget that adjusts revenues and/or expenses based on service volume.

**Float** Time delays in the billing and collection process. There are four categories: billing, collection, transit, and disbursement. An organization's goal is to optimize it for incoming revenues and outgoing bills.

**For-profit** A type of organization whose profits can be distributed outside the organization and must pay taxes. Also called "investor-owned organizations."

**Free cash flow** Typically used in the discounted cash flow calculation, it refers to those cash flows that are available to stakeholders (e.g., equity and debt holders) after consideration for taxes, capital expenditures, and working capital needs. Cash flow should be considered as the cash flow contribution the target is expected to make to the acquiring company. The following formula is used to calculate free cash flows: [EBIT × (1 − t) + noncash expenses − capital expenditures − incremental working capital].

**FTE** Full-time equivalent employees. Two half-time employees equal one FTE.

**FTEs per adjusted patient day** This is one measure used to help show how many revenue dollars are generated with a given number of full-time equivalent employees.

**Fully allocated costs** The costs of a service after taking into account its direct and fair share of allocated costs.

**Fund balance** Term used for residual interest by not-for-profit healthcare organizations. Used interchangeably with net assets.

**Future value** What an amount invested today (or a series of payments made over time) will be worth at a given time in the future using the compound interest method. This accounts for the time value of money. *See also* Present value.

**Future value factor (FVF)** A factor that, when multiplied by a present amount, yields the future value of that amount. It is calculated using the formula $(1 + i)^n$, where $i$ is the interest rate and $n$ is the number of periods. *See also* Present value factor (PVF).

**Future value factor of an annuity (FVFA)** A factor that, when multiplied by a stream of equal payments, equals the future value of that stream.

**Future value of an annuity** What a series of equal payments will be worth at some future date using compound interest. *See also* Future value factor of an annuity (FVFA) *and* Present value of an annuity.

# G

**Gain or loss** (1) The difference between the amount received in selling a capital asset and its book value. (2) The difference between the purchase price of a stock and its sale price.

**Gatekeepers** Persons who must preapprove the care received by a patient, such as a primary care physician who must approve a patient visiting a specialist. Gatekeepers are used in most point-of-service and HMO plans.

**General and administrative (G & A) expenses** Operating expenses that are not contained in the labor or supplies budgets.

**Generally accepted accounting principles (GAAP)** Term often used to describe the body of rules and requirements that shape the preparation of the four primary financial statements created by the financial accountants.

**General obligation bonds** Bonds for which the tax revenue of a government entity is pledged.

**Geographic adjustment factor (GAF)** A measure of the effect of geographic location on the cost of a service. It is used in calculating Medicare physician payments.

**Geographic practice cost index (GPCI)** A measure of the differences in resource costs among physician fee schedule areas. There are three GPCIs, one for each relative value unit component: a work GPCI, an overhead GPCI, and a malpractice GPCI.

**Global payments** Payments in which the fees for all providers and suppliers (hospitals, physicians, nurses, home healthcare agencies, drugs, etc.) are included in a single negotiated amount. Often called "bundling of services."

**Going private** Shares are owned exclusively by the acquiring party (e.g., management) rather than by third-party investors, and there is no market for trading its shares.

**Goodwill** Defined as the price or value paid for a business less the fair market value of the tangible assets acquired.

**Governing board** A committee that oversees and provides direction to the senior management of an organization that provides the goals, objectives, and approved programs used as the basis for budgetary development. In many cases it formally approves the finalized budget, especially the cash budget and budgeted financial statements.

**Grants** Funds given to a healthcare organization for special purposes, usually for a limited time.

**Gross patient revenue** The total amount the healthcare organization charges for services before discounts and allowances.

**Grouper** Computer software that translates variables such as age, diagnosis, and surgical codes into the diagnosis-related group under which the Medicare payment amount is determined.

**Growth rate in equity (GRIE)** An amount defined as (return on equity (ROE)/reported income index).

# H

**HC–general price level adjusted (HC-GPL)** Alternative method of financial reporting. Often referred to as constant dollar accounting.

**Healthcare Common Procedure Coding System (HCPCS)** The HCPCS is a coding system for all services performed by a physician or supplier. It is based on the American Medical Association Physicians' *Current Procedural Terminology* codes and is augmented with codes for physician and nonphysician services (such as ambulance and durable medical equipment), which are not included in CPTs.

**Health maintenance organization (HMO)** Entities that receive premium payments (fixed periodic prepayment) from enrollees with the understanding that the HMO will be financially responsible for all predefined health care required by its enrollees for a specified period of time. The health care is provided through the HMO's provider network.

**Health savings accounts (HSAs)** Accounts created by individuals and funded with pretax dollars that can be used to pay for a variety of healthcare expenses, including large deductibles and copayments.

**Hedge** A transaction that reduces the risk of an investment.

**High–low method** A technique that can be used to estimate the variable and fixed-cost coefficients of a semivariable cost function.

**Home health agency (HHA)** A public agency or private organization that is primarily engaged in providing skilled nursing services and other therapeutic services in the patient's home. Service examples are physical, occupational, or speech therapy; medical social services; and home health aide services.

**Home health resource groups** Eighty case-mix groups available for patient classification using three classification criteria: clinical severity, functional severity, and service utilization severity. The Home Health Resource Grouping system in the proposed rule uses data from a large-scale case-mix research project conducted between 1997 and 1999.

**Home value program (HVP)** Fundraising effort designed for senior citizens, aged 70 or older, who own mortgage-free homes. The homeowners sign a revocable agreement that, upon their deaths, transfers the title to their homes to the hospital. In return, they receive a monthly payment that is based on a loan from the hospital.

**Horizontal merger** A merger of two firms that operate in the same kind of business.

**Hospice** Palliative care, such as medical relief of pain, provided to patients who are certified to be terminally ill.

**Hospital insurance (HI, Medicare)** Medicare HI, also referred to as Part A, covers expenses of inpatient, hospice, skilled nursing facility, or home health agency services for individuals who are age 65 or older and are eligible for retirement benefits under the Social Security or Railroad Retirement systems. Coverage is also provided for individuals under age 65 who have been entitled for not less than 24 months to benefits under the Social Security or Railroad Retirement systems on the basis of disability and for certain other individuals who are medically determined to have end-stage renal disease and are covered by the Social Security or Railroad Retirement systems.

**Hurdle rate** *See* Cost of capital *and* Discount rate *and* Weighted average cost of capital (WACC).

# I

**ICD-10** A diagnosis and procedure classification system published by the World Health Organization (WHO). ICD-10-CM codes are the basis for grouping patients into diagnosis-related groups and is the successor of the ICD-9-CM.

**Income** The excess of revenue over expenses, from a large number of individual operations within a healthcare entity, it is aggregated in the statement of revenues and expenses.

**Increase in unrestricted net assets** The bottom line in the statement of operations. It includes items such as operating and nonoperating income, contributions of long-lived assets, transfers to parent company, and extraordinary items.

**Incremental cash flows** Cash flows that occur solely as a result of undertaking a project. Basically, the marginal difference between alternatives.

**Incremental decremental approach** An approach to budgeting that begins with what exists and applies a slight increase, no change, or a slight decrease to various line items, programs, or departments. *See also* Zero-base budgeting.

**Incurred but not reported (IBNR)** When services have been delivered but no claim has been received to date.

**Indenture** Legal document that states the conditions and terms of a bond.

**Indirect costs** Costs that are not traced to a cost object but must eventually be allocated across cost objects. *See also* Direct costs.

**Indirect department** A department that may provide services, but they are usually not directly traceable to a specific patient encounter.

**Indirect medical education** Medicare add-on payment to a teaching hospital. This allowance is related to the numbers of interns and residents at the hospital and the hospital's bed size.

**Individual practice associations (IPA) model HMO** Loose affiliation of providers who agree to cover the healthcare needs of a covered population on a capitated basis, usually through a per-member-per-month payment arrangement.

**Inflation** The rise in an economy's general level of prices.

**Institutional services** Services provided by hospitals (outpatient and inpatient), home health agencies, hospices, comprehensive outpatient rehabilitation facilities, end-stage renal disease facilities, rural health clinics, and skilled nursing facilities.

**Interest** (1) The cost to borrow money. It can be expressed in dollars or as a percentage. (2) Payment to creditors for the use of money on credit.

**Interim claim** A request for payment that does not cover a complete stay in a hospital or skilled nursing facility that is submitted by a provider when a beneficiary is still receiving services (i.e., has not yet been discharged).

**Internal claims processing** Reviewing claims sent to payers to ensure that care has been appropriately described and decrease the chances that the claims will be denied. This process usually includes utilization review.

**Internal rate of return (IRR)** The percentage return on an investment. It is the rate of return at which the net present value equals zero. Often used as a comparison to cost of capital.

***International Classification of Diseases*, 9th Revision, *Clinical Modification* (ICD-9-CM)** The ICD-9-CM is a diagnosis and procedure classification system. ICD-9-CM codes are the basis for grouping patients into diagnosis-related groups.

**Inventories** In a healthcare facility, these are items that are to be used in the delivery of healthcare services. They may range from normal business office supplies to highly specialized chemicals used in a laboratory.

**Investment banker** One who advises corporate clients on their financial strategy and/or is primarily involved in the distribution of securities from the issuing organization to the public.

**Investment centers** Responsibility centers responsible for making a certain return on investments.

**Investment grade** Bonds that have received a rating ranging from AAA to BBB (at S&P) or Aaa to Bbb (Moody's), of which the highest are called quality ratings.

**Investor-owned** Firms owned by risk-based equity investors who expect the managers of the corporation to maximize shareholder wealth. *See also* For-profit.

**IRS Form 990** All not-for-profit firms with annual revenues greater than $25,000 and who are exempt from federal income tax are required to file this form on an annual basis. The form contains a variety of financial information, including balance sheet and income statement data. The form also contains information on compensation for the highest paid executives.

**Issuance costs** Expenditures that are essential to consummate the financing arrangement.

**Issuer** An entity that sells bonds to raise money.

# J

**Joint ventures** An arrangement that involves the joining together of two or more firms in a project or even in a new company founded jointly by the two companies.

**Junk bonds** Bonds rated BB and below by S&P or Ba and below by Moody's. These are considered high risk and usually have a high default rate.

# L

**Labor budget** That part of the expense budget that forecasts the cost of fixed and variable labor.

**Labor productivity** A figure that shows how many revenue dollars are generated with a given number of full-time equivalent employees.

**Land and improvements** A long-term asset that indicates the cost of the land or constructed improvements to land, such as driveways, walkways, lighting, and parking lots.

**Lease** A contract in which the lessee (user) agrees to pay the lessor (owner) a specific amount over a period of time for the use of an asset.

**Least-squares regression** *See* Simple linear regression method.

**Lender** An entity that temporarily grants the use of money or an asset to another in return for compensation, usually in the form of interest.

**Length of stay** How much time a patient spends in a facility for services rendered or recuperation. One of the factors that determine the service intensity.

**Level-debt service** The amount of interest and principal repaid each year that remains fairly constant. Also called level-debt principal.

**Leveraged buyouts** The purchase of the entire public stock interest of a firm, or division of a firm, financed primarily with debt.

**Liabilities** The organization's legal obligations to pay its creditors. Liabilities are classified as current and noncurrent. Liabilities are one of the three major categories on the balance sheet and are part of the fundamental accounting equation.

**Lien** A security interest in one or more assets granted to lenders in a secured loan.

**Lifecycle costing** A method for estimating the cost of a capital project that reflects total costs, both operating and capital, over the project's estimated useful life.

**Lifetime reserve days, Medicare** A beneficiary is entitled to 60 lifetime reserve days for inpatient hospital care. When more than 90 days of inpatient care are required in a benefit period, a patient may choose to draw on the reserve days. Patients are required to pay a daily coinsurance amount equal to one-half of the inpatient hospital deductible for each reserve day.

**Limited liability company (LLC)** A business entity that combines the tax flow-through treatment characteristics of a partnership (i.e., no double taxation) with the liability protection of a corporation.

**Limited liability partnership (LLP)** Another name for a limited liability company.

**Limited partnership** Limited partnerships offer limited liability to the limited partners along with tax flow-through treatment. There is at least one general partner who has unlimited liability for the partnership's debts and obligations.

**Line-item budget** The budget format that lists revenues and expenses by category, such as labor, travel, and supplies. Categories are sometimes broken down into subcategories. *See also* Performance budget *and* Program budget.

**Line of credit** A contract between a lender and a potential borrower preauthorizing the potential borrower's right to borrow up to a specific amount on request as long as they fulfill the terms and conditions of the contract. Also called a letter of credit.

**Liquidity** The ease and speed with which an asset can be turned into cash.

**Liquidity ratios** Ratios that answer the question: How well is the organization positioned to meet its short-term obligations?

**Loan amortization schedule** A schedule detailing the principal and interest payments required to repay a loan. Typically, the periodic payments remain unchanged, but the proportion used to pay off the principal increases over time.

**Lockbox** A mailbox directly accessible by a bank that deposits receipts directly into the healthcare provider's account.

**Longitudinal data** Information that covers multiple periods. Used in horizontal and ratio analysis.

**Long-term debt** The amount owed for obligations that exceed 12 months past the date of the balance sheet.

**Long-term debt, net of current portion** The total amount of multiyear debt due in future years.

**Long-term debt to net assets ratio** (long-term debt/ net assets) A measure of the proportion of an organization's assets that are financed by debt as opposed to equity. In for-profit organizations, it is called the long-term debt to equity ratio and is calculated using the formula (long-term debt/ owners' equity).

**Long-term financing** Debt to be paid off in a period longer than 1 year.

**Long-term investments** A category of noncurrent assets not intended to be used for operations but only for capital appreciation and dividends that will be held for a period longer than 1 year.

# M

**Man-hours per equivalent discharge** A key performance indicator that measures average staffing hours per a calculated equivalent patients unit which reflects inpatient and outpatient activity adjusted for case intensity.

**Managed care** Any of a number of arrangements designed to control healthcare costs through monitoring, prescribing, or proscribing the provision of health care to a patient or population. *See also* Health maintenance organizations (HMOs).

**Managed-care organization (MCO)** A prepaid or capitated health plan that is a state-licensed legal entity that provides health care directly or under arrangements for its members and participates under agreement or contract in a federal Medicare managed-care program.

**Management buyout** The purchase of the entire public stock interest of a firm, or division of a firm, financed primarily with debt when the transaction is made by management.

**Management information system** A system designed to gather, store, manipulate, and analyze data in order to provide information for management decision making.

**Managerial accounting** The process of preparing management reports and accounts that provide financial and statistical information to managers.

**Mandatory services** Those services that each state Medicaid program is required to cover, including hospital, physician, and skilled nursing facility services.

**Marketable securities** Short-term claims that can be bought and sold through a capital market. Examples are treasury bills, commercial paper, and certificates of deposit.

**Market power** Results from increased market share.

**Market share** The most critical measure of performance in the market factor category. High market share often leads to higher realized prices and lower cost per unit.

**Market rate of interest** The current traded rate for similar risk securities.

**Market structure** Most healthcare markets are regional in nature, and there are travel limits beyond which most consumers will not venture. Greater market share leads to greater leverage when negotiating health plan contracts.

**Market value (MV)** The price at which something, such as bonds and stocks, could be bought or sold today on the open market.

**Mark-up ratio** The percentage of gross patient revenues over total expenses.

**Master indenture financing** Debt that is guaranteed by all members who are a part of the master indenture.

**Maturity** The end of a bond's life.

**Means tested program** A government-sponsored program in which beneficiaries become eligible through specific means testing. Medicaid is the largest and best known example.

**Medicaid** A joint federal–state entitlement program intended to provide basic medical services for certain groups of low-income and disabled persons.

**Medical Service Organization (MSO)** Organizations whose main purpose is to provide administrative services (claims management, utilization review, etc.) to or for healthcare organizations.

**Medicare beneficiary** An individual who is enrolled for coverage under the Medicare program.

**Medicare case-mix index (CMI)** An index that provides an indication of the average complexity of Medicare inpatients seen.

**Medicare eligibility** A determination of whether an individual meets the legal requirements for Medicare coverage (age 65 or older, disabled, or requiring kidney transplant or renal dialysis due to chronic kidney disease).

**Medicare provider** A facility, supplier, or physician who furnishes Medicare services.

**Medicare severity diagnosis-related group (MS-DRG)** The payment classification system used by Medicare for inpatient hospital services.

**Merger** The combination of two or more companies, with one continuing as a legal entity while all others cease to exist; the former company's assets and liabilities become part of the continuing company.

**Mission statement** A statement intended to guide the organization into the future by identifying the unique attributes of the organization, why it exists, and what it hopes to achieve.

**Monetary assets** Items that reflect cash or claims to cash that are fixed in terms of the number of dollars, regardless of changes in prices.

**Monetary liabilities** Items that reflect cash or claims to cash that are fixed in terms of the number of dollars, regardless of changes in prices.

**Money-market mutual funds** Pooling of investors' funds for the purchase of a diversified portfolio of short-term financial instruments, such as treasury bills and certificates of deposit. This pooling of funds allows small investors, such as small healthcare facilities, to earn short-term money market rates on their investments.

**Mortgage** A note payable that has as collateral real assets and that requires periodic payments.

**Mortgage bonds** Bonds that hold the healthcare provider's real property and equipment as security or collateral in case of default.

**Multiyear budget** Budgets that typically cover 2 to 5 years.

**Municipal bond insurance** Guarantee of municipal debt by an insurance firm. Collapsed in 2008–2009 as a result of the mortgage loan securitization debacle.

# N

**Negotiable certificates of deposit (CDs)** A type of certificate of deposit that an investor may sell before maturity.

**Net accounts receivable** The amount expected to be collected from payers. It is calculated as (gross accounts receivable – discounts and allowances – allowance for uncollectibles).

**Net assets** Assets minus liabilities. One of the three major categories on the balance sheet. Traditionally known as stockholders' equity in investor-owned organizations and fund balance in not-for-profit organizations. In not-for-profit healthcare organizations, net assets must be categorized into three categories: unrestricted, temporarily restricted, and permanently restricted.

**Net assets released from restriction** Previously restricted assets no longer restricted because the terms of the restriction have been met.

**Net assets to total assets** (net assets/total assets) A ratio that reflects the proportion of total assets financed by equity. In for-profit organizations it is called the equity to total asset ratio and is calculated using the formula (owners' equity/total assets).

**Net increase (decrease) in cash and cash equivalents** The section of the statement of cash flows that reports the total change in cash and cash equivalents over the accounting period.

**Net patient revenue** The revenue that the organization has a right to collect. It is computed as (gross patient service revenues – contractual allowance and charity care).

**Net patient revenue per equivalent discharge™** This metric determines the average amount of revenue realized per equivalent discharge and is affected by payer mix.

**Net patient revenue per FTE** This is one measure used to help show how many revenue dollars are generated with a given number of full-time-equivalent employees.

**Net present value (NPV)** The difference between the initial amount paid for an investment and the related future cash inflows after they have been adjusted (discounted) by the cost of capital.

**Net proceeds from a bond issuance** Gross proceeds less the underwriter's fee and other issuance fees.

**Net working capital** The difference between current assets and current liabilities.

**Nominal (unadjusted) dollars** From an accounting perspective, a dollar of one year is no different from a dollar of another year. No recognition is given to changes in the purchasing power of the dollar because purchasing power is not measured.

**Noncurrent assets** Assets that provide service for a period exceeding 1 year. Sometimes referred to as long-term assets.

**Noncurrent liabilities** Financial obligations paid off over a time period longer than 1 year.

**Nongovernment payers' percentage** One of several measures for contract negotiation assessment. It helps to assess any possible weakness in current contract terms. Specifically, it represents the percentage of revenues not derived from Medicare or Medicaid patients. A high number indicates greater relative importance of effective contract negotiation.

**Nonoperating expenses** Expenses of the organization incurred in non-healthcare-related activities.

**Nonoperating gains and losses** Result from peripheral or incidental transactions. The definitions of peripheral and incidental transactions are not exactly clear, and the terms could be treated inconsistently. In general, the following are categorized as nonoperating gains and losses: contributions or donations that are unrestricted income from endowments, income from the investment of unrestricted funds, gains or losses on sale of property, and net rentals of facilities not used in the operation of the facility.

**Nonoperating income** The income (operating revenues – operating expenses) earned in non-healthcare-related activities.

**Nonoperating ratio** (nonoperating revenues/total operating revenues) A ratio that reflects how dependent the organization is on nonpatient care–related net income.

**Nonoperating revenues** Revenues of the organization earned in areas not related to normal operations.

**Nonparticipating physician** Can choose to accept assignment on a case-by-case basis and has a lower Medicare fee schedule. The limiting charge is equal to 95% of the approved fee schedule.

**Notes payable** A legal obligation to pay the holder of the note or lien.

**Not-for-profit** (1) Organizations that have a special designation because they provide goods or services that result in needed community benefit. In turn, such organizations are not required to pay most taxes. (2) The designation of an organization as one that is not generally required to pay taxes and may not distribute its profits.

**Notes to the financial statements** Key information not available in the body of the statements, such as organization's structure, accounting practices, how charity is determined, the position of investments, which assets are restricted, and the depreciation method used.

# O

**Offering memorandum** A document that outlines the terms of the offering of a private placement security.

**Opening inventory** The cost of the supplies on hand at the beginning of the year.

**Operating budget** The revenue and expense budgets of an organization.

**Operating cash flows** The cash flows derived from an organization's operating activities.

**Operating endowments** Funds whose purpose is to provide a dependable flow of investment earnings that can be used to supplement expected weaknesses in operating earnings.

**Operating expenses** The expenses incurred from an organization's operating activities.

**Operating income** A measure of the income earned from operating activities. It is calculated as (unrestricted revenues, gains, and other support – expenses and losses).

**Operating lease** A lease for a period shorter than the equipment's economic life, usually cancelable.

**Operating margin** The proportion of profit remaining after subtracting total operating expenses from operating revenues. It is calculated as (operating income/total operating revenues).

**Operating revenues** Revenues generated from an organization's operating activities.

**Opportunity cost** Proceeds lost by forgoing other opportunities.

**Ordinary annuity** A series of payments made or received at the end of each period.

**Other assets** Those that are neither current nor involve property and equipment. Typically, they are either investments or intangible assets.

**Other expenses** A catch-all category for miscellaneous expenses and losses not included in other categories (telephone, travel, meals, etc.).

**Other income** Nonoperating income.

**Other revenue** Operating income not reported elsewhere under revenues, gains, and other support.

**Outlier** An extremely long or unusually high-cost inpatient hospital stay when compared with most stays classified in the same diagnosis-related group.

**Outlier provision** A provision that specifies that the hospital may pay on a basis other than per diem or case if charges exceed a specific limit. Also known as stop-loss provision.

**Output levels** Influence the level of costs in one of two ways: First, the absolute level of output provided may affect the quantity of resources necessary to produce the output level. Second, service intensity may affect resource requirements.

**Overhead costs** Costs in non-revenue-producing departments.

**Owner's equity** Residual interest for entities with ownership interest.

# P

**Patient services revenue** Revenue that results from the provision of services to patients.

**Parent organization** An entity that owns other companies.

**Part A** *See* Hospital insurance (HI).

**Part B** *See* Supplementary medical insurance (SMI).

**Participating physician** One who agrees to accept Medicare's payment for a service as payment in full and bills the patient for the copayment portion only.

**Partnerships** Unincorporated businesses with two or more owners.

**Par value** Amount that a bondholder is paid at the time of the bond's maturity. Also called face value.

**Pass-through payment** Payments to hospitals for costs that are excluded from the prospective payment system, including bad debt, kidney acquisition costs, and direct costs of medical education.

**Payback** A method to evaluate the feasibility of an investment by determining how long it would take until the initial investment is recovered. As it is usually applied, this method does not account for the time value of money.

**Payment basis** Describes the manner by which a payer (Medicare, Medicaid, commercial health plans, and others) determines the amount to be paid for a specific healthcare claim. There are three payment bases: cost, fee schedule, and price related.

**Penalties (out-of-network)** Charging patients a penalty for seeking care from out-of-network providers.

**Per diem rates** A set reimbursement per inpatient day based on the type of case.

**Performance budget** A budget that presents not only line items and programs but also the performance goals that each program can be expected to attain. *See also* Line-item budget *and* Program budget.

**Performance measure** Financial and nonfinancial standards against which organizational performance is measured.

**Periodic payments** Series of payments over time, such as interest paid to bondholders.

**Permanently restricted net assets** Donated assets that have restrictions on their use that will never be removed.

**Per member per month (PMPM)** The most common way in which providers receive capitated payments.

**Perpetuity** An investment that generates an annuity for an indefinite period of time.

**Planning/control cycle** A classification of the activities of the organization into four major components, with budgeting being the focus: strategic planning, planning, implementing, and controlling.

**Plant, property, and equipment** The category of assets summarizing the amount of the major capital investments of the facility. Plant means buildings, property is land, and equipment includes a wide variety of durable items from beds to computed tomographs. Property, plant, and equipment are recorded on the organization's books at cost and, over time, plant and equipment (but not land) are subject to depreciation.

**Plant replacement and expansion funds** Funds restricted for use in plant replacement and expansion.

**PMPM** *See* Per member per month (PMPM).

**Point of service (POS)** A hybrid between an HMO and a PPO in which patients are given the incentive to see providers participating in a defined network but may see non-network providers, though usually at some additional cost.

**Pooled equipment financing programs** Programs often sponsored by the state hospital association or a regional association in which individual hospitals are involved in the financing and can obtain funds from the pool. The interest rate is usually much lower because the risk is spread across several hospitals.

**Preadmission certification and second opinions** A requirement that prior approval or review of service takes place before care is delivered.

**Precertification** The process through which a patient obtains authorization from their insurer to receive a particular prescription drug or healthcare service.

**Preferred provider organization (PPO)** An independent provider or provider network preselected by the payer to provide a specific service or range of services at predetermined (usually discounted) rates to the payer's covered members.

**Premium** (1) An amount paid by an employee or employer to pay for healthcare insurance. (2) When the market rate is lower than the coupon rate, a bond is said to be selling at a premium.

**Premium revenues** Revenues earned from capitated contracts.

**Prepaid asset** A benefit paid for in advance (rent, insurance, etc.). Also called prepaid expense.

**Prepaid expenses** Expenditures already made for future service, such as prepayment of insurance premiums for the year, rents on leased equipment, or other similar items.

**Prepayment provision** A provision that specifies the point in time at which a debt can be retired and the penalty imposed for early retirement.

**Present value** The value today of a payment (or series of payments) to be received in the future taking into account the cost of capital. It is calculated using the formula: future value × present value factor [PV × FV × PVF *or* PV = FV × $1/(1 + i)^n$]. *See also* Future value.

**Present value factor (PVF)** A factor used to discount future cash flows. It is the reciprocal of the future value factor and is calculated by the formula $1/(1 + i)^n$. *See also* Future value factor (FVF).

**Present value of an annuity** What a series of equal payments in the future is worth today taking into account the time value of money. *See also* Future value of an annuity.

**Price elasticity** Concept that describes the relationship between a change in price and demand for the service or product.

**Price-related payment basis** When the provider is paid for services based on some relationship to its total charges or price for the services delivered to the patient.

**Price setting** The process of establishing specific prices for the services provided by the healthcare provider.

**Primary care gatekeeper** Primary care physician serves as a central triage point for the referral and approval of services.

**Principal** Amount invested.

**Principal diagnosis** The medical condition that is chiefly responsible for the admission of a patient to a hospital or for services provided by a physician or other provider. It is determined after the patient has been examined.

**Privately held** Shares of the company are held by relatively few investors and are not available to the general public.

**Private placement** The sale of securities directly to investors without a public offering.

**Processing float** The elapsed time between processing a payment once received and depositing it in the bank.

**Productivity of inputs** The relationship of physical resources to the outputs that are produced through the use of those resources.

**Product margin** The amount that a service contributes to cover all other costs after it has covered those costs that are there solely because the service is offered (its total variable cost and avoidable fixed costs) and would not be there if the service were dropped. Computed as (total contribution margin – avoidable fixed costs).

**Product margin rule** If a service's product margin is positive, the organization will be better off financially if it continues with the service, all other things equal. Conversely, if a service's product margin is negative, the organization will be better off financially if it discontinues the service, all else being equal.

**Products** Outputs or services.

**Professional corporation (PC)** A corporate form for professionals who want to have the advantages of incorporation, also called a professional association.

**Professional fees** Fees paid to contract clinicians such as physicians, social workers, and physical therapists. Nursing expenses are usually reported under a category such as labor expenses.

**Profitability index** Attempts to compare rates of return. The numerator is the net present value of the project, and the denominator is the investment cost.

**Profitability ratios** Ratios designed to answer the question: How profitable is the organization?

**Profit centers** Organizational units responsible for controlling their costs and earning revenues. There are three types of profit centers: traditional profit centers, capitated profit centers, and administrative profit centers.

**Pro-forma financial statements** Customized financial statements that do not necessarily conform to generally accepted accounting principles (GAAP). When they are prepared before the accounting period, they present what the organization's financial statements will look like if all budgets are met exactly as planned. They also can be prepared for historical statements. In that case, the financial statements are remade to illustrate the effect of a proposed transaction, such as a business combination, acquisition, or proposed issue of securities. Their role is to present underlying assumptions and events that permit investors to understand the potential effect of a proposed transaction.

**Program budget** A budget in which line items are presented by program. *See also* Line-item budget *and* Performance budget.

**Programming** The phase of management control that determines the nature and size of programs an organization provides to accomplish its stated goals and objectives. It is the first phase of the management control process and interrelates with planning.

**Prospective payment system (PPS)** System used by Medicare to reimburse hospitals a set amount based on the patient's diagnosis-related group (DRG) or ambulatory patient classification (APC).

**Provider networks** A preselected list of providers from which a patient can choose without being liable for additional costs beyond any deductibles and copayments.

**Provision for bad debt** A statement of operations account that estimates the portion of receivables that are not likely to be collected. The provision for bad debt is the cost recognized in a particular period only. The related allowance for uncollectibles on the balance sheet is a cumulative account.

**Public benefit organization** An organization in which the assets (and accumulated earnings) belong to the public or to the charitable beneficiaries the trust was organized to serve.

**Public offering**  A bond sold to the investing public through an underwriter (sometimes called an investment banker).

**Publicly traded companies**  For-profit firms that buy and sell shares of their company stocks on the open market.

**Purchasing**  Relates to the acquisition of supplies and labor.

# Q

*Qui tam*  An abbreviation of a Latin phrase that means "he who as well for the king as for himself sues in this matter." The technical legal term for the mechanism in the Federal False Claims Act that allows persons and entities with evidence of fraud against federal programs or contracts to sue the wrongdoer on behalf of the government.

**Quick ratio**  A measure of the organization's liquidity. Calculated as [(cash + marketable securities + net accounts receivable)/current liabilities].

# R

**Ratio analysis**  An approach to analyzing the financial condition of an organization based on ratios calculated from line items found in the financial statements. There are four major categories of ratios: liquidity, profitability, capitalization, and activity.

**RBRVS**  *See* Resource-based relative value scale (RBRVS). *See also* Relative value unit.

**Realized gains and losses**  The increases or decreases in the value of a stock from the time it was purchased until the time it is sold.

**Reasonable cost**  A qualification introduced by the payer to limit its total payment by excluding certain categories of cost or placing limits on costs that the payer deems reasonable.

**Reasonable return on investment (ROI)**  The level of ROI that will permit the firm to maintain its financial viability.

**Refinancing**  When the issuer buys back the outstanding bonds from the investors.

**Refunding**  When the outstanding bonds are not acquired by the issuer, and the present bondholders continue to maintain their investment.

**Relative value unit (RVU)**  A standard for measuring the value of a medical service provided by physicians relative to other medical services provided by physicians that has three components: the physician work component (reflecting physician time and intensity), the overhead component (reflecting all categories of practice expenses, exclusive of malpractice insurance costs), and the malpractice expense component (reflecting the cost of obtaining malpractice insurance).

**Relative weighting system**  A system used with relative value unit (RVU) costing in which weights are assigned for each of the commonly produced outputs. These assigned weights can be used to cost individual procedures.

**Relevant range**  The range over which fixed costs in total and variable costs per unit do not change.

**Replacement cost**  The valuation of assets measured by the money value required to replace them.

**Reserve requirements**  Some types of financing require the creation of fund balances in escrow accounts under the custody of the bond trustee.

**Resource-based relative value scale (RBRVS)**  A system for measuring physician input to medical services for the purpose of calculating a physician fee schedule. The relative value of each service is the sum of relative value units (RVUs) representing physician work, practice expenses, and the cost of malpractice insurance.

**Resource utilization groups IV (RUG IV)**  Per diem payments for each admission are case-mix adjusted using this resident classification for skilled nursing care.

**Responsibility center**  Organizational unit given the responsibility to carry out one or more tasks and/or achieve one or more outcomes.

**Restricted donation**  A donation with conditions that must be satisfied. *See also* Temporarily restricted net assets.

**Retained earnings**  The portion of the profits the organization keeps in-house to use in support of its mission.

**Retrospective review**  A review of all services after they have been performed and only reimbursing for those services deemed medically necessary by the payer.

**Return on equity (ROE)**  The ratio of net income divided by total equity. The primary financial criterion that should be used to evaluate and target financial performance in any organization.

**Return on net assets**  (excess of revenues over expenses/ net assets) In not-for-profit healthcare organizations, a measure of the rate of return for each dollar in net assets. In for-profit organizations, a measure of the rate of return for each dollar in owners' equity; called return on equity and has the formula (net income/owners' equity).

**Return on total assets**  (excess of revenues over expenses/ total assets) A measure of how much profit is earned for each dollar invested in assets. In for-profit organizations it is called return on assets and is calculated as (net income/ assets).

**Revenue**  Amounts earned by the organization from the provision of service or sale of goods.

**Revenue budget**  The budget that forecasts the operating and, in some cases, the nonoperating revenues that will be earned during the budget period.

**Revenue enhancement**  Supplementing traditional sources of revenue with new sources.

**Revenue rate variance**  The amount of the total revenue variance that occurs because the actual average rate charged varies from that originally budgeted. It can be calculated using the formula [(actual rate − budgeted rate) × actual volume].

**Revenue volume variance**  The portion of total variance in revenues due to the actual volume being either higher or lower than the budgeted volume. It can be computed using the formula [(actual volume – budgeted volume) × budgeted rate].

**Revolving line of credit** A contract that requires a lender to fulfill the borrower's credit request up to the prenegotiated limit.

**Rolling budgets** Budgets updated on an ongoing basis, continually forecasting a given time frame, for example, 3 years in advance.

**RVUs** *See* Relative value units.

# S

**Salaries and wages** The amount paid to staff (either salaried or hourly workers).

**Salvage value** The amount an organization would receive by selling a fixed asset, usually either at the end of a project or at the end of its useful life.

**Schedule H** Form that must be filed with IRS 990 forms by all not-for-profit hospitals starting in 2010. Primary purpose of this form is to collect information regarding the provision of charity care by not-for-profit hospitals.

**Secondary diagnosis** A medical condition other than the principal diagnosis that affected the treatment received or length of stay in a hospital, or services rendered by a physician or other provider.

**Secondary market** Markets that deal in the buying and selling of bonds that have already been issued.

**Secured loan** A loan in which specific assets are pledged as collateral.

**Securities and Exchange Commission (SEC)** The governmental agency charged with ensuring that market trading is fair, among other things.

**Sell-offs** Considered the opposite of mergers and acquisitions. The two major types are spin-offs and divestitures.

**Semiaverages method** Similar to the high–low method regarding its mathematical solution. To derive the estimate of variable cost, the difference between the mean of the high-cost points and the mean of the low-cost points is divided by the change in output from the mean of the high-cost points to the mean of the low-cost points.

**Semifixed (also called "step fixed")** A change regarding changes in output, which is not proportional. Considered variable or fixed, depending on the size of the steps relative to the range of volume under consideration.

**Semivariable** Costs that include elements of both fixed and variable costs.

**Serial bonds** Bonds issued at various maturities and coupon rates.

**Service centers** Organizational units primarily responsible for ensuring that services are provided to a population in a manner that meets the volume and quality requirements of the organization. The most basic type of responsibility centers.

**Service intensity** One of several factors that drive total healthcare costs; also referred to as services/encounters. Intensity is determined by how long a patient is in a facility and how much care they require.

**Service mix** (1) The range of services offered by a provider. (2) Issues focusing on the appropriateness of care.

**Service units (SUs)** Services produced by a department within the production (or treatment) process.

**Short-term financing** Financing paid back in less than 1 year.

**Short-term investments** Investments liquidated within 1 year, such as certificates of deposit, commercial paper, and treasury bills.

**Simple interest method** Financing in which only the interest on the principal is calculated each period. *See also* Compound interest method.

**Simple linear regression method** A method that produces estimates of variable cost and fixed cost that minimize the variance between predicted and actual observations. In essence, it is a more precise version of the visual-fit method. Also called least-squares regression.

**Simultaneous-equations** Method of cost allocation is used in an attempt to calculate the exact cost allocation amounts. A system of equations is established, and mathematically correct allocations are computed.

**Sinking fund** Funds paid periodically to the bond trustee, who maintains the fund for the healthcare provider as part of the bond contract. A covenant may establish that part of the principal be paid each year, earmarked for the orderly retirement or the redemption of bonds before maturity. It is analogous to the principal repayment of a mortgage.

**Skilled nursing facility (SNF)** An institution that meets specified regulatory certification requirements and is engaged primarily in providing inpatient skilled nursing care and rehabilitative services.

**Sole proprietorships** Unincorporated businesses owned by a single individual. They do not necessarily have to be small businesses. Solo practitioner physicians often are sole proprietors.

**Specific-purpose funds** Funds donated by individuals or organizations and restricted for purposes other than plant replacement and expansion or endowment.

**Specific services** Payment method in which the individual services provided to a patient in an encounter of care are not aggregated.

**Speculative bonds** Relatively high-return, high-risk bonds. Sometimes called junk bonds.

**Spin-off** A separate new legal entity that is formed with its shares distributed to existing shareholders of the parent company in the same proportions as in the parent company.

**Spread** The difference between the price paid for a security by an investment banker and its sale price. Usually quoted in terms of basis points.

**Staff model HMO** A HMO in which the providers are employees of the HMO.

**Standard cost profile (SCP)** Used in manufacturing cost accounting systems to accurately cost historical or future encounters of care.

**Standard volume** Critical in cost variance analysis. Equal to actual volume, unless there is some indication that not all output was necessary.

**Statement of cash flows** One of the four major financial statements. It answers the questions: Where did our cash come from and where did it go during the accounting period?

**Statement of changes in net assets** One of the four major financial statements. It explains the changes in net assets from one period to the next on the balance sheet. Also called statement of changes in owners' equity in a for-profit business.

**Statement of operations** One of the four major financial statements. It summarizes the organization's revenues and expenses during an accounting period as well as other items that affect its unrestricted net assets. It is analogous to, but different from, an income statement in a for-profit organization.

**Static budgets** Budgets that forecast for a single level of activity.

**Static coding** Direct coding of HCPCS codes into the charge master. Also referred to as "hard coding."

**Statistical forecasts** Predictions of future activity based on a mathematical model extrapolated from historical data. They can be determined from major econometric studies to simple time-series techniques.

**Statistics budget** The budget that identifies the amount of services provided, usually by payer type.

**Steerage discounts** Agreements by which payers agree to send patients to selected providers in return for discounts.

**Step-down method** A method of allocating costs that are not directly paid for (utilities, rent, administration) into those products or services to which payment is attached (day of care, a brief visit). *See also* Activity-based costing (ABC).

**Step-fixed costs** Fixed costs that increase in total at certain points as the level of activity increases, such as labor costs that increase when a new employee is added after certain volumes of service are reached.

**Stop-loss limit** A method used by providers to limit the risk in cases where costs incurred are significantly greater than standard reimbursements for those services.

**Stop-loss provision** This provision specifies that the hospital may pay on a basis other than per diem or case if charges exceed a specific limit. Also known as outlier provision.

**Strategic business units** Refer to areas of activity that may stand alone.

**Strategic financial planning** A method by which the organization develops its strategies and budgets to meet future financial targets.

**Strategic planning** First, a statement of mission or goals (or both) is required to provide guidance to the organization. Second, a set of programs or activities to which the organization will commit resources during the planning period is defined. There is not agreement among leading experts regarding the definition of strategic planning.

**Subjective forecasts** A prediction whose reliability is based on the wisdom and understanding of the forecaster. Often referred to as a "seat of the pants" method. They may have a place in the estimation of product line volumes.

**Subsidiary** An organization owned and/or managed by another organization.

**Substandard bonds** Very risky "junk bonds."

**Sunk cost** Costs already incurred. They should not be included in cost analyses of future projects.

**Supplementary medical insurance (SMI)** Medicare SMI, also referred as Part B, is a voluntary insurance program that covers physician services (inside or outside of the hospital), outpatient hospital services, ambulatory services, and certain medical supplies and other services for all persons age 65 or older and persons eligible for Part A due to disability or chronic renal disease.

**Supplies budget** The expense budget that forecasts fixed and variable supplies.

**Sustainable growth** Principle that states that no business entity can generate a growth rate in assets that is greater than its growth rate in equity for a prolonged period.

**SWOT analysis** A technique to evaluate an organization's *s*trengths, *w*eaknesses, *o*pportunities, and *t*hreats. This technique often is used as part of the strategic planning process.

# T

**Tangible assets** Assets that have a physical presence.

**Tax-exempt bonds (tax-exempt revenue bonds)** Bonds in which the interest payments to the investor are exempt from Internal Revenue Service (IRS) taxation. These bonds must be issued by an organization that has received tax exemption from the IRS and be used to fund projects that qualify as "exempt uses." Tax-exempt revenue bonds are backed by the organization's revenues. They offer lower interest rates than do taxable bonds.

**Tax shield** An investment that reduces the amount of income tax to be paid, often because interest and depreciation expenses are tax deductible.

**Temporarily restricted net assets** Assets that have restrictions on their use that will be removed with either the passage of time or the occurrence of some event. *See also* Restricted donation.

**Tender option** An option that permits investors to redeem their bonds at some predetermined interval—perhaps daily—at the face value. Also called a "put."

**Term** A specified amount of time.

**Term loans** A form of long-term financing that typically must be paid off within 10 years. They require the borrower to pay off or amortize the principal value of the loan over its life.

**Terminal value** The value of a bond at maturity.

**Third-party payer** An agent that agrees to pay on behalf of a patient or group of patients. Examples include Medicare, Medicaid, indemnity insurance companies, and HMOs.

**Time value of money** The idea that a dollar today is worth more than a dollar in the future.

**Times interest earned** [(excess of revenues over expenses + interest expense)/interest expense] A ratio that enables creditors and lenders to evaluate an organization's ability to generate earnings necessary to meet interest expense requirements. In for-profit organizations the ratio is calculated using the formula [(net income + interest expense)/interest expense]. The ratio answers the question: For every dollar in interest expense, how many dollars are there in profit before interest?

**Top-down approach** An approach to carrying out organizational tasks (e.g., budgeting) that relies heavily on higher management decision making with little employee input.

**Total asset turnover** (total revenues/total assets) A ratio that measures the overall efficiency of the organization's assets to produce revenue. It answers the question: For every dollar in assets, how many dollars of revenue are being generated?

**Total margin** The ratio of net income to total revenue, provides information on the level of profitability at a hospital.

**Total revenue** Price times total quantity.

**Traceability** The most basic classification of cost. Two major categories of costs classified in this manner are direct costs and indirect costs.

**Trade credit** Credit granted by one firm to another firm for the purchase of services or products.

**Transfer to parent** Transfer of assets from a subsidiary to its parent company.

**Transit float** The time elapsed between the time a check is deposited in the banking system and when the funds are available.

**Treasury bills (T-bills)** Financial instruments that can be purchased from the government and are considered default-free. They are among the most liquid short-term investments available. Rather than earning interest directly, they are purchased at a discount rate and redeemed at face value when they mature.

**Trend analysis** A type of horizontal analysis that looks at changes in line items compared to a base year. It is calculated as [(any subsequent year – base year)/base year] × 100.

**Trustee** An agent for bondholders who performs two primary functions: making the principal and interest payments to the bondholders and ensuring that the healthcare provider complies with the legal covenants of the bond.

# U

**Unadjusted historical cost (HC)** An alternative financial reporting method that represents the present method used by accountants.

**Uncompensated care percentage** The cost of care provided to indigent patients after subtracting any payment.

**Underwrite** A firm that brings out new securities issues, agreeing to purchase and resell them. They often work together on a given issue and help healthcare facilities issue bonds and advise management on the terms of the structure of the bonds. They sometimes guarantee the proceeds to the firm from a future security sale, in effect taking ownership of the securities.

**Unfavorable variance** (1) When actual revenues are lower than budgeted revenues. (2) When actual expenses are lower than budgeted expenses. *See also* Favorable variance.

**Uniform Bill–Form 92 (UB-92)** A Medicare claim form used by institutional providers.

**Unit of payment** The collection of services that will be combined or bundled to trigger a payment amount.

**Unrealized gains and losses** The change, since the last balance sheet, in the market value of stocks held for investment. Recognized as realized gains and losses only when the stocks are sold.

**Unrestricted net assets** All net assets (including those that have been restricted by management, the governing board, contractual agreements, or other legal documents) not restricted by donors.

**Unsecured bank loan** A short-term loan not backed by collateral.

**Utilization variance** Results from a difference between actual volume and standard volume, or the quantity of volume actually needed.

# V

**Variable costs** Costs that stay the same per unit but change directly in total with a change in activity over the relevant range: (total variable cost = variable cost per unit × number of units of activity).

**Variable labor budget** The expense budget that forecasts labor costs that vary as additional personnel or overtime hours are needed.

**Variable-rate debt** A security whose interest rate changes based on market conditions.

**Variable supplies budget** The expense budget that forecasts the costs of supplies that vary with the number of patients seen, such as disposable syringes, disposable gloves, and x-ray films. Also called the nonfixed supply budget.

**Vertical analysis** A method used to analyze financial statements that answers the general question: What percentage of one line item is another line item? Also called common-size analysis because it converts every line item to a percentage, thus allowing comparisons among the financial statements of different organizations.

**Vertical mergers**   A merger between a manufacturer and a supplier. This is different from a horizontal merger between two companies that manufacture similar products.

**Virtual corporations**   Corporations that save cash and limit their financial risk by hiring a limited number of employees, owning few physical assets, and contracting out for most services.

**Visual-fit method**   Cost estimation method. Individual data points are plotted on graph paper. A straight line is then drawn through the points to provide the best fit. Visual fitting of data is a good first step in any method of cost estimation.

**Volume variance**   The product of the difference between budgeted and actual volume ($Q^a - Q^b$) and the average fixed cost budgeted ($F/Q^b$).

**Voluntary health and welfare organizations**   Nonbusiness-oriented organizations that perform voluntary services in their communities. They are tax exempt and rely primarily on public donations for their funds.

# W

**Weighted average cost of capital (WACC)**   The cost of capital or required rate of return to undertake a project. Calculated as [debt/(debt + equity) × cost of debt] + [equity/(equity + debt) × cost of equity]. *See* Discount rate, Hurdle rate, *and* Cost of capital.

**Wire transfer**   An approach used to eliminate mail and transit float by electronically depositing payments in the bank. Related techniques are zero-balance accounts and sweep accounts, where the bank automatically removes any excess from subsidiaries and places it in the account of the parent corporation.

**Working capital**   Current assets. Calculated as (net working capital = current assets – current liabilities).

**Working capital cycle**   The activities of the organization that encompass (1) obtaining cash; (2) turning cash into resources, such as inventories and labor, and paying bills; (3) using the resources to provide services; and (4) billing patients for the services and collecting revenues so that the cycle can be continued.

# Y

**Yield to maturity (YTM)**   Market interest rate of a bond. The rate at which the market value of a bond is equal to the bond's present value of future coupon payments plus par value.

# Z

**Zero-base budgeting**   An approach to budgeting that regularly questions both the need for existing programs and their level of funding and the need for new programs. *See also* Incremental/decremental approach.

**Zero-coupon bonds**   Bonds issued with a very low coupon value or with no coupon at all.

# Common Healthcare Financial Management Acronyms

## A

**A/P** accounts payable

**A/R** accounts receivable

**AAAHC** Accreditation Association for Ambulatory Health Care

**AAE** affirmative action employer

**AAHAM** American Association of Healthcare Administrative Management

**AAHP** American Association of Health Plans

**AAMA** American Academy of Medical Administration

**AAMC** Association of American Medical Colleges

**AAPA** American Academy of Physician Assistants

**AAPCC** adjusted average per capita cost

**ABA** American Bar Association

**ABC** activity-based costing

**ABM** activity-based management

**ABN** advance beneficiary notice

**ACC** ambulatory care center

**ACHE** American College of Healthcare Executives

**ACPE** American College of Physician Executives

**ACPPD** average cost per patient day

**ACR** adjusted community rate

**ACS** ambulatory care services

**AD** admitting diagnosis

**ADA** American Dietetic Association; American Dental Association

**ADC** average daily census

**ADFS** alternative delivery and financing systems

**ADP** automatic data processing

**ADPL** average daily patient load

**ADS** alternative delivery system

**ADSC** average daily service charge

**ADT** admission/discharge/transfer

**AEP** appropriate evaluation protocol

**AFDC** Aid to Families with Dependent Children

**AFDS** alternative financing and delivery systems

**AG** affiliated group

**AHA** American Hospital Association

**AHCA** American Health Care Association (long-term care)

**AHIMA** American Health Information Management Association

**AHIP** assisted health insurance plan

**AICPA** American Institute of Certified Public Accountants

**ALOS** average length of stay

**AMA** American Medical Association

**AMGA** American Medical Group Association

**ANSI** American National Standards Institute

**APA** American Psychiatric Association; American Psychological Association

**APC** ambulatory payment classification

**APG** ambulatory patient group

**APHA** American Public Health Association

**APPAM** Association for Public Policy Analysis and Management

**APR** annual percentage rate

**ASC** ambulatory surgical/surgery center

**ASCII** American Standard Code for Information Interchange

**ASO** administrative services only

**AVG** ambulatory visit group

**AWI** area wage index

**AWP** average wholesale price

## B

**BBA** Balanced Budget Act of 1997

**BBRA** Balanced Budget Refinement Act (1999)

**BCD** binary code decimal

**BLS** Bureau of Labor Statistics

**BOL** bill of lading

**BQA** Bureau of Quality Assurance

## C

**CAH** critical access hospital

**CBA** cost-benefit analysis

**CBO** Congressional Budget Office

**CC** complications and/or comorbidities

**CCH** Commerce Clearing House

**CCI** correct coding initiative

**CCMU** critical care medical unit

**CCR** cost-to-charge ratio

**CCRC** continuing care retirement community

**CD** chemical dependency

**CDC** Centers for Disease Control and Prevention

**CE** continuing education

**CEA** cost-effectiveness analysis

**CEO** chief executive officer

**CER** capital expenditure review

**CEU** continuing education unit

**CFO** chief financial officer

**CFR** Code of Federal Regulations

**CHAMPUS** Civilian Health and Medical Program of the Uniformed Services

**CHAMPVA** Civilian Health and Medical Program of the Veterans Affairs

**CHC** community health center

**CHFP** certified healthcare financial professional

**CHIP** comprehensive health insurance plan, Children's Health Insurance Program; Consumer Health Information Program

**CHP** comprehensive health planning

**CIO** chief information officer

**CIS** computer information system

**CM** case mix

**CME** continuing medical education

**CMHC** community mental health center

**CMI** case-mix index; chronic mental illness

**CMN** certificate of medical necessity

**CMP** competitive medical plan

**CMS** Centers for Medicare and Medicaid Services (formerly known as the Health Care Financing Administration)

**CNH** community nursing home

**CNHI** Committee for National Health Insurance

**CNS** clinical nurse specialist

**COB** coordination of benefits; close of business

**COLA** cost-of-living adjustment

**CON** certificate of need

**COO** chief operating officer

**CORF** comprehensive outpatient rehabilitation facility

**CPA** certified public accountant

**CPEHS** Consumer Protection and Environmental Health Service

**CPEP** Carrier Performance Evaluation Program

**CPI** consumer price index

**CPR** customary, prevailing, and reasonable

**CPT** current procedural terminology

**CPT-4™** *Current Procedural Terminology*, Fourth Edition

**CPU** central processing unit

**CQI** continuous quality improvement

**CWF** common working file

**CY** calendar year


# D

**D/A** date of admission

**DBMS** database management system

**DC** diagnostic code

**DDR** discharge during referral

**DEFRA** Deficit Reduction Act

**DHHS** Department of Health and Human Services

**DI** disability insurance

**DIB** disability insurance benefit

**DISA** Data Interchange Standards Association

**DJIA** Dow Jones Industrial Average

**DME** durable medical equipment

**DMEPOS** durable medical equipment, prosthetics, orthotics, and supplies

**DMS** *See* DBMS

**DNR** do not resuscitate

**DOA** date of admission; dead on arrival

**DOD** Department of Defense

**DOE** Department of Energy; Department of Education

**DOH** Department of Health

**DOJ** Department of Justice

**DOL** Department of Labor

**DOS** date of service

**DOT** Department of Transportation

**DP** data processing

**DPH** Department of Public Health

**DRA** Deficit Reduction Act

**DRC** diagnosis-related category

**DRG** diagnosis-related group

**DSH** disproportionate share hospital

**DSM-IV** *Diagnostic and Statistical Manual of Mental Disorders*, Fifth Edition

**DSO** debt service obligation


# E

**E&A** evaluate and advise

**E&M** evaluation and management

**EBCDIC** extended binary coded decimal information code

**EBRI** Employee Benefit Research Institute

**ECF** extended care facility

**ECHO** electronic computing, health-oriented

**ECI** employment cost index

**EDI** electronic data interchange

**EDIFACT** EDI for administration, commerce, and trade

**EDP** electronic data processing

**EEO** equal employment opportunity

**EEOC** Equal Employment Opportunity Commission

**EFT** electronic funds transfer

**EGHP** employer group health plan

**EHIP** employee health insurance plan

**EMTALA** Emergency Medical Treatment and Active Labor Act

**EO** executive order

**EOB** explanation of benefits

**EOC** episode of care

**EOMB** explanation of medical benefits; Executive Office of Management and Budget; explanation of Medicare benefits

**EOQ** economic order quantity

**EPA** Environmental Protection Agency

**EPEA** expense per equivalent admission

**EPFT** electronic payment funds transfer

**EPO** exclusive provider organization

**ER** emergency room

**ERISA** Employment Retirement Income Security Act

**ERTA** Economic Recovery and Taxation Act

**ES** emergency service

**ESA** Employment Standards Administration

**ESRD** end-stage renal disease

**EVA** economic value added

# F

**F&A** fraud and abuse

**FAC** freestanding ambulatory care

**FAHS** Federation of American Health Systems

**FASB** Financial Accounting Standards Board

**FDA** Food and Drug Administration

**FDO** formula-driven overpayment

**FEC** freestanding emergency center

**FFC** federal funding criteria

**FFP** federal financial participation

**FFS** fee for service

**FFSS** fee-for-service system

**FFY** federal fiscal year

**FHA** Federal Housing Administration

**FHFMA** Fellow of Healthcare Financial Management Association

**FI** fiscal intermediary

**FICA** Federal Insurance Contributions Act

**FIFO** first in, first out

**FIG** fiscal intermediary group

**FOIA** Freedom of Information Act

**FPR** Federal Procurement Regulations

**FQHC** federally qualified health center

**FR** *Federal Register*

**FSI** Financial Strength Index

**FTC** Federal Trade Commission

**FTE** full-time equivalent

**FWHF** Federation of World Health Foundations

**FY** fiscal year

# G

**GAAP** generally accepted accounting principles

**GAF** geographic adjustment factor

**GAO** General Accounting Office

**GDP** gross domestic product

**GME** graduate medical education

**GNP** gross national product

**GPCI** geographic practice cost index

**GPM** gross profit margin

**GPO** Government Printing Office; group purchasing organization

# H

**H-B** Hill-Burton Act

**HAP** hospital accreditation program

**HAR** hospital associated representatives

**HAS** hospital administration services

**HB** hospital based

**HBO** hospital benefits organization

**HBP** hospital-based physician

**HC** health care; home care

**HCC** healthcare corporation

**HCD** healthcare delivery

**HCFA** Health Care Financing Administration, previous name for CMS. *See* CMS.

**HCFAR** Health Care Financing Administration ruling

**HCPCS** Healthcare Common Procedure Coding System

**HCRIS** Hospital Cost Reporting Information System

**HCTA** healthcare trust account

**HCUP** hospital cost and utilization project

**HDS** health delivery system

**HEAL** Health Education Assistance Loan

**HEDIS** Health Plan Employer Data and Information Set

**HEF** Health Education Foundation

**HFMA** Healthcare Financial Management Association

**HFPA** health facilities planning area

**HFSG** healthcare financing study group

**HH** hold harmless

**HHO** home health organization

**HHRG** home health resource groups

**HHS** Health and Human Services (Department of)

**HI** Hospital Insurance (refers to Medicare Part A)

**HIAA** Health Insurance Association of America

**HIBAC** Health Insurance Benefits Advisory Council

**HIBCC** Health Insurance Business Communications Council

**HIC** health information center; health insurance claim; health insurance company

**HINN** hospital-issued notice of noncoverage

**HIP** health insurance plan

**HIPAA** Health Insurance Portability and Accountability Act of 1996

**HIS** hospital information system

**HITF** health insurance trust fund

**HMO** health maintenance organization

**HMO/CMP** health maintenance organization/competitive medical plan

**HMPSA** health manpower shortage area

**HOPD** hospital outpatient department

**HPAC** Health Policy Advisory Center

**HPB** historic payment basis

**HPC** Health Policy Council

**HPR** hospital peer review

**HR** House of Representatives; House Resolution

**HRET** Hospital Research and Education Trust

**HRSA** Health Resources and Services Administration

**HSA** Health Services Administration

**HSQB** Health Standards and Quality Bureau

**HSR** health services research

**HSRC** Health Services Research Center

**HUD** Housing and Urban Development (Department of)

**HURA** Health Underserved Rural Area

**HURT** hospital utilization review team

**HV** hospital visit

# I

**I/O** input/output

**IBNR** incurred but not reported

**ICD** *International Classification of Diseases*

**ICD-9** *International Classification of Diseases*, 9th revision

**ICD-9-CM** *International Classification of Diseases*, 9th revision, *Clinical Modification*

**ICD-10** *International Classification of Diseases and Related Health Problems*, 10th revision

**ICD-10-CM** *International Classification of Diseases and Related Health Problems,* 10th revision, *Clinical Modification*

**ICF** intermediate care facility

**IDS** integrated delivery system

**IG** Inspector General

**IHS** Indian Health Service

**IME** indirect medical education

**IMS** information management system

**IO** investor owned

**IOL** intraocular lens

**IOV** initial office visit

**IP** inpatient

**IPA** individual practice association

**IPS** interim payment system

**IRS** Internal Revenue Service

**ITC** investment tax credit

# J

**JCAHO** Joint Commission on Accreditation of Healthcare Organizations

**JIT** just in time

**JUA** Joint Underwriting Association

# L

**LBO** leveraged buyout

**LIFO** last in, first out

**LOS** length of stay

**LPN** licensed practical nurse

**LTC** long-term care

**LTAC** long-term acute care facility

**LTCF** long-term care facility

**LTCU** long-term care unit

**LTD** long-term debt

**LVN** licensed vocational nurse

# M

**M&A** merger and acquisition

**M+C** Medicare+Choice

**MAC** major ambulatory category; maximum allowable charge

**MADC** mean average daily census

**MADRS** Medicare Automated Data Retrieval System

**MB** market basket; Medicare Bureau

**MCO** managed-care organization

**MDC** major diagnostic category

**MDS** minimum data set

**MEDISGRPS** Medical Illness Severity Grouping System

**MEDLARS** Medical Literature Analysis and Retrieval System

**MedPAC** Medicare Payment Advisory Commission

**MedPAR** Medicare Provider Analysis and Review file

**MEI** Medicare economic index

**MET** multiple employer trust

**MHB** maximum hospital benefit

**MIS** management information system

**MLP** mid-level practitioner

**MPFS** Medicare physician fee schedule

**MR** management review

**MRA** medical record administrator

**MRD** medical record department

**MRDF** machine-readable data file

**MRI** magnetic resonance imaging; mortality risk index

**MRP** maximum reimbursement point

**MSA** metropolitan statistical area

**MSO** medical service organization

**MSP** Medicare secondary payer

**MUA** medically underserved area

**MVPS** Medicare volume performance standard

# N

**NACHA**  National Automated Clearing House Association
**NAHC**  National Association for Home Care
**NAIC**  National Association of Insurance Commissioners
**NAPH**  National Association of Public Hospitals
**NAR**  net accounts receivable
**NAS**  National Academy of Sciences
**NBS**  National Bureau of Standards
**NCAHC**  National Council on Alternative Health Care
**NCCBH**  National Council for Community Behavior Healthcare
**NCHS**  National Center for Health Services
**NCI**  National Cancer Institute
**NCQA**  National Committee for Quality Assurance
**NF**  nursing facility
**NFA**  net fixed assets
**NFP**  not for profit
**NH**  nursing home
**NHC**  National Health Council
**NHCT**  National Health Care Trust
**NHF**  National Health Federation
**NHI**  national health insurance
**NIH**  National Institutes of Health
**NOA**  notice of admission
**NOI**  net operating income
**NOL**  net operating loss
**NonPAR**  nonparticipating physician
**NOR**  nonoperating revenue
**NP**  nurse practitioner
**NPI**  national provider identifier
**NPO**  nonprofit organization
**NPPR**  notice of proposed rulemaking
**NPR**  notice of program reimbursement
**NPSR**  net patient service revenue
**NRHA**  National Rural Health Association
**NSF**  not sufficient funds
**NTIS**  National Technical Information Services
**NUBC**  National Uniform Billing Committee

# O

**OASDHI**  Old Age Survivors, Disability, and Health Insurance Program
**OASIS**  Outcome and Assessment Information Set
**OBRA**  Omnibus Budget Reconciliation Act
**OD**  organizational development
**ODR**  Office of Direct Reimbursement
**OHTA**  Office of Health Technology Assessment
**OIG**  Office of Inspector General

**OJT**  on-the-job training
**OMB**  Office of Management and Budget
**OOP**  out of pocket
**OP**  outpatient
**OPD**  outpatient department
**OPM**  Office of Personnel Management
**OR**  operating room
**OSG**  Office of the Surgeon General
**OSHA**  Occupational Safety and Health Act; Occupational Safety and Health Administration
**OTA**  Office of Technology Assessment
**OTC**  over the counter
**OWCP**  Officer of Workers' Compensation Programs

# P

**PA**  physician assistant
**PAC**  preadmission certification
**PAM**  patient accounts manager
**PAR**  participating (provider or supplier)
**PCP**  primary care physician
**PE**  physician extender
**PHO**  physician hospital organization
**PL**  public law
**PM**  program memorandum
**PMPM**  per member per month
**PO**  physician organization
**POS**  point of service
**PPA**  preferred provider arrangement
**PPD**  per patient day; prepaid
**PPM**  physician practice management
**PPO**  preferred provider organization
**PPS**  prospective payment system
**PR**  peer review
**PRO**  peer review organization
**ProPAC**  Prospective Payment Assessment Commission
**PRP**  prospective reimbursement plan
**PRRB**  Provider Reimbursement Review Board
**PSO**  provider-sponsored organization

# Q

**QA**  quality assurance
**QAM**  quality assurance monitor/monitoring
**QAP**  quality assurance program
**QAS**  quality assurance standards
**QA/RM**  quality assurance/risk management
**QA/UR**  quality assurance/utilization review
**QM**  quality management

# R

**R&D** research and development
**RBRVS** resource-based relative value scale
**RCC** ratio of cost to charges
**REIT** real estate investment trust
**RFI** request for information
**RFP** request for proposal
**RFQ** request for quotation
**RHA** regional health administrator
**RHC** rural health clinic
**RHP** regional health planning
**RIF** reduction in force
**RM** risk management
**RMIS** risk management information systems
**ROE** return on equity
**ROI** return on investment
**RPCH** rural primary care hospital
**RRC** rural referral center
**RTU** relative time unit
**RUG** resource utilization group
**RVS** relative value scale/schedule/study
**RVU** relative value unit

# S

**S&P** Standard and Poor's
**SB** Senate Bill (National)
**SBU** strategic business unit
**SCH** sole community hospital
**SCP** sole community provider
**SD** standard deviation
**SE** standard error
**SEC** Securities and Exchange Commission
**SG** Surgeon General
**SGO** Surgeon General's Office
**SGR** sustainable growth rate
**SHA** state health agency
**SHC** state health commissioner
**SI** severity index
**SMI** Supplementary Medical Insurance (refers to Medicare Part B)
**SNF** skilled nursing facility
**SOB** statement of benefits
**SOC** standard of care
**SOI** severity of illness
**SOP** standard operating procedures
**SP** standard of performance
**SPA** state planning agency

**SR** Senate resolution
**SSA** Social Security Administration
**SSDI** Social Security Disability Insurance
**SSI** Supplemental Security Income
**SSOP** Second Surgical Opinion Program
**STD** short-term disability
**SUBC** State Uniform Billing Committee

# T

**T&E** travel and expense; trial and error
**TAAC** Technology Assessment Advisory Council
**TDA** tax-deferred annuity
**TEFRA** Tax Equity and Fiscal Responsibility Act
**TPA** third-party administrator
**TQM** total quality management
**TR** turnover rate
**TSA** tax-sheltered annuity

# U

**UB** uniform billing
**UB-92** Uniform Billing–Form 92
**UBI** unrelated business income
**UCAS** Uniform Cost Accounting Standards
**UCR** usual, customary, and reasonable
**UHCIA** Uniform Health Care Information Act
**UHDDS** Uniform Hospital Discharge Data Set
**UM** utilization management
**UPC** Uniform Product Code
**UR** utilization review
**USDA** U.S. Department of Agriculture
**USDT** U.S. Department of Transportation
**USFMG** U.S. foreign medical graduate
**USFMSS** U.S. foreign medical school student
**USMG** U.S. medical graduate
**USPCC** U.S. per capita cost
**USPHS** U.S. Public Health Service
**USSG** U.S. Surgeon General

# V

**VA** Veterans' Affairs
**VAH** Veterans' Affairs Hospital

# W

**WC** Workers' Compensation

**WHF-USA** World Health Foundation, United States of America
**WHO** World Health Organization
**WIC** Women, Infants, and Children

# X

**XR** x-ray

# Y

**YTD** year-to-date

# Z

**ZBB** zero-base budgeting
**ZPG** zero population growth

# Index

## A